THE
SKULL

VOLUME
1

THE
SKULL

VOLUME
1

Development

EDITED BY

JAMES HANKEN and BRIAN K. HALL

THE UNIVERSITY OF CHICAGO PRESS

Chicago and London

James Hanken is associate professor in the Department of Environmental, Population, and Organismic Biology at the University of Colorado, Boulder.
Brian K. Hall is Izaak Walton Killam Research Professor and professor of biology at Dalhousie University.

The University of Chicago Press, Chicago 60637
The University of Chicago Press, Ltd., London
© 1993 by The University of Chicago
All rights reserved. Published 1993
Printed in the United States of America

02 01 00 99 98 97 96 95 94 93   1 2 3 4 5

ISBN: 0-226-31566-5(cloth)
0-226-31567-3(paper)

Library of Congress Cataloging-in-Publication Data

The Skull / edited by James Hanken and Brian K. Hall.
    p.   cm.
    Includes bibliographical references and index.
    Contents: v. 1. Development—v. 2. Patterns of structural and
systematic diversity—v. 3. Functional and evolutionary
mechanisms.
    1. Skull—Anatomy. 2. Skull—Evolution. 3. Anatomy, Comparative.
I. Hanken, James. II. Hall, Brian Keith, 1941–   .
    [DNLM: 1. Skull—anatomy & histology. 2. Skull—growth &
development. 3. Skull physiology. WE 705 S629]
QL822.S58   1993
596'.04'71—dc20
DNLM/DLC   92-49119
for Library of Congress

CONTENTS

VOLUME 1

Development

VOLUME 2

Patterns of Structural and Systematic Diversity

VOLUME 3

Functional and Evolutionary Mechanisms

GENERAL INTRODUCTION

JAMES HANKEN AND BRIAN K. HALL

This is the first of three volumes on the vertebrate skull. The last decade has witnessed a resurgence of interest in cranial development, anatomy, function, and evolution, a rekindling of interest that may be traced to several sources. First, technological advances in the study of vertebrate development—such as the widespread use of the scanning electron microscope, sophisticated genetic and cell markers, in vitro culture methods, and a variety of molecular analyses—have allowed resolution of embryonic events at a scale that could not be approached by earlier investigators. Results of these studies have forced reevaluation of many long-held beliefs concerning the fundamental organization of the skull and of the vertebrate head generally, such as segmentation and the origin of the cranial skeleton and musculature. They have also underscored the primary role of developmental processes—both as a constraint and as a source of morphological novelty—in the evolution of cranial diversity. Second, the tremendous ferment in vertebrate systematics, following innovations in techniques (e.g., the use of molecular data in phylogeny reconstruction) and methodology (e.g., cladistics), has led vertebrate biologists both to return to the skull as a source of additional characters for phylogenetic inference and to reexamine trends in skull evolution in the light of revised hypotheses of vertebrate relationships. Third, the increased popularity of functional morphological analysis finds investigators asking questions about dynamic as well as static aspects of skull structure, and their bearing on skull evolution, that received little or no attention in the past.

Slightly more than 50 years ago, Sir Gavin de Beer (1937) published his monumental tome, *The Development of the Vertebrate Skull,* which culminated almost a century of intense examination of cranial structure, development, and evolution. The present series was first envisioned, then organized, and finally completed with an occasional rearward glance at de Beer's book and the high standards for scholarship that it established for this field. However, our series is far different in scope and content from de Beer's book, and is intended as a complement to it, not a successor. This reflects the changing nature of fundamental problems being addressed and the information deemed necessary to resolve them. For example, functional aspects of skull design and their implications for patterns of cranial evolution were rarely considered in more than a cursory manner in de Beer's time, whereas they are subject to intense scrutiny at present. And while this series is primarily concerned, as was de Beer, with features of the vertebrate skull per se, in many instances this requires detailed consideration of the complex of nervous, sensory, vascular, muscular, connective, and other cranial tissues that lie adjacent to the skull or otherwise influence its development, function, and evolution. Similarly, aspects of behavior and ecology are included in cases where they are important determinants of skull form, and vice versa. One feature that we have retained from de Beer is the ample use of high-quality illustrations, many published here for the first time.

The Development of the Vertebrate Skull suffered a curious fate. Although de Beer hoped his book would "serve as a starting-point for further work" (1937, 512) and, in fact, closed it with an agenda outlining specific problems he considered especially worthy of investigation, such was not the case. Interest in the skull waned in the decades following the book's publication, reflecting a general decline in the study of vertebrate morphology that has been reversed only in the last 10–15 years (Hall and Hanken 1985; Wake 1982). Thus, it is with a certain trepidation that we admit the same aim for this series, viz., that it will "serve as a starting-point for further work." We hope that it does not suffer the same fate.

There still is a tremendous amount of valuable and fundamental information concerning the skull left to be discovered, information with broad implications for many areas of vertebrate biology. To quote Thomas Henry Huxley (slightly out of context) from his famous Croonian lecture to the Royal Society of London on the question of head segmentation, "at the present day, the very questions regarding the composition of the skull, which were mooted and discussed so long ago by the ablest anatomists of the time, are still unsettled" (1858, 383).

The work comprises three volumes, reflecting the current intense interest in the skull. Our aims in assembling these volumes were (1) to organize and present the results of recent studies of skull development and structure in such a way as to interest specialists as well as vertebrate biologists generally; (2) to evaluate the implications of these results for fundamental questions in vertebrate structure and evolution; (3) to examine current studies of the functional bases and constraints of skull form; (4) to use the vertebrate skull to illustrate evolutionary patterns and processes and to test hypotheses that purport to account for them; and (5) to promote further interest and research in these and related issues.

The first (present) volume concerns cranial development and growth. The second volume (*Patterns of Structural and Systematic Diversity*) addresses the phylogenetic origin of the skull, its fundamental structure and histology, and patterns of cranial diversity in extant classes. The final volume (*Function and Evolutionary Mechanisms*) considers aspects of skull function and evolutionary mechanisms for cranial diversity. Authors were asked to present the conceptual bases of their respective topics, illustrated with appropriate examples, while highlighting areas of current interest and controversy and identifying prominent questions for future research. Thus, individual chapters are not intended to be comprehensive reviews of the topic at hand; such reviews would be well beyond the scope and size of the volumes. In a few instances, however, a more comprehensive treatment was the only effective way to synthesize a widely scattered literature that never before had been focused on a particular problem.

Reflecting the integrated, multidisciplinary approach that is being used to answer many contemporary questions in cranial biology, certain topics receive substantial treatment in more than one volume. Thus, while general aspects of skull development are considered in volume 1, more detailed accounts and specialized aspects of skull development in particular taxa are presented in several chapters in volume 2, and cranial ontogeny returns as a dominant theme in some chapters in volume 3. Similarly, we attempted to balance the treatments afforded different vertebrate classes in the three volumes, although for many topics a distinct taxonomic bias was inevitable given the narrow array of groups considered in earlier studies. Readers are therefore urged to consult more than one volume when using the series as a general reference source for information about a particular topic or taxonomic group.

A large number of people deserve thanks for their efforts in bringing these volumes to completion. We acknowledge two groups in particular. First and foremost we thank all the authors, who agreed to tackle the ambitious tasks we set before them and did so with a high degree of professionalism. Second, we thank our editors at the University of Chicago Press for their guidance, perseverance, and patience in working with us to bring this project to fruition.

REFERENCES

de Beer, G. R. 1937. *The Development of the Vertebrate Skull.* Oxford: Oxford University Press. Paperback reprint. Chicago: University of Chicago Press, 1985.

Hall, B. K., and J. Hanken. 1985. Foreword to G. R. de Beer, *The Development of the Vertebrate Skull,* pp. vii–xxviii. Chicago: University of Chicago Press.

Huxley, T. H. 1858. On the theory of the vertebrate skull. Proceedings of the Royal Society of London 9: 381–457.

Wake, D. B. 1982. Functional and evolutionary morphology. Perspectives in Biology and Medicine 25: 603–620.

PREFACE

JAMES HANKEN AND BRIAN K. HALL

This volume of *The Skull* deals with cranial development, and in this regard takes its lead from de Beer's (1937) classic work, *The Development of the Vertebrate Skull*. Many of the ten chapters concern topics that are of contemporary as well as classical interest, such as head segmentation (chap. 2), differentiation and morphogenesis of cranial cartilage and bone (chap. 4), metamorphosis (chap. 8), and later stages of ontogeny (chap. 9). Most of the remaining chapters, however, address topics that have come to be regarded as critical to a comprehensive understanding of cranial development only since de Beer's time. Perhaps the most obvious of these is the neural crest (chap. 3), a topic which received only brief mention by de Beer, who only reluctantly conceded its potential importance to understanding the embryonic origins of cranial tissues (Hall and Hanken 1985). Additional topics of this nature are the mechanisms of axis specification and cephalization (chap. 1), skull growth (chap. 5), and quantitative and developmental genetics (chaps. 6 and 7). An additional factor that sets virtually all these treatments apart from earlier considerations is their focus on underlying causal mechanisms rather than patterns of development. That many of these mechanisms operate at the molecular level is evident in several chapters. The volume concludes with a bibliography of comparative developmental studies since de Beer (1937), which attempts to bridge the exhaustive, indexed bibliography provided by de Beer and the computerized bibliographic data bases which have been made available in the last few years.

Together, these chapters provide an overview of many fundamental aspects of vertebrate skull development. In doing so, they establish the developmental context for considerations of cranial diversity, function, and evolution which make up subsequent volumes, and which make frequent use of ontogenetic data. They also provide an entrée to current literature and outstanding problems.

Contemporary research in cranial developmental biology is burgeoning. Mechanisms which are only beginning to be explored in the context of head development may very well assume a predominant position in the field within only a few years. As described in several chapters in this volume, an excellent candidate is homeobox genes, which, following from a series of recent studies (e.g., Hunt, Gulisano et al. 1991; Hunt, Whiting et al. 1991), are increasingly believed to play a critical role in the specification of morphogenetic patterning of cranial tissues and branchial segment identity. Consequently, this is an extremely exciting and rewarding time for those involved in cranial development, from experienced investigators to beginning students. We hope that this volume helps to sustain their enthusiasm far into the future.

REFERENCES

de Beer, G. R. 1937. *The Development of the Vertebrate Skull.* Oxford: Oxford University Press. Paperback reprint. Chicago: University of Chicago Press, 1985.

Hall, B. K., and J. Hanken. 1985. Foreword to G. R. de Beer, *The Development of the Vertebrate Skull,* pp. vii–xxviii. Chicago: University of Chicago Press.

Hunt, P., M. Gulisano, M. Cook, M.-H. Sham, A. Faiella, D. Wilkinson, E. Boncinelli, and R. Krumlauf. 1991. A distinct *Hox* code for the branchial region of the vertebrate head. Nature 353: 861–864.

Hunt, P., J. Whiting, S. Nonchev, M.-H. Sham, H. Marshall, A. Graham, R. Allemann, P. W. J. Rigby, M. Gulisano, A. Faiella, E. Boncinelli, and R. Krumlauf. 1991. The branchial *Hox* code and its implications for gene regulation, patterning of the nervous system and head evolution. Development 2 (suppl.): 63–77.

1

Axis Specification and Head Induction in Vertebrate Embryos

RICHARD P. ELINSON AND KENNETH R. KAO

MOST VERTEBRATE EGGS are spherical with radial symmetry. The vertebrate body, however, is bilaterally symmetric with three polarized axes: dorso-ventral, antero-posterior, left-right. The change from radial symmetry with one axis to the vertebrate body plan with three axes involves the specification of a second axis. The plane defined by the two axes is the plane of bilateral symmetry, separating the right side from the left, so the third axis is produced automatically (fig. 1.1). The vertebrate skull represents the most anterior portion of the antero-posterior axis as well as the most dorsal portion of the dorso-ventral axis. Obviously, its development is intimately involved with axis specification.

We will consider two questions: (1) What event breaks radial symmetry? And (2) How is this axial information carried through early development to the formation of a head? These questions have been analyzed mostly in reference to amphibians, so we will discuss this class first. The other classes will be reviewed comparatively, although except for birds, little is known for other vertebrates.

AMPHIBIANS

Breaking Radial Symmetry

The Radial Egg and Grey Crescent Formation. The full-grown amphibian egg is radially symmetric with an animal-vegetal axis (fig. 1.2). The animal half is marked by pigment in many species. The pigment granules are found throughout the cytoplasm of the animal half but are concentrated in the cortex. The vegetal half has little pigment but many large yolk platelets. The animal-vegetal axis forms during oogenesis, but its origin is not known. Prior to yolk uptake, the vegetal half is marked by the mitochondrial cloud, a dense accumulation of mitochondria and filaments (Heasman et al. 1984). During vitellogenesis, yolk is preferentially translocated

1

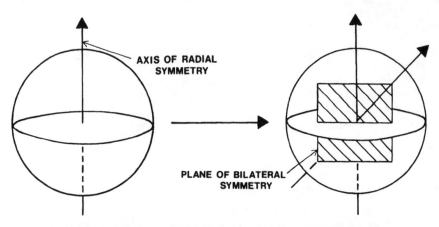

Fig. 1.1. Radial and bilateral symmetry. Vertebrate eggs are initially radially symmetric. Radial symmetry is broken by the formation of a second axis, and this event is called axis specification. The plane defined by the two polarized axes is the plane of bilateral symmetry, separating the embryo's body into right and left halves.

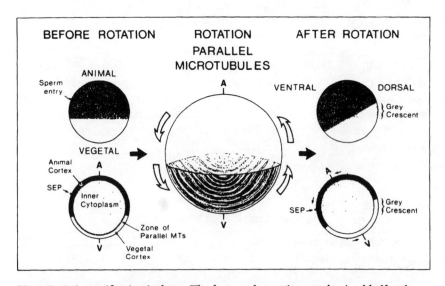

Fig. 1.2. Axis specification in frogs. The frog egg has a pigmented animal half and a nonpigmented, yolky vegetal half. During the first cell cycle, the outer cortex rotates by 30° relative to the inner cytoplasm. The direction of the rotation is correlated with the sperm entry point (SEP), so that the grey crescent forms equatorially opposite the sperm entry point. The grey crescent marks the future dorsal side of the embryo. A zone of parallel microtubules at the interface between the vegetal cortex and cytoplasm is involved in the cortical rotation. (From Elinson and Rowning 1988)

to the vegetal half and this sets up the yolk gradient (Danilchik and Gerhart 1987).

During the first cell cycle of the fertilized egg, there is a rearrangement of the cytoplasm which breaks the radial symmetry. The rearrangement consists of a 30 degree rotation of the outer cortex relative to the inner cytoplasm (Ancel and Vintemberger 1948; Vincent et al. 1986; Gerhart et al. 1989), with a concomitant swirling of the animal cytoplasm (Danilchik and Denegre 1991). In many species, the grey crescent results from the visibility of pigmented animal cytoplasm through the rotated vegetal cortex (fig. 1.2). The grey crescent marks the dorsal side of the embryo.

The unidirectional cortical rotation provides a second axis, yielding bilateral symmetry. More than that, cortical rotation is necessary for specifying dorsal and anterior structures. The consequences of cortical rotation are best illustrated by fate maps of the embryo's surface before and after rotation (fig. 1.3). Before rotation, the surface is fated to be featureless epidermis and endoderm. After rotation, the ectodermal fates include the central nervous system, the sense organs, and the epidermis of the body. It is easy to picture frog development based on this fate map. During gastrulation, the endoderm moves inside, and during neurulation, the central nervous system forms and is covered by epidermis. Of course, the actual movements are more complicated, particularly the important movements of the internal mesoderm, which is not portrayed (Keller 1975, 1976; Keller et al. 1985).

The importance of the cortical rotation in the establishment of bilateral symmetry and the specification of dorso-anterior structures is demonstrated by two types of experiments: inhibition of rotation and cutting of eggs. When the vegetal half of the egg is irradiated with ultraviolet (UV) light before rotation, cortical rotation does not occur (Manes and Elinson 1980; Vincent and Gerhart 1987). The resulting embryos cleave normally and gastrulate, but they remain radially symmetric and develop no dorsal or anterior structures (Malacinski et al. 1975; Scharf and Gerhart 1980, 1983). These ball-shaped embryos have ciliated epidermis, and produce blood cells with hemoglobin, a normal fate of ventral mesoderm. They lack striated muscle and fail to synthesize α-actin mRNA (Jamrich et al. 1985) or myosin (Cooke and Smith 1987) indicative of muscle cell differentiation.

With lower doses of UV, progressively more dorso-anterior development occurs (fig. 1.4). The head, which occupies the most extreme dorso-anterior area, is the structure most sensitive to UV. The mildest inhibition yields embryos with small heads (microcephaly) or only one eye (cyclopia). The conclusions that can be drawn from the UV inhibition experiments are first, that the ground state of the embryo is ventral, and second, that

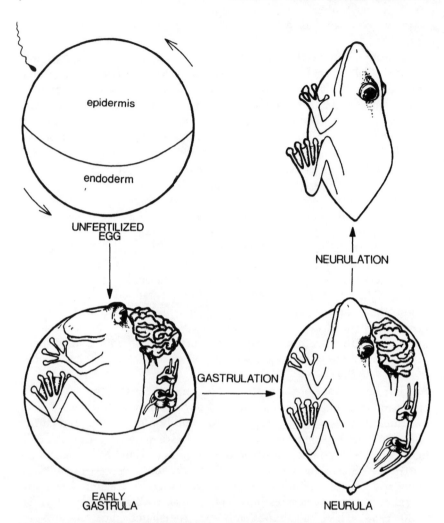

Fig. 1.3. Frog development. Before fertilization, the surface of the egg is fated to be epidermis and endoderm with no axial structures. As a result of the cortical rotation, the axes are specified so that the dorsal (grey crescent) side is fated to be central nervous system while the animal pole area is fated to be head epidermis, sense organs, and brain. Note that the neural and epidermal structures depicted in the early gastrula are fated to form there; their actual formation depends on the subsequent movements of gastrulation and neural induction. During gastrulation, the endoderm moves inside; during neurulation, the central nervous system becomes internal. The mesoderm is not depicted, since, at least in *Xenopus*, it forms internally. The mesodermal fate map is shown in fig. 1.7.

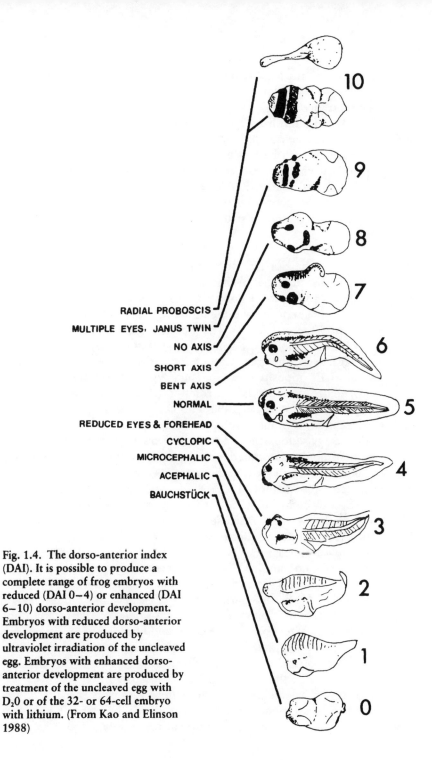

RADIAL PROBOSCIS
MULTIPLE EYES, JANUS TWIN
NO AXIS
SHORT AXIS
BENT AXIS
NORMAL
REDUCED EYES & FOREHEAD
CYCLOPIC
MICROCEPHALIC
ACEPHALIC
BAUCHSTÜCK

Fig. 1.4. The dorso-anterior index (DAI). It is possible to produce a complete range of frog embryos with reduced (DAI 0–4) or enhanced (DAI 6–10) dorso-anterior development. Embryos with reduced dorso-anterior development are produced by ultraviolet irradiation of the uncleaved egg. Embryos with enhanced dorso-anterior development are produced by treatment of the uncleaved egg with D_2O or of the 32- or 64-cell embryo with lithium. (From Kao and Elinson 1988)

the specification of the head requires the greatest change from the ground state. The change is the cortical rotation.

The importance of the rotation is further illustrated when eggs are cut into pieces. When a fertilized egg is bisected before rotation, both halves, if they have a nucleus, can develop dorso-anterior structures. Presumably, rotation occurs in each half. When an egg is cut after rotation, one half will frequently develop a head and other dorso-anterior structures while the other half lacks a head (Render and Elinson 1986). The cortical rotation produces a situation where one side of the egg is more capable of developing dorso-anterior structures, the head in particular, than the other side.

The Direction of the Cortical Rotation. The very first embryological experiments demonstrated that in the frog, there is a relation between where the sperm enters and how the body plan is laid out (Newport 1854; Roux 1887). The side of sperm entry is the future ventral side, and the face looks toward the entry point (fig. 1.3). The meridian including the sperm entry point and the animal pole is the dorso-ventral midline separating the future right and left halves. The grey crescent, indicative of the cortical rotation, forms equatorially opposite to sperm entry (fig. 1.2), and the sperm entry point is correlated with the axis of rotation (Vincent and Gerhart 1987).

The sperm entry point itself plays no causal role in specifying the direction of rotation. It simply marks where the sperm nucleus starts its migration in the egg cytoplasm. Rather, the growing sperm aster, a radial array of microtubules associated with the nucleus, specifies the direction. When asters are made to grow in the egg, the grey crescent forms opposite to the induced asters (Kubota 1967; Manes and Barbieri 1977). The aster exerts its effect by contributing to the formation of a cortical array of parallel microtubules, which as discussed later, is likely part of the mechanism for rotation (Houliston and Elinson 1991b).

While the aster biases the rotation, the aster's effect can be overcome, and indeed, it is not needed. Tilting or centrifuging eggs can provide stronger biases than the sperm aster (Ancel and Vintemberger 1948; Gerhart et al. 1981; Black and Gerhart 1985; Zisckind and Elinson 1990). Eggs with two or more sperm asters show a single axis of rotation and symmetry, with no aster dominant (Render and Elinson 1986; Vincent and Gerhart 1987). Artificially activated eggs have no sperm aster; nonetheless, they undergo a cortical rotation which specifies dorso-anterior development (Gerhart et al. 1986; Satoh and Shinagawa 1990).

The picture that emerges from these observations is that the nonrotated state becomes very unstable midway through the first cell cycle. The egg is programmed to undergo the cortical rotation which breaks radial symmetry, and the egg will use any cues available to it to specify direction. Given the fundamental importance of establishing bilateral symmetry and dorso-ventral polarity, it is no wonder that the cortical rotation is so automatic.

The Mechanism of the Cortical Rotation. The rotation moves the outer cortex, which is 1 to 3 μ thick, relative to the inner cytoplasm of the egg, which is 1,300 to 2,000 μ in diameter (fig. 1.2). Gravity can be used experimentally to move the inner cytoplasm relative to the cortex, but the normal rotation is not due to gravity. When the cortex is held in place, the rotation still occurs, indicating that the dense, vegetal yolk mass is being driven against gravity (Vincent et al. 1986). There must be an energy-requiring rotation motor.

Cellular motors usually employ a cytoskeletal track along which an ATPase moves, and in the case of the frog egg, microtubules appear to be the tracks. Inhibitors of microtubules, but not of actin filaments, prevent rotation (Manes et al. 1978; Vincent et al. 1987), and microtubules polymerize at the start of rotation and depolymerize upon its completion (Elinson 1985). An array of parallel microtubules has been found that is likely the tracks for rotation (Elinson and Rowning 1988; Elinson 1989). The parallel microtubules cover the interface between the cortex and the inner cytoplasm (fig. 1.2). They appear at the start of rotation, become indistinct at its completion, and run parallel to the axis of the rotation.

The parallel microtubules have a common polarity, with their "+" ends pointed toward the future dorsal side (Houliston and Elinson 1991a). They are associated with endoplasmic reticulum and kinesin, an ATPase which moves organelles toward the "+" ends of microtubules. One hypothesis for the cortical rotation is that a kinesin-like ATPase transports the cortex along the parallel microtubules which are anchored in the cytoplasm (Houliston and Elinson 1991a).

The Threshold Nature of Head Specification. Ventral development can be considered the ground state since only ventral development occurs when the cortical rotation is prevented (Manes and Elinson 1980; Vincent and Gerhart 1987). This statement implies simply that something must be done, namely the rotation, in order for dorsal and anterior structures to develop. Dorsal structures may result from inhibition of ventral development, however, as easily as from activation of dorsal development.

Specification of the head by the rotation appears to be a threshold effect, since over-rotation does not lead to larger heads (macrocephaly) (Chung and Malacinski 1983; Neff et al. 1984; Black and Gerhart 1985, 1986). Macrocephaly has been produced both experimentally (Huff

1962; Malacinski 1974) and by species hybridization (Porter 1941; Elinson 1977), but it results from alterations of induction patterns and cell movements during gastrulation (Kao and Elinson 1985; Elinson 1991). Over-rotation has also not led to embryos with obvious novel head or dorso-anterior structures, which we will call supraheads. This possibility is raised by the intriguing hypothesis on the evolutionary origin of the vertebrates; namely, a vertebrate is a protochordate to which a head was added at the anterior end (Gans and Northcutt 1983). Supraheads would provide structures on which to base speculations of evolution beyond vertebrates.

It is possible to obtain more head specification by treatment with heavy water (D_2O) before rotation, but this leads to multiple-headed embryos (Scharf et al. 1989). A frequent result of D_2O treatment is the Janus twin, which has two more or less normal heads joined to a common body with reduced posterior structures. The Janus morphology is carried to an extreme in radial proboscis embryos, which have radial symmetry with radial head structures including the eye and the cement gland (figs. 1.4, 1.5). Similar embryos can be produced by lithium treatment during cleavage (Kao et al. 1986), so this morphology will be discussed later. Rather

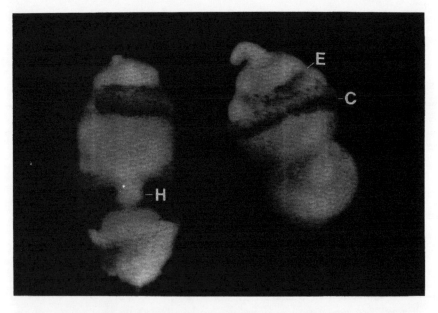

Fig. 1.5. Radial proboscis embryos. These DAI 10 embryos (fig. 1.4) were produced by treatment of 32-cell embryos with lithium. They have radial pigmented retinas (E) and cement glands (C), a central beating heart (H), some brain tissue, and a mass of notochord.

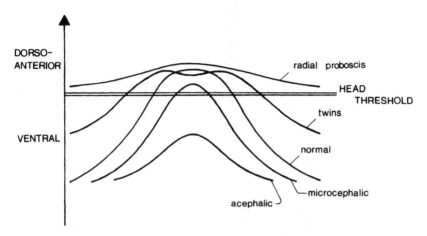

Fig. 1.6. The head threshold. The ground state of the frog embryo, and probably all vertebrate embryos, is ventral. When radial symmetry is broken, the head and other dorso-anterior structures are specified. When specification is insufficient, the head is reduced (microcephalic) or absent (acephalic). With overspecification, twins and radial proboscis embryos result.

than yield larger heads or supraheads, D_2O treatment produces multiple heads whose extreme state is the radial head.

The threshold concept of head specification is illustrated in figure 1.6. Normal embryos receive a sufficient stimulus from the rotation to produce a head, while a reduced stimulus yields microcephaly and acephaly. Attempts to increase the stimulus to above normal collapses the peak of the curve into two peaks, producing twinning. With radial proboscis embryos, the whole of the curve is above the threshold. The amount of dorso-anterior specification and, as a result, the amount of head produced, are a function of the organizer as discussed next.

Axial Information in Early Development

Overview. Following the cortical rotation which specifies the dorso-ventral axis, the amphibian egg divides many times to produce the blastula. This is followed by a period of cell movements known as gastrulation which grades into the differentiation of tissues and morphogenesis of the body. The fates of individual cells, or blastomeres, in the early embryo have been carefully mapped (Dale and Slack 1987a; Moody 1987; Takasaki 1987). These maps, combined with ones of later stages (Keller 1975, 1976), enable us to visualize how the body arises (figs. 1.3, 1.7). The fate maps, however, represent what we know about a cell's fate in normal development; they do not tell us what the cells know. In fact, most cells in the early embryo know very little.

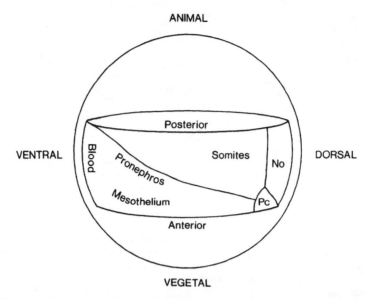

Fig. 1.7. Mesodermal fate map. In *Xenopus*, the cells fated to form mesoderm lie as an internal ring. During gastrulation, the ring turns itself inside out. Prechordal plate mesoderm (Pc) ends up near the former animal pole, where it induces the ectoderm to form the brain. The notochord (No) underlies and induces the ectoderm to form the spinal cord.

A few cells carry dorso-anterior information in the embryo during cleavage (Elinson and Kao 1989), and a series of cell interactions, known as inductions, convert this information into the dorsal axial structures of the embryo. The first induction occurs in the blastula stage and is called mesoderm induction (Hopwood 1990; Green and Smith 1991), since the mesoderm is specified at this time. Mesoderm has a dorso-ventral polarity, with the notochord and somitic muscle specified on the dorsal side (figs. 1.7, 1.8). The second induction is called dorsalization and affects the dorsal-to-ventral specification of the mesoderm (Dale and Slack 1987b). The third induction, known as primary or neural induction, occurs during gastrulation and produces the central nervous system as its major outcome (fig. 1.8). Here, the ectoderm is induced by the presumptive notochord and dorsal mesoderm (Sharpe 1990; Guthrie 1991). The region which causes dorsalization as well as neural induction is the organizer, discovered by Spemann and Mangold (1924). Neural induction is regionally different so that the brain forms at the anterior end and the spinal cord and tail mesoderm forms at the posterior end. The mechanism of embryonic induction has been an intractable problem for over 60 years, but renewed attacks have revived hopes for solutions. It should be noted, however, that almost

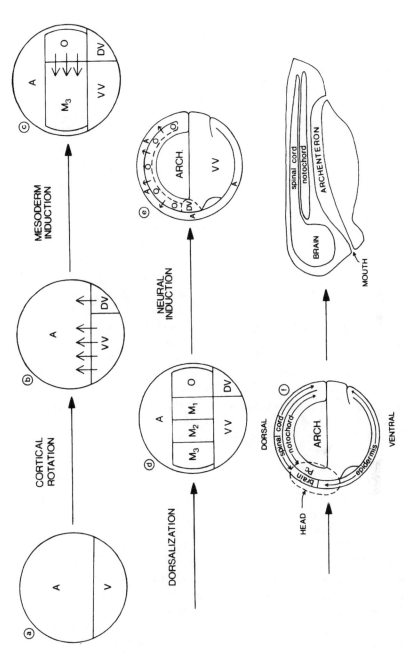

Fig. 1.8. The sequence of inductions. a. The egg has animal (A) and vegetal (V) parts. b. As a result of the cortical rotation following fertilization, the vegetal part acquires dorsal (DV) and ventral (VV) polarity. Vegetal cells later induce animal cells to form mesoderm. c. Dorsal vegetal cells induce the formation of the organizer (O); ventral vegetal cells induce the formation of ventral mesoderm (M_3). d. The organizer dorsalizes the mesoderm (M_1, M_2) to yield the notochord-to-blood spectrum of tissues (fig. 1.7). e. During gastrulation, the organizer becomes the roof of the archenteron (Arch.) and induces the overlying animal cells to form the central nervous system.f. Prechordal plate mesoderm (Pc) underlies the brain while the notochord underlies the spinal cord. Subsequent antero-posterior elongation yields the familiar tadpole. (Modified from Slack et al. 1984)

all of the recent work on early amphibian development has been done on only one species, the South African clawed toad, *Xenopus laevis*.

Location of Dorso-anterior Information. The formation of the head requires the correct specification and differentiation of dorso-anterior structures. Information for dorso-anterior development (Elinson and Kao 1989) is originally found on one side of the egg after rotation (Render and Elinson 1986), and is parceled out to a small number of cells during cleavage (Kageura and Yamana 1983, 1986; Gimlich 1986; Kageura 1990; Gallagher et al. 1991). The molecular nature of dorso-anterior information in these cells is unknown, but there exists a UV-labile component in full-grown oocytes which is required for later dorso-anterior development (Elinson and Pasceri 1989). There is also a cytoplasmic component in dorsal cells at the 16-cell stage which can generate a dorsal axis when injected into ventral cells (Yuge et al. 1990).

At the 32-cell stage, eight cells carry dorso-anterior information, but in different ways (fig. 1.9). The two dorsal vegetal cells can induce other cells to form dorsal mesodermal structures but do not themselves form those structures (Gimlich 1986; Dale and Slack 1987b). The six other dorsal cells themselves can differentiate into dorsal mesodermal tissues, notochord and somites, and can function as the organizer (Gimlich 1986; Kageura 1990). Dorsal equatorial cells are most active in this regard, with dorsal animal cells having less activity (Kageura 1990). Removal of the dorsal, equatorial cells leads to a deficiency of head structures (Takasaki 1987).

The progeny of the dorsal, equatorial cells improve in their ability to function as Spemann's organizer as development proceeds (Nakamura 1978; Gimlich 1986). Spemann's organizer, defined by transplantation experiments, is the region of the embryo which can organize the rest of the embryo to yield the full complement of dorso-anterior axial structures.

Mesoderm Induction. The early blastula consists of animal and vegetal cells (fig. 1.8), which in isolation differentiate into epidermis and endoderm respectively. When in contact, vegetal cells induce animal cells to form the mesoderm, the third primary germ layer (Nieuwkoop 1969a; Sudarwati and Nieuwkoop, 1971; Nieuwkoop et al. 1985). The original experiments have been confirmed and extended with the help of molecular markers and lineage tracers (Dale et al. 1985; Gurdon et al. 1985; Dale and Slack 1987b).

Mesoderm induction takes about two hours and occurs during the blastula stage (Gurdon et al. 1985). Induction does not require gap junctions (Warner and Gurdon 1987), and direct contact between the animal and vegetal cells is not necessary (Grunz and Tacke 1986). Nieuwkoop (1969b) showed that ventral vegetal cells induced the formation of ventral mesodermal tissues, including blood and mesothelium, while dorsal vege-

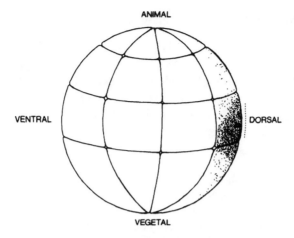

Fig. 1.9. Location of dorso-anterior information. In the 32-cell *Xenopus* embryo, eight cells carry dorso-anterior information, with the highest activity equatorially. The dotted line indicates where the dorsal lip of the blastopore will form at gastrulation. Spemann's organizer arises animal to the dorsal lip.

tal cells induced the formation of dorsal mesodermal tissues, mainly no-tochord and muscle. This dorsal-to-ventral pattern of mesoderm induction (Nieuwkoop 1973) is an early consequence of the cortical rotation de-scribed earlier.

Attempts to define the chemical nature of the signals were spurred by the finding that basic fibroblast growth factor (FGF) at very low concen-trations causes mesoderm induction (Slack et al. 1987). Both the mRNA for FGF and FGF itself are found in eggs and early embryos, suggesting that FGF is an endogenous mesoderm inducer (Kimelman and Kirschner 1987; Kimelman et al. 1988; Slack and Isaacs 1989; Shiurba et al. 1991). FGF, however, primarily induces ventral mesoderm, implying that other factors are required for induction of dorsal mesoderm. In addition, inhi-bition of FGF function by disrupting the FGF receptor has little effect on head development, although the resulting embryos exhibit gross abnor-malities of the axis (Amaya et al. 1991).

The most effective inducer of dorsal mesoderm is activin, a growth factor which also affects pituitary function and blood cell differentiation (Asashima et al. 1990; Smith et al. 1990; van den Eijnden-Van Raaij et al. 1990; Thomsen et al. 1990). When animal cells from a blastula are treated with activin, they are induced to form notochord, somites, and even eyes and neural tissue (Smith 1987; Green and Smith 1990; Sokol and Melton 1991). The latter tissues probably arise by secondary induction; that is, animal cells are induced to dorsal mesoderm which in turn induces other animal cells to anterior neural structures.

The development of dorsal mesoderm and the later formation of head structures are tightly connected, as illustrated by the ability to describe dorsal and anterior development with a single dorso-anterior index (DAI, fig. 1.4). The ability of cells to induce head structures is directly proportional to how strongly they were previously induced toward dorsal mesoderm (Ruiz i Altaba and Melton 1989b). The amount of head development in the embryo increases, with increasing numbers of cells induced to be dorsal mesoderm (Kao and Elinson 1988; Stewart and Gerhart 1990).

Pattern Respecification. The embryo's axis is defined in early cleavage stages by the asymmetric location of dorso-anterior information (fig. 1.9). Despite this arrangement, it is possible to respecify pattern by treating 32- to 64-cell embryos with lithium (Kao et al. 1986; Kao and Elinson 1988). In the most extreme case, dorso-anterior enhanced embryos develop radial head structures such as a radial eye and cement gland (figs. 1.4, 1.5). An unusually large proportion of the embryo is notochordal tissue, indicating an overcommitment to dorsal structures. The same phenotype can be produced by treating fertilized eggs with D_2O (Scharf et al. 1989). This extreme phenotype is due to dorso-anteriorization of the entire mesoderm, so that it all behaves like the organizer (Kao and Elinson 1988).

Lithium treatment represents entry into the normal pathways of commitment to dorso-anterior differentiation. Microinjection of lithium into single vegetal cells at the 32-cell stage causes formation of an extra head and axial structures, and this same treatment causes axis-deficient embryos to form a head and an axis (Kao et al. 1986). Lithium acts on animal cells, so that these cells respond to a ventral mesodermal induction signal by producing dorsal mesoderm with organizer activity (Slack et al. 1988; Kao and Elinson 1989; Cooke et al. 1989).

One effect of lithium is to inhibit the phosphatidylinositol (PI) cycle, an important second messenger system that affects Ca^{2+} levels, pH, and phosphorylation in cells (Berridge et al. 1989). The ability of inositol to counteract lithium's dorsalizing effect in the embryo suggests that this signal transduction mechanism is part of the biochemical pathway leading to organizer activity (Busa and Gimlich 1989). Induction of notochord and dorsal muscle by a viral oncogene, known to activate phosphorylation, further implicates signal transduction mechanisms in the generation of the organizer (Whitman and Melton 1989).

The lithium/D_2O phenotype can be reproduced by overexpression in embryos of *Xenopus* proteins related to the mammalian *int-1* (*wnt*) proto-oncogene (Christian et al. 1991). Cells derived from overexpression of *Xwnt* genes later behave like Spemann's organizer, suggesting that *Xwnt* proteins are related to the natural inducers of the organizer in the embryo

(Sokol et al. 1991). *Xwnt* and other mRNA's with dorsalizing activity have been isolated using a cDNA library derived from lithium-treated embryos (Smith and Harland 1991). Such molecular analyses of embryonic phenotypes provide useful groundwork for the identification of genes involved in dorso-anterior patterning.

Neural Induction. The central nervous system is induced to form from ectoderm by the organizer (fig. 1.8) (Spemann and Mangold 1924; Gimlich and Cooke 1983; Smith and Slack 1983). During gastrulation, the organizer migrates along the inner surface of the overlying ectoderm, inducing it to form a keyhole-shaped area, known as the neural plate (figs. 1.8, 1.10). The neural plate folds longitudinally into a neural tube, which is the

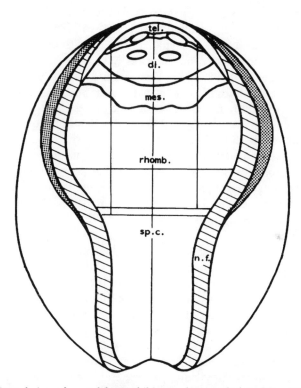

Fig. 1.10. Dorsal view of a urodele amphibian at the neural plate stage. Neural crest (hatched) is derived from the neural folds (n.f.), while placodal tissue (stippled) lies peripheral to the anterior neural plate. The neural plate is divided into the presumptive forebrain or prosencephalon, consisting of telencephalon (tel.) and diencephalon (di.); presumptive midbrain or mesencephalon (mes.); presumptive hindbrain or rhombencephalon (rhomb.); and presumptive spinal cord (sp.c.). (From Nieuwkoop et al. 1985)

precursor to the brain anteriorly and the spinal cord posteriorly (Jacobson and Gordon 1976; Eagleson and Harris 1990).

Recent observations have suggested two other means by which neural tissue can be specified. In one, the ectoderm on the dorsal side of the embryo is predisposed to neural differentiation (Sharpe et al. 1987). In the other, neural tissue is induced through the plane of the ectoderm, rather than from the underlying organizer. This induction occurs via a signal originating near the posterior end of the neural plate, which is contiguous with the posterior end of the dorsal mesoderm (London et al. 1988; Dixon and Kintner 1989; Phillips 1991). The experiments demonstrate that these alternative induction influences also contribute to the inductive influence provided by the organizer as it migrates along the ectoderm (Sharpe 1990; Guthrie 1991).

A major emphasis since Spemann's discovery has been to determine the nature of the neural inducing signals and to identify and isolate the induction molecules (Nakamura et al. 1978). As with dorsal mesoderm induction, signal transduction mechanisms have been implicated in neural induction (Otte et al. 1988, 1991; Durston and Otte 1991), but there has been little success in finding the natural inducer. Success has been reached, however, in identifying molecules expressed in response to neural induction (Jacobson and Rutishauser 1986; Kintner and Melton 1987; Sharpe 1988; Richter et al. 1988) and those expressed in the absence of induction (Jones and Woodland 1986; Akers et al. 1986; Jamrich et al. 1987). The use of probes for these and other molecules has proved useful in confirming and extending the original experiments on the induction and regional differentiation of the neural plate (Sharpe et al. 1987; Dixon and Kintner 1989; Sive et al. 1989; Sharpe and Gurdon 1990).

One path for the future is to see what is controlling the transcription of these genes in the neurectoderm versus the epidermis. This path would lead backward from the control elements of the genes to the factors that interact with those elements to the origin of those factors. Ultimately, the presence of the factors must depend on the interactions between the organizer and the ectoderm, and in this way, the natural inducing substances may be found.

Head Induction. It was recognized very early that there is regional specificity in neural induction, yielding, at one end, the brain and sense organs of the head, and at the other, the spinal cord and posterior mesoderm (Spemann 1931; Mangold 1933; Eyal-Giladi 1954; Takaya 1978). The region responsible for head induction is the anterior archenteron roof, which will become the pharyngeal endoderm, the prechordal plate or head mesoderm, and the anterior portion of the notochord. Pharyngeal endoderm forms mouth parts while the prechordal plate contributes to the loosely organized head mesenchyme. Both of these tissues are derived from animal cells by mesoderm induction (Nieuwkoop and Ubbels 1972). Many of the head mesodermal structures are derived from neural crest cells, a product of neural induction (Le Douarin 1980; Noden 1986). The posterior archenteron roof becomes the chordamesoderm which induces hindbrain and spinal cord.

Prechordal plate mesoderm and chordamesoderm differ in their morphogenetic behavior during gastrulation. Prechordal plate mesoderm undergoes anterior and lateral spreading after involution and induces the wide anterior neural plate (Hama et al. 1985; Keller et al. 1985; Keller and Tibbetts 1989). In contrast, the more posterior chordamesoderm continues a convergent extension after involution and does not undergo lateral spreading. The appearance of the prechordal plate during gastrulation in *Xenopus* is unremarkable, consisting of loosely organized cells of irregular shapes (Keller and Schoenwolf 1977). Analysis of molecular markers expressed in prechordal plate, such as the mRNA for a retinoic acid receptor (Ellinger-Zeigelbauer and Dreyer 1991), will help to determine the origin and properties of this mesoderm which is so important in head formation.

The difference between the anterior and posterior archenteron roofs in their inductive activities develops during gastrulation. When the anterior roof is transplanted before it has involuted, it induces trunk and tail structures. When the equivalent tissue is transplanted after involution, it induces head structures. The developmental change in the anterior roof depends on time, since the same change occurs when the preinvolution roof is cultured in vitro (Takaya 1978).

The apparent anterior-to-posterior shift in the organizer suggests the existence of separate inducers or a change in the inductive capacity of the organizer through time. Several hypotheses have been proposed to explain how the interaction of two inducers could generate the head-to-tail regional differentiation of the nervous system (reviewed by Nakamura et al. 1978; Toivonen 1978; Yamada 1981; Nieuwkoop et al. 1985). The double-gradient theory of Toivonen and Saxén (1955; Toivonen et al. 1963; Toivonen 1978) proposes gradients of neuralizing and mesodermalizing activities at right angles to each other. The neuralizing activity is highest at the dorsal midline and diminishes laterally, while the mesodermalizing activity is highest at the posterior end and diminishes anteriorly. Formation of the forebrain, eye, and nose results from neuralizing activity with no mesodermalizing activity; the spinal cord results from both activities.

Nieuwkoop et al. (1985) review the argument that instead of two gradients, there are two activities that act sequentially. The activating factor in the anterior organizer causes anterior neural development while the later transforming factor in the more posterior organizer leads to regionalization of the neural area. This hypothesis is supported by recent experiments which show that anterior mesoderm, when combined with undifferentiated ectoderm, induces expression of anterior-specific neural genes, while posterior mesoderm induces expression of anterior and posterior neural genes (Sharpe and Gurdon 1990).

Respecification of Neural Induction. An interesting feature of these theories is that the forebrain results from the simplest induction, either the activity of the neuralizing gradient without the mesodermalizing gradient or activation without transformation. The most anterior parts of the head represent those tissues which have escaped from any transforming influence.

The molecules responsible for the inducing activities are unknown, but retinoic acid is a candidate for the mesodermalizing or transforming activity. When pulsed with retinoic acid before neuralation, embryos lack forebrain, midbrain, eyes, and nose (Durston et al. 1989; Sive et al. 1990; Drysdale and Elinson 1991) and have alterations of dorso-anterior mesoderm (Ruiz i Altaba and Jessell 1991; Sive and Cheng 1991). Retinoic acid is present in the embryo in sufficient quantities to prevent the formation of head neural structures (Durston et al. 1989), but no specific anterior-posterior distribution of retinoic acid has been reported. On the other hand, the expression of the gene for a retinoic acid receptor has been localized to the prechordal plate (Ellinger-Zeigelbauer and Dreyer 1991), suggesting a direct action of retinoic acid on this tissue.

The effects of retinoic acid can be mimicked by the overexpression of a *Xenopus* homeobox gene *Xhox 3* that is normally expressed at low levels in dorso-anterior mesoderm and high levels in posterior mesoderm (Ruiz i Altaba and Melton 1989a). Overexpression by microinjection of *Xhox 3* RNA causes elimination of the antero-posterior gradient of *Xhox 3* and development of the head is inhibited (Ruiz i Altaba and Melton 1989c). This result raises the possibility that the *Xhox 3* gene is a key regulator of the antero-posterior pattern. The normal expression of *Xhox 3* in chordamesodermal cells may allow those cells to produce a mesodermalizing or transforming activity, which, in turn, suppresses head development posteriorly.

Neural Crest and Placodes. Neural crest and placodes are induced from the ectoderm and play important roles in head formation. The cephalic neural crest contributes to head mesenchyme along with the prechordal plate mesoderm, and the placodes form the anlagen of the nose, lens, and ear.

Although migration and differentiation of neural crest cells have been studied intensively, far less attention has been paid to their origin. Neural crest forms at the junction of neural plate and epidermis, the site of the neural folds (fig. 1.10). In many in vitro experiments on neural induction, pigment cells, a neural crest derivative, differentiate in the cultures (Leussink 1970; Barth and Barth 1974; Asashima and Grunz 1983). These casual observations related to neural crest induction should be extended in the future as more markers for neural crest cells become available.

Formation of neural crest at the periphery of the neural plate implies that its induction is intimately connected with neural induction. The neural inducing signal from the chordamesoderm to the ectoderm is strongest along the dorsal midline. The signal may then spread through the ectoderm, so that induced neural ectoderm itself induces neighboring ectoderm (Leussink 1970). The spreading of an inducing signal through a tissue is known as homoiogenetic induction (Mangold and Spemann 1927). Whether the neural inducing signal is derived from the chordamesoderm or spreads through the ectoderm, the boundaries of the neural plate appear to be defined by ectodermal competence. Competence is the ability of a tissue to respond to an inducing signal. The dividing line between neural plate and epidermis results from the loss of ectodermal competence before the inducing signal has spread to it (Albers 1987).

Neural crest, arising at the dividing line, may represent ectodermal cells barely competent to respond to the neural inducing signal. Alternatively, Nieuwkoop et al. (1985) hypothesize that a separate neural crest competence may persist longer than neural competence, so that the last ectoderm to be induced forms neural crest.

Placodes are local ectodermal thickenings found at the periphery of the anterior neural plate (fig. 1.10). They form owing to a series of inductions as the presumptive placodal areas contact different tissues during the movements of gastrulation. The presumptive lens is induced sequentially by the endoderm, the heart mesoderm, and the optic vesicle (Jacobson 1966; Henry and Grainger 1987), while the presumptive ear and nose are induced by a different set of three tissues (Jacobson 1966). The final inducer in all cases is neural tissue. The inductions of the placodes illustrate the complex sequence of interactions which was involved in tissue determination during development.

Molecular probes that recognize specific anterior structures are useful in describing the morphogenesis of the face. For instance, the hatching gland can be visualized by two different antibodies and appears as a Y-shaped structure on the dorso-anterior surface of the head (Sato and Sargent 1990; Drysdale and Elinson 1991). It is induced to form from the anterior neural folds and delineates ciliated epidermis from the nonciliated faceplate (Drysdale and Elinson 1991). Cement gland marks the ventral margin of the face and forms by a progressive series of inductions (Sive et al. 1989). The appearance of placodes, hatching gland, and cement gland are early events leading to the final modeling of the face.

BIRDS

Breaking Radial Symmetry

The bird egg is radially symmetric with a small disc of cytoplasm at one pole sitting on a huge mass of yolk. Specification of an antero-posterior axis and the plane of bilateral symmetry differs from the amphibian with respect to the timing and the force involved (reviewed by Eyal-Giladi 1984). The antero-posterior axis is specified in the chick at 14 to 16 hours in the uterus when the blastoderm consists of many cells overlying a cavity above the yolk (fig. 1.11) (Clavert 1962; Eyal-Giladi and Fabian 1980). Axis specification is correlated with the formation of the area pellucida which results from the shedding of cells from the blastoderm into the sub-blastoderm cavity. The blastoderm is thinner initially on the posterior side, and this is the first indication of the antero-posterior axis (Eyal-Giladi and Kochav 1976; Kochav et al. 1980). Axis specification in the chick occurs in the multicellular blastoderm and not in the single-celled zygote as in the frog.

The force involved in axis specification in the chick is gravity (Kochav and Eyal-Giladi 1971). When the blastoderm in vitro is held with one end higher than the other, the upper end becomes the tail and the lower end becomes the head. Tilting with respect to gravity is necessary in the quail blastoderm for development symmetry in vitro. A blastoderm cultured in a horizontal position does not form a primitive streak (Olszanska et al. 1984), and this embryo may be equivalent to the Bauchstück in amphibians (fig. 1.4).

Gravity also functions in vivo and this explains a rule of von Baer (1828, cited in Kochav and Eyal-Giladi 1971). This rule says that when you hold a chick egg with the pointed end of the shell to your right, the antero-posterior axis of the embryo is perpendicular to the long axis of the shell and the head is furthest from you. These relations result from the rotation of the egg in the uterus with the pointed end toward the cloaca in the chick (Clavert 1962). The blastoderm attempts to maintain a horizontal position on top of the yolk, but owing to the rotation, the blastoderm is tilted. The lower end becomes the head end, as in the in vitro situation (Kochav and Eyal Giladi 1971).

While gravity can cause axis specification in both chicks and amphibians, the action of gravity is different. In chicks, gravity appears to be the normal cause of axis specification. In amphibians, the normal

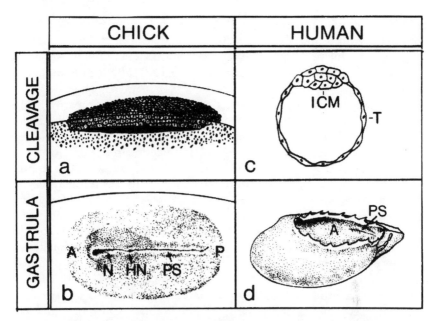

Fig. 1.11. Cleavage stages and gastrulae of chicks and humans. a. The chick blastoderm consists of many cells overlying a cavity above the mass of yolk. During axis specification, cells are shed into the cavity starting at the future posterior end. The resulting thinning of the upper layer of cells appears as the area pellucida. b. A view of the epiblast during gastrulation shows the primitive streak (PS), Hensen's node (HN), and neural folds (N). The chick embryo has an anterior (A) to posterior (P) progression in development so the neural folds for the brain are already well formed while presumptive notochord and mesoderm continue to ingress at Hensen's node and the primitive streak. c. The mammalian blastocyst consists of the thin trophoblast (T) surrounding a cavity and the inner cell mass (ICM). The amniotic cavity forms between the inner cell mass and the trophoblast, and that surface of the inner cell mass becomes the dorsal surface of the embryo. d. Removal of the amnion (jagged line) reveals the surface of the epiblast during gastrulation. As in chicks, a primitive streak (PS) is present which defines the anterior end (A). (Modified from Elinson 1987)

cause is the microtubule-dependent cortical rotation which gravity can override in experimental situations.

Axial Information in Early Development

The chick embryo develops two layers of cells: the surface epiblast, which will form the embryo's body as well as extraembryonic ectoderm and mesoderm, and the lower hypoblast, which becomes extraembryonic endoderm (Vakaet 1984). Later, the primitive streak forms in the epiblast and is the site where surface epiblast cells move between the epiblast and hypoblast to form mesoderm. The most anterior part of the streak is the primitive pit and the area surrounding the pit is Hensen's node (fig. 1.11). Presumptive notochord cells move into the middle layer at the pit, and the analogy is frequently made between Hensen's node and the dorsal lip of the amphibian blastopore (Selleck and Stern 1991). Both have organizer activity.

Information for antero-posterior polarity is carried primarily in the hypoblast and transferred to the epiblast by induction. When the hypoblast is rotated relative to the epiblast, the primitive streak is oriented according to the polarity of the hypoblast (Waddington 1933; Azar and Eyal-Giladi 1981; Eyal-Giladi 1984). The ability of the hypoblast to promote the formation of the primitive streak originally lies in the posterior marginal zone, which contributes cells to the developing hypoblast (Azar and Eyal-Giladi 1979; Khaner and Eyal-Giladi 1989, but see Stern 1990 for an alternative view). The epiblast also carries information for the polarity of the primitive streak, but it requires the hypoblast for its expression. An epiblast without a hypoblast does not form a primitive streak. When a reaggregated hypoblast lacking polarity is cultured with an epiblast, a primitive streak forms in the epiblast, and the streak is oriented according to the polarity of the epiblast (Mitrani and Eyal-Giladi 1981).

As in amphibians, growth factors have been implicated in the inductions which transmit axial information in early development. Treatment of epiblasts with activin generates axial structures, including notochord, somites, and neural plate, and activin mRNA is present in the hypoblast before gastrulation (Mitrani and Shimoni 1990; Mitrani, Ziv et al. 1990). These findings suggest that activin plays a major role in axis formation of the chick embryo. FGF is also present in chick embryos (Mitrani, Gruenbaum et al. 1990), so it likely is involved in early signaling events.

Transplantation of Hensen's node from the anterior end of the primitive streak to another place in the blastoderm leads to the induction of a secondary embryo. This experiment demonstrates the organizer activity of Hensen's node (Waddington and Schmidt 1933; Gallera 1971; Hara 1978; Vakaet 1984). Using a chick-quail nuclear marker, Hornbruch et al. (1979) demonstrated the induction of somites by the transplanted Hensen's node as well as the induction of a neural plate. As with amphibians, there is regional specificity of induction of the nervous system. The prechordal plate induces forebrain, the anterior head-process induces mid- and hindbrain, and the posterior head-process induces spinal cord (Gallera 1971; Hara 1978). Neural crest forms at the boundary between the neural plate and the epidermis as in amphibians (Rosenquist 1981).

An entertaining but difficult exercise has been to identify homologies between amphibian and chick fate maps and cell movements (Waddington

1952; Ballard 1981). A more profitable way to uncover homologies may be to see which tissues are involved in the inductions yielding the axial structures. Hensen's node is like the organizer, while the posterior marginal zone of the chick epiblast may function like the dorsal vegetal cells in the amphibian embryo. As the inductive events are defined more carefully with molecular markers, lineage tracers, and identification of natural inducers, homologies between amphibian and chick developmental patterns will become clearer.

FISH, REPTILES, MAMMALS

Almost everything known about axis specification has been found in chicks or in various amphibians, urodeles previously and *Xenopus laevis* more recently. There is very little information in any other species. Among fish, development of sturgeon (Ballard and Ginsberg 1980) and lungfish (Wourms and Kemp 1982) appears similar to that of amphibians through gastrulation. This raises the possibility that axis specification is also similar. Dettlaff and Ginsberg (1954, cited in Clavert 1962; Nieuwkoop et al. 1985) report that the sturgeon egg has a clear crescent that marks the plane of bilateral symmetry and that the position of the clear crescent can be specified by the rotation of the whole egg. It would be interesting to see whether the sturgeon egg has the parallel microtubules thought to be the motor for grey crescent formation in the frog egg.

Development of teleosts is very different from that of sturgeons and amphibians through cleavage and gastrulation (Ballard 1973, 1981, 1982; Kimmel et al. 1991). Long (1983) indicated that in the trout, information for bilateral symmetry resided in the yolk syncytial layer and could be transferred to the blastodisc where the embryonic axis forms. Although gravity has been suggested as the cause (Clavert 1962), Long and Speck (1984) found no effect of gravity on symmetrization in medaka. The plane of bilateral symmetry was not correlated with the initial cleavage furrows as it frequently is for amphibians (Long and Speck 1984; Kimmel and Law 1985).

In several reptiles, the eggs rotate in the uterus, and the embryos follow von Baer's rule as described for chicks (reviewed by Clavert 1962). This suggests that the axis is specified, as in chicks, owing to action of gravity during the cellular blastoderm stage (Kochav and Eyal-Giladi 1971).

Our knowledge of mammalian early development has advanced rapidly, but virtually nothing is known about axis specification. Initially, the egg is radially symmetric as indicated by the site of polar body formation, and in the mouse, by the area where sperm entry occurs (Nicosia et al. 1977). The radial symmetry of the egg is not carried to the embryo, since at the eight-cell stage, each cell appears to be equivalent in terms of developmental potential. Within a few cell divisions, the embryo develops into the blastocyst. The blastocyst consists of an outer, thin epithelium, the trophoblast, enclosing a small clump of cells, the inner cell, mass, and a fluid-filled cavity (fig. 1.11). The inner cell mass divides into an epiblast (primitive ectoderm) and a hypoblast (primitive endoderm) analogous to those in the chick, and as in the chick, the epiblast gives rise to the fetus as well as extraembryonic structures. The surface of the epiblast closest to the trophoblast is dorsal and the surface of epiblast closest to the hypoblast is ventral.

A primitive streak and Hensen's node develop on the dorsal surface of the epiblast (fig. 1.11), and gastrulation and axis development appear similar to those in the chick. Smith (1980, 1985) has shown that the embryonic axes are correlated with the position of attachment of the blastocyst to the uterine wall. The basis for these correlations is not known, although gravity acting on a tilted inner cell mass would be one possibility. There is no information on which cells carry the axial information. Based on the chick, one would predict that the hypoblast would become specified first.

The transmission of information for head and axial development probably involves many of the same molecules as have been identified in amphibians. FGF and other growth factors are present before and during gastrulation in mouse embryos (Rappolee et al. 1988; Haub and Goldfarb 1991; Hebert et al. 1991), suggesting that they are involved in mesoderm induction. Retinoic acid is present posterior to Hensen's node as early as the neural plate stage, and is conspicuously absent from the head of later embryos (Rossant et al. 1991). This localization contributes to the hypothesis that retinoic acid plays a role in antero-posterior patterning.

Molecular and genetic analysis has identified other genes whose expression is important for head and axial development. Mutations of *Brachyury* produce characteristic defects of mesoderm and notochord, and this gene is normally expressed early in the formation of those cell types (Wilkinson et al. 1990). A large number of homeobox-containing genes (*Hox* genes) are expressed in the developing hindbrain of the mouse. Their precise spatial pattern of expression suggests that they function in antero-posterior patterning of this region (Holland and Hogan 1988; Hunt et al. 1991; Lufkin et al. 1991).

Once a gene in mouse is identified as interesting, its function can be tested by targeted gene disruption. In effect, a mutation of that gene is created. Disruptions to *Hox* genes caused specific abnormalities to hindbrain, face, and other structures (Lufkin et al. 1991; Chisaka and Capecchi 1991). These results indicate that *Hox* genes are critical links in the chain of events, generating structures of the head.

ABNORMALITIES OF AXIS SPECIFICATION AND HEAD INDUCTION

A complete range of abnormalities of axis specification have been generated in amphibians (fig. 1.4). UV irradiation of the zygote before cleavage produces dorso-anterior reduced embryos, while treatment with D_2O before cleavage or with lithium during early cleavage produces dorso-anterior enhanced embryos. The reduced embryos show progressive loss of structures, from a reduced head to cyclopia (one eye) to no head to a radial embryo with no nervous system, notochord, somites, or other dorso-anterior structures. The enhanced embryos have progressively more dorso-anterior structures and fewer posterior structures, culminating in a radial embryo with a radial eye, a mass of notochordal and neural tissue, and a heart, but with no trunk or tail. These morphologies are abnormalities of axis specification and result from differences in quantity of Spemann's organizer (Kao and Elinson 1988; Elinson and Kao 1989).

The mildest dorso-anterior reduced abnormalities, including cyclopia, can be produced later in development by treatments during gastrulation. Curiously, lithium, which causes dorso-anterior enhancement when applied during early cleavage, is a potent agent for causing cyclopia when applied later (Adelman 1934, 1936; Lehman 1938; Yamaguchi and Shinagawa 1989). The target of the late treatments was thought to be prechordal plate mesoderm which induces the brain to form, since surgical removal of the prechordal plate causes head reduction and cyclopia (Adelman 1937; Neff et al. 1987). However, Masui (1956, 1960) demonstrated that lithium also exerts an effect on the ectoderm, suppressing its ability to form forebrain in response to an inducing signal. Abnormal development of the brain and head can be due to abnormalities in either the prechordal plate mesoderm or in the responding ectoderm.

Many cases of abnormal head induction have been reported in humans (Cohen 1982; Bixler et al. 1985; Carles et al. 1987) and other mammals (Wright and Wagner 1934; Juriloff et al. 1985). These are classified as holoprosencephaly, a reduction of the prosencephalon or forebrain. Cyclopia is a severe form, and agnathia, a reduction or absence of the lower jaw, is frequently associated with holoprosencephaly. The term "otocephaly" is used to describe the fusion or close approach of the ears as a result of agnathia, but many cases of otocephaly are part of the holoprosencephalic series (fig. 1.12).

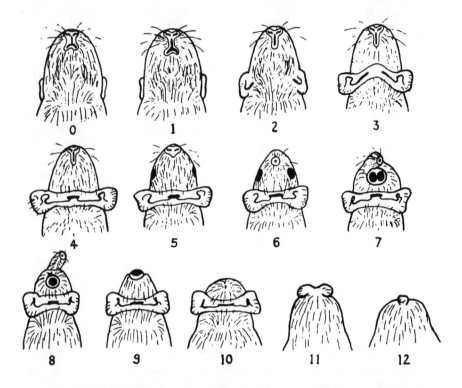

Fig. 1.12. Holoprosencephaly in guinea pigs. A mutation causes progressive loss of the brain and lower jaw. As the lower jaw disappears, the ears approach each other and fuse at the ventral midline (otocephaly). Grades 8 and 9 are cyclopic. These twelve grades correspond to DAI 2-4 in frogs (fig. 1.4). (From Wright 1934)

The heterogeneous collection of holoprosencephalic syndromes has been considered a reflection of abnormalities of the prechordal plate mesoderm during gastrulation based on amphibians (Bixler et al. 1985; Juriloff et al. 1985). As suggested above, this need not be the case. Head deficiencies are equally likely to result from defects in the responding ectoderm as compared to the mesoderm (Masui 1956, 1960). While careful histological analysis may distinguish a defect acting in the mesoderm from one in the ectoderm, the necessary experiment is to transplant ectoderm and mesoderm between mutant and normal animals.

The conjunction of the head abnormalities in humans and other mammals and the experimental analysis in amphibians and chicks raises some intriguing questions. Analysis of head induction would be greatly facilitated by methods to identify prechordal plate mesoderm. The presence of mutations that yield holoprosencephaly in guinea pigs (fig. 1.12; Wright

1934) and mice (Juriloff et al. 1985) suggests that there are genes that act either in the prechordal plate or in the responding ectoderm. Identification of those genes and isolation of their products may provide the necessary molecular markers for these tissues.

Another question is whether cases of holoprosencephaly in mammals are abnormalities of head induction per se or whether they are the only surviving abnormalities of axis specification. Holoprosencephaly in mammals is usually lethal; yet, it represents only the two or three mildest grades of dorso-anterior reduction in amphibians (compare figs. 1.4 and 1.12). Mammalian or bird embryos corresponding to the amphibian acephalic or Bauchstück (fig. 1.4) have not been identified. It is possible that the more severe mammalian defects result in early embryonic lethality. The mouse mutation that reduces the prosencephalon does seem to be a mutation of head induction rather than of axis specification since there is little evidence for high early mortality (Juriloff et al. 1985).

Finally, dorso-anterior enhancement has been found in amphibians, but we are unaware of its recognition in birds or mammals. Conjoined twins with anterior duplications are likely to arise during axis specification, and they may represent the expression of enhanced specification in amniotes. There may also be classes of mammalian abnormalities, analogous to dorso-anterior enhanced amphibians, where some facial or head abnormality is coupled to posterior reduction.

A good place to look for these human syndromes would be cases of hypertelorism, where the eyes are widely separated and which is sometimes associated with a cleft face. A quite different syndrome is iniencephaly, where the back is greatly shortened, bringing the base of the skull near the lower back (Salmon 1978). An interesting exercise would be to see which human head abnormalities fall into the dorso-anterior enhanced series defined on amphibians. This might provide an etiology for those abnormalities.

FINAL COMMENTS

The radial symmetry of the vertebrate egg is broken early in development by an event known as axis specification. Axial information is carried by a sequence of inductive cell interactions in which the key player is Spemann's organizer. The organizer dorsalizes the mesoderm, induces the ectoderm to form neural tissue, and itself differentiates into notochord and mesoderm. Neural induction is regionally specific, so that a wide neural plate, the presumptive brain, is induced anteriorly and is bordered by cephalic neural crest and placodes. These tissues, plus prechordal plate mesoderm and anterior endoderm, make up the head. While the head is specified very early, its eventual appearance results from a series of inductions.

There is optimism resulting from new approaches that the problem of embryonic induction can be solved. The use of modern lineage tracers and molecular markers allows the close monitoring of inductive events. These techniques have led to advances in the analysis of mesoderm induction and are providing insights into neural induction. The discovery that molecules like FGF, activin, and retinoic acid can cause or affect induction has aroused considerable interest. Although many artificial inducers were identified previously, the current crop of molecules can be found in the embryo and provides links to known signal transduction mechanisms in cells.

The rapid progress of the last few years promises to provide a molecular and cellular explanation for axis specification and head induction in the near future.

ACKNOWLEDGMENTS

We thank Richard Fong for his drawings, and NSERC, Canada, for funding during the writing of this chapter.

REFERENCES

Adelmann, H. 1934. A study of cyclopia in *Amblystoma punctatum*, with special reference to the mesoderm. Journal of Experimental Zoology 67: 217–281.

Adelmann, H. B. 1936. The problem of cyclopia. Parts I and II. Quarterly Review of Biology 11: 161–182, 284–304.

———. 1937. Experimental studies on the development of the eye. IV. The effect of the partial and complete excision of the prechordal substrate on the development of the eyes of *Ambystoma punctatum*. Journal of Experimental Zoology 75: 199–237.

Akers, R. M., C. R. Phillips, and N. K. Wessells. 1986. Expression of an epidermal antigen used to study tissue interaction in the early *Xenopus laevis* embryo. Science 231: 613–616.

Albers, B. 1987. Competence as the main factor determining the size of the neural plate. Development, Growth, and Differentiation 29: 535–545.

Amaya, E., T. J. Musci, and M. W. Kirschner. 1991. Expression of a dominant negative mutant of the FGF receptor disrupts mesoderm formation in *Xenopus* embryos. Cell 66: 257–270.

Ancel, P., and P. Vintemberger. 1948. Recherches sur le déterminisme de la symétrie bilatérale dans l'oeuf des amphibiens. Bulletin biologique de France et de Belgique 31 (suppl.): 1–182.

Asashima, M., and H. Grunz. 1983. Effects of inducers on inner and outer gastrula ectoderm layers of *Xenopus laevis*. Differentiation 23: 206–212.

Asashima, M., H. Nakano, K. Shimada, K. Kinoshita, K. Ishii, H. Shibai, and N. Ueno. 1990. Mesodermal induction in early amphibian embryos by activin A (erythroid differentiation factor). Roux's Archives for Developmental Biology 198: 330–335.

Azar, Y., and H. Eyal-Giladi. 1979. Marginal zone cells—the primitive streak-inducing component of the primary hypoblast in the chick. Journal of Embryology and Experimental Morphology 52: 79–88.

———. 1981. Interaction of epiblast and hypoblast in the formation of the primitive streak and the embryonic axis in chick, as revealed by hypoblast-rotation experiments. Journal of Embryology and Experimental Morphology 61: 133–144.

Ballard, W. W. 1973. A new fate map for *Salmo gairdneri*. Journal of Experimental Zoology 184: 49–74.

———. 1981. Morphogenetic movements and fate maps of vertebrates. American Zoologist 21: 391–399.

———. 1982. Morphogenetic movements and fate map of the cypriniform teleost, *Catostomus commersoni* (Lacepede). Journal of Experimental Zoology 219: 301–321.

Ballard, W. W., and A. S. Ginsberg. 1980. Morphogenetic movements in acipenserid embryos. Journal of Experimental Zoology 213: 69–103.

Barth, L. G., and L. J. Barth. 1974. Ionic regulation of embryonic induction and cell differentiation in *Rana pipiens*. Developmental Biology 34: 1–22.

Berridge, M. J., P. Downes, and M. R. Hanley. 1989. Neural and developmental actions of lithium: A unifying hypothesis. Cell 59: 411–419.

Bixler, D., R. Ward, and D. D. Gale. 1985. Agnathia-holoprosencephaly: A developmental field complex involving the face and brain; report of three cases. Journal of Craniofacial Genetics and Developmental Biology 1 (suppl.): 241–249.

Black, S. D., and J. C. Gerhart. 1985. Experimental control of the site of embryonic axis formation in *Xenopus laevis* eggs centrifuged before first cleavage. Developmental Biology 108: 310–324.

———. 1986. High-frequency twinning of *Xenopus laevis* embryos from eggs centrifuged before first cleavage. Developmental Biology 116: 228–240.

Busa, W. B., and R. L. Gimlich. 1989. Lithium-induced teratogenesis in frog embryos prevented by a polyphosphoinositide cycle intermediate or a diacylglycerol analog. Developmental Biology 132: 315–324.

Carles, D., F. Serville, M. Mainguene, and J. P. Dubecq. 1987. Cyclopia-otocephaly association: A new case of the most severe variant of agnathia-holoprosencephalic complex. Journal of Craniofacial Genetics and Developmental Biology 7: 107–113.

Chisaka, O., and M. R. Capecchi. 1991. Regionally restricted developmental defects resulting from targeted disruption of the mouse homeobox gene *hox-1.5*. Nature 350: 473–479.

Christian, J. L., J. A. McMahon, A. P. McMahon, and R. T. Moon. 1991. *Xwnt-8*, a *Xenopus Wnt-1/int-1* related gene responsive to mesoderm-inducing growth factors, may play a role in ventral mesodermal patterning during embryogenesis. Development 111: 1045–1055.

Chung, H. M., and G. M. Malacinski. 1983. Reversal of developmental competence in inverted amphibian eggs. Journal of Embryology and Experimental Morphology 73: 207–220.

Clavert, J. 1962. Symmetrization of the egg of vertebrates. Advances in Morphogenesis 2: 27–60.

Cohen, M. M. 1982. An update on the holoprosencephalic disorders. Journal of Pediatrics 101: 865–869.

Cooke, J., and J. C. Smith. 1987. The midblastula cell cycle transition and the character of mesoderm in u.v.-induced nonaxial Xenopus development. Development 99: 197–210.

Cooke, J., K. Symes, and E. J. Smith. 1989. Potentiation by the lithium ion of morphogenetic responses to a Xenopus inducing factor. Development 105: 549–558.

Dale, L., and J. M. W. Slack. 1987a. Fate map of the 32-cell stage of Xenopus laevis. Development 99: 527–551.

———. 1987b. Regional specification within the mesoderm of early embryos of Xenopus laevis. Development 100: 279–295.

Dale, L., J. C. Smith, and J. M. W. Slack. 1985. Mesoderm induction in Xenopus laevis: A quantitative study using a cell lineage label and tissue-specific antibodies. Journal of Embryology and Experimental Morphology 89: 289–312.

Danilchik, M. V., and J. M. Denegre. 1991. Deep cytoplasmic rearrangements during early development in Xenopus laevis. Development 111: 845–856.

Danilchik, M., and J. C. Gerhart. 1987. Differentiation of the animal-vegetal axis in Xenopus laevis oocytes. I. Polarized intracellular translocation of platelets establishes the yolk gradient. Developmental Biology 122: 101–112.

Dixon, J. E., and C. R. Kintner. 1989. Cellular contacts required for neural induction in Xenopus embryos: Evidence for two signals. Development 106: 749–757.

Drysdale, T. A., and R. P. Elinson. 1991. Development of the Xenopus laevis hatching gland and its relationship to surface ectoderm patterning. Development 111: 469–478.

Durston, A. J., and A. P. Otte. 1991. A hierarchy of signals mediates neural induction in Xenopus laevis. In Cell-Cell Interactions in Early Development, J. Gerhart, ed. New York: Wiley-Liss, pp. 109–127.

Durston, A. J., J. P. M. Timmermans, W. J. Hage, H. F. J. Hendricks, N. J. de Vries, M. Heideveld, and P. D. Nieuwkoop. 1989. Retinoic acid causes an anteroposterior transformation in the developing central nervous system. Nature 340: 140–144.

Eagleson, G. W., and W. A. Harris. 1990. Mapping of the presumptive brain regions in the neural plate of Xenopus laevis. Journal of Neurobiology 21: 427–440.

Elinson, R. P. 1977. Macrocephaly and microcephaly in hybrids between the bullfrog Rana catesbeiana and the mink frog Rana septentrionalis. Journal of Herpetology 11: 94–96.

———. 1985. Changes in levels of polymeric tubulin associated with activation and dorso-ventral polarization of the frog egg. Developmental Biology 109: 224–233.

———. 1987. Change in developmental patterns: Embryos of amphibians with large eggs. In *Development as an Evolutionary Process,* R. A. Raff and E. C. Raff, eds. New York: Alan R. Liss, pp. 1–21.

———. 1989. Microtubules and specification of the dorsoventral axis in frog embryos. BioEssays 11: 124–127.

———. 1991. Separation of an anterior inducing activity from development of dorsal axial mesoderm in large headed frog embryos. Developmental Biology 145: 91–98.

Elinson, R. P., and K. R. Kao. 1989. The location of dorsal information in frog early development. Development, Growth, and Differentiation 31: 423–430.

Elinson, R. P., and P. Pasceri. 1989. Two UV-sensitive targets in dorsoanterior specification of frog embryos. Development 106: 511–518.

Elinson, R. P., and B. Rowning. 1988. A transient array of parallel microtubules in frog eggs: Potential tracks for a cytoplasmic rotation that specifies the dorsoventral axis. Developmental Biology 128: 185–197.

Ellinger-Zeigelbauer, H., and C. Dreyer. 1991. A retinoic acid receptor expressed in the early development of *Xenopus laevis.* Genes and Development 5: 94–104.

Eyal-Giladi, H. 1954. Dynamic aspects of neural induction in amphibia. Archives de biologie 65: 179–259.

———. 1984. The gradual establishment of cell commitments during the early stages of chick development. Cell Differentiation 14: 245–255.

Eyal-Giladi, H., and B. C. Fabian. 1980. Axis determination in uterine chick blastodiscs under changing spatial positions during the sensitive period for polarity. Developmental Biology 77: 228–232.

Eyal-Giladi, H., and S. Kochav, 1976. From cleavage to primitive streak formation: A complementary normal table and a new look at the first stages of the development of the chick. I. General morphology. Developmental Biology 49: 321–337.

Gallagher, B. C., A. M. Hainski, and S. A. Moody. 1991. Autonomous differentiation of dorsal axial structures from an animal cap cleavage stage blastomere in *Xenopus.* Development 112: 1103–1114.

Gallera, J. 1971. Primary induction in birds. Advances in Morphogenesis 9: 149–180.

Gans, C., and R. G. Northcutt. 1983. Neural crest and the origin of vertebrates: A new head. Science 220: 268–274.

Gerhart, J., G. Ubbels, S. Black, K. Hara, and M. Kirschner. 1981. A reinvestigation of the role of the grey crescent in axis formation in *Xenopus laevis.* Nature 292: 511–516.

Gerhart, J. C., M. Danilchik, T. Doniach, S. Roberts, B. Rowning, and R. Stewart. 1989. Cortical rotation of the *Xenopus* egg: Consequences for the anteroposterior pattern of embryonic dorsal development. Development 107 (suppl.): 37–51.

Gerhart, J. C., M. Danilchik, J. Roberts, B. Rowning, and J. P. Vincent. 1986. Primary and secondary polarity of the amphibian oocyte and egg. In *Game-*

togenesis and the Early Embryo, J. G. Gall, ed. New York: Alan R. Liss, pp. 305–319.

Gimlich, R. L. 1986. Acquisition of developmental autonomy in the equatorial region of the *Xenopus* embryo. Developmental Biology 115: 340–352.

Gimlich, R. L., and J. Cooke. 1983. Cell lineage and the induction of second nervous systems in amphibian development. Nature 306: 471–473.

Green, J. B. A., and J. C. Smith. 1990. Graded changes in dose of a *Xenopus* activin A homologue elicit stepwise transitions in embryonic cell fate. Nature 347: 391–394.

———. 1991. Growth factors as morphogens: Do gradients and thresholds establish body plan? Trends in Genetics 7: 245–250.

Grunz, H., and L. Tacke. 1986. The inducing capacity of the presumptive endoderm of *Xenopus laevis* studied by transfilter experiments. Roux's Archives of Developmental Biology 195: 467–473.

Gurdon, J. B., S. Fairman, T. J. Mohun, and S. Brennan. 1985. Activation of muscle-specific actin genes in *Xenopus* development by an induction between animal and vegetal cells of a blastula. Cell 41: 913–922.

Guthrie, S. 1991. Horizontal and vertical pathways in neural induction. Trends in Neuroscience 14: 123–126.

Hama, T., H. Tsujimura, T. Kaneda, K. Takata, and A. Ohara. 1985. Inductive capacities for the dorsal mesoderm of the dorsal marginal zone and pharyngeal endoderm in the very early gastrula of the newt, and presumptive pharyngeal endoderm as an initiator of the organization center. Development, Growth, and Differentiation 27: 419–433.

Hara, K. 1978. "Spemann's organizer" in birds. In *Organizer: A Milestone of a Half-Century from Spemann*, O. Nakamura and S. Toivonen, eds. Amsterdam: Elsevier/North Holland Biomedical Press, pp. 221–265.

Haub, O., and M. Goldfarb. 1991. Expression of the fibroblast growth factor-5 gene in the mouse embryo. Development 112: 397–406.

Heasman, J., J. Quarmby, and C. C. Wylie. 1984. The mitochondrial cloud of *Xenopus* oocytes: The source of germinal granule material. Developmental Biology 105: 458–469.

Hebert, J. M., M. Boyle, and G. R. Martin. 1991. mRNA localization studies suggest that murine FGF-5 plays a role in gastrulation. Development 112: 407–415.

Henry, J. J., and R. M. Grainger. 1987. Inductive interactions in the spatial and temporal restriction of lens-forming potential in embryonic ectoderm of *Xenopus laevis*. Developmental Biology 124: 200–214.

Holland, P. W. H., and B. L. M. Hogan. 1988. Expression of homeo box genes during mouse development: A review. Genes and Development 2: 773–782.

Hopwood, N. D. 1990. Cellular and genetic responses to mesoderm induction in *Xenopus*. Bioessays 12: 465–471.

Hornbruch, A., D. Summerbell, and L. Wolpert. 1979. Somite formation in the early chick embryo following grafts of Hensen's node. Journal of Embryology and Experimental Morphology 51: 51–62.

Houliston, E., and R. P. Elinson. 1991a. Evidence for the involvement of microtubules, endoplasmic reticulum, and kinesin in the cortical rotation of fertilized frog eggs. Journal of Cell Biology 114: 1017–1028.

——. 1991b. Patterns of microtubule polymerization related to cortical rotation in *Xenopus laevis* eggs. Development 112: 107–117.

Huff, R. E. 1962. The developmental role of material derived from the nucleus (germinal vesicle) of mature ovarian eggs. Developmental Biology 4: 398–422.

Hunt, P., J. Whiting, I. Muchamore, H. Marshall, and R. Krumlauf. 1991. Homeobox genes and models for patterning the hindbrain and branchial arches. Development 1 (suppl.): 187–196.

Jacobson, A. G. 1966. Inductive processes in embryonic development. Science 152: 25–34.

Jacobson, A. G., and R. Gordon. 1976. Changes in shape of the developing nervous system analyzed experimentally, mathematically, and by computer simulation. Journal of Experimental Zoology 197: 191–246.

Jacobson, M., and U. Rutishauser. 1986. Induction of neural cell adhesion molecule (NCAM) in *Xenopus* embryos. Developmental Biology 116: 524–531.

Jamrich, M., T. D. Sargent, and I. B. David. 1985. Altered morphogenesis and its effect on gene activity in *Xenopus laevis* embryos. Cold Spring Harbor Symposia on Quantitative Biology 50: 31–35.

——. 1987. Cell-type-specific expression of epidermal cytokeratin genes during gastrulation of *Xenopus laevis*. Genes and Development 1: 124–132.

Jones, E. A., and H. R. Woodland. 1986. Development of the ectoderm in *Xenopus:* Tissue specification and the role of cell association and division. Cell 44: 345–355.

Juriloff, D. M., K. K. Sulik, T. H. Roderick, and B. K. Hogan. 1985. Genetic and developmental studies of a new mouse mutation that produces otocephaly. Journal of Craniofacial Genetics and Developmental Biology 5: 121–145.

Kageura, H. 1990. Spatial distribution of the capacity to initiate a secondary embryo in the 32-cell embryo of *Xenopus laevis*. Developmental Biology 142: 432–438.

Kageura, H., and K. Yamana. 1983. Pattern regulation in isolated halves and blastomeres of early *Xenopus laevis*. Journal of Embryology and Experimental Morphology 74: 221–234.

——. 1986. Pattern formation in 8-cell composite embryos of *Xenopus laevis*. Journal of Embryology and Experimental Morphology 91: 79–100.

Kao, K. R., and R. P. Elinson. 1985. Alteration of the anterior-posterior embryonic axis: The pattern of gastrulation in macrocephalic frog embryos. Developmental Biology 107: 239–251.

——. 1988. The entire mesodermal mantle behaves as Spemann's organizer in dorsoanterior enhanced *Xenopus laevis* embryos. Developmental Biology 127: 64–77.

——. 1989. Dorsalization of mesoderm induction by lithium. Developmental Biology 132: 81–90.

Kao, K. R., Y. Masui, and R. P. Elinson. 1986. Lithium-induced respecification of pattern in *Xenopus laevis* embryos. Nature 322: 371–373.

Keller, R. E. 1975. Vital dye mapping of the gastrula and neurula of *Xenopus laevis*. I. Prospective areas and morphogenetic movements of the superficial layer. Developmental Biology 42: 222–241.

———. 1976. Vital dye mapping of the gastrula and neurula of *Xenopus laevis*. II. Prospective areas and morphogenetic movements of the deep layer. Developmental Biology 51: 118–137.

Keller, R. E., M. Danilchik, R. Gimlich, and J. Shih. 1985. The function and mechanism of convergent extension during gastrulation of *Xenopus laevis*. Journal of Embryology and Experimental Morphology 89 (suppl.): 185–209.

Keller, R. E., and G. C. Schoenwolf. 1977. An SEM study of cellular morphology, contact, and arrangement as related to gastrulation in *Xenopus laevis*. Roux's Archives of Developmental Biology 182: 165–186.

Keller, R. E., and P. Tibbetts. 1989. Mediolateral cell intercalation in the dorsal, axial mesoderm of *Xenopus laevis*. Developmental Biology 131: 539–549.

Khaner, O., and H. Eyal-Giladi. The chick's marginal zone and primitive streak formation. I. Coordinative effect of induction and inhibition. Developmental Biology 134: 206–214.

Kimelman, D., J. A. Abraham, T. Haaparanta, T. M. Palisi, and M. Kirschner. 1988. The presence of fibroblast growth factor in the frog egg: Its role as a natural mesoderm inducer. Science 242: 1053–1056.

Kimelman, D., and M. Kirschner. 1987. Synergistic induction of mesoderm by FGF and TGF-β and the identification of an mRNA coding for FGF in the early *Xenopus* embryo. Cell 51: 869–877.

Kimmel, C. B., D. A. Kane, and R. K. Ho. 1991. Lineage specification during early embryonic development of the zebrafish. In *Cell-Cell Interactions in Early Development*, J. Gerhart, ed. New York: Wiley-Liss, pp. 203–225.

Kimmel, C. B., and R. D. Law. 1985. Cell lineage of zebrafish blastomeres. III. Clonal analyses of the blastula and gastrula stages. Developmental Biology 108: 94–101.

Kintner, C. R., and D. A. Melton. 1987. Expression of *Xenopus* N-CAM RNA in ectoderm is an early response to neural induction. Development 99: 311–325.

Kochav, S., and H. Eyal-Giladi. 1971. Bilateral symmetry in chick embryo determination by gravity. Science 171: 1027–1029.

Kochav, S., M. Ginsburg, and H. Eyal-Giladi. 1980. From cleavage to primitive streak formation: A complementary normal table and a new look af the first stages of the development of the chick. Developmental Biology 79: 296–308.

Kubota, T. 1967. A regional change in the rigidity of the cortex of the egg of *Rana nigromaculata* following extrusion of the second polar body. Journal of Embryology and Experimental Morphology 17: 331–340.

Le Douarin, M. 1980. Migration and differentiation of neural crest cells. Current Topics in Developmental Biology 16: 31–85.

Lehmann, F. E. 1938. Regionale Verschiedenheiten des Organisators von *Triton*, inbesondere in der vorderen und hinteren Kopfregion, nachgewiesen durch phasenspezifische Erzeugung von Lithiumbedingten und operativ bewirkten Regionaldefekten. Wilhelm Roux' Archiv für Entwicklungsmechanik der Organismen 138: 106–158.

Leussink, J. A. 1970. The spatial distribution of inductive capacities in the neural plate and archenteron roof of urodeles. Netherlands Journal of Zoology 20: 1–79.

London, C., R. Akers, and C. Phillips. 1988. Signals from the dorsal blastopore lip region during gastrulation bias the ectoderm toward a non-epidermal pathway in *Xenopus laevis*. Developmental Biology 133: 157–168.

Long, W. L. 1983. The role of the yolk syncytial layer in determination of the plane of bilateral symmetry in the rainbow trout, *Salmo gairdneri* Richardson. Journal of Experimental Zoology 228: 91–97.

Long, W. L., and N. A. Speck. 1984. Determination of the plane of bilateral symmetry in the teleost fish, *Oryzias latipes*. Journal of Experimental Zoology 229: 241–245.

Lufkin, T., A. Dierich, M. LeMeur, M. Mark, and P. Chambon. 1991. Disruption of the *Hox-1.6* homeobox gene results in defects in a region corresponding to its rostral domain of expression. Cell 66: 1105–1119.

Malacinski, G. M. 1974. Biological properties of a presumptive morphogenetic determinant from the amphibian oocyte germinal vesicle nucleus. Cell Differentiation 3: 31–44.

Malacinski, G. M., H. Benford, and H. M. Chung. 1975. Association of an ultraviolet irradiation sensitive cytoplasmic localization with the future dorsal side of the amphibian egg. Journal of Experimental Zoology 191: 97–110.

Manes, M. E., and F. D. Barbieri. 1977. On the possibility of sperm aster involvement in dorso-ventral polarization and pronuclear migration in the amphibian egg. Journal of Embryology and Experimental Morphology 40: 187–197.

Manes, M. E., and R. P. Elinson. 1980. Ultraviolet light inhibits grey crescent formation on the frog egg. Roux's Archives of Developmental Biology 189: 73–76.

Manes, M. E., R. P. Elinson, and F. D. Barbieri. 1978. Formation of the amphibian egg grey crescent: Effects of colchicine and cytochalasin B. Roux's Archives of Developmental Biology 185: 99–104.

Mangold, O. 1933. Über die Induktionsfähigkeit der verschiedenen Bezirke der Neurula von Urodelen. Naturwissenschaften 21: 761–766.

Mangold, O., and H. Spemann. 1927. Über Induktion von Medullarplatte durch Medullarplatte im jüngeren Keim, ein Beispiel homöogenetischer oder assimilatorischer Induktion. Wilhelm Roux' Archiv für Entwicklungsmechanik der Organismen 111: 341–422.

Masui, Y. 1956. Effect of LiCl on the organizer and the presumptive ectoderm. Annotaciones zoologicae japonenses 29: 75–78.

———. 1960. Alteration of the differentiation of the gastrula ectoderm under the influence of lithium chloride Memoirs of the Konan University, Science Series 4: 79–104.

Mitrani, E., and H. Eyal-Giladi. 1981. Hypoblastic cells can form a disc inducing an embryonic axis in chick epiblast. Nature 289: 800–802.

Mitrani, E., Y. Gruenbaum, H. Shohat, and T. Ziv. 1990. Fibroblast growth factor during mesoderm induction in the early chick embryo. Development 109: 387–393.

Mitrani, E., and Y. Shimoni. 1990. Induction by soluble factors of organized axial structures in chick epiblasts. Science 247: 1092–1094.

Mitrani, E., T. Ziv, G. Thomsen, Y. Shimoni, D. A. Melton, and T. Bril. 1990. Activin can induce the formation of axial structures and is expressed in the hypoblast of the chick. Cell 63: 495–501.

Moody, S. A. 1987. Fates of the blastomeres of the 32-cell stage Xenopus embryo. Developmental Biology 122: 300–319.

Nakamura, O. 1978. Epigenetic formation of the organizer. In Organizer: A Milestone of a Half-Century from Spemann, O. Nakamura and S. Toivonen, eds. Amsterdam: Elsevier/North Holland Biomedical Press, pp. 179–220.

Nakamura, O., Y. Hayashi, and M. Asashima. 1978. A half-century from Spemann: Historical review of studies on the organizer. In Organizer: A Milestone of a Half-Century from Spemann, O. Nakamura and S. Toivonen, eds. Amsterdam: Elsevier/North Holland Biomedical Press, pp. 1–47.

Neff, A. W., F. Briggs, and H. M. Chung. 1987. Craniofacial development mutant pi (Pinhead) in the axolotl (Ambystoma mexicanum) which exhibits reduced interocular distance. Journal of Experimental Zoology 241: 309–316.

Neff, A. W., M. Wakahara, A. Jurand, and G. M. Malacinski. 1984. Experimental analysis of cytoplasmic rearrangements which follow fertilization and accompany symmetrization of inverted Xenopus eggs. Journal of Embryology and Experimental Morphology 80: 197–224.

Newport, G. 1854. Researches on the impregnation of the ovum in the amphibia; and on the early stages of development of the embryo. Philosophical Transactions of the Royal Society of London 144: 229–244.

Nicosia, S. V., D. P. Wolf, and M. Inoue. 1977. Cortical granule distribution and cell surface characteristics in mouse eggs. Developmental Biology 57: 56–74.

Nieuwkoop, P. D. 1969a. The formation of the mesoderm in urodelean amphibians. I. Induction by the endoderm. Wilhelm Roux' Archiv für Entwicklungsmechanik der Organismen 162: 341–373.

———. 1969b. The formation of the mesoderm in urodelean amphibians. II. The origin of the dorso-ventral polarity of the mesoderm. Wilhelm Roux' Archiv für Entwicklungsmechanik der Organismen 163: 298–315.

———. 1973. The "organization center" of the amphibian embryo: Its origin, spatial organization, and morphogenetic action. Advances in Morphogenesis 10: 1–39.

Nieuwkoop, P. D., A. G. Johnen, and B. Albers. 1985. The Epigenetic Nature of Early Chordate Development. Cambridge: Cambridge University Press.

Nieuwkoop, P. D., and G. A. Ubbels. 1972. The formation of the mesoderm in urodelean amphibians. IV. Qualitative evidence for the purely "ectodermal" origin of the entire mesoderm and of the pharyngeal endoderm. Roux's Archives für Entwicklungsmechanik der Organismen 169: 185–199.

Noden, D. 1986. Origins and patterning of craniofacial mesenchymal tissues. Journal of Craniofacial Genetics and Developmental Biology 2 (suppl.): 15–31.

Olszanska, B., E. Szolajska, and Z. Lassota. 1984. Effect of spatial position of uterine quail blastoderms cultured in vitro on bilateral symmetry formation. Roux's Archives of Developmental Biology 193: 108–110.

Otte, A. P., C. H. Koster, G. T. Snoek, and A. J. Durston. 1988. Protein kinase C mediates neural induction in *Xenopus laevis*. Nature 334: 618–620.

Otte, A. P., I. M. Kramer, and A. J. Durston. 1991. Protein kinase C and regulation of the local competence of *Xenopus* ectoderm. Science 251: 570–573.

Phillips, C. R. 1991. Effects of the dorsal blastopore lip and the involuted dorsal mesoderm on neural induction in *Xenopus laevis*. In *Cell-Cell Interactions in Early Development*, J. Gerhart, ed. New York: Wiley-Liss, pp. 93–107.

Porter, K. R. 1941. Diploid and androgenetic haploid hybridization between two forms of *Rana pipiens* Schreber. Biological Bulletin 80: 238–264.

Rappolee, D. A., C. A. Brenner, R. Schultz, D. Mark, and Z. Werb. 1988. Developmental expression of PDGF, TGF-α, and TGF-β genes in preimplantation mouse embryos. Science 241: 1823–1825.

Render, J., and R. P. Elinson. 1986. Axis determination in polyspermic *Xenopus laevis* eggs. Developmental Biology 115: 425–433.

Richter, K., H. Grunz, and I. B. Dawid. 1988. Gene expression in the embryonic nervous system of *Xenopus laevis*. Proceedings of the National Academy of Science, U.S.A. 85: 8086–8090.

Rosenquist, G. C. 1981. Epiblast origin and early migration of neural crest cells in the chick embryo. Developmental Biology 87: 201–211.

Rossant, J., R. Zirngibl, D. Cado, M. Shago, and V. Giguère. 1991. Expression of a retinoic acid response element-*hsplacZ* transgene defines specific domains of transcriptional activity during mouse embryogenesis. Genes and Development 5: 1333–1344.

Roux, W. 1887. Beiträge zur Entwicklungsmechanik des Embryo. 4. Die Richtungsbestimmung der Medianebene des Froschembryos durch die Copulationsrichtung des Eikernes und Spermakernes. Archiv für mikroskopische Anatomie 29: 157–212.

Ruiz i Altaba, A., and T. Jessell. 1991. Retinoic acid modifies mesodermal patterning in early *Xenopus* embryos. Genes and Development 5: 175–187.

Ruiz i Altaba, A., and D. A. Melton. 1989a. Bimodal and graded expression of the *Xenopus* homeobox gene *Xhox 3* during embryonic development. Development 106: 173–183.

———. 1989b. Interaction between peptide growth factors and homeobox genes in the establishment of anteroposterior polarity in frog embryos. Nature 341: 33–38.

———. 1989c. Involvement of the *Xenopus* homeobox gene *Xhox 3* in pattern formation along the anterior-posterior axis. Cell 57: 317–326.

Salmon, M. A. 1978. *Developmental defects and syndromes*. Aylesbury, England: HM + M Publishers.

Sato, S. M., and T. D. Sargent. 1990. Molecular approach to dorsoanterior development in *Xenopus laevis*. Developmental Biology 137: 135–141.

Satoh, H., and A. Shinagawa. 1990. Mechanism of dorso-ventral axis specification in nuclear transplanted eggs of *Xenopus laevis*. Development, Growth, and Differentiation 32: 609–617.

Scharf, S. R., and J. C. Gerhart. 1980. Determination of the dorso-ventral axis in eggs of *Xenopus laevis:* Complete rescue of UV-impaired eggs by oblique orientation before first cleavage. Developmental Biology 79: 181–198.

Scharf, S. R., and J. C. Gerhart. 1983. Axis determination in eggs of *Xenopus laevis:* A critical period before first cleavage, identified by the common effects of cold, pressure, and UV-irradiation. Developmental Biology 99: 75–87.

Scharf, S. R., B. Rowning, M. Wu, and J. C. Gerhart. 1989. Hyperdorsoanterior embryos from *Xenopus* eggs treated with D_2O. Developmental Biology 134: 175–188.

Selleck, M. A. J., and C. D. Stern. 1991. Fate mapping and cell lineage analysis of Hensen's node in the chick embryo. Development 112: 615–626.

Sharpe, C. R. 1988. Developmental expression of a neurofilament-M and two vimentin-like genes in *Xenopus laevis.* Development 103: 269–277.

———. 1990. Regional neural induction in *Xenopus laevis.* BioEssays 12: 591–596.

Sharpe, C. R., A. Fritz, E. M. DeRobertis, and J. B. Gurdon. 1987. A homeobox-containing marker of posterior neural differentiation shows the importance of predetermination in neural induction. Cell 50: 749–758.

Sharpe, C. R., and J. B. Gurdon. 1990. The induction of anterior and posterior neural genes in *Xenopus laevis.* Development 109: 765–774.

Shiurba, R. A., N. Jing, T. Sakakura, and S. F. Godsave. 1991. Nuclear translocation of fibroblast growth factor during *Xenopus* mesoderm formation. Development 113: 487–494.

Sive, H. L., and P. F. Cheng. 1991. Retinoic acid perturbs the expression of *Xhox.lab* genes and alters mesodermal determination in *Xenopus laevis.* Genes and Development 5: 1321–1332.

Sive, H. L., B. W. Draper, R. M. Harland, and H. Weintraub. 1990. Identification of a retinoic acid-sensitive period during primary axis formation in *Xenopus laevis.* Genes and Development 4: 932–942.

Sive, H. L., K. Hattori, and H. Weintraub. 1989. Progressive determination during formation of the anteroposterior axis in *Xenopus laevis.* Cell 58: 171–180.

Slack, J. M. W., L. Dale, and J. C. Smith. 1984. Analysis of embryonic induction by using cell lineage markers. Philosophical Transactions of the Royal Society of London B307: 331–336.

Slack, J. M. W., B. G. Darlington, J. K. Heath, and S. F. Godsave. 1987. Mesoderm induction in early *Xenopus* embryos by heparin-binding growth factors. Nature 326: 197–200.

Slack, J. M. W., and H. V. Isaacs. 1989. Presence of basic fibroblast growth factor in the early *Xenopus* embryo. Development 105: 147–153.

Slack, J. M. W., H. V. Isaacs, and B. G. Darlington. 1988. Inductive effects of fibroblast growth factor and lithium ion on *Xenopus* blastula ectoderm. Development 103: 581–590.

Smith, J. C. 1987. A mesoderm-inducing factor is produced by a *Xenopus* cell line. Development 99: 3–14.

Smith, J. C., B. M. J. Price, K. Van Nimmen, and D. Huylebroeck. 1990. Identification of a potent *Xenopus* mesoderm-inducing factor as a homolog of activin A. Nature 345: 729–731.

Smith, J. C., and J. M. W. Slack. 1983. Dorsalization and neural induction: Properties of the organizer in *Xenopus laevis*. Journal of Embryology and Experimental Morphology 78: 299–317.

Smith, L. J. 1980. Embryonic axis orientation in the mouse and its correlation with blastocyst relationships to the uterus. Part 1. Relationships between 82 hours and 4¼ days. Journal of Embryology and Experimental Morphology 55: 257–277.

———. 1985. Embryonic axis orientation in the mouse and its correlation with blastocyst relationships to the uterus. II. Relationships from 4.5 days to 9.5 days. Journal of Embryology and Experimental Morphology 89: 15–35.

Smith, W. C., and R. M. Harland. 1991. Injected Xwnt-8 RNA acts early in *Xenopus* embryos to promote formation of a vegetal dorsalizing center. Cell 67: 753–765.

Sokol, S., J. L. Christian, R. T. Moon, and D. A. Melton. 1991. Injected Wnt RNA induces a complete body axis in *Xenopus* embryos. Cell 67: 741–752.

Sokol, S., and D. A. Melton. 1991. Pre-existent pattern in *Xenopus* animal pole cells revealed by induction with activin. Nature 351: 409–411.

Spemann, H. 1931. Über den Anteil von Implantat und Wirtskeim an der Orientierung und Beschaffenheit der induzierten Embryonalanlage. Wilhelm Roux' Archiv für Entwicklungsmechanik der Organismen 123: 389–517.

Spemann, H., and H. Mangold. 1924. Über Induktion von Embryonalanlagen durch Implantation artfremder Organisatoren. Wilhelm Roux' Archiv für Entwicklungsmechanik der Organismen 100: 599–638.

Stern, C. D. 1990. The marginal zone and its contribution to the hypoblast and primitive streak of the chick embryo. Development 109: 667–682.

Stewart, R. M., and J. C. Gerhart. 1990. The anterior extent of dorsal development of the *Xenopus* embryonic axis depends on the quantity of organizer in the late blastula. Development 109: 363–372.

Sudarwati, S., and P. D. Nieuwkoop. 1971. Mesoderm formation in the anuran *Xenopus laevis* (Daudin). Wilhelm Roux' Archiv für Entwicklungsmechanik der Organismen 166: 189–204.

Takasaki, H. 1987. Fates and roles of the presumptive organizer region in the 32-cell embryo in normal development of *Xenopus laevis*. Development, Growth, and Differentiation 29: 141–152.

Takaya, H. 1978. Dynamics of the organizer. A. Morphogenetic movements and specificities in induction and differentiation of the organizer. In *Organizer: A Milestone of a Half-Century from Spemann*, O. Nakamura and S. Toivonen, eds. Amsterdam: Elsevier/North Holland Biomedical Press, pp. 49–70.

Thomsen, G., T. Woolf, M. Whitman, S. Sokol, J. Vaughan, W. Vale, and D. A. Melton. 1990. Activins are expressed early in *Xenopus* embryogenesis and can induce axial mesoderm and anterior structures. Cell 63: 485–493.

Toivonen, S. 1978. Regionalization of the embryo. In *Organizer: A Milestone of a Half-Century from Spemann*, O. Nakamura and S. Toivonen, eds. Amsterdam: Elsevier/North Holland, pp. 119–156.

Toivonen, S., and L. Saxén. 1955. The simultaneous inducing action of liver and bone-marrow of the guinea-pig in implantation and explantation experiments with embryos of *Triturus*. Experimental Cell Research 3 (suppl.): 346–357.

Toivonen, S., L. Saxén, and T. Vainio. 1963. Über die Natur der deuterenkephalen Leistung in der embryonalen Induktion. Wilhelm Roux' Archiv für Entwicklungsmechanik der Organismen 154: 293–307.

Vakaet, L. 1984. Early development of birds. In *Chimeras in Developmental Biology*, N. Le Douarin and A. McLaren, eds. London: Academic Press, pp. 71–88.

van den Eijnden-Van Raaij, A. J. M., E. J. J. van Zoelent, K. van Nimmen, C. H. Koster, G. T. Snoek, A. J. Durston, and D. Huylebroeck. 1990. Activin-like factor from a *Xenopus laevis* cell line responsible for mesoderm induction. Nature 345: 732–734.

Vincent, J. P., and J. C. Gerhart. 1987. Subcortical rotation in *Xenopus* eggs: An early step in embryonic axis specification. Developmental Biology 123: 526–539.

Vincent, J. P., G. F. Oster, and J. C. Gerhart. 1986. Kinematics of gray crescent formation in *Xenopus* eggs: The displacement of subcortical cytoplasm relative to the egg surface. Developmental Biology 113: 484–500.

Vincent, J. P., S. R. Scharf, and J. C. Gerhart. 1987. Subcortical rotation in *Xenopus* eggs: A preliminary study of its mechanochemical basis. Cell Motility and Cytoskeleton 8: 143–154.

Waddington, C. H. 1933. Induction by the endoderm in birds. Wilhelm Roux' Archiv für Entwicklungsmechanik der Organismen 128: 502–521.

————. 1952. Modes of gastrulation in vertebrates. Quarterly Journal of Microscopical Science 93: 221–229.

Waddington, C. H., and G. A. Schmidt. 1933. Induction by heteroplastic grafts of the primitive streak in birds. Wilhelm Roux Archiv für Entwicklungsmechanik der Organismen 128: 522–563.

Warner, A. E., and J. B. Gurdon. 1987. Functional gap junctions are not required for muscle gene activation by induction in *Xenopus* embryos. Journal of Cell Biology 104: 557–564.

Whitman, M., and D. A. Melton. 1989. Induction of mesoderm by a viral oncogene in early *Xenopus* embryos. Science 244: 803–806.

Wilkinson, D. G., S. Bhatt, and B. G. Herrmann. 1990. Expression pattern of the mouse *T* gene and its role in mesoderm formation. Nature 343: 657–659.

Wourms, J. P., and A. Kemp. 1982. SEM of gastrulation and development of the lungfish *Neoceratodus*. American Zoologist 22: 876.

Wright, S. 1934. On the genetics of subnormal development of the head (otocephaly) in the guinea pig. Genetics 19: 471–505.

Wright, S., and K. Wagner. 1934. Types of subnormal development of the head from inbred strains of guinea pigs and their bearing on the classification and interpretation of vertebrate monsters. American Journal of Anatomy 54: 383–447.

Yamada, T. 1981. The concept of embryonic induction in the passage of time. Netherlands Journal of Zoology 31: 78–98.

Yamaguchi, Y., and A. Shinagawa. 1989. Marked alteration of midblastula transition in the effect of lithium on formation of the larval body pattern of *Xenopus laevis*. Development, Growth, and Differentiation 31: 531–541.

Yuge, M., Y. Kobayakawa, M. Fujisue, and K. Yamana. 1990. A cytoplasmic determinant for dorsal axis formation in an early embryo of *Xenopus laevis*. Development 110: 1051–1056.

Zisckind, N., and R. P. Elinson. 1990. Gravity and microtubules in dorsoventral polarization of the *Xenopus* egg. Development, Growth, and Differentiation 32: 575–581.

2

Somitomeres: Mesodermal Segments of the Head and Trunk

ANTONE G. JACOBSON

INTRODUCTION

THE VERTEBRATE EMBRYO is considered segmented because of the early appearance of somites in the trunk, the subsequent arrangement of somite derivatives such as muscles, bones, and dermis, and the secondary segmental arrangement of associated spinal nerves and other structures.

Somites appear in the trunk and tail, and in the caudal parts of the head, but whether they exist in the regions of the head rostral to the ears and result in segmentation of the head has long been controversial (see, e.g., Goodrich 1930; de Beer 1937; Jarvik 1980; Jollie 1984). Many of the past arguments have invoked criteria for segmentation that are most likely secondary. These criteria include the neuromeric segmentation of the brain and the numbers and positions of cranial nerves.

Kingsbury (1926, 83) stated, "It must, of course, be recognized that, if the head is really segmented in its composition, each segment must at least embody a neuromere, a nerve, and a mesodermal somite." This somewhat transcendental view is an improvement over the earlier view of Haeckel that a segment or metamere was a morphological individual.

Kingsbury and Adelmann (1924) are cited frequently as giving embryological evidence against segmentation of the head. They say, "No support is found for the 'segmentation of the head'" (p. 278), but they also say, "While the head cannot be considered as composed of a succession of segments however modified, it is fully recognized that the paraxial mesoderm of the head, like that of the trunk, is characteristically segmented" (p. 279).

Since development of the vertebrates is largely epigenetic, it is reasonable to look for segmentation in one system and the effects of that segmentation on other systems. I will argue in this chapter that the primordial segmentation is in the paraxial mesoderm and that other systems, such as the nervous system, are secondarily affected by the primordial segmentation.

42

Segmentation of the entire head mesoderm has been described in embryos of sharks by several people (Balfour 1878, 1881; de Beer 1922; Goodrich 1930), but in the amniotes, segmentation of the head mesoderm has been more controversial.

This chapter reviews the evidence that paraxial mesoderm in both the head and the trunk is segmented during gastrulation in vertebrate embryos in general; that these initial mesenchymal segments—the somitomeres—condense into somites in the trunk, but not in the head rostral to the ears; and that the segmental pattern of the nerves of the trunk, and perhaps in the head as well, is imposed by the segmented mesoderm. Segmentation of the central nervous system into brain compartments and neuromeres follows in time the segmentation of the paraxial mesoderm and appears to be related to the mesodermal pattern.

Patterson (1907) did experiments on chick embryos that resolved a debate as to whether somites formed rostral to the "first" one that appears in the hind part of the head. He marked the mesoderm just rostral to the first-appearing somite, either with a small cautery or by pinning with a tiny glass needle. Later, when many somites had formed, the injury or pin was located just rostral to the most anterior somite, i.e., no additional somites were delineated in front of the first one seen to form. Patterson did notice, as have others, that a rudimentary somite begins rostral to the first somite, but this rudiment never separates from the head mesoderm by forming a rostral cleft. In the course of his study, Patterson observed shallow transitory depressions in the head mesoderm rostral to the first somite. Patterson states (p. 132), "Since these shallow transitory depressions are situated at regular intervals, I might suggest that they lend themselves to another interpretation, namely, as vestigial clefts separating the cephalic mesoblastic somites." He further states (p. 132), "In fact, if these vestigal clefts are studied in connection with the various conditions seen in the myotomes, the above interpretation becomes evident, for in passing backwards from the anterior end of the embryo one finds that the clefts become more and more pronounced. This is evidenced by (1) the vestigal clefts, (2) the rudimentary somite, whose anterior cleft fails to separate it from the head mesoderm, (3) the slowness of the first clefts in cutting off the anterior protovertebrae [In those days "protovertebrae" was synonymous with "somites"], (4) and finally the sharpness and rapidity with which all succeeding protovertebrae are cut off. In other words the influence of the process which has completely obliterated or greatly modified the anterior cephalic somites, gradually becomes weaker in passing posteriorly, and finally ceases altogether."

With the discovery by Meier (1979) that all somites begin as patterned groups of loose mesenchymal cells, which he named "somitomeres," and that the sequence of somitomeres begins at the tip of the head, segmenting the entire paraxial mesoderm of the head, as well as the trunk, the question of whether the head is in some sense segmented seems settled. Patterson may have seen the head somitomeres in 1907.

In this chapter, I will review the evidence for segmentation of the head into somitomeres in six vertebrate classes, relate head somitomeres to trunk somitomeres, give the evidence that head somitomeres may retain the ability to form somites under some experimental circumstances, and discuss various embryological processes that may have participated in the many modifications of the head region.

SOMITOMERES

The discovery of somitomeres by Meier (1979) was serendipitous. In a study of the forming otic placode, he fixed chick embryos in glutaraldehyde, stripped off the head ectoderm, postfixed in osmium tetroxide, then examined with stereo scanning electron microscopy the mesodermal regions that underlie the otic ectoderm. Meier observed that the paraxial head mesoderm was clearly segmented into patterned arrays of mesenchymal cells. Segmental units consisted of loose mesenchymal cells concentrically arranged into a bull's-eye pattern. The pattern was most apparent in the interlocking cellular processes between adjacent rings of cells, which often center on a single cell. When first formed, somitomeres are not condensed masses as seen in the somites that form from them later, but are loosely arranged. They appear to have been formed by expansion, not condensation. The use of stereo pairs of scanning electron micrographs best revealed the pattern; the patterned and interlocking cellular processes are three-dimensional, and the unit as a whole is often concave or convex, centering on the central cell of the group. Most somitomeres are bisected by a line of interlocking cellular processes that lies perpendicular to the long axis of the body, thus dividing the somitomere into rostral and caudal halves (fig. 2.1). Interfaces between concave units are particularly apparent in stereo. Each of these segmental units is bilaminar, having a dorsal and a ventral layer. The appearance of somitomeres is similar in dorsal and ventral views.

The somitomeres, when recently formed, extend laterally exactly to the position of the lateral border of the neural plate, which will form later. Somitomere boundaries match the lateral extent of the plate in both brain and spinal cord regions. Since the somitomeres are present before the plate is formed, it is possible that the lateral boundary of the somitomeres has some role in defining the plate boundary, or that both systems are responsive to the same or similar defining events. When the neural plate, which is initially wide, condenses toward the midline, the underlying somito-

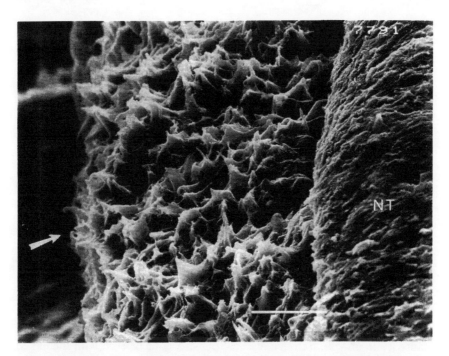

Fig. 2.1. An oblique view by scanning electron microscopy of a somitomere in the segmental plate of a quail embryo. The epidermis has been removed to reveal the patterned loose mesenchymal cells in the paraxial mesoderm lateral to the neural tube (NT). The processes of the cells of the somitomere are arranged in concentric circles, and a line of processes (arrow) divides the somitomere into rostral and caudal halves. Bar, 50 μm.

meres condense toward the midline with it (Lipton and Jacobson 1974). When the neural plate begins to roll into a tube, the correspondence of the lateral boundaries of plate and somitomeres is lost.

Partly because the ability to perceive pattern varies from person to person, some have found more difficulty in seeing somitomeres than others. Meier's pattern perception was excellent, and his analyses of these segmental units were based on examination of thousands of stereo scanning electron micrographs. The same patterns of segmentation were seen in different animals of the same species at the same stages. Somitomeres seen on one side of the axis were matched in mirror image by similar units on the other side of the axis. Further, there was a consistent relationship between the positions of head somitomeres and the positions of brain compartments and neuromeres. Somitomeres, first discovered in the chick embryo, have now been described in embryos of six classes of vertebrates.

In every form studied, somitomeres first appear during gastrulation at the tip of the head, and are laid down in tandem array through the head, trunk, and then the tail. This orderly appearance of somitomeres is especially clear in the flat embryos of chick and quail. The most anterior first pair of somitomeres is formed while the primitive streak is still elongating (Triplett and Meier 1982). The second pair is in place by the time the streak is fully elongated, and the third pair has formed when the streak begins to regress. The rest follow (Meier 1982a, b).

In the chick embryo, the most recently formed pair of somitomeres always appears just slightly caudal and lateral to Hensen's node, once the streak is established (Triplett and Meier 1982). These same positions near Hensen's node were called the "somite forming centers" by Spratt (1954, 1955) because when he purturbed these areas experimentally somite formation was impaired. Spratt placed the somite forming centers at 0.05 mm caudal to Hensen's node on either side of the primitive streak.

A number of pairs of somitomeres are established, typically occupying the entire length of the embryo from the tip of the head to the hindmost parts. Then one of these somitomeres (in the chick embryo the eighth, located caudal to the ear placodes) condenses and forms clefts, both cranially and caudally. Thenceforth this segment is called the first somite because it can now be seen in a dissecting microscope or even with the naked eye. In the chick embryo, subsequent somites then condense in order from somitomeres caudal to the first somite (fig. 2.2). In some other species, the first few somites appear in a more complex order that will be discussed below. In all forms studied, after the first several somites are established, the next somite to form always appears immediately caudal to the last one that formed. By this time in the embryo, two regions of uncondensed somitomeres can now be seen: one group in the head, the rostral regions of which do not normally produce somites; the other group in the trunk, caudal to the last-formed somites and stretching to the tail bud. This caudal expanse of paraxial mesoderm that is not overtly condensed into somites is called the "segmental plate" in avian embryos and the "presomitic mesoderm" in mammalian embryos. Somites continually condense from the rostral end of the segmental plate, while somitomeres are continually added by the primitive streak or by the tail bud at the caudal end.

The Formation of Somites in the Segmental Plate

When the segmental plate is isolated, it eventually produces somites from one end to the other (Sandor and Amels 1970; Packard and Jacobson 1976; Packard 1978, 1980a, b; Sandor and Fazakas-Todea 1980). Packard and Jacobson (1976) showed that the isolated chick segmental plate usu-

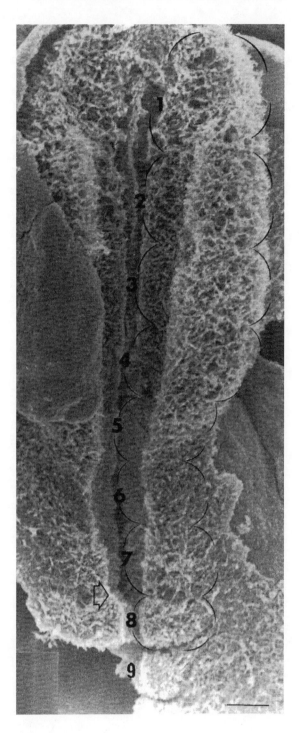

Fig. 2.2. Scanning electron micrograph of a dorsal view of the cranial end of a stage-8 chick embryo. The neural plate and epidermis have been removed on the right side to reveal the underlying somitomeres and somites of the head (brackets, 1–9). The borders indicated were verified in stereo views. The first segmental cleft (open arrow) lies between segments 7 and 8. Segments 8 and 9 are the two most rostral somites. Bar, 100 μm. (From Meier 1981)

ally forms 10 to 12 somites. Meier (1979) examined chick segmental plates with stereo scanning electron microscopy (SEM) and found them to be organized into 10 to 12 somitomeres. By making parallel transverse cuts across both segmental plates, examining the plate on one side with SEM to count the number of somitomeres, culturing the opposite plate until it formed some somites, and then comparing the numbers of somitomeres in the one with the number of somites plus somitomeres in the other, it was found that the numbers were the same. It was clear that the somitomeres had formed into somites (Packard and Meier 1983, 1984; Tam et al. 1982).

The gradual epithelialization and compaction of the somitomeres of the segmental plate into somites has been described by Meier (1979) and by others (Cheney and Lash 1984; Lash 1985). As the somitomere becomes epithelial, the interface between the two lamina that compose the somitomere enlarges into a cavity which is the prospective myocoel. Cells of the epithelium that comprises the mature somitomere and the nascent or maturing somite have their apical surfaces toward the myocoel and their basal ends pointing outward.

COMPARATIVE ANALYSIS OF SOMITOMERES

Somitomeres were first discovered and described in white leghorn chick embryos (Meier 1979, 1980, 1981, 1982a, b, 1984; Meier and Jacobson 1982; Anderson and Meier 1981; Packard and Meier 1983; Triplett and Meier 1982). The appearance of somitomeres is essentially identical in another avian species, *Coturnix coturnix japonica,* the Japanese quail (Meier 1982a, 1984; Packard and Meier 1983; Triplett and Meier 1982). Like the chick, the quail embryo has seven pairs of head somitomeres cranial to the first somites and 10 to 12 pairs of somitomeres in the segmental plates. The somitomeres appear during gastrulation next to the regressing Hensen's node. In short, the somitomeres of the quail embryo are almost identical to those of the chick embryo.

Patrick Tam brought his expertise with embryological studies of the laboratory mouse (*Mus domesticus,* CF-1 albino strain) to Texas in order to collaborate with Meier; several papers examined somitomeres in this mammal (Tam and Meier 1982; Meier and Tam 1982; Tam et al. 1982; Meier 1982a, 1984). When the curious topology of the mouse embryo is taken into account, mouse somitomeres are reasonably similar to those of the bird with respect to their time and order of appearance, their relationships to the neuromeres and brain compartments, and the number of somitomeres cranial to the first somites (they too have seven) (fig. 2.3). They

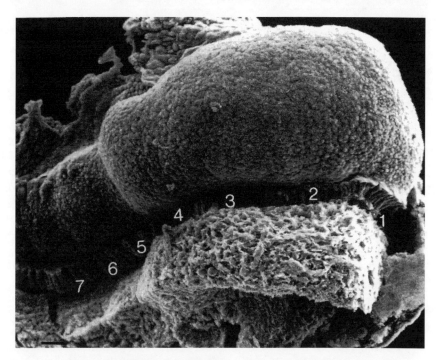

Fig. 2.3.a. Dorsal view (SEM) of the head of an eight-day-old mouse embryo. The open neural plate on the right half of the embryo (bottom) has been removed to reveal the underlying somitomeres and somites. Bulges and furrows already mark positions of neuromeres in the intact neural plate (top), and the first seven somitomeres are numbered. Bar, 10 μm. (From Meier 1982a)

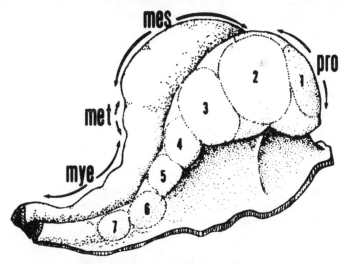

Fig. 2.3.b. Drawing of brain parts (top) and somitomeres (1–7, bottom) relate to parts in fig. 2.3.a. pro, prosencephalon; mes, mesencephalon; met, metencephalon; mye, myelencephalon. (From Meier 1982a)

differ somewhat in the segmental plate (called presomitic mesoderm in the mouse embryo). When the chick and quail embryos have 10 to 12 somitomeres in each segmental plate, the mouse embryo has but six somitomeres in the equivalent presomitic mesoderm.

Chester Yntema had passed on to David Packard the use of snapping turtle embryos, and this form (*Chelydra serpentina*) was chosen as a representative reptile to examine somitomeres (Packard and Meier 1984; Meier and Packard 1984; Meier 1982a, 1984). The snapping turtle embryo has seven somitomeres cranial to the first somite, and the relationships of these somitomeres to brain regions and to neural crest distribution is very similar to that in bird and mouse embryos (fig. 2.4). The turtle embryo has six to seven somitomeres in its segmental plate and in this respect more closely resembles the mouse than the bird embryo (Packard and Meier 1984).

Insofar as the forms cited above can be considered representative of the three classes of amniotes, it would appear that the amniotes all form the same numbers of somitomeres cranial to the first somite, all form them during gastrulation, and all have similar relationships between cranial somitomeres and brain parts, and between cranial somitomeres and cranial crest distribution. The only differences of note were that the bird embryos have 10 to 12 somitomeres in their segmental plates, whereas mammal and reptile embryos have six to seven.

Since all the amniotes examined gastrulate using something resembling a primitive streak, it seemed possible that somitomere organization could be restricted to embryos that gastrulate in this way. That was one reason that somitomeres were studied in amphibian embryos. Amphibians gastrulate in quite a different way, using a blastopore, and among amphibians there are major differences in details of gastrulation between the anurans and the urodeles. Representatives of both of these groups have now been examined for somitomeres. As a representative urodele, the California newt, *Taricha torosa,* was chosen (Jacobson and Meier 1984). This form has but four somitomeres cranial to the first somite (that is, cranial to the somite that is eventually most rostral). In contrast to the bird em-

---

Fig. 2.4. Dorso-lateral view of the left side of the head of a snapping turtle embryo (*Chelydra serpentina*). In this scanning electron micrograph, the epidermis and portions of the brain have been removed from the left side to reveal the underlying somitomeres (1–7) and somites (8–10). Neural crest from the mesencephalon (MES) has migrated onto the second somitomere. The other brain parts are prosencephalon (PRO) and rhombencephalon (RHOM). The otic placode (removed) centers above the boundary between the sixth and seventh somitomeres. Bar, 100 μm. (From Meier and Packard 1984)

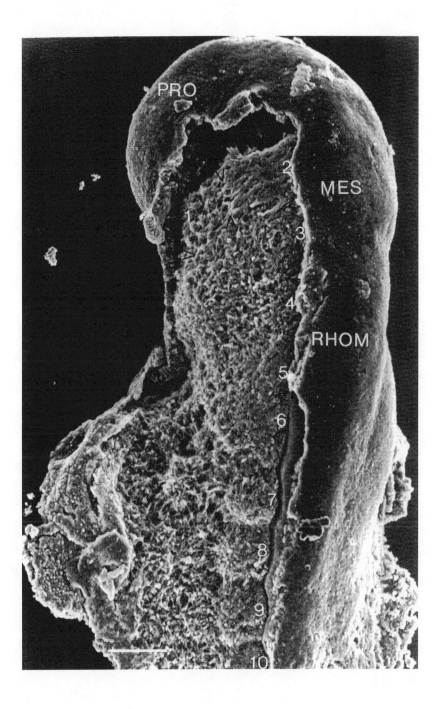

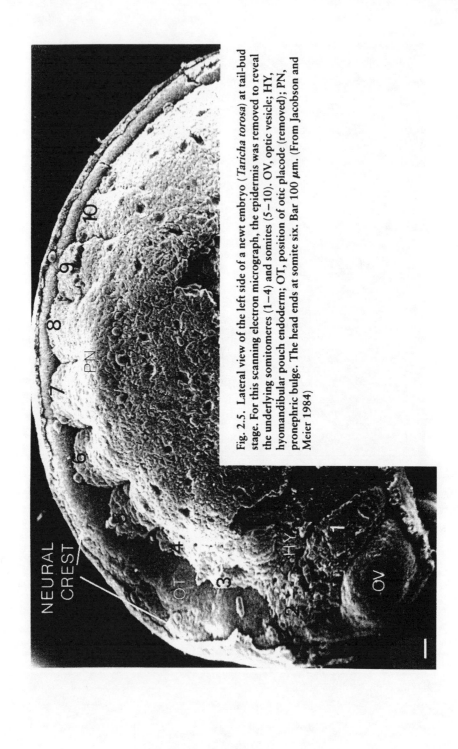

Fig. 2.5. Lateral view of the left side of a newt embryo (*Taricha torosa*) at tail-bud stage. For this scanning electron micrograph, the epidermis was removed to reveal the underlying somitomeres (1–4) and somites (5–10). OV, optic vesicle; HY, hyomandibular pouch endoderm; OT, position of otic placode (removed); PN, pronephric bulge. The head ends at somite six. Bar 100 μm. (From Jacobson and Meier 1984)

bryo, the first somite to appear is not the most cranial somite. The first somite visible with light microscopy appears at midneurula stage 17, and forms from segment seven. Two additional somites then condense cranial to this one (from segments six and five), and from then on somites form caudally in order. The order of formation of the first few somites is thus seven, six, five, eight, nine, etc. (fig. 2.5).

Before any somites form, the entire length of the embryo is already segmented into somitomeres. When the first somite appears at stage 17, there are already about 18 somitomeres in the newt embryo, and additional somitomeres are subsequently added from the tail bud. The first four somitomeres do not normally condense into somites. The first somitomere lies beneath and adjacent to the prosencephalon (just as in the amniote embryos), but for the rest of the somitomeres, where the newt embryo has one somitomere, the amniote embryo has two.

After several somites have formed, there are about seven somitomeres in the segmental plate of the newt embryo until well into late tail-bud stages, when the number may be as few as five. The cranial neural crest migrates out in a patterned way that appears quite similar to the pattern seen in amniote embryos with respect to relationships to the brain parts and the otocyst, but is modified with respect to the somitomeres that occur in different numbers in the newt (Jacobson and Meier 1984).

An anuran embryo, that of *Xenopus laevis,* has also been studied (Jacobson and Meier 1986; and unpublished). Like the newt embryo, this form has only four somitomeres cranial to the first somite, and it too first forms somitomere seven into a somite, followed by six and five, then eight, etc. The fifth segment is thus the most cranial somite and the four somitomeres that lie more rostral in the head do not normally go on to condense into somites. The relationships of the head somitomeres to brain parts and neural crest distribution are as seen in the newt embryo. The segmental plate of the *Xenopus* embryo, once a few somites have condensed, appears to contain about five to seven somitomeres.

With the disparity now discovered between the numbers of preotic somitomeres in the amniote and the amphibian embryos, it seemed a good idea to look at a representative teleost. For this study, we chose the convenient laboratory cyprinodont, *Oryzias latipes,* the Japanese medaka (Jacobson and Meier 1986; Martindale et al. 1987). This form has seven somitomeres in the head cranial to the first somite, and about 10 somitomeres in its segmental plate (fig. 2.6).

In the embryos of the newt and of *Xenopus,* the first somitomeres are associated with the entire prosencephalon as in the amniotes, but caudad to that, where the amniote has two somitomeres, the amphibia have but

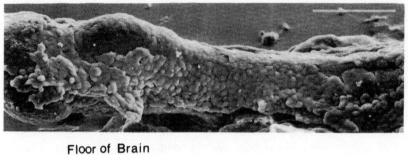

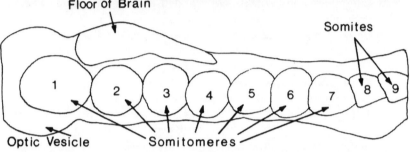

Fig. 2.6. Ventral view of the right side of a teleost embryo (*Oryzias latipes*).
Top: Scanning electron micrograph of an embryo with the epidermis removed. Bar,
100 μm. *Bottom:* The drawing indicates the positions of the seven head somitomeres
(1–7) and two of the head somites (8–9). (From Jacobson and Meier 1986)

one. The teleost embryo is like the amniotes. These relationships are dia-
gramed in figure 2.7.

The characteristics of somitomeres in the species reviewed above are
summarized in table 2.1. Besides the representatives of five classes of vertebrates (mammals, birds, reptiles, amphibia, and bony fishes) reviewed
above, a sixth class, the cartilaginous fishes (in this case a shark) has also
been studied by others.

Much of the early literature on head segmentation was concerned with
studies of head segmentation in shark embryos (Balfour 1878, 1881; de
Beer 1922; Goodrich 1930). The sharks are similar to the amphibia in that
they have but three preotic segments, and a fourth beneath the otocyst, but
they have four to five postotic segments in the head compared to but two
in the amphibia. Gilland (1985), who is doing a study with scanning electron microscopy of the embryo of the shark, *Squalus acanthias,* has identified somitomeres in the head of this shark and confirmed or modified
some aspects of the older literature, but this study is still in progress and
must await completion for more details.

In amphioxus and in larval lampreys, the parachordal mesoderm is
completely segmented from dorsal to ventral edges (Jarvik 1980). In ver-

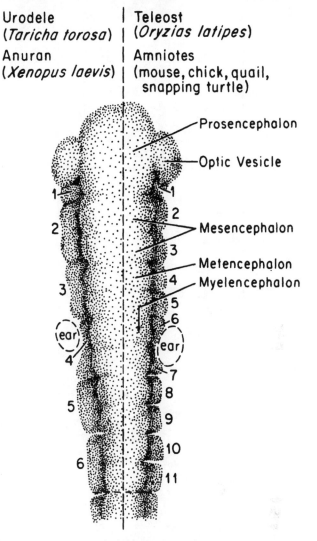

Fig. 2.7. Dorsal view of the brain and the somitomeres and somites of the head. The first (most rostral) somite is number five in the amphibia and number eight in the teleost and amniotes. In all the forms indicated, the first somitomere is associated with the prosencephalon. Caudal to the first somitomere, wherever amphibia have one mesodermal segment, amniotes and the teleost have two. The arrangement in shark embryos is similar to that of the amphibia. Note the relation of the somitomeres to the brain parts and the neuromeres.

TABLE 2.1. Characteristics of somitomeres in different vertebrate embryos

Example	Number of head somitomeres	Diameter of somitomere (μm)	Area of dorsal face (μm)^2	Number of cells on somitomere face	Number of somitomeres in segmental plate	Reference
Laboratory mouse	7	80	5,027	100	5–7	Meier and Tam 1982
Chick and quail	7	175	24,045	200–300	10–12	Meier 1979, 1982a
Snapping turtle (Chelydra serpentina)	7	90	6,362	230	6–7	Meier and Packard 1984
Urodele (newt) (Taricha torosa)	4	285	63,796	38	5–7	Jacobson and Meier 1984
Anuran (Xenopus laevis)	4	207	33,655	35	5–7	Jacobson and Meier 1986
Teleost (medaka) (Oryzias latipes)	7	32	804	56	10	Martindale et al. 1987

tebrates with jaws, except in the branchial region, the hypomere or lateral plate mesoderm is not obviously segmented in adults or in embryos previously examined. Meier (1980) examined chick embryos with scanning electron microscopy and detected segmentation of the intermediate and lateral plate mesoderm in a pattern continuous laterally with that of the somitomeres. He has described segmentally arranged bands of lateral plate mesoderm. The center of each band is raised and there are grooves where the bands abut one another. These grooves are in register with the intersegmental clefts of the paraxial mesoderm.

The Different Somitomere Patterns in Sharks and Amphibia Compared to Amniotes and Teleosts

An important point that emerges from the information discussed above is that the numbers of somitomeres in the head that do not disperse (pre- and subotic somitomeres) fall into two categories: the sharks and amphibia with four, and the amniotes and teleosts with seven. This difference appears to continue caudally among the somitomeres that condense into somites so that, for example, one amphibian somite is equivalent to two amniote somites.

Getting from one condition to the other seems most likely to have been by means of the splitting of each somitomere (except the first) into two (fig. 2.8); or alternatively, adjacent somitomeres may have fused into one (fig. 2.9). This suggests that the arrangement of head segments of amniotes in relation to brain parts and ear position cannot be explained by adding segments from the trunk or by crushing fewer around the ear as others have argued (cf. Goodrich 1930).

The positioning of limbs is quite variable among species (Goodrich 1913), but there is a rather consistent impression that the forelimb is anchored more rostrally in amphibia than in amniotes, or at least in mammals. In at least one case, that of a human being (Williams and Warwick 1980) and a salamander (Detwiler 1934), the disparity in position of the brachial plexus in the two forms can be accounted for by the two-for-one relationship of mesodermal segments and thus of spinal nerves in these species (table 2.2).

The areas of newly formed somitomeres are rather consistent within a species, but differ by 30-fold among the species examined (table 2.1). Areas are difficult to visualize from numbers, so the different-sized somitomeres are shown to scale in figure 2.10. The two amphibia examined have the largest somitomeres, and the teleost the smallest. The number of cells that compose a somitomere face varies greatly among the species, as does the size of the cells (estimated by dividing the area of a somitomere by the number of cells that compose it). The largest somitomere, that of *Taricha torosa,* is composed of 38 cells, and the next largest, that of *Xeno-*

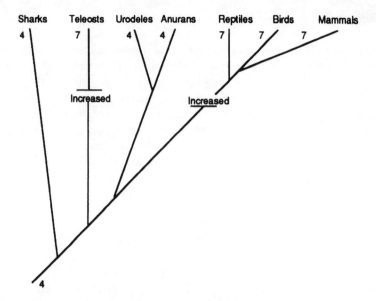

Fig. 2.8. For the various groups shown, the numbers indicate the number of head somitomeres rostral to the first somite. If the vertebrate line began with four cranial somitomeres, then two different lines, the teleosts and the amniotes, must have increased this number.

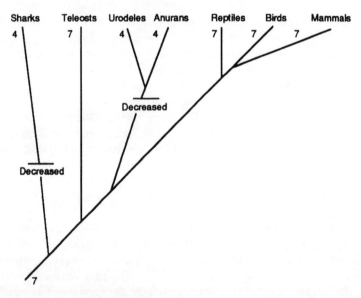

Fig. 2.9. If the vertebrate line began with seven cranial somitomeres rostral to the first somite (numbers), then two different lines, the sharks and the amphibia, have decreased this number. A third, equally parsimonious possibility is that four was the ancestral number, increasing to seven between the sharks and the teleosts, then decreasing to four again in the amphibian line.

TABLE 2.2. Comparison of a salamander and human mesodermal segments and associated nerves through the brachial region

	Ambystoma segments	Human segments	
	1	1	
	2	2	
Head		3	
somitomeres	3	4	
		5	
	4	6	
		7	
Head	5	8	
somites		9	
	6	10	
		11	
Spinal nerve 1	7	12	C1
		13	C2
Spinal nerve 2	8	14	C3
		15	C4*
Spinal nerve 3*	9	16	C5*
		17	C6*
Spinal nerve 4*	10	18	C7*
		19	T1*
Spinal nerve 5*	11	20	T2*
		21	T3
Spinal nerve 6	12	22	T4

* = Brachial plexus

pus laevis, is composed of just 35 cells. There is not a consistent correlation between nuclear size (DNA/nucleus) and cell size. The amphibian cells are large at the time of somitomere formation partly because they are still packed with yolk platelets. It could be that the small number of cells in a somitomere face in the amphibia is about as few cells as together can make a somitomere pattern.

Comparison of Somitomeres in the Head and in the Segmental Plate

Somitomeres are formed in a continuous series starting at the tip of the head. Head somitomeres have the same appearance as somitomeres formed later in the segmental plate. The principal difference that is seen is that segmental plate somitomeres go on to condense into somites and head somitomeres normally do not. Later, the products of the somites, such as muscle masses and bones, are distinctly segmented in a pattern related to that of the original somites, but the products of the head somitomeres are not obviously segmented. Head somitomeres are initially larger than trunk somitomeres, and their sizes match the width of the neural plate in those

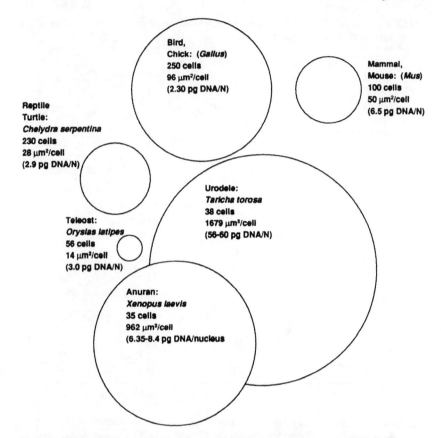

Fig. 2.10. The areas of newly formed somitomeres are compared among several forms. The numbers of cells that compose the dorsal faces of the somitomeres are indicated, as well as an approximation of cell size, derived by dividing the total area by the number of cells. The picograms of DNA per nucleus are given to show that cell size does not correlate well with nuclear size. The very large cells of the amphibian embryos are still packed full of yolk platelets when somitomeres form.

regions. The head somitomeres that do not condense into somites become more dispersed as the brain elongates and expands.

What information there is on the fates of the head somitomeres comes from the work of Noden (1983a, b). He transplanted somitomeres between quail and chick embryos and used the quail nucleolar marker to identify the cells from the quail transplants (Noden 1983a). He found that all the voluntary muscles of the head come from somitomeres, but the connective tissue associated with these muscles is of cranial neural crest origin. His experiments indicate that the sixth and seventh somitomeres form jaw-opening and hyobranchial muscles, the fifth somitomere forms lateral rectus and palpebral depressor muscles, the fourth somitomere forms jaw-closing muscles, and the third somitomere forms the dorsal oblique muscle. While the experiments have not been done to demonstrate it, the first and second somitomeres are the likely sources of the extrinsic eye muscles innervated by the oculomotor nerve. The somitomeres also make contributions to the cranial skeleton, including most of the sphenoid, otic, and occipital complexes and the petrous temporal bone (Noden 1982, 1983a). Finally, some dermis and meningeal cells of the head are of somitomeric origin (Noden 1983a). The somitomeres thus make the same sorts of contributions in the head that somites make in the trunk according to the results of Noden. More recent studies (Couly et al. 1992) concluded that somitomeres do not contribute to the dermis.

Noden (1983a, b) found with his quail-chick transplant experiments that the pattern of myogenesis followed by the mesenchyme derived from the somitomeres is determined by the association with prospective connective tissue of cranial neural crest origin. This seems to be a characteristic that differs between the head and trunk. This patterning ability of the cranial crest cells reflects a programming that occurs prior to the onset of neural crest migration, when the precursors of these cells are still part of the neuroepithelium (Noden 1983b). Thus, the cells that form the voluntary muscles of the head are derived from the somitomeric segments, but the pattern of muscle condensation is directed by the cranial neural crest. This is one of the ways that the neural crest, a tissue new to the vertebrate line, has participated in the development of the vertebrate head.

SOMITOMERES AS PART OF THE MIGRATION PATHWAY OF THE CRANIAL NEURAL CREST CELLS

A regular pattern of migration of cranial neural crest in relation to the positions of the somitomeres has been observed (Meier 1982a; Meier and Packard 1984; Jacobson and Meier 1984), but this pattern is quite different from the pattern of neural crest migration in the trunk, and cranial neural crest forms many more tissues than does the trunk crest.

The prosencephalic region does not appear to contribute much to the cranial neural crest; the most rostral crest cells arise at the posterior border of the prosencephalon. The mesencephalic region produces a large shelf of cranial neural crset cells that migrate in a general rostro-ventral direction. The mesencephalic crest invests above and below the optic vesicle. Neural crest arises all along the mid- and hindbrain regions, but there are gaps in lateral crest migration near where cranial ganglion V forms and where the otocyst forms. Besides its relationship to the overlying epidermis, the crest migrates first over the neural tube for some distance, and then encounters

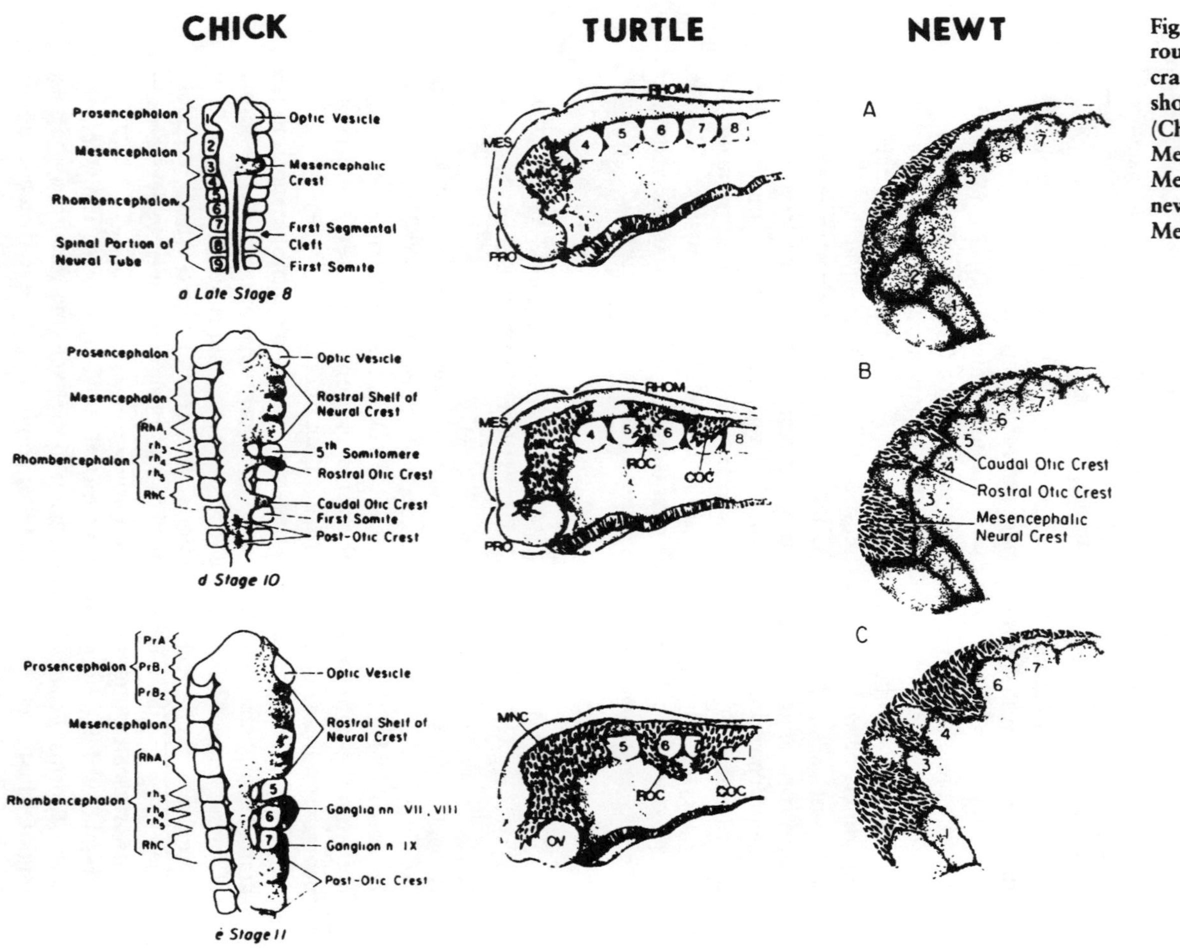

Fig. 2.11. The similar routes of migration of the cranial neural crest are shown in three species. (Chick from Anderson and Meier 1981; turtle from Meier and Packard 1984; newt from Jacobson and Meier 1984)

and migrates over the paraxial mesodermal somitomeres. The migration of the cranial neural crest may be guided by a segmentally arranged pattern of differences in the neural tube, in the somitomeres, and even in the overlying ectoderm. Couly and Le Douarin (1990) have used quail-chick transplants to define what they term "ectomeres" in the epidermis of the heads of chick embryos. These ectomeres angle rostrally and ventrally at 45°, and they are related to segmentation of the neuromeres and the somitomeres. Since the somitomeres are the first segmentally arranged structures to appear, their pattern is likely imposed on the ectodermal structures, both neural and epidermal.

In the amniotes, the mesencephalic crest associates with somitomeres two, three, and one. The most anterior rhombencephalic crest joins the mesencephalic shelf of crest cells and covers somitomere four and some of the rostral position of five. Much of somitomere five is left bare of crest. A stream of rostral otic crest migrates down the border between somitomeres five and six. Most of somitomeres six and seven, which lie beneath the otic vesicle, remain bare of migrating crest. A caudal otic crest migrates ventrally over the caudal part of somitomere seven and over somitomere eight and the more caudal ones (fig. 2.11, chick and turtle; the mouse is similar). In the amphibian embryos studied, where the amniote has two somitomeres (except for the first), the amphibian embryos have but one (see fig. 2.7). The pattern of crest migration is the same in the amphibian embryo, but the numbers of the somitomeres encountered differ. The gaps in lateral migration occur as in the amniote embryo, but the somitomeres left exposed are much of numbers three and four. The rostral otic crest migrates laterally along the border between somitomeres three and four (equivalent to the border between somitomeres five and six in the amniote embryo) (fig. 2.11, newt). In all the forms studied, the streams of rostral and caudal otic crest converge beneath the otocyst.

SOMITES AND THE SEGMENTAL DISTRIBUTION OF SPINAL NERVES

There are other segmental characteristics in both head and trunk that are imposed by the mesodermal metameric pattern. Detwiler (1934) did transplantation experiments on amphibian embryos that purturbed the numbers and positions of somites in relation to the neural tube. He demonstrated that the spinal nerves form in accord with the positions of the somites. More recently it has been shown that motor axons emerge from the neural tube and migrate laterally only through the rostral half of the sclerotome of each maturing somite (Keynes and Stern 1984; Rickman et al. 1985; Bronner-Fraser 1986). Reversing the axis of the spinal cord has no effect on the position of outgrowth of ventral roots, so the segmentation is not intrinsic to the cord. If the axis of a file of somites is reversed, then axons grow out only through the former rostral halves of the somites, now positioned caudally (Keynes and Stern 1984). Migration of neural crest that forms the spinal dorsal root ganglia also is restricted to the rostral compartment of the sclerotome of the somite. The spinal dorsal root ganglia are composed from neural crest cells that arise above both the rostral and caudal halves of the somite, but the caudal crest cells migrate axially and then move laterally only at the level of the rostral half of the somite (Teillet et al. 1987). It is clear that the arrangement of the spinal nerves in a segmental pattern is secondary to the metameric pattern of the somites, which in turn was derived from the somitomeres.

As noted above, one frequently can see in somitomeres an overlapping of cell processes that define a seam that divides the somitomere into anterior and posterior compartments (fig. 2.1). These seams are seen in somitomeres of both the head and the trunk. It is possible that the differences that emerge in the somite between rostral and caudal parts may have arisen in the somitomeres.

RELATIONSHIPS BETWEEN SOMITOMERES AND NEUROMERES

Another characteristic of vertebrate embryos that is often considered segmental or metameric is the appearance of bulges and furrows in the neural tube. These have been called "neuromeres" and were described by von Baer (1928) in the chick embryo. They have since been described in several species (e.g., Berquist 1952), and in much more detail in the chick embryo (Vaage 1969). There is a consistent relationship between neuromeres and the somitomeres (fig. 2.7). In all species studied, the first (the most rostral) somitomere underlies the entire prosencephalon. In the amniotes, the second somitomere is beneath the first mesencephalic neuromere and the third somitomere is beneath the second mesencephalic neuromere. The fourth somitomere is beneath the metencephalon, and subsequent somitomeres are associated one to one with early rhombencephalic neuromeres. Such a relationship continues between somites and neuromeres in the spinal cord. The pattern of neuromeres becomes modified through time (Vaage 1969). Some neuromeres subdivide, so that through time, the relationship of the neuromere pattern to the mesodermal segment pattern alters. When a neuromere that is apposed to a somitomere subdivides, it often does so along a line that is in register with the line of cell processes that subdivides the somitomere into rostral and caudal halves.

There is no direct information about whether the somitomeres specify the positions of neuromeres, or vice versa, or neither. However, one can speculate that it is more likely that the somitomeres influence the positions of the neuromeres because somitomeres appear in the embryo before the neural plate develops. Even in the mouse embryo, in which the bulging of the neuromeres is present already in the open neural plate (Jacobson and Tam 1982), the somitomeres have formed long before the neural plate reaches this stage. The neuromeres are most likely secondary to the segmentation of the paraxial mesoderm into somitomeres.

Interesting molecular and cellular events now have been related to neuromeric segments, so it is important to relate the neuromeres to the mesodermal segments. In figure 2.12, the central part of the diagram shows cranial ganglia, motor roots, and motor nuclei in relation to the neuromeres (rhombomeres) in the hindbrain of an advanced (stage 21) chick embryo (from Lumsden and Keynes 1989). The left of the diagram shows how expression of some homeobox-containing genes (HOX 2 series), and the zinc-finger gene Krox 20, is related to neuromere boundaries in the mouse embryo (from Wilkinson, Bhatt, Cook et al. 1989; Wilkinson, Bhatt, Chavrier et al. 1989). At the top of the diagram, I have symbolized, rather than drawn accurately, the forebrain and midbrain to show their relations to the first three pairs of somitomeres. On the right of the diagram, I have positioned the head somitomeres (segments one to seven) and the four head somites (segments eight to eleven) in relation to the brain parts and rhombomeres at these advanced stages of development. The first pair of somitomeres is associated with the prosencephalon; the second and third pairs are associated with the two neuromeres of the mesencephalon. The fourth somitomere lies adjacent to the metencephalon of the hindbrain (R1). Earlier in development, the remaining more caudal somitomeres were adjacent to successive rhombomeres, but by these advanced stages, some of the neuromeres have subdivided (Vaage 1969), and in the more caudal reaches, the neuromeres are no longer clear.

A good landmark is the position of the otic vesicle. It lies over the boundary between somitomeres six and seven, which coincides with the boundaries of the current rhombomeres numbered five and six. The rhombomeres opposite somitomeres five, six, and seven have subdivided. The rhombomeres labeled seven and eight have vague boundaries at the stage shown, where earlier a neuromere lay opposite each of somitomeres eight, nine, ten, and eleven that occupy that position.

It appears that cranial motor roots emerge in association with the cranial halves of somitomeres, just as motor roots of spinal nerves emerge into cranial halves of trunk somites. Similarly, the cranial ganglia are arranged in association with cranial portions of the somitomeres and head somites. Nerve III emerges from the mesencephalon and could be in the rostral part of one of the somitomeres located at that position. Nerve IV arises in the base of rhombomere one (R1), but emerges from its top.

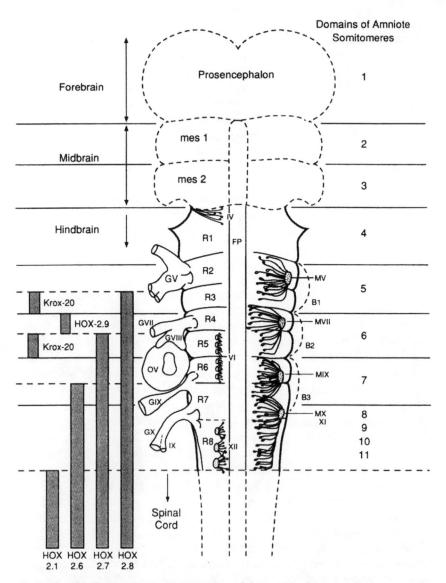

Fig. 2.12. This diagrammatic representation of the amniote brain combines cytological data relating cranial nerve roots and ganglia to brain neuromeres in the stage-21 chick embryo (central part of the figure from Lumsden and Keynes 1989), the positional levels of expression of homeobox-containing genes (*HOX* 2 series) and a zinc-finger gene (*Krox*-20) in the 9.5-day mouse embryo (data at left from Wilkinson, Bhatt, Cook et al. 1989), and the positions of the head somitomeres of the amniote embryo (1–11, right). Somitomeres eight to eleven condense to become the four occipital somites. The mesencephalic neuromeres (mes 1, 2) and the rhombomeres

Rhombomere one coincides with the rostral part of somitomere four. Somitomeres five, six, and seven coincide with the positions of branchial
arches one, two, and three. Both the ventral root and ganglion of nerve V
emerge in the rostral part of somitomere five. Nerve VI emerges near the
border of rhombomeres four and five and could be associated with the
rostral part of somitomere six. The motor root of nerve VII and the ganglia
of nerves VII and VIII are associated with the rostral part of somitomere
six. The motor root and the ganglion of nerve IX are associated with the
rostral part of somitomere seven. The roots and ganglia of nerves X and
XI emerge in the rostral parts of somitomere eight. It seems likely that the
head somitomeres serve the same function as the trunk somites in limiting
nerve formation to the rostral parts of each mesodermal segment.

HEAD SOMITOMERES AND THE FORMATION OF SOMITES

Some experiments have suggested that head somitomeres can be caused to
form somites (Meier and Jacobson 1982). We cut the chick embryo transversely just caudal to Hensen's node at the fully elongated streak stage
(stage 4). The rostral and caudal fragments were then separated and cultured separately on agar for 15 hours. The caudal fragment was also slit
longitudinally down the midline, and the resulting fragments separated
before culturing. At the time of the experiment, the rostral fragment contained the prechordal plate, the node, and the first two pairs of somitomeres (cf. Meier 1984). The caudal fragments contained the rest of the
primitive streak and the positions that the rest of the somitomeres and
somites would occupy. The prospective somitomeres would still be in the
streak and the epiblast, the most recently formed pair (the second pair)
having just been established next to the node and removed with the rostral
fragment. It is not known for certain whether some of the prospective
somitomere material in the epiblast would have been removed with the
rostral fragment.

Somites formed in the caudal fragments, beginning at the most rostral
end of the isolate. The first of these somites appeared at the rostral end by

(R1–8) are numbered. The cranial sensory ganglia (GV–X), branchial and somatic
motor nuclei (IV–XII), and the combined roots of the sensory and branchial motor
nerves (MV–MXI) are shown. The prosencephalon and mesencephalon are
symbolized rather than accurately drawn to show the relation of these parts to the
first three somitomeres. The branchial arches (B1–3) coincide with the positions of
somitomeres five, six, and seven. Note that the roots and ganglia of the cranial nerves
appear to be positioned in the rostral halves of somitomeres. FP = floor plate. OV =
otic vesicle.

four hours of incubation, and seven to eight somites formed by 15 hours. At 15 hours the isolates were fixed and examined with stereo SEM. The whole medial edge of each caudal fragment consisted of somites or, more caudally, of somitomeres. The most rostral somites that formed in these split isolates must have been prospective cranial somitomeres. Cranial somitomeres three to seven could be expected to form in these isolates, but in their places one finds definitive somites.

The uncertainty as to the exact position of the prospective somitomeres while still in the epiblast leaves some doubt about this interpretation of these experiments. We saved the rostral fragments and cultured them as well, as they made, in some cases, nipplelike extensions at the midline that contained notochord and small somites. I suspect that the node has made notochord that has then regulated to produce rows of small somites. In any event, these extensions contained somites, not somitomeres. The present best interpretation is that the prospective somitomeres numbers three to seven have been converted to somites in these experiments. This hidden ability to form somites suggests that head somitomeres retain some ancestral abilities that are modified in normal development in modern vertebrate embryos.

In some experiments, the caudal fragment was not split down its midline. These intact fragments were cultured 15 hours and then fixed and examined with stereo SEM. They contained somitomeres from one end to the other. It seems that in some way the development into somites requires shearing, either by the regressing node, or by cutting.

These experiments are reviewed more fully in Jacobson and Meier (1986).

EMBRYOLOGICAL PROCESSES THAT MAY HAVE MODIFIED THE METAMERIC PROPERTIES OF THE HEAD REGION

It is noted above that trunk somites have rostral and caudal sclerotomal compartments, that the rostral compartment is the only one that allows motor nerve outgrowth from the neural tube, and that neural crest cells migrate only through the rostral compartments to give rise to the spinal ganglia. Spinal nerves thus assume the segmental properties of the somites. It now appears that the head somitomeres may have the same role in positioning and limiting cranial nerve development.

The brain elongates and expands before cranial nerves are established. If the more rostral head somitomeres condensed to becomes somites rather than remain dispersed as a patterned mesenchymal group, they could not embrace the expanding brain. Stretching of the head somitomeres has been noted during head development (Jacobson and Meier 1984). The somito-meres are closely associated with the overlying brain plate, and the brain plate elongates considerably during neural tube closure (Jacobson 1984). This is a likely source of the stretching of the somitomeres that is observed. Stretching of the rostral component of a head somitomere would expand the region that may be capable of positioning cranial nerves.

The flexing of the head, found in every vertebrate embryo (Goodrum and Jacobson 1981), would also distort the positions of the rostral por-tions of the head somitomeres and thus might modify the sites of cranial nerve formation. Head flexure appears to be driven forcefully by the bend-ing of the brain (Jacobson et al. 1979). It may be that the stretching and flexing seen in the head would allow several ventral roots to emerge next to a single rostral portion of a head segment, just as lining up two rostral components of trunk somites next to the spinal cord allows emergence of a broad band of ventral roots there (Stern and Keynes 1987).

In contrast to the mesodermal segments of the head, the columns of somites in the trunk region, and at least the anterior end of the seg-mental plate, are under compression (Packard and Jacobson 1979). We also showed that isolated segmental plates, without neural tube or noto-chord, formed long oval somites. The normal compression of the segmen-tal plate and somites thus appears to result from the close association with the neural plate (and notochord). A great increase in the length of the neural plate occurs in that part of the neural plate that is closing, and that overlies the caudal end of the segmental plate (Jacobson 1981). Assuming that the underlying caudal segmental plate is attached, the rapid elongation of the closing neural plate could compress the rostral segmental plate and somite column to some extent. Compression of the trunk somites in the rostro-caudal axis also results from growth of the so-mites (Packard and Jacobson 1979). The effects of the moderate elongation of the adjacent closed neural tube and notochord would be to stretch the somites somewhat, but this appears to be overcome by the rapid growth of the somites.

The head somitomeres begin to be distorted shortly after they are formed. Processes that produce these distortions include elongation of the brain area (Jacobson 1984), formation of head and lateral body folds, flex-ures and torsions of the brain (Goodrum and Jacobson 1981), and possibly the influx of other mesenchyme from the cranial neural crest and from epidermal placodes. If flexures and torsions are having a distorting effect on the head metameric pattern, one would expect to find the primordial pattern remaining best in those lower forms that have the least flexures and torsions—in sharks, teleosts, and amphibians, as opposed to am-niotes. This seems to be the case.

The ventral roots emerge from the basal plates of the central nervous system, and these plates do not extend into the prosencephalon. Thus, no ventral roots would be expected from the prosencephalon, and none are seen. The first pair of somitomeres, located adjacent to the prosencephalon in all embryos studied, would thus not be expected to host any ventral roots.

The cranial ganglia are composed in a way that is quite different from the formation of spinal dorsal root ganglia. In the trunk, neural crest cells accumulate opposite the rostral portion of each somite and form the spinal ganglia. In the head, epidermal placodes are formed, some of which make the nose, lens, and inner ear mechanism, and others of which contribute the mesenchymal cells from which the cranial ganglia partly are formed. Cranial neural crest cells also contribute to the cranial ganglia. How mesenchymal cells derived from epidermal placodes are combined with neural crest cells in certain positions to form the cranial ganglia is not known. Quite different rules could apply to the migration of these mesenchymal cell types as compared to the situation in the trunk, or the rules could be similar and the cells could accumulate opposite the rostral portions of the head somitomeres in their much-distorted positions.

Two findings of Noden may give some clues as to how the controlling factors of patterning have diverged in head and trunk. Noden (1983b) found that repositioning of neural crest in the head region (which contributes the connective tissues associated with the voluntary muscles of the head) produced voluntary muscle patterns that were appropriate for the region from which the neural crest was taken, not for the somitomeres from which the myoblasts arose. The programming for this patterning was present in the crest before it had begun to migrate. Therefore, unlike the trunk region where the axial muscles are segmentally arranged in the same pattern as the somites, the voluntary muscles of the head are patterned by the cranial neural crest (but the cranial neural crest may have been patterned by the somitomeres that formed earlier).

A second finding was that quail-to-chick transplantation of trunk somites or somitomeres to the head region produced myoblasts from these transplanted trunk somites or somitomeres that frequently were integrated into normal voluntary muscles of the head (Noden 1986). The head neural crest apparently is able to pattern these foreign myoblasts into normal head patterns. However, in some cases the transplanted trunk somites or somitomeres interfered with normal migration of the cranial neural crest. In the same paper, Noden reports preliminary results of transplantation of head somitomeres into the trunk region. These transplanted head somitomeres were able to give rise to appendicular muscles. Thus, head and trunk somitomeres appear to have the same potentials, but are controlled in their patterns of expression by other tissues in the local environment that differ in head and trunk.

The head and trunk thus differ in a number of ways. The head has a larger neural plate (the brain plate), different morphogenetic movements (including elongations and flexures that distort the somitomeres), epidermal placodes, and an expanded amount of, and role for, the neural crest. Together these produce a pattern of head morphogenesis that obscures, yet retains, the original orderly metameric pattern of the somitomeres.

SUMMARY AND CONCLUSIONS

There have been centuries of agreement that the trunk of vertebrates is segmented, but there has been equally long controversy as to whether the head is segmented. Until recently, segmentation was thought to begin with the division of the paraxial mesoderm of the trunk into somites, and it has been known at least since the 1930s that the somites then influenced the metameric patterning of the spinal nerves. There have been conflicting reports as to whether the head is segmented into somites.

In 1979, Meier discovered that the entire paraxial mesoderm of the chick embryo, from the tip of the head to the hindmost parts, is patterned into metamerically arranged segmental units of organized mesenchymal cells. He called these units "somitomeres." They have now been described in examples of embryos of six vertebrate classes, from sharks to mammals. In each case somitomeres appear first during gastrulation, always form first at the tip of the head, and then progressively, pair by pair, more caudad.

Somitomeres have remarkable similarities in appearance and in relation to other axial structures in all the species examined. The lateral borders of somitomeres coincide with the lateral boundary of the neural plate when that structure becomes evident, and the somitomeres condense toward the midline in concert with the condensation of the neural plate. Specific neuromeres in the neural tube are associated with specific somitomeres. It is possible that the somitomeres impose patterning onto the central nervous system.

All somites begin as somitomeres. Eventually, some somitomeres in the caudal head region condense, become bilaminar epithelial bags with their apical surface at the interior, and form deep clefts between themselves and their neighboring somitomeres both rostrally and caudally. These clefts make the units more easily seen and they are now recognized as somites.

After the first few somites have condensed, each vertebrate embryo has a characteristic number of head somitomeres rostral to the first-formed somite, and another characteristic number of somitomeres occupying the segmental plate caudal to the last-formed somite. Somitomeres in the segmental plate progressively condense into somites, while new somitomeres are added from the primitive streak or the tail bud.

The head somitomeres normally do not condense into somites (but can be made to, experimentally), and represent the primordial metameric segmentation of the head. They contribute tissues to the head that are similar to parts formed by somites in the trunk, that is, voluntary muscles and bones. The metameric pattern of these head parts is greatly modified by (among other things) cranial neural crest, mesenchyme from the epidermal placodes, and elongation and flexure of the brain. The combined effects of these head tissues and processes is to distort greatly the metameric pattern of the head somitomeres.

Transplantation of somitomeres into the trunk, and somites into the head, showed that these metameric units will contribute parts appropriate for their new environments. The environment of the trunk allows retention of most of the original metameric pattern, where in the head the parts that form are much less obviously segmented, even when they form from a transplanted somite. The environment of the head alters the metameric pattern. The cranial neural crest, a tissue new to the vertebrate line, is certainly one of the tissues responsible for the changes in the head metameric pattern.

Is the vertebrate head segmented? Yes it is, in the embryo. In all vertebrate embryos examined, the head is segmented metamerically into somitomeres. This primordial segmental pattern is then distorted by other tissues and processes that have appeared in vertebrate heads. Such distortions are less evident in the trunk. The adult head has many of the parts that are segmentally arranged in the trunk, but arrangement in the head is greatly distorted from the ideal.

Some of the arguments about head segmentation persist in the face of these facts because the arguments contain a vestigal transcendentalism, an insistence on comparing the finished product in the adult to some idealized concept of "segment" rather than accepting the clear metamerism of the early embryo and noting how the embryo then modifies this pattern.

Traits such as the segmentation of the paraxial mesoderm into somitomeres that appear very early in the development of vertebrate embryos may represent primordial characteristics of the group. The subsequent modification of these early traits should give insights into vertebrate evolution.

ACKNOWLEDGMENTS

The discovery of somitomeres and the majority of the work on the subject was by my late colleague, Stephen Meier. Mark Martindale provided the photographs of teleost somitomeres. Research reported here was supported by National Institutes of Health grants DE-05616, NS-16072, and HD-25902, and National Science Foundation grant DCB-8420014.

REFERENCES

Anderson, C. L., and S. Meier. 1981. The influence of the metameric pattern in the mesoderm on migration of cranial neural crest cells in the chick embryo. Developmental Biology 85: 383–402.

Baer, K. E. von. 1828. *Über die Entwicklungsgeschichte der Thiere*, pt. 1. Königsberg.

Balfour, F. M. 1878. *A Monograph on the Development of Elasmobranch Fishes*. Journal of Anatomy and Physiology, 1876–1877 and 1878. London: Macmillan.

———. 1881. *A Treatise on Comparative Embryology*, vol. 2. London: Macmillan.

Berquist, H. 1952. Studies on the cerebral tube in vertebrates: The neuromeres. Acta zoologica 33: 117–187.

Bronner-Fraser, M. 1986. Analysis of the early stages of trunk neural crest migration in avian embryos using monoclonal antibody HNK-1. Developmental Biology 115: 44–55.

Cheney, C. M., and J. W. Lash. 1984. An increase in cell-cell adhesion in the chick segmental plate results in a meristic pattern. Journal of Embryology and Experimental Morphology 79: 1–10.

Couly, G., and N. M. Le Douarin. 1990. Head morphogenesis in embryonic avian chimeras: Evidence for a segmental pattern in the ectoderm corresponding to the neuromeres. Development 108: 543–558.

Couly, G., P. M. Coltey, and N. M. Le Douarin. 1992. The developmental fate of the cephalic mesoderm in quail-chick chimeras. Development 114: 1–15.

de Beer, G. R. 1922. The segmentation of the head in Squalus acanthias. Quarterly Journal of Microscopical Science 66: 457–474.

———. 1937. *The Development of the Vertebrate Skull*. New York: Oxford University Press.

Detwiler, S. R. 1934. An experimental study of spinal nerve segmentation in *Amblystoma* with reference to the pleurisegmental contribution to the brachial plexus. Journal of Experimental Zoology 67: 395–441.

Gilland, E. H. 1985. Morphology and development of head mesoderm in early embryos of *Squalus acanthias*. American Zoologist 25: 93A. Abstract.

Goodrich, E. S. 1913. Metameric segmentation and homology. Quarterly Journal of Microscopical Sciences, n.s., 59: 227–248.

———. 1930. *Studies on the Structure and Development of Vertebrates*. London: Macmillan. Reprint. New York: Dover, 1958.

Goodrum, G. R., and A. G. Jacobson. 1981. Cephalic flexure formation in the chick embryo. Journal of Experimental Zoology 216: 399–408.

Jacobson, A. G. 1981. Morphogenesis of the neural plate and tube. In *Morpho-

genesis and Pattern Formation, T. G. Connelly, L. L. Brinkley, and B. M. Carlson, eds. New York: Raven Press, pp. 233–263.

————. 1984. Further evidence that formation of the neural tube requires elongation of the nervous system. Journal of Experimental Zoology 230: 23–28.

Jacobson, A. G., and S. Meier. 1984. Morphogenesis of the head of a newt: Mesodermal segments, neuromeres, and distribution of neural crest. Developmental Biology 106: 181–193.

————. 1986. Somitomeres: The primordial body segments. In *Somites in Developing Embryos,* R. Bellairs, D. A. Ede, and J. W. Lash, eds. New York: Plenum Publishing Co.

Jacobson, A. G., D. M. Miyamoto, and S.-H. Mai. 1979. Rathke's pouch morphogenesis in the chick embryo. Journal of Experimental Zoology 207: 351–366.

Jacobson, A. G., and P. P. L. Tam. 1982. Cephalic neurulation in the mouse embryo analyzed by SEM and morphometry. Anatomical Record 203: 375–396.

Jarvik, E. 1980. *Basic Structure and Evolution of Vertebrates,* vol. 2. New York: Academic Press.

Jollie, M. 1984. The vertebrate head: Segmented or a single morphogenetic structure? Journal of Vertebrate Paleontology 4: 320–329.

Keynes, R. J., and C. D. Stern. 1984. Segmentation in the vertebrate nervous system. Nature 310: 786–789.

Kingsbury, B. F. 1926. Branchiomerism and the theory of head segmentation. Journal of Morphology 42: 83–109.

Kingsbury, B. F., and H. B. Adelmann. 1924. The morphological plan of the head. Quarterly Journal of Microscopical Science 68: 239–285.

Lash, J. W. 1985. Somitogenesis: Investigations on the mechanism of compaction in the presomitic mass and a possible role for fibronectin. In *Developmental Mechanisms: Normal and Abnormal.* New York: Alan R. Liss, pp. 45–60.

Lipton, B. H., and A. G. Jacobson. 1974. Analysis of normal somite development. Developmental Biology 38: 73–90.

Lumsden, A., and R. Keynes. 1989. Segmental patterns of neuronal development in the chick hindbrain. Nature 337: 424–428.

Martindale, M. Q., S. Meier, and A. G. Jacobson. 1987. Mesodermal metamerism in the teleost, *Oryzias latipes* (the medaka). Journal of Morphology 193: 241–252.

Meier, S. 1979. Development of the chick mesoblast: Formation of the embryonic axis and establishment of the metameric pattern. Developmental Biology 73: 25–45.

————. 1980. Development of the chick mesoblast: Pronephros, lateral plate, and early vasculature. Journal of Embryology and Experimental Morphology 55: 291–306.

————. 1981. Development of the chick embryo mesoblast: Morphogenesis of the prechordal plate and cranial segments. Developmental Biology 83: 49–61.

————. 1982a. The development of segmentation in the cranial region of vertebrate embryos. Scanning Electron Microscopy/1982, pt. 3: 1269–1282.

————. 1982b. The distribution of cranial neural crest cells during ocular morphogenesis. In *Clinical, Structural, and Biochemical Advances in Hereditary Eye Disorders*, D. L. Daentl ed. New York: Alan R. Liss, pp. 1–15.

————. 1984. Somite formation and its relationship to metameric patterning of the mesoderm. Cell Differentiation 14: 235–243.

Meier, S., and A. G. Jacobson. 1982. Experimental studies of the origin and expression of metameric pattern in the chick embryo. Journal of Experimental Zoology 219: 217–232.

Meier, S., and D. S. Packard, Jr. 1984. Morphogenesis of the cranial segments and distribution of neural crest in embryos of the snapping turtle, *Chelydra serpentina*. Developmental Biology 102: 309–323.

Meier, S., and P. P. L. Tam. 1982. Metameric pattern development in the embryonic axis of the mouse. I. Differentiation of the cranial segments. Differentiation 21: 95–108.

Noden, D. M. 1982. Patterns and organization of craniofacial skeletogenic and myogenic mesenchyme: A perspective. In *Factors and Mechanisms Influencing Bone Growth*, A. D. Dixon and B. Sarnat, eds. New York: Alan R. Liss, pp. 167–203.

————. 1983a. The embryonic origins of avian cephalic and cervical muscles and associated connective tissues. American Journal of Anatomy 168: 257–276.

————. 1983b. The role of the neural crest in patterning of avian cranial, skeletal, connective, and muscle tissues. Developmental Biology 96: 144–165.

————. 1986. Patterning of avian craniofacial muscles. Developmental Biology 116: 347–356.

Packard, D. S., Jr. 1978. Chick somite determination: The role of factors in young somites and the segmental plate. Journal of Experimental Zoology 203: 295–306.

————. 1980a. Somite formation in cultured embryos of the snapping turtle, *Chelydra serpentina*. Journal of Embryology and Experimental Morphology 59: 113–130.

————. 1980b. Somitogenesis in cultured embryos of the Japanese quail, *Coturnix coturnix japonica*. American Journal of Anatomy 158: 83–91.

Packard, D. S., Jr., and A. G. Jacobson. 1976. The influence of axial structures on chick somite formation. Developmental Biology 53: 36–48.

————. 1979. Analysis of the physical forces that influence the shape of chick somites. Journal of Experimental Zoology 207: 81–92.

Packard, D. S., Jr., and S. Meier. 1983. An experimental study of the somitomeric organization of the avian segmental plate. Developmental Biology 97: 191–202.

————. 1984. Morphological and experimental studies of the somitomeric organization of the segmental plate in snapping turtle embryos. Journal of Embryology and Experimental Morphology 84: 35–48.

Patterson, J. T. 1907. The order of appearance of the anterior somites in the chick. Biological Bulletin 13: 121–133.

Rickman, M., J. W. Fawcett, and R. J. Keynes. 1985. The migration of neural crest cells and the growth of motor axons through the rostral half of the chick somite. Journal of Embryology and Experimental Morphology 90: 437–455.

Sandor, S., and D. Amels. 1970. Researches on the development of axial organs. VI. The role of the neural tube in somitogenesis. Revue roumaine d'embryologie et de cytologie, Série embryologie 7: 49–57.

Sandor, S., and I. Fazakas-Todea. 1980. Researches on the formation of axial organs in the chick embryo X: Further investigations on the role of ecto- and endoderm in somitogenesis. Revue roumaine de morphologie, d'embryologie, et de physiologie 26: 29–32.

Spratt, N. T. 1954. Studies on the organizer center of the early chick embryo. In *Aspects of Synthesis and Order in Growth*. Thirteenth Symposium of the Society for the Study of Development and Growth. Princeton, N.J.: Princeton University Press, pp. 209–231.

———. 1955. Analysis of the organizer center in the early chick embryo. I. Localization of prospective notochord and somites cells. Journal of Experimental Zoology 128: 121–164.

Stern, C., and R. J. Keynes. 1987. Interactions between somite cells: The formation and maintenance of segment boundaries in the chick embryo. Development 99: 261–272.

Teillet, M.-A., C. Kalcheim, and N. Le Douarin. 1987. Formation of the dorsal root ganglia in the avian embryo: Segmental origin and migratory behavior of neural crest progenitor cells. Developmental Biology 120: 329–347.

Tam, P. P. L., and S. Meier. 1982. The establishment of a somitomeric pattern in the mesoderm of the gastrulating mouse embryo. American Journal of Anatomy 164: 209–225.

Tam, P. P. L., S. Meier, and A. G. Jacobson. 1982. Differentiation of the metameric pattern in the embryonic axis of the mouse. II. Somitomeric organization of the presomitic mesoderm. Differentiation 21: 109–122.

Triplett, R. L., and S. Meier. 1982. Morphological analysis of the development of the primary organizer in avian embryos. Journal of Experimental Zoology 220: 191–206.

Vaage, S. 1969. The segmentation of the primitive neural tube in chick embryos. Advances in Anatomy, Embryology, and Cell Biology 41: 7–87.

Wilkinson, D. G., S. Bhatt, P. Chavrier, R. Bravo, and P. Charnay. 1989. Segment-specific expression of a zinc-finger gene in the developing nervous system of the mouse. Nature 337: 461–464.

Wilkinson, D. G., S. Bhatt, M. Cook, E. Bonicelli, and R. Krumlauf. 1989. Segmental expression of HOX-2 homeobox-containing genes in the developing mouse hindbrain. Nature 341: 405–409.

Williams, P. L., and R. Warwick, eds. 1980. *Gray's Anatomy*. 36th British ed. Philadelphia: W. B. Saunders, p. 1094.

3

Pattern Formation and the Neural Crest

ROBERT M. LANGILLE AND BRIAN K. HALL

INTRODUCTION

ONE HUNDRED YEARS AGO to claim that an ectodermal derivative such as the neural crest was in any way involved with the formation of skeletal structures was the embryological and evolutionary equivalent of nailing an additional thesis to the cathedral door. That skeletal structures were mesodermal in origin was dogma, known and accepted by all; an ectodermal origin was heresy. The germ layer theory was an impregnable barrier that could not be breached, either in the embryo, by tissues developing from other than their predestined layer, or in theory, by those who studied those embryos (Oppenheimer 1940; de Beer 1947). Ectoderm formed neural and epidermal derivatives. Endoderm formed the alimentary canal and any organs, such as the pancreas, that arose by budding from the gut. Mesoderm formed the remainder of the tissues and organs in the vertebrate body, including the skeleton. The embryo was united from head to tail by the uniform and unitarian origin of its tissues from these fundamental germ layers.

What a contrast this is to the situation we find ourselves in today, for it is not the germ layers but the cellular organization that arises from them that preoccupies our thinking. Previously, it was thought that mesenchyme (meshworks of cells embedded in an extracellular matrix) arose only from mesoderm, and that epithelia (sheets of connected cells resting on a basement membrane) arose only from ecto- and endoderm. However, epithelia or mesenchyme can arise from all three germ layers, and epithelial-to-mesenchymal and mesenchymal-to-epithelial transitions occur, not only in vitro, which is an artificial circumstance, but also in the embryo (Greenburg and Hay 1982; Hay 1982, 1989).

Thus, cellular organization is neither confined to, nor defined by, germ layer of origin. The vertebrate axial skeleton is not unified from head to tail through its construction on a unified plan, either because of germ layer origin, or as transformations and fusions of vertebrae as Goethe thought.

While all the postcranial skeleton is mesodermal in origin, as are the roof and base of the cranial vault, the remainder of the skull and all the facial and visceral skeleton are derived from those ubiquitous ectodermal derivatives, the neural crest cells.

In this chapter we will not be concerned with documenting or detailing the fate-mapping studies that have demonstrated the neural crest origin of the skull and craniofacial skeleton. Such maps have been created for representative agnathans (*Petromyzon marinus,* the lamprey), fish (*Oryzias latipes,* the Japanese medaka), birds (*Gallus domesticus,* the common fowl), and amphibians (numerous species of urodeles, and, for the tadpole skeleton, of frogs) and are assumed to apply to other members of these groups and to groups not yet studied (reptiles, mammals). As the details of these maps have been reviewed recently, we do not repeat them here; rather we refer you to Le Douarin (1982), Hall (1987), Noden (1986), and Hall and Hörstadius (1988) and to the chapters by Thorogood in this volume and by Hanken and Hall in volume 3. Nor do we discuss the differentiation of neural crest cells in any depth, for that topic is also treated by Thorogood in this volume.

Our concern is with the role that the neural crest cells play in patterning the vertebrate head. Therefore, this chapter should be read in association with Jacobson's chapter in this volume on segmentation of the head mesoderm into somitomeres, with Thomson's chapter in volume 2 on the consequences of embryonic segmentation for adult cranial structure, and with Thorogood's chapter in this volume on differentiation and morphogenesis of cranial skeletal tissues.

We begin with a discussion of the history of the discovery, acceptance, and realization of the importance of the neural crest. Then the subdivision of the neural crest into cranial (skeletogenic) and trunk (nonskeletogenic?) regions is discussed, followed by a longer section dealing with the embryonic behavior of neural crest cells. Two shorter sections follow: one presents evidence of rostro-caudal polarity of neural crest cells and the influence of these cells on the differentiation of associated tissues; the other presents an overview of head segmentation and patterning. The final section deals with the mechanism of craniofacial pattern formation and the possible role homeobox-containing genes play coordinating the interrelationships and differentiation of neural crest, mesoderm (somitomeres), neural tube (neuromeres) and ectoderm (ectomeres).

THE DISCOVERY OF THE NEURAL CREST

The first report of a distinctive band of cells lying along the developing neural tube close to the ectoderm was made by His (1868), who named this band of cells *Zwischenstrang,* the neural crest. It was in light micro-scopic serial sections of the early chick embryo that His discovered this cell band. From such sections he reconstructed the behavior of these cells, re-porting their translocation from their initial association with the neural tube, ventro-laterally to form the spinal ganglia.

Within eight to ten years other reports of the presence and possible role of these cells began to appear. The dorsal roots of the spinal ganglia were described as arising from these cells associated with the spinal cord in sharks (Balfour 1876b; Sagemehl 1882; Kastschenko 1888) and these cells were claimed to contribute to the cranial mesenchyme in sharks, te-leosts, and birds (Kastschenko 1888; Goronowitsch 1892, 1893a, b). Pig-ment cells were also shown to arise from these neural crest cells (Borcea 1909). The first to document that the neural crest separated from the neu-ral ectoderm and therefore had a separate existence from very early in embryonic development was Brachet (1908) in his studies on the frog *Rana.*

His's discovery of the neural crest origin of the spinal ganglia was controversial because the spinal ganglia were regarded as mesodermal, originating from the myotomes that produced the axial musculature. The suggestion that cranial mesenchyme arose from the neural crest was equally controversial, for mesenchyme was regarded as mesodermal, and indeed, was required by the germ layer theory to be mesodermal.

The initial claims by Kastschenko and Goronowitsch for a neural crest origin of cranial mesenchyme in sharks, teleosts, and birds were followed by Platt's (1893, 1897) announcement that not only mesenchyme but also visceral arch cartilage and dentine of the teeth were ectodermal in origin. Platt thought that these tissues arose from placodal lateral cra-nial ectoderm. It was Platt who coined the terms "mesectoderm" and "mesentoderm" for mesenchyme of ecto- and mesodermal origin respec-tively. As discussed by Landacre (1921), Stone (1922b), Holmdahl (1928), de Beer (1947), Hörstadius (1950), and Hall and Hörstadius (1988), these claims of an ectodermal origin of skeletal and dental tissues created great controversy.

It would be 30 to 40 years before the detailed descriptive study of Landacre (1921) and the experimental studies of Stone (1922a, b, 1926, 1927, 1929, 1932) would provide additional evidence for the neural crest origin of cranial mesenchyme and visceral arch skeletal elements. Landacre took advantage of cytological differences between neural crest and other cells in the urodele, *Ambystoma jeffersonianum,* differences such as size, and amount of yolk and pigment, to follow, in serial sections, the migra-tion of neural crest cells into the visceral arches and their appearance in the visceral arch cartilages. Stone extirpated regions of the amphibian neu-ral crest and used the resulting deficiencies to map the neural crest origin of the cranial skeleton. Similar techniques were used by Raven, Reisinger, Ichikawa, and Harrison (see Hörstadius 1950 for details and references). These results were then confirmed by the transplantation of vitally stained blocks of neural crest by Hörstadius and Sellman (1946). These pioneering studies led to our current extensive knowledge of the contribution of the neural crest to the craniofacial skeleton, a contribution that is confined to cells of the cranial neural crest.

CRANIAL AND TRUNK NEURAL CREST

That neural crest cells migrate both from the future brain and from the future spinal cord gave rise to the designations of cranial and trunk neural crest cells. These terms are not merely geographical; there is much evidence that only cells of the cranial neural crest can form skeletal and dental tissues, i.e., are skeleto- and odontogenic. The only connective tissue components that arise from cells of the trunk neural crest are the connective tissues of the median fins of amphibians and fishes (Raven 1931, 1936; Du Shane 1935). Although migrating neural crest cells are associated with migrating scleratomal cells in the region of future vertebral development, Detwiler and van Dyke (1934) and Raven (1931, 1936) demonstrated that the vertebral neural arches were not formed from neural crest cells.

Hörstadius and Sellman (1946) identified the skeletogenic cranial neural crest in *A. mexicanum* as that region extending caudad from the midprosencephalon to the rostral rhombencephalon. Skeletogenesis could be obtained neither from the most rostral prosencephalon nor from the trunk neural crest. More recent experiments with avian embryos bear out the same conclusion (Nakamura and Ayer-LeLièvre 1982). However, although not skeletogenic, the most caudad trunk neural crest of both urodele and rodent embryos is odontogenic, capable of forming both odontoblasts that deposit dentine and the alveolar bone that is associated with the roots of the teeth (Chibon 1970, 1974; Lumsden 1987, 1988). Smith and Hall (1990), in discussing this issue in the context of the formation of the dermal exoskeleton in both Recent and in fossil fishes, concluded that dermal skeletal units that consist of a layer of dentine overlying bone of attachment and that are found in the trunk are, in all probability, derivatives of the trunk neural crest.

Given that an important aspect of the role of the neural crest in cranial patterning relates to neural crest cell migration and migration pathways, we devote the following section to the embryonic behavior of neural crest cells before moving on to discuss neural crest polarity and influence on associated tissues during head development, head segmentation, and possible mechanisms of patterning in the vertebrate head.

EMBRYONIC BEHAVIOR OF NEURAL CREST CELLS

Overview

The behavior of neural crest cells continues to be a prolific area of research, owing to their highly migratory capabilities and the observation that these cells are an embryonic microcosm encapsulating most of the events of development. They begin as an apparently homogeneous population of cells, although this is in dispute. (See Hall and Hörstadius 1988 for a discussion of the heterogeneity within the neural crest, but also see Bagnara 1987 and, recently, Dupin et al. 1990 for evidence in support of pleuropotentiality of neural crest "stem cells.") Nevertheless, the neural crest as a whole exhibits the capability of differentiating into at least 10 different cellular phenotypes (more, if you consider cementocytes as distinct from osteocytes and even more if you consider the different neuronal and pigment cell types derived from neural crest; see Noden 1978c; Le Douarin 1982; Hall and Hörstadius 1988). From their point of origin, they migrate over varying distances, during which time they receive signals from the external environment which guide them, produce increasing restrictions on their phenotypic fates, and ultimately determine where they will settle within the craniofacial region. At this point the crest cells themselves begin to assert an influence over their final environmental neighbors and begin an elaborate exchange of alternating influences over and from neighboring tissues (the widest studied and most prominent neighboring tissue being epithelia) as differentiation proceeds.

All neural crest cells originate at the neural tube–ectodermal junction and, as just stated, must therefore migrate variable distances to reach their final destinations. Thus we begin with a brief account of neural crest migration. (For more exhaustive reviews, the reader is directed to a number of comprehensive articles; see Newgreen and Erikson 1986; pertinent chapters in Maderson 1987; and Hall and Hörstadius 1988.) However, two events must first proceed before the cells begin their migration, namely epithelial-mesenchymal transition and escape from the epithelium through the basal lamina.

Epithelial-Mesenchymal Transition

Epithelial-mesenchymal transition of neural crest cells has been extensively analyzed in the chick (Bancroft and Bellairs 1976; Tosney 1982; Newgreen and Gibbins 1982; Tosney 1982) and mouse (Nichols 1981, 1985; Chan and Tam 1988) and involves a loss of cell junctions and cell polarity, as well as a change in the orientation of the cells. In relation to the future regionalization of neural crest cells, there is as yet little evidence to support or refute the possibility that neural crest cells receive signals at this very early stage which specifically direct the pattern of their early migration. However, studies currently in progress on homeobox genes suggest that this may well be a particularly sensitive time in the "programming" of neural crest and associated tissues (see below in section on mechanism of patterning).

At one time the basal lamina was thought to pose a possible barrier that neural crest cells had to remove in some manner before migration could begin and which might influence the migration pathways. However, detailed studies of the basal lamina under neural crest cells have revealed holes (Tosney 1982) or absence of a basal lamina (Martins-Green and Erikson 1987) in some instances. Chan and Tam (1988) have demonstrated breakdown of mouse basal lamina of the cranial neural crest coincident with the onset of migration (which in rodents studied to date amounts to a largely lateral displacement as the separation of crest occurs during the neural fold stage (Smits-van Prooije et al. 1985; Nichols 1981; Tan and Morriss-Kay 1985) so that in fact the basal lamina provides no obstacle for the neural crest cells.

Migration

As stated in the introduction, the migration of neural crest proceeds along somewhat segmented routes and there is a good antero-posterior correlation between the origin and destination of neural crest cells within the head (Langille and Hall 1988a, b). The precise routes of migration for cranial neural crest depend in part on the species; nevertheless a generalized pattern can be obtained. Unlike the posterior cranial (cardiac and myencephalic neural crest), most of the cranial neural crest does not have somites to negotiate, but instead paraxial mesoderm which is organized more subtly into somitomeres (see the chapter by Jacobson in this volume). Noden (1987) and Chan and Tam (1988) have demonstrated that a subpopulation of cranial neural crest cells does migrate into/through somitomeric mesoderm; however, to date, it is not known whether any interaction between this mesoderm and the migrating neural crest influences the route of migration (possible interactions between the somitomeres, ectomeres, and neural crest cells will be detailed below). In birds, the most intensively studied and therefore best-known group, most of the migrating neural crest cells move along the dorsal route between the ectoderm and underlying paraxial mesoderm to the level of the first branchial gangliogenic neural crest, which emigrates from the metencephalic level (see Fig. 3.1).

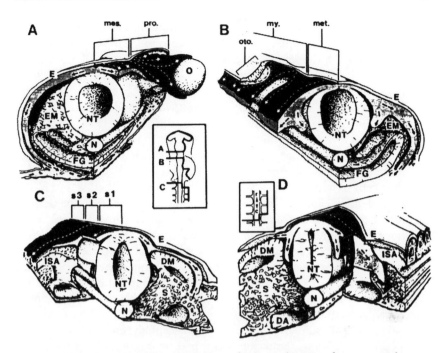

Fig. 3.1. Three-dimensional representations of avian embryos to demonstrate the major routes of neural crest cell migration (black and hatched). Arrows indicate the direction of migration. The orientations of A to D are shown in the insets. A. A view rostrad from the mesencephalon to the prosencephalon. Neural crest cells migrate beneath the ectoderm toward the foregut at the level of the mesencephalon. Cells from the diencephalon invest the optic vesicle. B. A view caudad from the metencephalon to the anterior myelencephalon showing neural crest cell migrations laterally and ventrally. Note the unoccupied zones caudal to the metencephalon and around the otocyst. C. A view caudad over the first fully formed somites; neural crest cells are shown migrating beneath the ectoderm. D. A view rostrad in the trunk region; neural crest cells migrate between the neural tube and somites. Abbreviations: c, caudal; DA, dorsal aorta; DM, dermomyotome; E, ectoderm; EM, cranial endomesenchyme; FG, foregut; ISA, intersegmental artery; mes, mesencephalon; met, metencephalon; my, myelencephlon; N, notochord; NT, neural tube; O, optic vesicle; oto, otocyst; pro, prosencephalon; r, rostral; S, sclerotome; s1–s3, somites 1–3. Reproduced from Newgreen and Erikson (1986), with the permission of the publisher.

To date, this appears to be the case for all other studies of neural crest migration (teleosts: Sadaghiani and Vielkind 1990; *Xenopus:* Sadaghiani and Theibaud 1987; rat or mouse: Nichols 1985, 1986, 1987; Smits-van Prooije et al. 1985; Tan and Morriss-Kay 1986; Chan and Tam 1988). The rest of the cranial crest caudad to the metencephalon migrates primarily by the ventral pathway (fig. 3.1).

We shall now briefly review the destinations of cranial neural crest cells as detailed in compilations of Newgreen and Erikson (1986) and Erikson (1986) of the extensive chick-quail chimera data of Le Lièvre, Le Douarin, Noden, and colleagues (Le Lièvre 1971a, b, 1974, 1978; Le Lièvre and Le Douarin 1975; Noden 1975, 1978a, b, c, 1980, 1982a, b, 1983a, b; D'Amico-Martel and Noden 1980, 1983) and the more limited data available for mammals (Nichols 1981, 1985, 1986, 1987; Smits-van Prooije et al. 1985; Tan and Morriss-Kay 1985, 1986; Chan and Tam 1988). No cells leave from the telencephalic level; the most rostral migration commences instead from the anteriormost edge of the diencephalic level, the cells of which end up in the frontonasal region (Le Lièvre 1971b, 1974; Noden, 1978a, c). Caudal prosencephalic neural crest migrates to the ocular region, ending up in the endothelium and corneal matrix with a minor component ending up in the frontonasal region (Johnston 1966; Noden 1975). Mesencephalic neural crest translocates to the eye and contributes to the ciliary ganglion and maxillary portion of the first branchial arch (Noden 1975, 1978c) while the mandibular portion of the first arch is populated by metencephalic crest (Le Lièvre 1974; Noden 1978c), which also contributes to the trigeminal ganglion (Noden 1975; D'Amico-Martel and Noden 1980) as described above. Myelencephalic crest is divided into pre- and postotic crest, the more rostral preotic migrating into the hyoid arch and contributing cells to the facial (VII) ganglia and the more caudal postotic migrating into arches III and IV as it contributes cells to the superior (IX), jugular (X), petrosal (IX), and nodose (X) ganglia (Narayana and Narayana 1980; D'Amico-Martel and Noden 1983) and the superior cervical ganglia (Newgreen 1979).

Clearly as described above the cranial neural crest is segmented, inasmuch as it migrates into and forms the cores of a series of segmented pouches, the visceral arches. As revealed by several authors using light microscopy (Johnston 1966; Noden 1980) and more graphically using scanning electron microscopy (Meier 1982, 1984; Meier and Jacobson 1982; Meier and Packard 1984; Tan and Morriss-Kay 1985), the migration route of cranial neural crest is also segmented in the amphibian, bird, and mammalian representatives studied to date, with two gaps occurring consistently. A rostral gap occurs between the metencephalic and myelencephalic crest, a caudal gap between pre- and postotic crest. A further gap seems to occur where the neural crest migrates around the optic vesicle, but as Noden has shown (1975, 1978c), this is only a delay in migration as the neural crest subsequently enters the cornea of the eye, and does not represent true segmentation of migration route. Despite this segmentation of migration the neural crest does not remain segmented, but instead fills the entire ventral region of the head (see fig. 3.2). Therefore the segmentation of the neural crest route does not

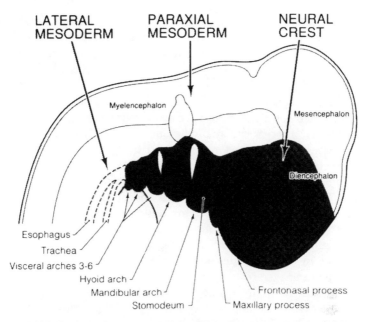

LATERAL
MESODERM

PARAXIAL
MESODERM

NEURAL
CREST

Myelencephalon

Mesencephalon

Diencephalon

Esophagus
Trachea
Visceral arches 3-6
Hyoid arch
Mandibular arch
Stomodeum

Frontonasal process
Maxillary process

Fig. 3.2. A lateral schematic view of the developing craniofacial region of the embryonic chick illustrating the distribution of mesenchyme derived from neural crest, paraxial mesoderm, and lateral mesoderm. Note that mesenchyme derived from the neural crest fills the entire ventral region of the head. Reproduced from Noden (1988), with the permisssion of the publisher.

match the visceral arch segmentation pattern, and at present, the implications of the segmentation of the cranial neural crest migration route remain moot.

Control of Migration

The glycoproteins fibronectin and laminin have been put forward as molecules which neural crest cells use to locate pathways during migration, since neural crest cells in vitro migrate well on both, and both of these molecules are found along some of the neural crest routes (Newgreen and Thiery 1980; Duband and Thiery 1982; Newgreen 1984; Bilozur and Hay 1988). In particular, the blocking of fibronectin with antibody or competative inhibitors disrupts migration (Boucat et al. 1984; Bronner-Fraser 1985). Additionally, glycosaminoglycans (GAGs) such as hyaluronic acid and chondroitin sulfate, associated with the glycoproteins mentioned above, are implicated in facilitating neural crest cell migration. Hyaluronic acid (HA) is thought to increase cell-free space in the matrix, thereby allowing passage (Tucker and Erikson 1984); and cessation of migration of crest cells into the corneal stroma has been shown to occur concomitantly with the local secretion of hyaluronidase (Toole and Trelstad 1971). Nevertheless, although injection of hyaluronidase at the appropriate time has been shown to decrease neural crest migration, it did not eliminate it (Anderson and Meier 1982). Chondroitin sulfate (CS) on the other hand has been shown to retard neural crest migration in vitro and appears to predominate in areas where neural crest cells do not migrate (see Newgreen and Erikson 1986 for a review of specific evidence and see Perris and Johansson 1990 for a recent explanation of mechanism). Recently, Perris and Bronner-Fraser and colleagues have been critically analyzing the role of GAGs, particularly HA and CS and heparin sulfate, as they interact with collagens and other matrix constituents in modulating crest cell migration (Perris and Johansson 1990; and see Perris and Bronner-Fraser 1989) and although such studies are revealing the full extent of the permissiveness (both +ve and −ve) of matrix molecules to neural crest cell migration, there is as yet no concrete evidence to suggest that the matrix is laid out in a specific pattern which dictates neural crest migration and hence patterning within the head.

One fundamental point which is still unclear is why neural crest cells migrate primarily in the ventral direction. A great many possibilities such as haptotaxis and galvanotaxis have been ruled out (see Newgreen and Erikson 1986, and especially Erikson 1986) and in fact Erikson (1985) has shown that trunk neural crest cells placed ventrally will migrate dorsally, utilizing the correct pathway. In addition to the matrix, cell-cell interactions also play a role, since one aspect of developmental regulation displayed by crest cells is the limited ability to migrate antero-posteriorly or even dorso-laterally to the opposite side of the embryo and compensate for adjacently extirpated crest cells (Hall and Hörstadius 1988). Thus the control of migration and implications for patterning in the craniofacial region remain to be fully explained.

Interactions: Cell-Cell/Cell-Matrix

Cell-cell and cell-matrix interactions occur at various times during migration as well as after. One of the most striking examples of the impact of matrix–neural crest interactions which occur during migration is the discovery that ventral route (or perhaps more properly, medio-ventral route) matrix of the axolotl greatly enhances neurogenesis while lateral route matrix enhances pigment cell differentiation when neural crest cells migrate from extirpated neural tubes onto these extirpated matrices in culture (Perris et al. 1988). Transient expression (or lack of expression) of particular matrix molecules can also affect crest cell migration and hence pattern formation. Löfberg et al. (1980, 1989) have shown that the failure of pigment cell migration in the white mutant of the axolotl is due to the inability of the matrix to support crest cell migration at the appropriate stage. Interestingly, the matrix from older, mutant axolotls will support crest cell migration. Thus, control of pigment pattern in the white axolotl, which is due to a single recessive gene, d, occurs through a heterochronic shift in the matrix composition of the migratory route of the crest-derived pigment cells.

Examples of cell interactions resulting in commitment of neural crest cells at the onset or after migration can also be found. Hall and Tremaine (1979) demonstrated that the commitment to chondrogenic (Meckel's cartilage) differentiation of chick mandibular crest was induced at the commencement of migration (presumably by interaction with either the perineural epithelia and/or its basal lamina or adjacent nonepithelial matrix). It is equally important to note, however, that osteogenic mandibular crest, which will populate mandibular regions immediately adjacent to the chondrogenic crest, is not committed until well after migration has ceased, the induction to osteogenic differentiation occurring via mandibular epithelium (Tyler and Hall 1977). Thus migration is not always the venue of neural crest cell commitment. From the point of view of craniofacial patterning, this plasticity in time and place of neural crest cell commitment must surely allow for increased modification of the vertebrate skull.

The end point for migration will be only briefly discussed here. Unlike the trunk, where most of the crest cells form discrete structures (e.g., dorsal root ganglia, enteric neurons) among a wider array of mesodermal and endodermal derivatives, the neural crest of the face fills the entire ventral region of the head (fig. 3.2). Thus neural crest cells migrating from a zone of high concentration atop the neural tube into a zone of lower concentration in the adjacent matrix apparently stop migration when the two crest populations of either side meet in the ventral margin or in some instances stop temporarily at obstacles they will later populate, such as described above for the eye. Cessation becomes an issue only in the case of neural crest structures such as ganglia, which in some instances are surrounded by mesodermal mesenchyme and which cease migration in relatively dorsal locations, or in the case of the patterning of subpopulations of crest cells (such as the cells committed to form Meckel's cartilage outlined above). The latter is considered in the next chapter by Thorogood, particularly in the discussion of his flypaper model for the cessation of neural crest migration. In the case of ganglia, as Perris et al. (1988) have shown, the matrix of the medial migration route induces gangliogenesis, which presumably would arrest the migration of the induced cells.

Once neural crest cells have reached their end point, differentiation of

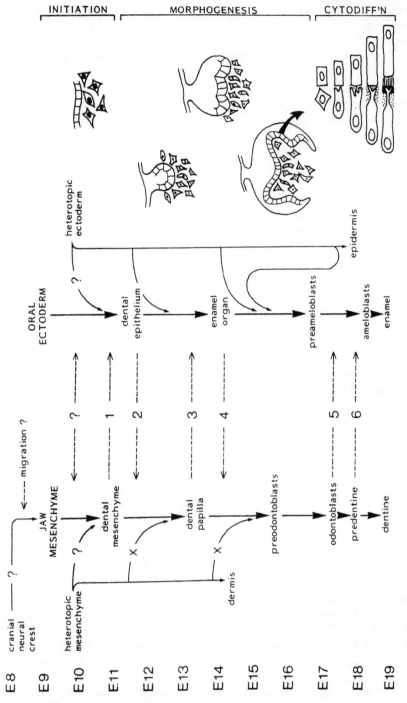

Fig. 3.3. An overview of the interactions which occur between oral epithelium and neural crest–derived mesenchyme during odontogenesis and amelogenesis in the formation of the murine tooth. E8–E19 refer to embryonic age in days postconception. Solid arrows indicate cell or tissue differentiations; dashed arrows indicate tissue interactions. The major cellular changes in dental epithelium and mesenchyme are shown diagrammatically on the right. Reproduced from Lumsden (1988), with the permission of the publisher.

the cells and morphogenesis of craniofacial structures begins. Cell-cell and/ or cell-matrix interactions play a major role in controlling or regulating these processes in those subpopulations which are not already as fully determined as the cells from Meckel's cartilage of the chick (but even for these, cell-matrix interactions may align the cells in correct formation to produce the appropriate structure, as proposed by Thorogood; see next chapter). There are ample descriptions of the interactions neural crest cells are involved in during the differentiative stage, and the reader is directed to other, more comprehensive reviews (Hall 1987; Noden 1988; Hall and Hörstadius 1988; and Thorogood, this volume) for thorough treatments of the subject. Here, the following example of neural crest–epithelial interactions during odontogenesis from the review of Lumsden (1987) will suffice to illustrate the complexity of epigenetic interactions which can be (but not in every case are) required for the differentiation of neural crest cells at this comparatively late embryonic stage. Figure 3.3 details the set of interactions which occur between oral epithelium and neural crest–derived mandibular mesenchyme during odontogenesis. The neural crest–derived dental mesenchyme becomes committed to forming a particular tooth type by embryonic day E11 or E12, yet still requires further epithelial interaction up to E18, when predentin and enamel matrix deposition begin. What this illustrates, for the purposes of the present analysis, is the plasticity which is still present at the differentiative phase for certain subpopulations of cranial neural crest cells. With respect to patterning of the vertebrate head it is thus obvious that control of such interactive patterns does not lie within one of the differentiating tissues and that repatterning, as it occurs in evolution, is possible via many routes.

EMBRYONIC BEHAVIOR AND PATTERN FORMATION

The embryonic behavior of neural crest cells provides the potential for the extensive interactions of these cells with their environment: the ectoderm, mesoderm, and endoderm they migrate past and the extracellular matrices these latter tissues produce which the crest cells pass through. Any alteration in the pathway can thus alter the pattern, and therefore initial control of pattern would seem to reside within these tissues/structures. As interactions occur and crest cells become more and more restricted, control of differentiation and subsequent pattern formation passes to the crest cells themselves. In the next section (before addressing patterning specifically), we shall briefly discuss the evidence suggesting that neural crest or portions of neural crest receive sufficient restrictive programming to control pattern formation prior to migration as well as the evidence for the dominance of crest cells over certain cell types during differentiation.

ROSTRO-CAUDAL POLARITY AND INFLUENCE ON TISSUES DURING DIFFERENTIATION

Several lines of evidence indicate that the cranial neural crest may be to some extent programmed prior to migration to produce specific structures in an antero-posteriorly graded fashion. Hörstadius and Sellman (1946) demonstrated the inability of large regions of axolotl neural crest to form appropriate structures if they were grafted after a 180° rotation. For example, when frontal regions of crest came to lie over and migrated into the gill arches, the skeletal elements which developed in the branchial region did not appear typical and possessed teeth, while the branchial crest which had migrated into the front of the head produced structures the authors identified as hyoid elements attached to the rostral end of the mandible. Likewise, 90° rotations also produced unusual skeletal structure, suggesting that the neural crest cells were differentiating in a manner more consistent with their anterio-posterior level of origin than with the antero-posterior positions to which they were actually migrating within the experimental embryos (Hörstadius and Sellman 1946; also see Hall and Hörstadius 1988, figs. 25, 26, and 29 for good examples). The other well-documented case of rostro-caudal polarity of crest is the heterotopic grafting experiments of Noden (1983b) in which presumptive frontonasal, maxillary, or mandibular quail or chick embryo crest was grafted in place of the presumptive hyoid crest of host chick embryos. In a majority of the cases a second ectopic mandible, including a hatching tooth, was produced in the hyoid arch region of the host chick (Noden 1983b). In the case of presumptive mandibular neural crest, the cells were clearly following the program of their point of origin rather than the place of their subsequent migration. In the case of the maxillary and frontonasal crest the interpretation of the data is more difficult. However, Noden (1983b) suggested that since under normal circumstances these two populations of crest come under the influence of neuroepithelia or neuroectoderm-derived structures (Hörstadius 1950; Benoit and Schowing 1970), this crest may not be irreversibly specified. It must also be recalled that the maxilla is part of the "first" or mandibular arch, and thus production of mandibular structures is less difficult to understand in this instance. Yet, it is still unclear why the most anterior level of crest should give rise to an ectopic mandible in the hyoid arch, unless, at least for the case of trabecular crest, it represents an evolutionary duplication of mandibular arch or mandible-like arch crest which has become associated with the neurocranium.

It is important to remember that in both of these cases a large piece of neural crest had to be perturbed to create these chimeric skeletons. It has long been observed (Hall and Hörstadius 1988) that a high degree of regulation from adjacent neural crest or mesoderm is possible to compensate for the removal or alteration of short segments of crest. Thus the crest is not a ridged mosaic down to the individual cell level, but does apparently contain some restrictions on the potential to differentiate into various cranial structures along the anterio-posterior axis. Further discussion of a possible controlling mechanism for antero-posterior postion is presented below.

We should also, at this point, discuss the limited evidence for neural crest control of developing tissues. This evidence again comes primarily from two sources. One, recently recounted by Jacobson and Sater (1988), is the ability of neural crest cells to suppress a variety of developing cell types, including lens induction in *Triton taeniatus* (Von Woellwarth 1961) and induction of mesonephros in the developing newt, *Taricha torosa;* frog, *Xenopus laevis;* and mouse (Etheridge 1968, 1972; Gans 1987). The second example is of neural crest control of morphogenesis of associated muscle, both during normal differentiation and especially during the formation of ectopic structures such as the hyoid-placed mandibles described above, which were also found, in a number of cases, to have received the appropriate muscle insertions (Noden 1983a, b, 1987, 1988). This form of patterning, primarily by differentiating skeletal tissue upon the associated musculature, has also been observed in the developing limb bud (Zwilling 1961) and again highlights the shift in patterning control, from tissues or epigenetic signals which permit neural crest migration and restrict neural crest subpopulations at earlier embryonic stages, to the neural crest itself, which subsequently acts as a pattern template, in an as yet unresolved manner, to direct muscle and associated tissue morphogenesis.

HEAD SEGMENTATION AND PATTERNING

Given that the trunk axial mesoderm is clearly segmented, similar evidence for segmentation has been sought in the head. Resolving this problem has obvious implications for understanding the mechanisms of craniofacial pattern formation.

That the vertebrate head is segmented is an old idea; see Russell (1916), de Beer (1937), Hall and Hanken (1985) for overviews. As summarized in 1985, "There is perhaps no topic pertaining to the fundamental organization and structure of the vertebrate head that is more 'classical' a problem than segmentation" (Hall and Hanken 1985, vii).

Goethe, after the famous scene in the Jewish cemetery in Venice in

1790, saw the skull as modeled on three vertebrae but did not publish his theory until 1820. In the meantime, numerous anatomists and morphologists (Oken, Spix, Bojanus, Geoffroy, Meckel, Vicq d' Azyr) between 1807 and 1820 saw the skull as a modification of the vertebrae (Russell 1916; de Beer 1937), with anywhere between three and seven vertebrae involved; four was apparently the favorite number (de Beer 1937). De Beer was especially scathing of this theory, commenting that "among these protagonists of anatomie philosophique or Naturphilosophie, the vertebral theory of the skull is almost the classical example of the fantastic lengths to which speculation, unchecked by scientific evidence, can go in a frantic effort to find, at all costs, the reflection in different parts of the body of some idealized form" (de Beer 1937, 7). Although Thomas Huxley demolished the vertebral theory of the skull in his Croonian lecture of 1858, the notion that the embryonic head, if not the skull, is built upon a segmented plan has persisted.

Balfour (1876a) argued most cogently for a segmented organization of the vertebrate head. A diversity of views has existed over the ensuing years. On the one hand, Kingsbury (1926) and Romer (1972) rejected any notion of cranial segmentation. On the other, Bjerring (1977) and Jarvik (1980) saw cranial and trunk segmentation as a continuum. De Beer (1937) wrote his monographic treatment on the development of the vertebrate skull against the background and in the context of segmentation.

The location of the posterior border of the skull across the vertebrates has been a subject of debate (de Beer, 1937). The scenario proposed by Northcutt and Gans (1983), in which the anterior portion of the skull, being of neural crest origin, has a fundamentally different embryological origin from the posterior, mesodermal, and segmented portion of the skull, implies that while the posterior portion of the skull may be segmented, the anterior region is not. Under this scenario, we have to consider the skull as a composite structure, and more important, we must examine each tissue or organ system separately for signs of segmentation. Interestingly, as recently pointed out by Lonai and Urtreger (1990), this division of anterior from posterior skull may have a genetic basis, as it roughly corresponds to the rostralmost limit of expression for the *Hox* 1 gene series in the mouse.

There is no a priori requirement for segmentation involving all the structures in the head; segmentation could be restricted to individual organs. Jacobson (this volume) summarizes the evidence for paraxial mesoderm being the primarily segmented system in the vertebrate head. Furthermore, as with parasegments in insects, segmentation need not be reflected in boundaries that present as morphological entities.

What have recent studies contributed to this classical problem?

We now know from the work initiated by Meier (1984) and summarized by Jacobson in this volume that the head (paraxial) mesoderm is segmented into somitomeres. The most caudal somitomeres become somites proper; the rostral somitomeres provide the head musculature (Noden 1983a). Furthermore, the neural crest, although unsegmented when it arises, is distributed in a segmented pattern through neural crest cell migration. Although unsegmented before migration, the skeletogenic cranial neural crest is regionalized rostro-caudally (Langille and Hall 1988a, b; Hall and Hörstadius 1988).

We now know that the brain develops from segmented neuromeres (Vaage 1969; Meier 1982; Lumsden and Keynes 1989; Fraser et al. 1990), that the cranial nerves are ordered segmentally, and that neuromeric segmentation is secondary, being imposed upon the neural ectoderm by the mesoderm (Hogan et al. 1985; Frohman et al. 1990). Moreover, at least for the embryonic chick, we now know that the cranial ectoderm is segmented into ectomeres, which correspond to the neuromeric boundaries (Couly and Le Douarin 1990); and work on homeobox genes, particularly in the mouse, has revealed a pattern of expression in overlapping domains in the developing nervous system (Holland 1988; Kessel and Gruss 1990; Lonai and Urtreger 1990) that parallels neuromeric segmentation (Wilkinson, Bhatt, Chavrier 1989; Wilkinson, Bhatt, Cook et al. 1989).

Clearly, the issue of head segmentation, this "classical" problem, is not dead and, indeed, should not be allowed to die. The data from these more recent studies will be expanded upon as we discuss the control of patterning of the craniofacial region and the role of the neural crest in this process in the next section.

PATTERNING MECHANISMS

We are, at the time of writing this chapter, just beginning to understand the mechanics of developmental pathways which convey patterning of the craniofacial region. We begin by assembling the data that suggest a possible mechanism of pattern control and then integrate these data with specific examples of craniofacial neural crest differentiation to show that the model both fits existing data and poses new problems to be solved.

Positional Information: Restriction of Neural Crest Cells

As stated earlier, it has been known for a long time that trunk neural crest cannot replace cranial neural crest, as it does not participate significantly in connective tissue differentiation either in situ or when heterotopically transplanted to the head region (Nakamura and Ayer-Le Lièvre 1982;

Le Douarin 1982; Hall and Hörstadius 1988). Thus, it is clear that neural crest cells receive some restrictive information polarizing the neural crest into cranial (anterior) and trunk (posterior) regions either prior to or during the separation of neural crest from the neurectoderm. Evidence of further restriction of the cranial neural crest into frontonasal, first arch, second arch, and so on has until recently relied soley on the evidence provided by Hörstadius and Sellman (1946) and Noden (1983b) of the rostro-caudal polarity of the crest as outlined above. However, more recently a variety of studies have pointed toward a mechanism by which rostro-caudal patterning of neural crest and indeed all of the cranial tissues is achieved, although it is still not clear when the restriction of neural crest occurs, or whether it is accomplished in one or a cascade of several steps.

Positional Information: Neuromeres

The first real evidence of a mechanism for producing positional information to restrict neural crest in a rostro-caudal sequence comes from the data of Lumsden and Keynes (1989) and Fraser et al. (1990), who demonstrated that the pattern of rhombomeres, morphologically distinct serial constrictions (neuromeres) of the hindbrain, corresponds directly with the arrangement of roots of the sensory and branchial motor nerves. The relationship consists of pairs of rhombomeres which (1) contribute the roots of specific sensory and branchial motor nerves, and (2) innervate the corresponding cranial sensory ganglion (containing neural crest derivatives) and the branchial arch (also containing neural crest derivatives) which lies immediately ventral to the pair; see figure 3.4 for details. Furthermore, these authors established that the rhombomere boundaries are indeed real, inasmuch as once established, cells within the hindbrain do not cross between rhombomeres. These data only hint at possible early control of anterio-posterior (A-P) restriction of neural crest since the crest which contributes to the segmentally arranged branchial arches originates from rhombomeric ectoderm and thus may be similarily patterned. And it should be pointed out that support for the closeness of neural crest and neurectoderm is not limited to geographic location of origin; Bronner-Fraser and Fraser (1989) have shown by cell marker studies that at least some cells in the early neural fold give rise to both neural tube and neural crest derivative cells.

Positional Information: Ectomeres

A second tissue which has been shown to have profound influence on neural crest is the epithelia with which it interacts (Hall 1987; Lumsden 1987, 1988). Noden (1984) was among the first to notice that the neural crest did not migrate through a static environment, but that associated morpho-

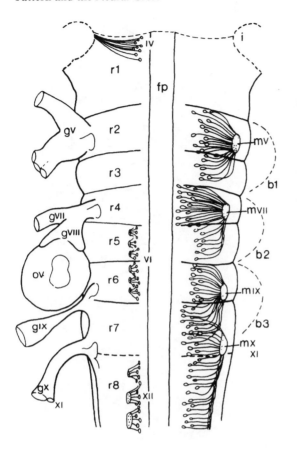

Fig. 3.4. A schematic diagram of the hindbrain of a stage-21 embryonic chick to illustrate the relationship between cranial sensory ganglia (g^v–g^x), branchial and somatic motor nuclei (IV–XII), and the combined roots of the sensory and branchial motor nerves (mv–mx) to the eight rhombomeres (r1–r8) and three branchial arches (b1–b3). Each pair of rhombomeres contributes the roots of specific sensory and branchial motor nerves and innervates the corresponding cranial sensory ganglia and adjacent branchial arch, each of which contains neural crest derivatives. Abbreviations: fp, floor plate; i, isthmus/midbrain-hindbrain boundary; ov, otic vesicle. Reproduced from Lumsden and Keynes (1989), with the permission of the publisher.

genetic movements caused a ventral displacement of the ectoderm. Couly and Le Douarin (1990) have greatly expanded on this observation in showing that, in aves, the ectoderm which lies adjacent to the neural crest at the commencement of migration follows the same pathways, thus remaining adjacent to the neural crest of the superficial craniofacial regions at their final destination. Although the ectoderm is not segmented, Couly and Le Douarin have coined the term "ectomeres" for the regions of epithelia which will line specific facial structures such as the branchial arches. These ectomeres are derived from dorsal sites that originate in register with specific neuromeres (fig. 3.5), although it is unclear whether the ectomere-neuromere relationship is equivalent to the rhombomere–branchial arch relationship outlined above and in figure 3.4. Nevertheless, the data of Couly and Le Douarin, combined with that of Lumsden, Keynes, and Fra-

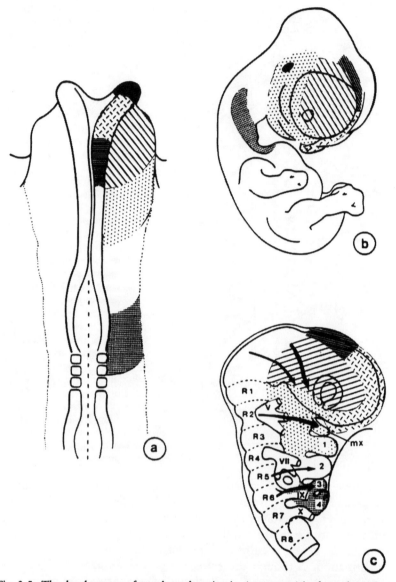

Fig. 3.5. The development of ectodermal territories (ectomeres) in the embryonic chick. Diagrammatic representation of the movement of the ectoderm from dorsal to ventro-lateral positions in a chick embryo, beginning from the 3-somite stage (a, dorsal view) to the eight-day embryo (b, lateral view). Nasal mucosa (■), upper beak ectoderm (⸪), ectoderm covering the anterior calvarium (▦), eyelids and cornea (\\\\ ), ectoderm of the first arch (⫶⫶), second arch (☐), third and fourth arches (▤). c. A lateral view of a 3.5-day-old embryo to show the eight

ser, provides strong support for an underlying mechanism driving the A-P polarity and positional information of the vertebrate head.

HOMEOBOX GENES AND COORDINATION OF CRANIOFACIAL DEVELOPMENT

The last data for the mechanism of control of A-P polarity and positional information are observations on the segmental expression of homeobox genes, particularly some recent data on the "transference" of homeobox expression in immediately postgastrula mouse embryos. Homeotic genes in *Drosophila* contain a 180 base-pair sequence (the homeobox); they are involved in the developmental regulation of segmental structures (Kessel and Gruss 1990). The discovery of homeobox-containing genes in a variety of vertebrates unleashed at first a slow and now exponentially increasing amount of data showing widespread distribution of subsets of these genes. A variety of functions have been proposed, either by implication of expression pattern or by abnormalities caused by overexpression; overexpression of *Xhox* 3 in *Xenopus* prevents normal anterior mesoderm development (Ruiz i Altaba and Melton 1989), and ectopic expression of *Hox* 1.1 in the mouse causes craniofacial abnormalities (Balling et al. 1989). Currently, the expression of homeobox and related, developmentally important genes has been analyzed to the greatest extent in the mouse. As demonstrated in figure 3.6, *Hox* families 1, 2, 3, and 4, the engrailed gene (En), paired-type homeobox (pax), and the zinc finger gene *Krox*-20 create a pattern of expression over the entire embryonic central nervous system (CNS) such that the anterior limits of expression coincide with various neuromeres, or, in the case of *Hox* 2.9 and *Krox*-20, the expression is restricted to specific neuromeres (Murphy et al. 1989; Wilkinson, Bhatt, Chavrier et al. 1989; Wilkinson, Bhatt, Cook et al. 1989; Lonai and Urtreger 1990; Kessel and Gruss 1990). This gives us a somewhat complex, but nevertheless highly suggestive argument for the involvement of these genes in the segmental arrangement of the vertebrate head.

Homeobox and related gene expression is also found in the adjacent, segmentally arranged paraxial mesoderm in a similar pattern of overlap,

---

rhombomeres (R1–R8) and the branchial arches that they innervate (see also fig. 3.4). R1 to R3 correspond to the trigeminal nerve (V) that innervates the first branchial arch (1). R4 and R5 correspond to the facial nerve (VII) that innervates the second branchial arch (2). R6 to R8 correspond to the glossopharyngeal (IX) and vagal (X) nerves that innervate branchial arches 3 and 4. Arrows indicate the direction of neural crest cell migration; mx, maxillary bud. Reproduced from Couly and Le Douarin (1900) with the permission of the publisher.

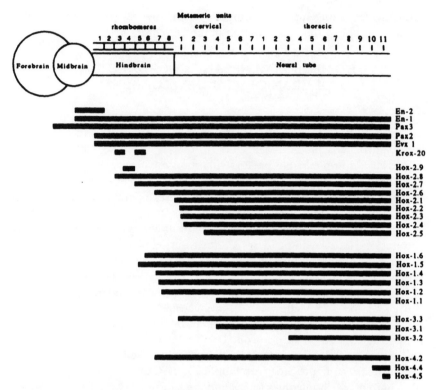

Fig. 3.6. A diagrammatic representation of anterior expression boundaries of the engrailed gene (En), paired type homeobox genes (Pax), zinc finger gene *Krox*-20 and *Hox* genes 1.1 to 4.5 in the mouse embryo. Anterior limits of expression either coincide with individual rhombomeres (e.g., *Hox* 2.8) or regions of the brain (e.g., En-1), or are restricted to specific rhombomeres (*Hox* 2.9, *Krox*-20). Note that the map indicates the boundaries of maximal expression for each gene and therefore represents a composite of various embryological stages. Reproduced from Kessel and Gruss (1990) with the permission of the publisher.

although not in register with expression over the CNS but rather displaced in a caudal, direction (Mahon et al. 1988; Duboule and Dollé 1989; Graham et al. 1989; Gaunt et al. 1989). Most of the studies of mesodermal expression have centered on provertebral mesoderm (Gaunt et al. 1988); some have also documented *Hox* expression in trunk neural crest derivatives, suggesting that further research may uncover the link which coordinates trunk patterning. As detailed below, such information is just coming to light in the case of the head.

Very early on, it was pointed out that neural crest may express some homeobox or related genes, owing to their initial association with the neurectoderm which displays elaborate *Hox* expression. And indeed recently, homeobox gene expression has been found in cranial neural crest cells. Examples are *Hox* genes 2.8, 2.9, and 2.1 (Wilkinson, Bhatt, Cook et al. 1989), *Hox* 1.1 (Mahon et al. 1988), *Hox* 2.9 (Frohman et al. 1990), and *Hox* 7 (Robert et al. 1989; Hill et al. 1989). The later examples of *Hox* 7 expression are especially significant in relation to craniofacial development, as the neural crest expression of the genes persists in crest-derived craniofacial mesenchyme.

The study by Frohman et al. (1990) has a special significance to the question of control of craniofacial development, for it is, to the authors' knowledge, the first report of the transference of *Hox* gene expression across a variety of tissues, beginning during late gastrulation. These authors report that on embryonic day 7.5 in the mouse (E7.5), which corresponds to late gastrulation, *Hox* 2.9 is expressed in the mesoderm adjacent and posterior to the region of ectoderm which will form hindbrain anlage. At neurulation, *Hox* 2.9 becomes expressed in the neural plate, but only in that region overlying mesoderm which also expresses the gene. As neurulation continues, *Hox* 2.9 becomes restricted to that portion of the neural floor plate cells, then neuromere B, which will form rhombomere four (also see Murphy et al. 1989; Wilkinson, Bhatt, Cook et al. 1989). At the same time, expression can be detected in the neural crest cells overlying that region (prootic crest which will migrate into the hyoid or arch two) and the thin ectoderm just lateral to the neural tube. Paraxial mesodermal expression is low by this time at the level of the second arch, but greater than background. Likewise, with time and migration, more ventral crest loses *Hox* 2.9 expression, while other ventral and posterior tissues, the endoderm and ectoderm of the third arch and cleft of the second arch and adjacent lateral plate mesoderm, all express elevated levels of the gene. By E9.5 *Hox* 2.9 gene expression is now limited to rhombomere four and dorsal (ganglionic) neural crest, but no further ventrally in arches two or three. The only ventral expression in the branchial arch region is now found in arch four in the same tissues in which expression was observed earlier in arch three.

Thus Frohman and colleagues have uncovered "coordinate expression of a Hox gene in multiple germ layers" and further describe the system in this fashion: "anteroposterior information is acquired by mesoderm, mesoderm induces positional values within (neuro-) ectoderm and endoderm, and both events occur within a restricted window of time."

A MECHANISM FOR CRANIOFACIAL PATTERNING

We can now put all the above information together to describe the possible mechanism of positional information transfer to cranial ectomesenchyme.

The work of Frohman et al. (1990) strongly supports the idea that developmental regulation genes are first switched on in the early mesoderm, possibly during the initial stages of gastrulation, that is, during primary induction. If this bears out with future studies, then primary induction not only specifies the bilateral symmetry of the vertebrate embryo (Langille and Hall 1989) but also antero-posterior positional information through *Hox* and related genes (we leave out any inclusion of dorso-ventral patterning through mesoderm inducing factors, as this goes beyond the scope of the present chapter, but see Langille and Hall 1989). This information is conveyed to the neurectoderm, neural crest anlage, and adjacent ectoderm, which Couly and Le Douarin (1990) have decisively shown will remain in direct association with the neural crest (see above). Obviously this mechanism may include other, as yet undiscovered, regulating genes.

If one assumes that homeobox genes are acting to coordinate development, then the data of Frohman and colleagues (1990) fit nicely with a variety of other experimental data revealing the often extensive cell-cell/cell-matrix interactions observed to take place during neural crest migration and differentiation as described above (and see Thorogood, this volume; Hall 1987; Noden 1988; Hall and Hörstadius 1988).

Control of craniofacial pattern formation thus appears complex and interactive, with increasing control being channeled through the crest cells themselves as restriction-differentiation proceeds. Thus, as neural crest cells are restricted in developmental fate, they become the dominant factor in the patterning of those craniofacial regions they invest. For example, neural crest mesenchyme within the avian sclera is still subject to specification by the adjacent epithelial papillae with respect to the location of sclera ossicle formation, yet the type and shape of bone the neural crest cells will lay down, once specified to do so, clearly reside within the crest cells themselves (Hall 1981; Fyfe and Hall 1983; Hall 1989). The same is also true for the dentary; it is dependent upon an epithelium for induction, but when induced by scleral epithelia, it produces jaw-like bone, not ossicle-like bone (Hall 1981, 1989). A final example is the odontogenic crest. The early induction of teeth, which also includes spatial patterning, is the result of a series of incompletely understood interactions between oral epithelium and underlying ectomesenchyme. However, once induced, tooth morphogenesis is under the control of the neural crest—derived dental papilla (see Lumsden 1987, 1988).

Interestingly, pattern formation of craniofacial neural crest derivatives may be fully understood only once we have established which genes and/or gene products are being coordinated (if indeed they are) by *Hox* and similar genes as well as what controls the *Hox* genes themselves. To illustrate the point let us return to the experiments of Noden (1983b) in which presumptive mandibular, maxillary, and frontonasal crest all give rise to ectopic mandibles if grafted heterotopically so that the cells migrate into the hyoid arch. Noden transplanted not only neural crest but also the associated neural tube and ectoderm, that is to say, three of the four tissues Frohman et al. (1990) have shown to display coordinating *Hox* expression. Since the ectoderm (ectomeres) migrate along with the crest as Couly and Le Douarin (1990) have shown, the formation of secondary mandibles by the mandibular neural crest is more easily understood; whether they would still form without the mandibular ectomere now becomes the question. More difficult to explain are the cases of the maxillary and frontonasal crest which should migrate along with maxillary and frontonasal ectomeres. Noden (1983b) had stated that in their normal migration these two populations of crest cells come under the influence of neuroepithelia and that lack of this influence in his transplants allowed the mandibular pattern to surface. Even though the more anterior regions of neuroepithelia were grafted back with the crest, the cells in the hyoid region move too far away to be influenced by the ectopic neural tissue, giving Noden's suggestion plausibility. But the discovery of ectomeres poses an additional twist, suggesting that maxillary or frontonasal crest cells and their ectomeres will interact and express a mandibular phenotype in an ectopic region. However, when under the influence of another tissue, for example forebrain neuroepithelia, these tissues interact as before but produce the appropriate maxillae or frontonasal structures. This suggests that although coordination of these tissues via homeobox genes may be occurring, there is still a hierarchy of signals, all set by the same *Hox* gene(s) which fine-tunes pattern formation. The resolution of the mechanism controlling craniofacial pattern formation will no doubt provide exciting insight not only into the differentiation of tissues within the head but also into the general principles of vertebrate differentiation and morphogenesis.

SUMMARY AND CONCLUSIONS

Although first identified over a century ago, the importance of the neural crest in vertebrate development, especially that of the head, has gained appreciation only over the last 50 years and wide acceptance over the last 20. This embryonic tissue is subdivided into two regions, trunk and cranial neural crest, not only on morphological grounds, but also on the basis of the cell types which derive from them. In particular, only the cranial neural crest has been demonstrated to give rise to skeletal structures. The cranial neural crest in fact makes a major contribution to the vertebrate head, differentiating into a wide variety of tissues, representing a veritable fourth germ layer. It therefore plays a very important role in pattern formation of the head. From its origin at the neural tube–ectodermal junction it migrates latero-ventral into the embryonic head, encountering both matrix and cell signals along the route. Cell-cell and matrix-cell signaling continue even after the cells have reached their destination and are vital in the differentiation of these cells. The epigenetic nature of neural crest migration and differentiation allows for variability in control of neural crest differentiation, but in general, with increasing time and as neural crest cells become more restricted, they acquire greater control of both their own differentiation and morphogenesis and that of adjacent tissues.

The pattern of *Hox* gene expression, coupled with neuromere, mesomere, and ectomere identification, all provide strong evidence for the segmented prepattern of the vertebrate head. The neural crest fits the model of the vertebrate head as a segmented structure inasmuch as it retains its antero-posterior position during migration. Yet the epigenetic nature of neural crest differentiation allows for the formation of a head without strict serial duplication of all structures as the crest cells are free to interact with different cell types or matrices both along their migration routes and at their destination points. And recent evidence for the coordinate expression, in the embryonic head, of a *Hox* gene in multiple germ layers, including the neural crest, suggests that these genes may indeed be acting to coordinate the epigenetic interactions which occur during neural crest differentiation and morphogenesis, thereby coordinating pattern formation in the vertebrate head.

ACKNOWLEDGMENTS

Brian K. Hall acknowledges the support of the Natural Sciences and Engineering Research Council of Canada through grant A-5056. Robert M. Langille acknowledges the support of the Natural Sciences and Engineering Research Council of Canada through a University Research Fellowship and the Medical Research Council of Canada through grant MT-10579.

REFERENCES

Anderson, L. G., and S. Meier. 1981. The influence of the metameric pattern in the mesoderm on migration. Developmental Biology 85: 385–402.
————. 1982. Effect of hyaluronidase treatment on the distribution of cranial neural crest cells in the chick embryo. Journal of Experimental Zoology 221: 329–335.
Bagnara, J. T. 1987. The neural crest as a source of stem cells. In *Developmental and Evolutionary Aspects of the Neural Crest*, P. F. A. Maderson, ed. New York: John Wiley and Sons, pp. 57–87.
Balfour, F. M. 1876a. On the development of elasmobranch fishes. Journal of Anatomy and Physiology, London 10: 377–410, 517–570.

———. 1876b. On the development of the spinal nerves in elasmobranch fishes. Philosophical Transactions of the Royal Society 166: 175–195.

Balling, R., G. Mutter, P. Gruss, and M. Kessel. 1989. Craniofacial abnormalities induced by ectopic expression of the homeobox gene Hox-1.1 in transgenic mice. Cell 56: 337–347.

Bancroft, M., and R. Bellairs. 1976. The neural crest cells of the trunk region of the chick embryo studied by SEM and TEM. Zoon 4: 73–85.

Beer, G. R. de. 1937. *The Development of the Vertebrate Skull.* Oxford: Oxford University Press. Reissued with a new foreword by B. K. Hall and J. Hanken. Chicago: University of Chicago Press, 1985.

———. 1947. The differentiation of neural crest cells into visceral cartilages and odontoblats in *Ambystoma,* and a reexamination of the germ-layer theory. Proceedings of the Royal Society of London B 134: 377–398.

Benoit, J. A., and J. Schowing. 1970. *Morphogenesis of the neurocranium.* In *Tissue Interactions during Organogenesis,* E. Wolff, ed. New York: Gordon Breach, pp. 105–130.

Bilozur, M. E., and E. D. Hay. 1988. Neural crest migration in 3D extracellular matrix utilizes laminin, fibronectin, or collagen. Developmental Biology 125: 19–33.

Bjerring, H. C. 1977. A contribution to structural analysis of the head of craniate animals. Zoologica scripta 6: 127–183.

Borcea, M. I. 1909. Sur l'origine du coeur, des cellules vasculaires migratrices et des cellules pigmentaires chez les Téléostéens. Comptes rendus Hebdomadaires des séances, Académie des sciences, Paris 149: 688–689.

Boucaut, J. C., T. Darribère, T. J. Poole, H. Aoyama, K. M. Yamada, and J. P. Thiery. 1984. Biologically active synthetic peptides as probes of embryonic development: A competitive peptide inhibitor of fibronectin function inhibits gastrulation in amphibian embryos and neural crest cell migration in avian embryos. Journal of Cell Biology 99: 1822–1830.

Brachet, A. 1908. Recherches sur l'ontogenèse de la tête chez les Amphibiens. Archives de biologie, Paris 23: 165–257.

Bronner-Fraser, M. 1985. Alterations in neural crest migration by a monoclonal antibody that affects cell adhesion. Journal of Cell Biology 101: 610–617.

Bronner-Fraser, M., and S. Fraser. 1989. Developmental potential of avian trunk neural crest cells in situ. Neuron 3: 755–766.

Chan, W. Y., and P. P. L. Tam. 1988. A morphological and experimental study of the mesencephalic neural crest cells in the mouse embryo using wheat germ agglutinin-gold conjugate as the cell marker. Development 102: 427–442.

Chibon, P. 1970. Capacité de régulation des excédents dans la crête neurale d'Amphibien. Journal of Embryology and Experimental Morphology 24: 479–496.

———. 1974. Un système morphogénétique remarquable: La crête neurale des vertébrés. Année biologique 13: 459–480.

Couly, G., and N. M. Le Douarin. 1990. Head morphogenesis in embryonic avian chimeras: Evidence for a segmental pattern in the ectoderm corresponding to the neuromeres. Development 108: 543–558.

D'Amico-Martel, A., and D. Noden. 1980. An autoradiographic analysis of the development of the chick trigeminal ganglion. Journal of Embryology and Experimental Morphology 55: 167–182.

———. 1983. Contributions of placodal and neural crest cells to avian peripheral ganglia. American Journal of Anatomy 166: 445–468.

Detwiler, S. R., and R. H. van Dyke. 1934. The development and functions of deafferented fore limbs in *Ambylstoma*. Journal of Experimental Zoology 68: 321–346.

Duband, J. L., and J. P. Thiery. 1982. Distribution of fibronectin in the early phase of avian cephalic neural crest migration. Developmental Biology 93: 308–323.

Duboule, D., and P. Dollé. 1989. The structural and functional organization of the murine HOX gene family resembles that of *Drosophilia* homeotic genes. European Molecular Biology Organization (EMBO) Journal 8: 1497–1505.

Dupin, E., A. Baroffio, C. Dulac, P. Cameron-Curry, and N. M. Le Douarin. 1990. Schwann-cell differentiation in clonal cultures of the neural crest as evidenced by the anti-Schwann cell myelin protein monoclonal antibody. Proceedings of the National Academy of Sciences, U.S.A. 87: 1119–1123.

Du Shane, G. P. 1935. An experimental study of the origin of pigment cells in Amphibia. Journal of Experimental Zoology 72: 1–31.

Erikson, C. A. 1985. Control of neural crest cell dispersion in the trunk of the avian embryo. Developmental Biology 111: 138–157.

———. 1986. *Morphogenesis of the neural crest.* In *Developmental Biology,* vol. 2, L. Browder, ed. New York: Plenum Publishing Corp., pp. 481–543.

Etheridge, A. L. 1968. Determination of the mesonephric kidney. Journal of Experimental Zoology 169: 357–370.

———. 1972. Suppression of kidney formation by neural crest cells. Wilhelm Roux' Archiv für Entwicklungsmechanik der Organismen 169: 268–270.

Fraser, S., R. Keynes, and A. Lumsden. 1990. Segmentation in the chick embryo hindbrain is defined by cell lineage restrictions. Nature 344: 431–435.

Frohman, M. A., M. Boyle, and G. R. Martin. 1990. Isolation of the mouse Hox-2.9 gene: Analysis of embryonic expression suggests that positional information along the anterior-posterior axis is specified by the mesoderm. Development 110: 589–608.

Fyfe, D. M., and B. K. Hall. 1983. The origin of the ectomesenchymal condensations which precede the development of the bony scleral ossicles in the eyes of embryonic chicks. Journal of Embryology and Experimental Morphology 73: 69–86.

Gans, C. 1987. The neural crest: A spectacular invention. In *Developmental and Evolutionary Aspects of the Neural Crest,* P. F. A. Maderson, ed. New York: John Wiley and Sons, pp. 361–379.

Gaunt, S. J., R. Krumlauf, and D. Duboule. 1989. Mouse homeo-genes within a subfamily, Hox-1.4, -2.6, and -5.1 display similar anteroposterior domains of expression in the embryo, but show stage- and tissue-dependent differences in their regulation. Development 107: 131–141.

Gaunt, S. J., P. T. Sharpe, and D. Duboule. 1988. Spatially restricted domains of homeo-gene transcripts in mouse embryos: Relation to a segmented body plan. Development 104 (suppl.): 169–179.

Goethe, J. W. 1820. *Zur Naturwissenschaften uberhaupt, besonders zur Morphologie.* Leipzig.

Goronowitsch, N. 1892. Die axiale und die laterale Kopfmetamerie der Vögelembryonen. Die Rolle der sog. "Ganglienleisten" im Aufbaue der Nervenstämme. Anatomische Anziger 7: 454–464.

———. 1893a. Untersuchungen über die Entwicklung der sogenannten "Ganglienleisten" im Kopfe der Vögelembryonen. Morphologisches Jahrbuch 20: 187–259.

———. 1893b. Weiters über die ektodermal Entstehung von Skeletanlagen im Kopfe der Wirbeltiere. Morphologisches Jahrbuch 20: 425–428.

Graham, A., N. Papalopulu, and R. Krumlauf. 1989. The murine and *Drosophila* homeobox gene complexes have common features of organization and expression. Cell 57: 367–378.

Greenburg, G., and E. D. Hay. 1982. Epithelia suspended in collagen gels can lose polarity and express characteristics of migrating mesenchymal cells. Journal of Cell Biology 95: 333–339.

Hall, B. K. 1981. Specificity in the differentiation and morphogenesis of neural crest–derived scleral ossicles and of epithelial scleral papillae in the eye of the embryonic chick. Journal of Embryology and Experimental Morphology 66: 175–190.

———. 1987. Tissue interactions in the development and evolution of the vertebrate head. In *Developmental and Evolutionary Aspects of the Neural Crest,* P. F. A. Maderson, ed. New York: John Wiley and Sons, pp. 215–259.

———. 1989. Morphogenesis of the skeleton: Epithelial or mesenchymal control? In *Trends in Vertebrate Morphology,* H. Splechtna and H. Hilgers, eds. Progress in Zoology 35. Stuttgart: Gustav Fischer Verlag, pp. 198–201.

Hall, B. K., and J. Hanken. 1985. Foreword. In *The Development of the Vertebrate Skull,* G. R. de Beer, ed. Chicago: University of Chicago Press, pp. vii–xxviii.

Hall, B. K., and S. Hörstadius. 1988. *The Neural Crest.* Oxford: Oxford University Press.

Hall, B. K., and R. Tremaine. 1979. Ability of neural crest cells from the embryonic chick to differentiate into cartilage before their migration away from the neural tube. Anatomical Record 194: 469–476.

Hay, E. D. 1982. Interaction of embryonic cell surface and cytoskeleton with extracellular matrix. American Journal of Anatomy 165: 1–12.

———. 1989. Extracellular matrix, cell skeletons, and embryonic development. American Journal of Medical Genetics 34: 14–29.

Hill, R. E., P. F. Jones, A. R. Rees, C. M. Sime, M. J. Justice, N. G. Copeland, N. A. Jenkins, E. Graham, and D. R. Davidson. 1989. A new family of mouse homeo box–containing genes: Molecular structure, chromosomal location, and developmental expression of Hox-7.1. Genes and Development 3: 26–37.

His, W. 1868. *Untersuchungen über die erste Anlage des Wirbeltierleibes.* Die erste Entwicklung des Hühnchens im Ei. Leipzig: F. C. W. Vogel.

Hogan, B., P. W. H. Holland, and P. Schofield. 1985. How is the mouse segmented? Trends in Genetics 1: 67–74.

Holland, P. W. H. 1988. Homeobox genes and the vertebrate head. Development 103 (suppl.): 17–24.

Holmdahl, D. E. 1928. Die Enstehung und weitere Entwicklung der Neuralleiste (Ganglienleiste) bei Vogeln und Saugetieren. Zeitschrift für Mikroskopische-Anatomische Forschung 14: 99–298.

Hörstadius, S. 1950. The Neural Crest: Its Properties and Derivatives in the Light of Experimental Research. Oxford: Oxford University Press.

Hörstadius, S., and S. Sellman. 1946. Experimentelle untersuchungen über die Determination des Knorpeligen Kopfskelettes bei Urodelen. Nova acta Regiae societatis scientiarum Upsaliensis, ser. 4, 13: 1–170.

Jacobson, A. G., and A. K. Sater. 1988. Features of embryonic induction. Development 104: 341–359.

Jarvik, E. 1980. Basic Structure and Evolution of Vertebrates, vols. 1 and 2. London: Academic Press.

Johnston, M. C. 1966. A radioautographic study of the migration and fate of cranial neural crest cells in the chick embryo. Anatomical Record 156: 143–156.

Kastschenko, N. 1888. Zur Entwicklungsgeschichte der Selachier-embryos. Anatomische Anziger 3: 445–467.

Kessel, M., and P. Gruss. 1990. Murine developmental control genes. Science 249: 374–379.

Kingsbury, B. F. 1926. Branchiomerism and the theory of head segmentation. Journal of Morphology 42: 83–109.

Landacre, F. L. 1921. The fate of the neural crest in the head of the Urodeles. Journal of Comparative Neurology 33: 1–43.

Langille, R. M., and B. K. Hall. 1988a. Role of the neural crest in development of the cartilaginous cranial and visceral skeleton of the medaka, Oryzias latipes (Teleostei). Anatomy and Embryology 177: 297–305.

———. 1988b. Role of the neural crest in development of the trabeculae and branchial arches in embryonic sea lamprey, Petromyzon marinus P (L). Development 102: 301–310.

———. 1989. Developmental processes, developmental sequences, and early vertebrate phylogeny. Biological Reviews, Cambridge Philosophical Society 64: 73–91.

Le Douarin, N. 1982. The Neural Crest. Cambridge: Cambridge University Press.

Le Lièvre, C. 1971a. Recherches sur l'origine embryologique des arcs viscéraux chez l'embryon d'Oiseau par la méthode des greffes interspécifiques entre Caille et Poulet. Comptes rendus de la Société de biologie 165: 395–400.

———. 1971b. Recherches sur l'origine embryologique du squelette viscéral chez l'embryon d'Oiseau. Comptes rendus d'Association d'anatomie 152: 575–583.

———. 1974. Rôle des cellules mésectodermiques issues des crêtes neurales céphaliques dans la formation des arcs branchiaux et du squelette viscéral. Journal of Embryology and Experimental Morphology 47: 17–37.

———. 1978. Participation of neural crest derived cells in the genesis of the skull in birds. Journal of Embryology and Experimental Morphology 47: 17–37.

Le Lièvre, C., and N. M. Le Douarin. 1975. Mesenchymal derivatives of the neural crest: Analysis of chimaeric quail and chick embryos. Journal of Embryology and Experimental Morphology 34: 125–154.

Löfberg, J., K. Ahlfors, and C. Fallstrom. 1980. Neural crest cell migration in relation to extracellular matrix organization. Developmental Biology 75: 148–167.

Löfberg, J., R. Perris, and H. H. Epperlein. 1989. Timing in the regulation of neural crest cell migration: Retarded "maturation" of regional extracellular matrix inhibits pigment cell migration in embryos of the white axolotl mutant. Developmental Biology 131: 168–181.

Lonai, P., and A. O. Urtreger. 1990. Homeogenes in mammalian development and the evolution of the cranium and central nervous system. FASEB Journal 4: 1436–1443.

Lumsden, A. G. S. 1987. The neural crest contribution to tooth development in the mammalian embryo. In Developmental and Evolutionary Aspects of the Neural Crest, P. F. A. Maderson, ed. New York: John Wiley and Sons, pp. 261–300.

———. 1988. Spatial organization of the epithelium and the role of neural crest cells in the initiation of the mammalian tooth germ. Development 103 (suppl.): 155–170.

Lumsden, A. G. S., and R. Keynes. 1989. Segmental patterns of neuronal development in the chick hindbrain. Nature 337: 426–428.

Maderson, P. F. A., ed. 1987. Developmental and Evolutionary Aspects of the Neural Crest. New York: John Wiley and Sons.

Mahon, K. A., H. Westphal, and P. Gruss. 1988. Expression of homeobox gene Hox 1.1 during mouse embryogenesis. Development 104 (suppl.): 187–195.

Martins-Green, M., and C. A. Erikson. 1987. Basal lamina is not a barrier to neural crest cell emigration: Documentation by TEM and by immunoflurescent and immunogold labelling. Development 101: 517–533.

Meier, S. 1982. The development of segmentation in the cranial region of vertebrate embryos. Scanning Electron Microscopy 3: 1269–1282.

———. 1984. Somite formation and its relationship to metameric patterning of the mesoderm. Cell Differentiation 14: 235–243.

Meier, S., and A. G. Jacobson. 1982. Experimental studies of the origin and expression of metameric pattern in the chick embryo. Journal of Embryology and Zoology 219: 217–232.

Meier, S., and D. S. Packard, Jr. 1984. Morphogenesis of the cranial segments and distribution of neural crest in embryos of the snapping turtle, Chelydra serpentina. Developmental Biology 102: 309–323.

Murphy, P., D. R. Davidson, and R. E. Hill. 1989. Segment-specific expression of a homeobox-containing gene in the mouse hindbrain. Nature 341: 156–159.

Nakamura, H., and C. S. Ayer-Le Lièvre. 1982. Mesectodermal capabilities of trunk neural crest of birds. Journal of Embryology and Experimental Morphology 70: 1–18.

Narayana, C. H., and Y. Narayana. 1980. Neural crest and placodal contributions in the development of the glossopharyngeal-vagal complex in the chick. Anatomical Record 196: 71–82.

Newgreen, D. F. 1979. The rostral level of origin of sympathetic neurons in the chick embryo, studied in tissue culture. American Journal of Anatomy 154: 557–562.

———. 1984. Spreading of explants of embryonic chick mesenchymes and epithelia on fibronectin and laminin. Cell and Tissue Research 227: 297–317.

Newgreen, D. F., and C. A. Erikson. 1986. The migration of neural crest cells. International Review of Cytology 103: 89–145.

Newgreen, D. F., and I. Gibbins. 1982. Factors controlling the time of onset of the migration of neural crest cells in the fowl embryo. Cell and Tissue Research 224: 145–160.

Newgreen, D. F., and J. P. Thiery. 1980. Fibronectin in early avian embryos: Synthesis and distribution along migratory pathways of neural crest cells. Cell and Tissue Research 211: 269–336.

Nichols, D. H. 1981. Neural crest formation in the head of the mouse embryo as observed using a new histological technique. Journal of Embryology and Experimental Morphology 64: 105–120.

———. 1985. The ultrastructure and immunohistochemistry of the basal lamina beneath the escaping neural crest mesenchyme in the head of the mouse embryo. Anatomical Record 211: 138A.

———. 1986. Formation and distribution of neural crest mesenchyme to the first pharnygeal arch region of the mouse embryo. American Journal of Anatomy 176: 221–231.

———. 1987. Ultrastructure of neural crest formation in the midbrain/rostral hindbrain and proetic hindbrain regions of the mouse embryo. American Journal of Anatomy 179: 143–154.

Noden, D. M. 1975. An analysis of the migratory behavior of avian cephalic neural crest cells. Developmental Biology 42: 106–130.

———. 1978a. The control of avian cephalic neural crest cytodifferentiation. I. Skeletal and connective tissues. Developmental Biology 67: 296–312.

———. 1978b. The control of avian cephalic neural crest cytodifferentiation. II. Neural tissues. Developmental Biology 67: 313–329.

———. 1978c. Interactions directing the migration and cytodifferentiation of avian neural crest cells. In The Specificity of Embryonical Interactions, D. Garrod, ed. London: Chapman Hall, pp. 4–49.

———. 1980. The migration and cytodifferentiation of cranial neural crest cells. In Current Research Trends in Prenatal Craniofacial Development, R. M. Pratt and R. L. Christiansen, eds. Amsterdam: Elsevier/North Holland, pp. 3–25.

———. 1982a. Patterns and organization of craniofacial skeletogenic and myogenic mesenchyme: A perspective. In Factors and Mechanisms Influencing Bone Growth, A. D. Dixon and B. G. Sarnat, eds. New York: Alan R. Liss, pp. 167–203.

———. 1982b. Periocular mesenchyme: Neural crest and mesodermal interactions. In *Ocular Anatomy, Embryology, and Teratology*, F. A. Jakobiec, ed. Philadelphia: Harper and Row, pp. 97–120.

———. 1983a. The embryonic origins of avian cephalic and cervical muscles and associated connective tissues. American Journal of Anatomy 168: 257–276.

———. 1983b. The role of the neural crest in patterning of avian cranial skeletal, connective, and muscle tissues. Developmental Biology 96: 144–165.

———. 1984. Craniofacial development: New views on old problems. Anatomical Record 208: 1–13.

———. 1986. Origins and patterns of craniofacial mesenchymal tissues. Journal of Craniofacial Genetics and Developmental Biology 2 (suppl.): 15–32.

———. 1987. Interactions between cephalic neural crest and mesodermal populations. In *Developmental and Evolutionary Aspects of the Neural Crest*, P. F. A. Maderson, ed. New York: John Wiley and Sons, pp. 89–119.

———. 1988. Interactions and fates of avian craniofacial mesenchyme. Development 103 (suppl.): 121–140.

Northcutt, R. G., and C. Gans. 1983. The genesis of neural crest and epidermal placodes: A reinterpretation of vertebrate origins. Quarterly Review of Biology 58: 1–28.

Oppenheimer, J. M. 1940. The non-specificity of the germ layers. Quarterly Review of Biology 15: 1–27.

Perris, R., Y. von Boxberg, and J. Löfberg. 1988. Local embryonic matrices determine region-specific phenotypes in neural crest cells. Science 241: 86–89.

Perris, R., and M. Bronner-Fraser. 1989. Recent advances in defining the role of the extracellular matrix in neural crest development. Comments on Developmental Neurobiology 1: 61–83.

Perris, R., and S. Johansson. 1990. Inhibition of neural crest cell migration by aggregating chondroitin sulfate proteoglycans is mediated by their hyaluronate-binding region. Developmental Biology 137: 1–12.

Platt, J. B. 1893. Ectodermic origin of the carilages of the head. Anatomischer Anzeiger 8: 506–509.

———. 1897. The development of the cartilaginous skull and of the branchial and hypoglossal musculature in Necturus. Morphologisches Jahrbuch 25: 377–464.

Raven, C. P. 1931. Zur Entwicklung der Ganglienleiste. 1. Die Kinematik der Ganglienleisten Entwicklung bei den Urodelen. Wilhelm Roux' Archive für Entwicklungsmechanik der Organismen 125: 210–293.

———. 1936. Zur Entwicklung der Ganglienleiste. V. Über die Differenzierung des Rumpfganglienleistenmaterials. Wilhelm Roux' Archiv für Entwicklungsmechanik der Organismen 134: 122–145.

Robert, B., D. Sassoon, B. Jacq, W. Gehring, and M. Buckingham. 1989. Hox-7: A mouse homeobox gene with a novel pattern of expression during embryogenesis. EMBO Journal 8: 91–100.

Romer, A. S. 1972. The vertebrate animal as a dual animal—somatic and visceral. In *Evolutionary Biology*, vol. 6, T. Dobzhansky, M. K. Hecht, and W. C. Steere, eds. New York: Appleton-Century-Crofts, pp. 121–156.

Ruiz i Altaba, A., and M. Melton. 1989. Involvement of the *Xenopus* homeobox gene Xhox3 in pattern formation along the anterior-posterior axis. Cell 57: 317–326.

Russell, E. S. 1916. *Form and Function: A Contribution to the History of Animal Morphology.* London: John Murray. Reprinted. Chicago: University of Chicago Press, 1982.

Sadaghiani, B., and C. H. Theibaud. 1987. Neural crest development in the *Xenopus* laevis embryo, studied by interspecific transplantation and scanning electron microscopy. Developmental Biology 124: 91–110.

Sadaghiani, B., and J. R. Vielkind. 1990. Distribution and migration pathways of HNK-1-immunoreactive neural crest cells in teleost fish embryos. Development 110: 197–209.

Sagemehl, M. 1882. *Untersuchingen über die Entwicklung der Spinal-nerven.* Dorpat.

Smith, M. M., and B. K. Hall. 1990. Development and evolutionary origins of vertebrate skeletogenic and odontogenic tissues. Biological Reviews 65: 277–374.

Smits-van Prooije, A. E., C. Vermeijs-Keers, R. E. Poelmann, M. M. T. Mentink, and J. A. Dubbeldam. 1985. The neural crest in presomite to 40 somite murine embryos. Acta morphologica neerlando-scandinavica 23: 99–114.

Stone, L. S. 1922a. Experiments on the development of the cranial ganglia and the lateral line sense organs in *Amblystoma punctatum.* Journal of Experimental Zoology 35: 421–496.

———. 1922b. Some notes on the migration of neural crest in *Rana palustris.* Anatomical Record 23: 39–40.

———. 1926. Further experiments on the extirpation and transplantation of mesectoderm in *Amblystoma punctatum.* Journal of Experimental Zoology 44: 95–131.

———. 1927. Further experiments on the transplantation of neural crest (mesectoderm) in amphibians. Proceedings of the Society for Experimental Biology and Medicine 24: 945–948.

———. 1929. Experiments showing the role of migrating neural crest (mesectoderm) in the formation of head skeleton and loose connective tissue in *Rana palustris.* Wilhelm Roux' Archiv für Entwicklungsmechanik der Organismen 118: 40–77.

———. 1932. Transplantation of the hyobranchial mesentoderm including the right lateral anlage of the second basibranchium in *Ambystoma punctatum.* Journal of Experimental Zoology 62: 109–123.

Tan, S. S., and G. Morriss-Kay. 1985. The development and distribution of the cranial neural crest in the rat embryo. Cell and Tissue Research 240: 403–416.

———. 1986. An analysis of cranial neural crest cell migration and early fates in postimplantation rat chimaeras. Journal of Embryology and Experimental Morphology 98: 21–58.

Toole, B. P., and R. Trelstad. 1971. Hyaluronate production and removal during corneal development in the chick. Developmental Biology 26: 28–35.

Tosney, K. W. 1982. The segregation and early migration of cranial neural crest cells in the avian embryo. Developmental Biology 89: 13–24.

Tucker, R. P., and C. A. Erickson. 1984. Morphology and behavior of quail neural crest cells in artificial three-dimensional extracellular matricies. Developmental Biology 104: 390–405.

Tyler, M. S., and B. K. Hall. 1977. Epithelial influences on skeletogenesis in the mandible of the embryonic chick. Anatomical Record 188: 229–240.

Vaage, S. 1969. The segmentation of the primitive neural tube in chick embryos. Advances in Anatomy, Embryology, and Cell Biology 41: 7–87.

Von Woellwarth, C. 1961. Die rolle des neuralleistenmaterials und der Temperatur bei der Determination der Augenlinse. Embryologia 6: 219–242.

Wilkinson, D. G., S. Bhatt, P. Chavrier, R. Bravo, and P. Charnay. 1989. Segment-specific expression of a zinc-finger gene in the developing nervous system of the mouse. Nature 337: 461–464.

Wilkinson, D. G., S. Bhatt, M. Cook, E. Bonicelli, and R. Krumlauf. 1989. Segmental expression of Hox-2 homeobox-containing genes in the developing mouse hindbrain. Nature 341: 405–409.

Zwilling, E. 1961. Limb morphogenesis. Advances in Morphogenesis 1: 301–338.

4

Differentiation and Morphogenesis of Cranial Skeletal Tissues

PETER THOROGOOD

Any particular developmental pathway probably represents an evolutionary compromise between maximizing the ease of ordering the spatial distribution of the·determinants of commitment and minimizing the need for migration of differentially committed embryonic cells.

—GUNTHER STENT (1985)

INTRODUCTION

TO A BIOLOGIST, as to the layman, the shape of even an idealized vertebrate skull is complex indeed. In order to describe it the morphologist resorts to analogy with architectural and geographical terminology and talks of arches, bridges, vaults, and ridges. But a precise terminology of form eludes us because a skull is not homeomorphic with any other form in the living world apart from the skulls of other vertebrate species (Thompson 1942); that homeomorphism reflects phylogenetic relationship and, presumably, a commonality of developmental mechanism. In spite of its topological complexity we might ask, perhaps with justification, if the development of the vertebrate skull is not basically a trivial problem. After all we must remember that this complex form arises from the growth and fusion of a number of separate and independent centers of ossification and chondrification, whose spatial distribution is much simpler. Is it not simply a problem of two familiar tissues, cartilage and bone, differentiating in a rather more complex pattern than we observe elsewhere in the vertebrate body? Is there any reason to believe that the factors controlling skeletal differentiation and morphogenesis in the head are necessarily any different from those operating elsewhere in, for example, the formation of a vertebral column, limb, or girdle? If not, then clearly there can be no justification for adding to the great bulk of literature on these tissue and cell types. But in fact there are unique challenges posed by the development of the skull, and problems exist at a multiplicity of conceptual levels (although whether or not the subcellular and molecular control mechanisms turn out to be intrinsically different from those operating elsewhere

112

in the body, or just organized in a more complex spatiotemporal way, remains to be seen).

At the level of cell differentiation we find that there are not simply endochondral bone and primary hyaline cartilage of the classic textbook phenotypes, but other types of skeletal tissues found almost exclusively in the head, principally membrane bone and secondary cartilage (Hall 1987a and see chapter by Beresford, vol. 2). Moreover, analysis of development is complicated by the fact that skeletogenic cells of all phenotypes in the developing head differentiate in mesenchyme coming from at least two distinct, broad-based lineages, namely mesoderm-derived and neural crest–derived (see chapter by Langille and Hall, this volume). At a higher organizational level, that of morphogenesis, we find that in addition to the aforementioned problem of morphological complexity and the inherent problems posed when trying to understand phenotypic change during evolution, metamorphosis, and dysmorphogenesis of the skull, there is the phenomenon of massive relocation of cells during cephalic development caused by active cell migration and passive displacement. This means that critically important events in development of lineally related cells can, and do, occur at spatially disparate points, rendering an analysis of determinative events, in relation to phenotypic expression of that determined state, difficult to achieve. Likewise, cells of different lineage may be brought into close proximity by such relocations and form composite tissues and organs, creating similar problems for analysis. Finally, we are left with the question of familial, sexual, and racial traits in skull form which demonstrate a strong genetic component in their specification. What are the genes which control this topological complexity and determine its subtle, heritable variations? What type of molecules do they code for and how are the spatiotemporal patterns of expression by these genes controlled during craniofacial development? It is in the context of these problems that this critical review of current thinking is presented.

SKELETAL DIFFERENTIATION IN THE HEAD

Origin of Cells, Lineage, and Potency

A variety of ablation and grafting experiments, in the fashion of traditional experimental embryology, have demonstrated that skeletal elements in the head are composed of mesenchyme which can be derived either entirely from neural crest (the so-called ectomesenchyme) or entirely from primary mesoderm (arising from the mesoblast at gastrulation) or which can, in a small number of cases, comprise cells derived from both of these sources. In the very limited number of "model" species which have been analyzed in sufficient detail, the broad distribution of the mesenchyme from the two lineages is surprisingly regular and consistent, to the extent that, by the use of cell marking techniques or the production of experimental chimeras, it has been possible to plot the interface between them (see fig. 4.1). In birds for example, the interface runs from the prosencephalic/mensencephalic border anteriorly, behind the adenohypophysis and back to the dorsal margin of the pharyngeal pouches, ending caudally at, but not beyond, the laryngotracheal diverticulum (see fig. 3 in Noden 1986). The greater part of the mesenchyme ventral to this interface is crest-derived, and dorsal to it, mesoderm-derived. Thus, analysis of heterospecific quail/chick chimeras provides direct evidence that the facial and visceral arch skeleton is crest-derived, that the membrane bones forming the vault of the cranium are largely mesoderm-derived, and that at the interface are found some mixed composition elements such as the rostral ossification center of the frontal bone and the otic capsule (Le Lièvre 1978; Noden 1978). Indirect evidence, mostly from neural crest ablation experiments, largely supports this interpretation for other vertebrate taxa (reviewed by Hörstadius 1950; Hall and Hörstadius 1988). As far as we can tell, again from a limited number of vertebrate species, there is a remarkable degree of constancy in derivation. This applies not only to major features such as the pan-vertebrate derivation of Meckel's cartilage from the neural crest but also in finer detail; for example, the second basibranchial or its homologue is always mesoderm-derived in amphibians and birds (Hörstadius and Sellman 1946; Chibon 1966; Le Lièvre 1978); reptiles and mammals await detailed analysis.

The mixed-composition elements (whose character can usually be detected only in experimental chimeras, created usually by grafting cephalic neural crest) pose an interesting problem in that skeletal tissues homogeneously composed of cells from one or other lineage (i.e., crest- or mesoderm-derived) will, in vitro, fuse only with skeletal tissues of like derivation and not with tissue derived from the other lineage (Chiakulas 1957; Fyfe and Hall 1979). However, mixed-composition elements developing in vivo reflect fusion of initially separate centers of skeletogenic differentiation, or the "entrapment" of one such center by another (Noden 1986). The failure of differentiated skeletal tissues of different lineage derivation to fuse with each other in vitro awaits explanation at the molecular level but suggests an underlying chemical difference (the phenomenon may also be not without relevance to maxillofacial surgeons). In fact crest-derived skeletal tissues are confined to the head, the rest of the axial skeleton and the entire appendicular skeleton being, as far as is known, entirely mesoderm-derived. (This comment applies to the endoskeleton; a neural crest derivation for the dermal skeleton of fishes, e.g., for the fin rays, is widely assumed but remains to be demonstrated conclusively; Smith and Hall 1990; Thorogood 1991.) This restriction of skeletogenic potential to the cephalic crest was the first recognized, and remains the best established, evidence for popu-

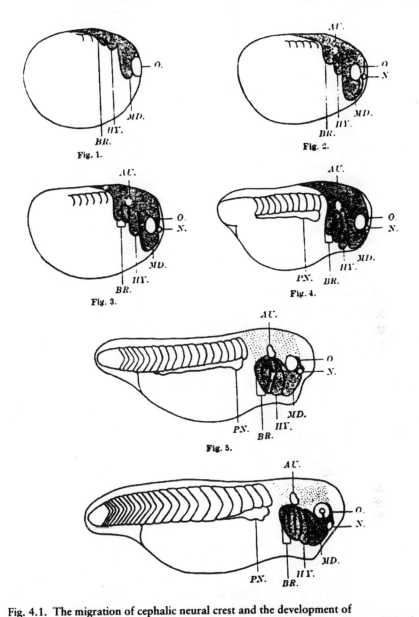

Fig. 1.

Fig. 2.

Fig. 3.

Fig. 4.

Fig. 5.

Fig. 4.1. The migration of cephalic neural crest and the development of ectomesenchyme in the head of *Rana palustris*. The bulk of the neural crest—derived cells migrate ventro-laterally as mandibular (MD), hyoid (HY), and branchial (BR) tongues of tissue; the branchial extension subsequently subdivides into four and forms the ectomesenchymal component of the visceral arches. Although produced some 60 years ago, the diagram illustrates clearly how ectomesenchyme does not become intermingled with head mesoderm but migrates to occupy a discrete region ventro-laterally on the head. There it forms most, if not all, of the facial and visceral arch skeleton. Au, Auditory placode; N, nasal placode; O, optic vesicle; PN, pronephros. (With permission, from Stone 1929)

lation heterogeneity within the neural crest. Trunk crest is unable to produce skeletogenic progeny; even when grafted to the head, it will produce only fibrous connective tissue (Nakamura and Ayer-Le Lièvre 1982). (In contrast, odontogenic potential may be differently distributed within the crest; see discussion in Lumsden 1987). Given this, one might expect some unique properties of the head skeleton arising from the cephalic crest contribution. However, skeletal tissues found in the head appear to be no different in composition from cartilage and bone found elsewhere in the body. Quantitative differences may, and do, occur; for example, the preponderance of elastin fibers in the nasal and auricular cartilages; and antigenic differences have been reported between cartilages from different sites (Brigham et al. 1977). But expression of the differentiated state seems essentially identical to skeletal tissues elsewhere (e.g., Luder et al. 1988) and cells of either lineage seem to respond identically to the same differentiation signals (Le Lièvre 1978; Thorogood 1988). What differences do exist reflect largely quantitative variations in the composition of the matrix (usually in relation to functional demand), cellularity, vascularity, turnover of matrix components, and responsiveness to mechanical factors (Hall 1987a; Marks and Popoff 1988; and the chapter by Beresford, vol. 2).

The biggest single obstacle to a clearer understanding of developmental events in this system remains our ignorance of the commitment state, potency, and precise lineage of the cells destined to give rise to the head skeleton. That is to say, we simply do not know enough about the developmental history of the cells concerned. For instance, is a committed skeletogenic progenitor population established in the cephalic crest before migration commences? Intrinsic differences between cephalic and trunk crest clearly do exist (see above). In vitro clonal analysis provides circumstantial evidence not only that the avian cephalic crest is highly heterogeneous in terms of proliferative ability and differentiative potential, but that such heterogeneity is established very early in crest development (Baroffio et al. 1988). Further clonal analysis of cultured cells revealed that only 3.3% of the clones were derived from a precursor cell common to both ectomesenchyme and neurogenic differentiation pathways (Baroffio et al. 1991). However, lineage analysis of individual, labeled trunk crest cells and their progeny in vivo (Bronner-Fraser and Fraser 1988; Serbedzija et al. 1989) demonstrates unequivocally that differentiative fate is established subsequent to, or during, but not prior to, migration. The corollary of this is that the premigratory crest, in the trunk at least, comprises a homogeneous population of multipotential cells. It has been suggested elsewhere (Heath et al. 1992) that the timing of each approach is critical in that the in vitro clonal analysis used cells already in the early stages of migration, whereas the in vivo lineage analysis was based upon the injection of a marker into individual cells which were still within the dorsal roof of the neural tube and clearly still to migrate. In fact, a third strategy deploying monoclonal antibodies against avian cephalic neural crest cells and adopting differential epitope expression as a criterion for detecting population heterogeneity, also demonstrates that subpopulations arise progressively during crest ontogeny rather than prior to migration (Heath et al. 1992). We may conclude from these various approaches that although there is evidence for a qualitative difference between head and trunk crest, in that ectomesenchyme arises only from the former and in that such ectomesenchyme may be established early, there is to date no unequivocal evidence for a committed skeletogenic subpopulation existing within the crest prior to migration.

There is strong evidence, however, that epitheliomesenchymal tissue interactions, operating locally, have some fundamental, but as yet undefined, role in causing head mesenchyme of either lineage to differentiate into cartilage and bone. For example, isolated premigratory cephalic neural crest, from amphibian or avian embryos, lacks the ability to form primary cartilage or membrane bone when isolated in vitro; and yet in association with certain epithelia, in vitro or in vivo, cephalic crest will differentiate chondrogenically (Wilde 1955; Drews et al. 1972; Epperlein and Lehmann 1975; Tyler and Hall 1977; Bee and Thorogood 1980; Graveson and Armstrong 1987; and see fig. 4.2) and, in rare cases, osteo-

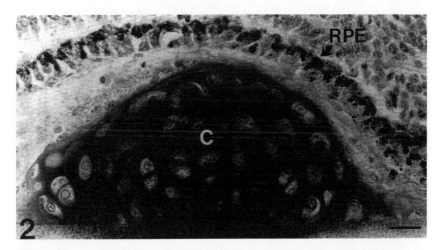

Fig. 4.2. Tissue combination culture of chick premigratory mesencephalic neural crest with retinal pigmented epithelium (RPE) generates the formation of cartilage (C) within the crest-derived mesenchyme. Whereas isolated crest cultured alone forms only an undifferentiated mesenchyme, the result illustrated demonstrates the consequence of interaction with an appropriate epithelium. Scale bar equals 20 μm. (From Bee and Thorogood 1980)

genically (Bee and Thorogood 1980). This suggests that factors extrinsic to the cells are causally involved, but lack of understanding over the commitment state of the responding cells obstructs further interpretation. Do such factors create a permissive environment within which the cells can express their commitment state or provide an instructive signal leading to a change in commitment and, concomitantly, a restriction in potency? Elsewhere it has been proposed that until a clearer understanding prevails, such interactions are best described in more neutral terms as "chondrogenesis-promoting" or "osteogenesis-promoting" (Thorogood et al. 1986; Thorogood 1987) rather than osteogenic or chondrogenic inductions. In this account, for reasons of space and developmental chronology, attention will be focused primarily on membrane bone and primary cartilage, since these are the skeletal tissues in which skull form is first laid down. (Endochondral bone and secondary cartilage differentiate somewhat later.)

Osteogenesis (Membrane Bone)

Various traditional experimental strategies have provided some understanding of the underlying mechanisms, but not a full appreciation of molecular events. (Surprisingly, the greater proportion of the mechanistic analyses have utilized avian systems and, in this respect, amphibian cephalic skeletogensis, where the phenomenology is equally well documented, has been largely neglected). Removal of ectoderm from the presumptive cranial aspect of the avian head, or ablation of underlying neuroepithelium, results in an absence of the mesodermally derived parietal, frontal, and supraoccipital, and the crest-derived squamosal, membrane bones (Schowing 1968), demonstrating the osteogenesis-promoting role of the prosencephalon, mesencephalon, and rhombencephalon. More recent studies have revealed that, additionally, overlying ectoderm is necessary for a full expression of osteogenesis in this system (Tyler 1983). Epitheliomesenchymal interactions underlying avian membrane bone formation have been thoroughly investigated in an extensive program of tissue dissociation/recombination experiments carried out in vitro by Hall and colleagues, working primarily on the differentiation of crest-derived avian mandibular mesenchyme (reviewed by Hall 1982b, 1984). Following their original demonstration that a mandibular epithelial presence is vital over a critical period if mandibular mesenchyme is to differentiate osteogenically at a later stage (Tyler and Hall 1977), three important conclusions emerged: (1) that osteogenesis-promoting interactions are matrix-mediated, (2) that the epithelium has to be mitotically active, and (3) that the interaction is apparently effected by a collagenous component of the mandibular ectodermal basal lamina (Hall et al. 1983).

The directionality of such interactions is demonstrated by the fact that treatment of the epithelial partner with agents blocking collagen synthesis impairs its ability to elicit an osteogenic response from the mesenchymal partner in any subsequent tissue recombination experiments; treated mesenchyme will recover and differentiate osteogenically when subsequently combined with untreated epithelium (Bradamante and Hall 1980). However, mandibular mesenchyme is capable of mounting an osteogenic response to epithelial from sites other than in the head, for example, limb bud and dorsal trunk ectoderms (Hall 1978), and therefore this interaction is not specific in the strictly instructive sense (Wessells 1979). Furthermore, although the presence of an epithelium is necessary for osteogenesis to ensue, the form or morphology of the developing bony element appears to be a property of the mesenchymal partner in the recombination and is not determined by the epithelium (Hall 1981). Thus, both mandibular and scleral papilla mesenchyme will differentiate osteogenically in tissue recombination experiments and display their origin-specific morphogenesis into bony rods and bony plates/ossicles respectively, even when combined heterotypically with the reciprocal epithelium (i.e., mandibular mesenchyme with scleral papilla epithelium; scleral papilla mesenchyme with mandibular epithelium).

The mechanism underlying osteogenesis-promoting tissue interactions remains to be elucidated but recent evidence indicates that epithelia, or epithelially derived basal laminae, might simply have a mitogenic effect on adjacent mesenchyme. Interestingly, sodium fluoride, known to stimulate mitosis and matrix production in cultured bone cells (Farley et al. 1983), is capable of substituting for epithelium in promoting in vitro osteogenesis of mandibular mesenchyme (Hall 1987c). However, the possibility that exogenous sodium fluoride might interact with a serum component in the culture medium to bring about this effect makes a precise interpretation of events at the molecular level difficult. Recent data reveal that not all osteogenesis-promoting interactions are necessarily matrix-mediated. The interaction promoting formation of the scleral ossicles, unlike its mandibular counterpart, is apparently diffusion-mediated, operating in vitro over distances of up to $150-300$ μm (Pinto and Hall 1991). How this observation integrates with earlier work is not clear, but it can now be concluded that osteogenesis-promoting interactions in the embryonic head are not uniform with regard to mechanism.

Chondrogenesis (Primary Cartilage)

Parallel investigations have been carried out on the developmentally earlier, chondrogenesis-promoting tissue interactions underlying the formation of the avian cartilaginous neurocranium (Bee and Thorogood 1980). Use of premigratory neural crest in transfilter culture with appropriate epithelia led to the elimination of any possibility of a diffusion-mediated mechanism being responsible (Smith and Thorogood 1983). Ultrastructural assessment of the in vivo epitheliomesenchymal interface revealed intact basal

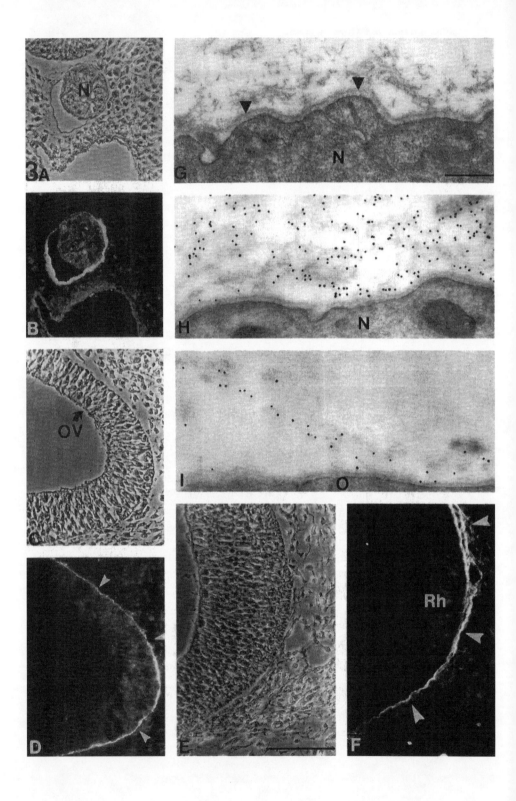

laminae and an absence of plasmalemmal contact between the cells of the epithelium and the crest-derived mesenchyme. Thus, a cell contact-mediated mechanism could also be discounted, leaving the possibility that these interactions might be matrix-mediated (Thorogood and Smith 1984). Subsequent immunocytochemical analysis of extracellular matrix at the interface between the two cell populations in one such chondrogenesis-promoting interaction, between presumptive pigmented retina and mesencephalic crest-derived periodular mesenchyme, revealed a compositional change correlated with the known duration of the interaction. (It should be noted that these in vivo interactions, like those promoting osteogenesis, are completed several days before the responding mesenchyme expresses its differentiated phenotype.) Type II collagen, the predominant collagen species of cartilage matrix and therefore generally regarded as a specific marker for chondrogenic differentiation, is transiently expressed at the interface, i.e., at the basal aspect of the epithelial tissue, against which the migrating crest cells come to lie. Further investigation revealed that type II collagen is expressed elsewhere in the head, in addition to previously reported ocular locations within the corneal stroma and vitreous (see fig. 4.3a, b, e, and f). Principally these locations are round the basolateral aspects of the

---

Fig. 4.3. Immunolocalization of type II collagen, at quail tissue interfaces where chondrogenesis-promoting interactions occur. Phase contract (A, C, and E) and immunofluorescent (B, D, and F) micrographs prepared by using affinity-purified, polyclonal rabbit antichick type II collagen, followed incubation with FITC-conjugated goat antirabbit. A, B. T.S. of cervical notochord (N) at stage 24; staining present in the perinotochordal sheath. C, D. T.S. of otic vesicle (OV) at stage 18; staining present basally on otic epithelium (arrowheads). E, F. T.S. of rhombencephalic wall at stage 16; staining present basally on the neuroepithelium (arrowheads).

G, H, and I are all transmission electron micrographs illustating pre-embedding immunogold staining. Tissue was lightly fixed in 4% paraformaldehyde/0.25% glutataraldehyde, incubated initially in affinity-purified, rabbit polyclonal antichick type II collagen, and subsequently in *Staphylococcal* protein A conjugated with 15 nm gold particles, before a standard 2.5% glutataraldehyde fixation, postosmication and resin embedding. G. lead citrate/uranyl acetate stained control section section showing the basal (i.e., outer) aspect of stage-16 quail notochord cell (N), basal lamina (arrowheads), and fibrillar components of the reticulate lamina upper half of the field of view. H. unstained, immunogold preparation of similar field, illustrating the abundance of gold particles located on electron-dense material with comparison with (G) reveals to be extracellular matrix fibrils. I. unstained, immunogold preparation of the basal aspect of the stage-16 quail otic vesicle epithelium, illustrating a similar, but sparser, distribution of gold particles in the reticulate lamina. In both (H) and (I) immunolocalization of type II collagen shows it to be confined to the reticulate lamina and not deep within surrounding mesenchyme.

Scale bar: for light micrographs (E) 30 μm; for transmission electron micrographs (G) 100 nm.

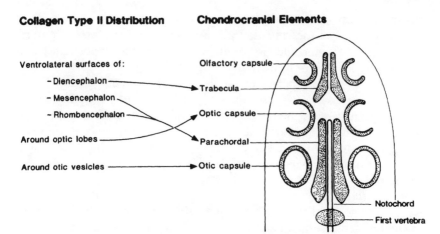

Collagen Type II Distribution   **Chondrocranial Elements**

Ventrolateral surfaces of: Olfactory capsule

  – Diencephalon   Trabecula

  – Mesencephalon

  – Rhombencephalon   Optic capsule

Around optic lobes   Parachordal

Around otic vesicles   Otic capsule

Notochord

First vertebra

Fig. 4.4. Diagram correlating the transient distribution of type II collagen to the component parts of the avian cartilaginous neurocranium which subsequently form as a result of tissue interactions at the sites listed on the left-hand side. Neurocranial organization has been idealized to a general vertebrate pattern. (From Thorogood et al. 1986)

diencephalon, mesencephalon, and rhombencephalon, around optic and otic vesicles (Thorogood et al. 1986; Fitch et al. 1989) and at rather later stages, around the nasal pits and olfactory conchi (Croucher and Tickle 1989). Distribution of this collagen type maps precisely with the sites of those interactions known to generate the constituent parts of the cartilaginous neurocranium (see fig. 4.4). Not only is the spatial pattern coincident, but so too is the timing of transient type II expression, which correlates with the duration of the interactions concerned (Thorogood et al. 1986). Thus, there is a strong spatial and temporal correlation between the transient expression of type II collagen and the sites and duration of matrix-mediated interactions which generate the component parts of the cartilaginous neurocranium.

Clearly a parallel exists between these interactions promoting cartilage formation in the head and those tissue interactions generating the formation of the cartilaginous primordia of the vertebral bodies. Sclerotomal cells, derived from the medial aspect of the (mesodermal) somite, migrate toward the midline, undergo a matrix-mediated interaction with the notochord, and differentiate chondrogenically in a regular segmental pattern. The vertebrate notochord is epithelial in character, albeit rather atypical in form, and in addition to typical basal lamina components, the perinotochordal or matrix or sheath contains two components characteristic of cartilage—type II collagen (see fig. 4.3c, d) and cartilage-specific proteoglycan, synthesized briefly by the notochord itself. In vitro exposure of sclerotome cells to perinotochordal sheath, or to either of these two components, elicits an enhanced sclerotomal synthesis of the same two molecules, the collagen and the proteoglycan (Kosher and Church 1975; Lash and Vasan 1978), assembled into a stable matrix as the chondrocytic phenotype becomes established (Vasan 1987). How far the parallel between the two systems can be taken is not known: in fact it is not yet clear if the two sets of data reflect a common underlying mechanism. In experiments to date, purified type II collagen apparently does not substitute for the type II–rich epithelial basal lamina in eliciting a chondrogenic response from premigratory neural crest cells in culture (Thorogood, work in progress). However, it is naive to assume that a single type of matrix molecule will necessarily be responsible, and it is more likely that several matrix components, assembled naturally into a native, three-dimensional matrix, will act together in such interactions (Bissell 1987; and see below). In this respect it should be noted that even in the Kosher and Church (1975) experiments mentioned above, the responding mesenchyme was a committed sclerotome which displayed an enhanced differentiative response, and therefore the purified matrix components, upon which the cells were cultured, were not initiating a chondrogenic response from a "naive" mesenchyme. Therefore, exposure to appropriate matrix molecules may not of itself be sufficient to promote chondrogenesis in cells so fated, and other factors, such as a critical mass threshold being attained by the responding mesenchyme, are likely to be prerequisities for chondrogenic differentiation of both mesodermal and crest cells (see useful discussions in Kratochwil 1983; Hall 1987b, 1991).

A fuller understanding of the causal sequence of events at the cellular level is dependent upon identifying the origin of the transient type II collagen detected at epitheliomesenchymal interfaces in the head. Is it epithelial or mesenchymal in origin, and if from the latter tissue, why is it only briefly expressed when the tissue is destined to differentiate into cartilage at a later stage? Current evidence indicates that the type II collagen is largely, if not entirely, derived from (neuro) epithelium. Firstly, circumstantial evidence emerges from the ultrastructural location of the type II collagen at the relevant tissue interfaces, as defined using TEM immunogold techniques. This reveals that, during the interactions, transiently expressed type II is located in the reticulate lamina, that is, it is closely associated with the basal lamina of the epithelium and is not around adjacent mesenchyme cells (Thorogood, Smith-Thomas, and Courtney, in preparation). If synthesized by the mesenchyme, a general distribution in the extracellular compartment of that tissue might be anticipated, but this is not seen, although a polarized secretion by these mesenchyme cells

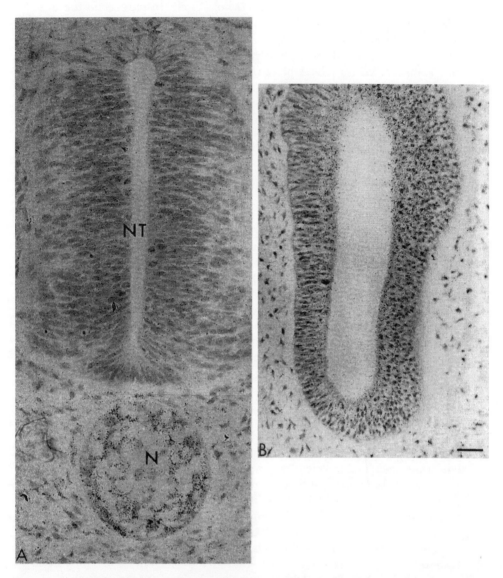

Fig. 4.5. Autoradiographs from in situ hybridization on chick tissue sections with a cDNA probe for chick type II collagen mRNA. A. Stage-14 neural tube with silver grains located over notochord (N) and, to a lesser extent, over the neuroepithelial wall of the neural tube (NT) and the most medial sclerotome. B. Stage-20 otic vesicle and periotic mesenchyme; silver grains are confined to the epithelial wall of the otic vesicle and very few can be detected within the mesenchyme. Both figures demonstrate clearly the presence of type II collagen mRNA in nonchondrogenic, epithelial tissues, at whose basal surface transient type II collagen can be detected immunocytochemically (micrographs kindly supplied by Masando Hayashi). Scale bar equals c.20 μm.

at the interface cannot be excluded. However, it is significant that the ultrastructural distribution of perinotochordal type II collagen, although more abundant at a comparable stage, is identical in relation to the basal lamina.

Secondly, unequivocal evidence comes from in situ hybridization experiments using a cDNA probe specific to chick type II collagen mRNA. Work in progress indicates that type II collagen message is detectable in cells of the notochord, otic vesicle, neuroepithelium, and neural tube before message is detectable in the responding mesenchyme (Hoffman and Thorogood, unpublished observations; Masando Hayashi, personal communication; and see fig. 4.5). Although type II is typically a stromal collagen and characteristically made by chondrocytes, there are in fact three precedents for epithelial synthesis: the notochord (see above), the corneal epithelium (Linsenmayer et al. 1977), and lastly, a true neuroepithelium—the neural retina (Smith et al. 1976). These synthesize the type II collagen found in the perinotochordal sheath, the primary corneal stroma, and the vitreous respectively. Recent molecular evidence demonstrates unequivocally that the type II collagen gene is indeed transcriptionally active in such epithelia (e.g., avian cornea: Hayashi et al. 1988; various tissue in mouse embryo: Cheah et al. 1991). Whereas the previously described immunocytochemical evidence defines only the patterns of the accumulated gene product, in situ hybridization techniques enable us to define just when and where the type II genes are transcriptionally active. It is clear from such approaches that epithelia can and do produce type II collagen, a type normally thought of as interstitial, at critical times during normal development. The possible roles of epithelially derived type II collage as a signaling molecule, or as a means of binding differentially a signaling molecule, at sites of chondrogenesis-promoting tissue interactions are discussed further below.

SKULL MORPHOGENESIS: GENETIC SPECIFICATION OR EPIGENETICS?

One of the principal questions currently under debate is at what developmental level specification of skull morphology occurs. In recent years discussion has become, to some extent, polarized between those who believe that form is specified in the initial stages of neurulation or at least prior to the migration of skeletogenic precursors from within the neural crest, and those who believe that form arises epigenetically as a result of cell/cell and tissue interactions subsequent to the onset of migration. This is not a trivial issue and consequently will be dealt with in some detail. I shall consider each interpretation, reviewing briefly its merits and disadvantages, and then discuss briefly whether or not these two interpretations are really mutually exclusive.

Specification of Skull Form Prior to Crest Migration

Over many years a number of workers have shown convincingly a very clear regionalization of skeletogenic precursors within the neural folds. That is to say, groups of crest cells giving rise to individual skeletal elements can be fate-mapped to discrete axial levels within the neural folds (e.g., agnathans: Langille and Hall 1988b; teleosts: Langille and Hall 1988a; amphibians: Hörstadius 1950; Chibon 1966; Aves: Le Lièvre 1978; Noden 1978). It is important to remember at this point that a fate map is not a map of cell commitment. In the late 1940s and early 1950s, a number of papers from a Swiss group described the craniofacial morphology of amphibian larvae which were experimentally produced, heterospecific chimeras (Andres 1949; Wagner 1949; 1955; reviewed by Baltzer 1952). Such chimeras were the result of neural crest grafts, or at least neural fold/plate grafts carried out between urodele and anuran early neurula stages. The most successful and best-reported combination of the experimental series was the *Bombina* cephalic neural fold grafted orthotopically into *Triturus* hosts. The two species have characteristically different head skeletons (see fig. 4 in Wagner 1949) and, in addition, *Triturus* possess true teeth. On allowing the neurula hosts to develop to larval stages and then examining the head skeleton, it is found that the branchial arches on the operated side are characteristic of the neural fold donor species (in this case, *Bombina*), whereas the unoperated "control" side is typical of the host pattern (see fig. 6 in Wagner 1949). Interestingly, chimeric teeth formed which were found to comprise *Triturus* ameloblasts and *Bombina* odontoblasts (Wagner 1955). This was a critically important result for students of tooth development. Anurans normally develop teeth only after metamorphosis and the teeth characteristically lack a true enamel. In these experiments the *Triturus* host environment has not only elicited *Bombina* odontoblasts to differentiate before metamorphosis but has also revealed that *Bombina* odontoblasts can "induce" ameloblast differentiation in the overlying ectoderm. (See Lumsden 1987 for a full discussion.)

These experiments were designed essentially to investigate the developmental background to homology (Baltzer 1952) and they constitute some of the first experiments carried out explicitly to explore the mechanism(s) controlling pattern in this system. The apparent autonomy of skeletal morphogenesis, by which the *Bombina* cells form species-specific skeletal elements in the *Triturus* host environment, was interpreted as reflecting an early specification of pattern before the graft was removed from the neural fold of the donor species. Little consideration was given to possible causal mechanisms and the interpretation of the experimental result is largely at the phenomenological level. The diagrammatic representations of the results (Wagner 1949) are striking, although it is unfortunate that there are no illustrations of the pattern following homospecific orthotopic grafts in order to eliminate surgical trauma and healing as a factor influencing skeletal pattern. Interpretation of what are assumed to be homologous skeletal elements is based entirely on shape and spatial relationship with other elements.

More recently this model of early specification has been extended to avian species as a result of a meticulous program of grafting experiments by Noden (1983; reviewed 1984, 1986, 1988; and see chapter by Langille and Hall, this volume). Although this model too is based on creation of heterospecific (quail/chick) chimeras, it is not a donor-specific pattern within the host head that reveals an apparently early specification of morphogenesis, but the fact that the grafts are heterotopic and that graft-derived cells differentiate in a donor site-specific pattern. Quail/chick chimerism is exploited simply to facilitate identification of graft-derived cells among host tissue (Le Douarin 1973).

Mesencephalic neural crest typically contributes to first arch skeletal elements, of the maxillary and mandibular facial processes; myelencephalic crest gives rise to skeletal tissue in the second and third branchial areas. This fate map is assumed to be identical for quail and chick species even though the former develops at a slightly faster rate. Whereas orthotopic grafting, used to establish such fate maps, leaves subsequent skeletal pattern unimpaired (Le Lièvre 1978; Noden 1978), certain heterospecific grafts produce striking and unpredicted results. Noden found that grafting of first arch crest to the axial level of second or third arch resulted in a graft-derived supernumary first arch skeleton developing in a second or third arch site; in addition, integumentary structures formed which cannot be considered first arch, such as a rudimentary upper beak and egg tooth, together with a secondary auditory meatus. Again, in the absence of any skeletal element-specific markers, identification of duplicated elements is based on shape and spatial relationships, but there is indeed a striking resemblance to a normal mandibular skeleton (see figs. 9 and 15, Noden 1983). Noden has concluded that "prior to the onset of migration neural crest populations have acquired a regional morphogenetic specification. This means that the patterns in which skeletal and connective tissues will form, and surface ectoderm be specified, result from programming that occurs before the crest population begins to disperse" (Noden 1983). Surprisingly, first arch rotated through 180° before grafting still gives a supernumerary skeleton with the normal orientation. Even more surprisingly, heterochronic grafts of the first arch, taken from donor embryos some 3–4 hours older and at a stage when a significant proportion of the crest cells have emigrated from the neural folds, still produced an entire supernumary skeleton comparable to that produced by a graft of the same developmental stage as the host. Clearly morphogenetic specification is not a programming of fate operating at the single-cell level. Nevertheless, these are striking and dramatic findings in need of an explanatory mechanism. Understandably, Noden has viewed the data as comparable to that of Andres and Wagner and thereby extends their conclusions to amniotes. However, it should be noted that prosencephalic (i.e., forebrain) neural crest and neural fold tissue from other axial levels all provide the same result when grafted, i.e., supernumerary first arch derivatives, and therefore the "programming" is not unique to any particular axial level. In fact, Noden has postulated that this is a kind of "default" fate—a basic branchial arch programming, expressed by crest from all cephalic axial levels under these experimental conditions (Noden 1983).

Although not explicitly stated in the earlier Swiss work or in the more recent work of Noden, it is implied that most, if not all, of the crest-derived branchial skeleton (i.e., viscerocranium) is determined in this way, by morphogenetic specification occurring before migration. Such an interpretation, if correct, has not only obvious developmental importance but also profound phylogenetic significance in terms of the evolutionary changes in the organization and function of the branchial arches (Gans and Northcutt 1983; Gans 1989).

An Assessment of Regional Morphogenetic Specification

If we seek support for the interpretation of the amphibian data made by Wagner and colleagues, then the conclusions to be drawn from other analyses are often equivocal in this respect. Harrison (1938) describes the creation of heterospecific chimeras made between *Ambystoma punctatum* and *A. mexicanum*, whose larvae characteristically differ in size. Unilateral grafts of neural fold, adjacent hindbrain, and overlying ectoderm are initially made from one species to the other and are left in situ for graft-derived crest cells to migrate into the host visceral arches, which are themselves then serially grafted into a second individual of the host species, so that finally only the ectomesenchyme of the visceral arches is derived from the original donor species. At the larval stage, the visceral arches on the operated side are always characteristic, in size, of the original donor species. Elegant though these experiments are (and the original intention was to demonstrate the crest derivation of the visceral arch skeleton), for our purposes they do not demonstrate premigratory specification of form but simply reflect species-specific differences in growth rates.

An alternative approach is to change the axial position of crest cells (as in Noden's heterotopic grafting experiments), thereby confronting crest cells with an axially inappropriate environment. In amphibians, this has been achieved by 180° rotation of neural plate or neural folds. Hörstadius and Sellman (1946) reported profound alterations in pattern following such rotation and concluded that there are intrinsic differences between "trabecular," "mandibular," and "visceral arch" crest. However, these are difficult experiments to interpret since rotation of the neural plate relocates the entire fore- and midbrain together with associated organ primordia (such as optic vesicles) which are all known to influence skeletal pattern. Also, the fact that in spite of a 180° rotation, mandibular structures still form rostral to (admittedly poorly developed) visceral arches should not be overlooked (see figs. 26b and f in Hörstadius 1950. More recent experiments, in which reciprocal heterotopic grafts of radioisotopically labeled "trabecular" and "posterior branchial arch" crest are made, result in normal skeletogenesis, with grafted cells contributing to structures which they do not normally form (Chibon 1966; see also fig. 4.6). Thus, for Amphibia the question of whether or not early morphogenetic specification of form occurs within the crest appears to remain unresolved. Given the importance of the phenomenon, the situation deserves reinvestigation.

In avian systems, as a result of Noden's careful experimentation, there are at least three items of experimental evidence clearly demonstrating that morphogenetic specification cannot be operating at the level of individual cells. Firstly, reversal of a neural crest graft through 180°, which reverses its anterio-posterior polarity prior to growth, does not change the polarity of the supernumerary first arch elements which subsequently form (Noden 1983). Secondly, grafting of neural crest from a range of axial levels gives rise to an identical set of supernumerary first arch elements (Noden 1983). Lastly, crest taken from slightly older donor embryos, at a stage when up to "between one half and two thirds of the crest cells had emigrated . . . and were not available for transplantation" (Noden 1983), gives an identical result to that obtained with an "intact" crest graft from a younger donor embryo. It is also perhaps significant that in these experiments graft-derived cells also contribute to a number of host skeletal elements all of which apparently have a relatively normal morphology and size (e.g., otic capsule). From these results Noden concludes that "morphogenetic specification does not mean that the premigratory neural crest is a mosaic population in which the fate of individual cells is determined . . . [but] refers instead to a mesenchymal population having the ability to develop in a patterned, well-organised manner. Such sub-populations, some of which may be skeletogenic, will form at discrete, defined locations and each will be programmed to aggregate and grow in an appropriate shape" (Noden 1983).

However, given that morphogenesis is a phenomenon displayed at the cell population level but driven by coordinated changes at the level of individual cells, it is still difficult to conceive a mechanism for such "pro-

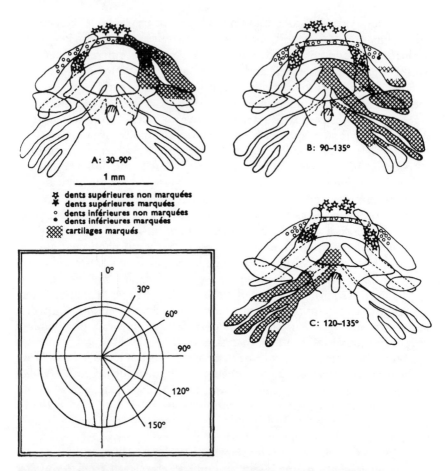

A: 30–90°

1 mm

✪ dents supérieures non marquées
✦ dents supérieures marquées
○ dents inférieures non marquées
● dents inférieures marquées
▨ cartilages marqués

B: 90–135°

C: 120–135°

0°
30°
60°
90°
120°
150°

Fig. 4.6. A clear demonstration of "negative" regulation is illustrated in these diagrams of the branchial arch skeleton (including teeth/*dents*) following orthotopic grafting of additional cephalic neural crest, in the urodele *Pleurodeles waltlii*. Grafts were taken from one of three sites in H-thymidine-labeled donor neurulae (see inset, lower left, for details of graft origin). The typical location and fate of graft-derived cells within the unlabeled hosts, as determined autoradiographically, is mapped for each of the three classes of graft using the symbols given in the key. Note that in spite of different graft origin, the form and pattern of the larval branchial arch skeleton is unequivocally identical among all three classes of graft, and indistinguishable from unoperated controls (not shown). Regulation for "excess" crest has occurred and there is no evidence of supernumary skeletal elements, which might be expected if morphogenetic fate was specified before crest migration. (With permission, from Chibon 1970)

gramming," especially given that any precise spatial arrangement of cells within the neural plate and/or neural fold is highly unlikely to be maintained during the de-epithelialization of the neural crest, cell emigration from the folds, and subsequent translocation through the head tissues. Furthermore, it is perhaps difficult to define the exact role of the undoubtedly important tissue interactions (see above) in this scenario. They might, conceivably, serve a simple permissive role in the expression of regional morphogenetic specification.

Perhaps more fundamental problems arise when we try to reconcile such a model with the widely reported regulative ability of the neural crest. Although in some experimental designs, "positive" regulation (i.e., compensation for ablation of tissue) seems to be minimal (e.g., Langille and Hall's recent work on neural crest ablation in lampreys and teleosts, 1988a, b), Amphibia display both positive regulation (e.g., Stone 1929; Hörstadius 1950) and "negative" regulation (i.e., compensation for excess tissue; e.g., Chibon 1970; and see fig. 4.6). Avian systems can either fail to show positive regulation (Johnston 1964; Hammond and Yntema 1964) or show it very convincingly (McKee and Ferguson 1984). A lack of uniformity in the results from a number of systems is incidentally of great interest and McKee and Ferguson suggest that it is the extent of crest ablation that determines whether or not positive regulation will occur. Thus, minor ablations which do not remove supporting tissues permit regulation from crest immediately rostral or caudal migrating to fill the defect within hours, whereas more extensive deletions of associated tissues eliminate components, such as extracellular matrix, which might facilitate infilling migration. A review of the literature reveals that indeed in many of those instances where positive regulation fails to occur, the ablation has included entire neural folds (e.g., Hammond & Yntema 1964), neural plate (e.g., Hörstadius 1950), or the neural tube at that axial level (e.g., Le Lièvre 1974). (This, in essence, is why ablation is an unsatisfactory strategy for fate-mapping the neural crest; a fate map derived from ablation experiments can, if undetected positive regulation occurs, only underestimate the destined fates of the ablated tissue. Ablation should be relied upon only when other approaches, such as heterotopic grafting or cell marking with retroviral labeling, are technically not possible.) Thus, the extent of regulation varies with both different taxa and different operative strategies but can be quite extreme. Hörstadius (1950) describes cases where the unilaterial ablation of the entire amphibian branchial arch crest did not prevent the formation of a complete viscerocranium, regulation having occurred as a result of crest cells migrating across the midline from the unoperated side. But whatever the extent of regulation, the fact remains that neither positive nor negative regulation should occur at all if morphogenetic specification of pattern has taken place within the population of cells comprising the undisturbed neural folds before de-epithelialization and crest migration.

We are left with several unanswered questions. For example, do other cephalic crest-derived tissues display an early morphogenetic specification of fate equivalent to that proposed for the crest-derived skeleton? Is the concept applicable to mesodermally derived skeletal tissues in the head, and, if so, when does the programming of mesodermal morphogenetic fate take place? On balance, the concept of regional morphogenetic specification taking place before crest migration raises several important issues. While none of the preceding discussion precludes the possibility that a skeletogenic lineage might be established prior to migration, no mechanism of morphogenetic programming that persists throughout crest cell migration and yet is compatible with the coordinated regulative events following experimental perturbation, has emerged to date. Much of the experimental data seems equally interpretable as evidence supporting an epigenetic control of skeletal pattern in the head, by cell and tissue interactions operating locally during and after crest migration.

Epigenetic Determination of Skull Form, During and After Crest Migration

Use of the word "epigenetic" does not, in any sense, diminish the role of genes, or imply that pattern is somehow outside genetic control. Epigenesis simply refers to the interplay that takes place among the components of a developmental system, whose consequences are not themselves under direct genetic control ("components" can be interpreted as molecular, cellular, or tissue levels of organization). Quite minor and sometimes quantitative changes within the "epigenetic domain" (Alberch 1982) can have morphogenetic consequences which at a trivial level constitute variation, but at more profound levels can result in dysmorphogenesis and, rarely, create novel phenotypes of phylogenetic significance (Hall 1992). Of the many examples which could be chosen from craniofacial development, I have selected two in which biomechanical factors have morphogenetic consequences (for further discussion of this topic, see chapter by Herring, this volume).

The first concerns the development of the ocular skeleton in many submammalian vertebrates. The developing optic cup, and subsequently the eye, is supported by a cartilaginous optic cartilage—the scleral cartilage (formed as a result of tissue interaction between mesencephalic crest-derived cells and the presumptive pigmented retina, see fig. 4.2). Later in development, a species-specific number of protective scleral ossicles, composed of membrane bone, form at the margin of the cornea (again as the result of crest-derived mesenchyme undergoing an interaction with, in this case, overlying conjunctival epithelium). Both of these skeletal systems can have their final form and pattern profoundly disturbed by perturbation of eye growth. For example, between the fourth and ninth day of incubation, the chick eye undergoes a 500-fold increase in volume as fluid accumulates in the vitreous. The introduction of a microcatheter into the developing optic cup allows that fluid to drain out rather than accumulate (Coulombre et al. 1962). The volume of the eye is dramatically reduced as a consequence but development and differentiation are, in other respects, normal. The ocular skeleton, however, displays considerable differences in form and pattern. The scleral cartilage forms on schedule but it is reduced in size, corresponding to the smaller eye which it now encapsulates; instead of being large and thin-walled it is small and thick-walled (Weiss and Amprino 1940). Furthermore, the scleral ossicles are reduced in number and the degree of reduction correlates directly with growth retardation of the eye (reviewed by Coulombre 1965). In both these systems, the necessary tissue interactions have taken place satisfactorily—otherwise there would be no skeletogenic differentiation—but the form and pattern of that differentiation are not programmed, and local influences, in this case growth of an adjacent organ, have fundamentally affected morphology.

One further example is the development of secondary or adventitious cartilage, a tissue which forms within the periosteum at points of articulation between membrane bones and provides an embryonic articulating surface. In fact, the potential to form secondary cartilage exists throughout the periosteum that covers membrane bones, but is normally expressed only at sites of their articulation (Thorogood 1979). The reason for this discrete distribution is that it is only at these points that shearing forces and pressure are exerted on the periosteum as the embryonic musculo-skeletal system begins to function. Paralysis of striated muscle contraction removes the stimulus for differentiation, and secondary cartilage is then absent from all articulations between membrane bones (Murray and Smiles 1965; Hall 1968). Thus, the patterned distribution of this skeletal tissue is determined indirectly by the interplay between the skeleton and the adjacent muscles. As in the previous examples, there is no evidence for prior specification or programming of pattern or form (other examples and further discussion can be found in Thorogood 1983; Hall 1984).

However, a more fundamental influence on events within the epigenetic domain is the location and timing of the all-important tissue interactions. In fact, epithelia in the head do differ regionally, and with time, in their ability to promote chondrogenesis and osteogenesis (Bee and Thorogood 1980; Hall 1982a; Smith and Thorogood 1983). Location of an interaction will also be affected by changing migration patterns of the crest cells, and therefore cell translocation becomes vitally important as a morphogenetic factor. Teratogenic perturbation of crest migration by retinoids, for example, does indeed change skeletal pattern (Morriss and

Thorogood 1979), in this particular case, by affecting cell/matrix interactions; migrating cells slough off surface fibronectin and, as a result, are unable to maintain cytoskeletal organization and probably lose the ability to interact with the matrices through which they normally migrate (Thorogood et al. 1982). Cell translocation is therefore critical for at least two major reasons. Firstly, it is the pathways of migration which create the opportunity for local interaction with epithelia or epithelially derived matrices. Secondly, the migration pathway (or circumstances of translocation) determines precisely where cells end up, i.e., where they express their phenotype.

An epigenetic model has been proposed which attempts to incorporate both location of tissue interactions and cell translocation/movement as causal factors in the determination of skull form (Thorogood 1987, 1988). As the "flypaper" model has been dealt with in depth elsewhere, I shall describe it here only in brief detail. At an anatomical level the shape of the vertebrate skull is determined in two major ways—cranially, by the mode and rate of growth of the developing brain, and facially, by the chondrocranium. Both brain and chondrocranium are operating epigenetically in that they act as structural templates around which, and on which, the membranous and endochondral bone elements, respectively, are formed. The flypaper model seeks to explain the morphogenesis of the neurocranial portion of the chondrocranium; some aspects are based on confirmed observations, others on predictions which can be experimentally tested.

It is proposed that the very early developing head be viewed as a complex of highly folded epithelia (e.g., neural tube, invaginating placodes, optic vesicle evaginating from the diencephalon, foregut). Within this bag of convoluted epithelia there is very extensive extracellular compartment comprising matrix occupied by a sparse population of mesodermally derived mesenchyme. As the cephalic neural tube forms, neural crest cells are released into this matrix, and given the pre-existing low mesodermal cell density, will migrate autonomously and opportunistically, wherever matrix exists that will permit migration. The real issue is what stops or arrests this migration, and it is proposed that certain epithelially derived matrices provide a trapping function, causing localized arrest of migrating crest cells, or at least a subpopulation of them. Following arrest of migration, cells accumulate and undergo a matrix-mediated interaction with the epithelium at that site, which promotes chondrogenic differentiation. Clearly, the existence and location of such trapping matrices is crucial. Regional differences in epithelially associated matrices have been described above with the transient presence of type II collagen in the reticulate lamina, at the sites of such interactions. Furthermore, cell-free native matrix from one such site, the pigmented retina, causes arrest of mesencephalic neural crest migration in vitro (Thorogood 1988). Our preliminary observations indicate that the two major matrix glycoproteins, laminin and fibronectin, promote active migration of cephalic crest cells in vitro, whereas pure type II collagen, in the same assay, very effectively inhibits it, providing the interesting possibility that certain molecules, in this case type II, might have dual roles—operating in both arrest of migration and the chondrogenesis-promoting interaction. It is highly probable that other matrix molecules active in this way remain to be identified.

A major corollary of the flypaper model is that control of neurocranial form can consequently be reduced to two major parameters operating at the cellular level: (1) how the epithelia fold up and create a pattern of trapping matrix, and (2) the parameter of cell migration—that is, for instance, how fast, or how many, cells migrate. Minor changes in these parameters, operating within the epigenetic domain, will alter neurocranial form in greater or lesser ways. Given the template function of the cartilaginous neurocranium, this will have further epigenetic consequences on the formation of the bony skull. If we seek to define genetic influence on skull form, then we must turn to the genes involved in these two parameters of extracellular matrix and cell movement. Thus, genes encoding for matrix molecules and their cell surface receptors, for cell adhesion molecules, and for cytoskeletal proteins are perhaps some of the best candidates. Indirectly, such gene activity will underpin the basic rules of cell behavior operating within this epigenetic domain; changing activity of the genes will alter events therein, with morphological consequences.

The Flypaper Model: An Assessment

The robustness of any theoretical model is measured by the experimental testing of predictions based upon that model. Several such predictions will be considered here (for more detail, see Thorogood 1988). First, if cell trapping by an extracellular matrix (component) does occur, then it must be mediated by a surface receptor or binding protein expressed by the responding cells. Recently a cell surface binding protein for type II collagen has been immunocytochemically identified on the surface of a subpopulation of cephalic neural crest cells (Hoffmann, Thorogood, and von der Mark, in preparation). Anchorin CII is a 34 Kd membrane protein of the lipocortin/calpactin family, a group of structurally related, membrane-associated proteins characterized by an ability to bind to phospholipids in a calcium-dependent manner and thought to mediate in certain signal transduction events (Moss and Crumpton 1990). It is typically expressed by chondrocytes and has a high binding affinity for the abundant type II collagen in the chondrocytes environment (von der Mark et al. 1986), but in early craniofacial development it may mediate trapping of migrating crest cells. Second, given the parallels with the sclerotome/notochord in-

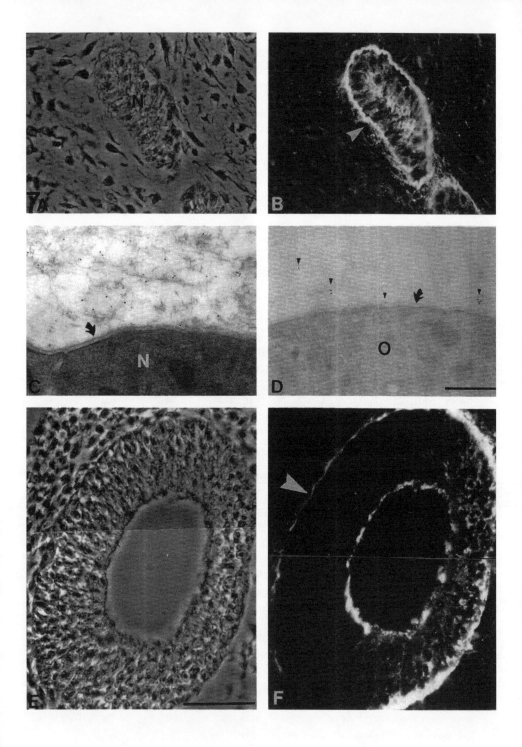

teraction, other cartilage-specific matrix molecules may be expressed at the tissue interfaces listed in fig. 4.4, just as cartilage-specific proteoglycan is codistributed with type II collagen in the perinotochordal sheath. Mapping of the collective distribution of all keratan sulfate–containing proteoglycans, including cartilage-specific proteoglycan (which has a number of keratan sulfate side-chains as well as abundant chondroitin sulfate), reveals an incomplete correlation with type II collagen at the relevant tissue interfaces. At some, such as the type II-positive basal aspect of the optic vesicle, there is a complete absence of keratan sulfate–containing proteoglycans and so there is no coexpression. In contrast, at the type II-positive basal aspect of the otic vesicle, there is an abundance of such proteoglycans (Heath and Thorogood 1989; and see fig. 4.7). Similarly, coexpression of types II and IX collagen, the latter being a minor cartilage collagen, is not observed at sites of such interactions (Fitch et al. 1989). Clearly, parallels with the sclerotome/notochord system are limited and cell/matrix relationships within this system are more complicated than previously thought (see below).

Third, although the flypaper model is based largely upon data emerging from studies on avian systems, if it is valid, then it should have wide application throughout the vertebrates (assuming that successful developmental mechanisms generating common anatomical patterns are highly conserved). Recent immunocytochemical studies of the mouse embryo have revealed a pattern of transient type II collagen at tissue interfaces similar to that described for the avian embryo (Wood et al. 1991). Moreover, the collagen at such interfaces appears to be derived from the epithelial partner in which coincident transcriptional activity of the type II

Fig. 4.7. Immunolocalization of keratan sulfate–containing proteoglycans at tissue interfaces where chondrogenesis-promoting interactions occur. Phase contrast (A and E) and immunofluorescence (B and F) micrographs were prepared by using the mouse monoclonal antibody MZ15 (Zanetti et al. 1985) followed by incubation in a sheep FITC–conjugated antimouse. A, B. Oblique, L.S. of stage-14 notochord at rhombencephalic level illustrating strong staining in the perinotochordal sheath (arrowhead). E, F. T.S. of stage-18 otic vesicle showing strong staining basally and some staining apically (i.e., luminal aspect). Interestingly, the basal staining becomes weaker on the medial side of the otic vesicle (arrowhead), but the significance of this differential distribution is not clear. C, D. Unstained, TEM pre-embedding immunogold preparations using MZ15 (see fig. 4.3 legend for technical details). C. The basal aspect of a stage-14 notochord (N) with abundant fold particles associated with the fibrillar elements in the reticulate lamina; basal lamina (arrow). D. The basal aspect of a stage-16 otic vesicle epithelial cell (O). A sparser, but nevertheless positive distribution of gold particles (arrowheads) indicating, like (C), the presence of keratan sulfate–containing proteoglycans in the reticulate lamina. Scale bars: for light micrographs (E) 30 μm; for transmission electron micrographs (D), 200 nm.

collagen gene has been demonstrated (Cheah et al. 1991). Immunocyto-chemical analyses of representatives of "lower" vertebrate taxa reveal comparable patterns of transient type II collagen (amphibians: Klymkowsky and Hanken 1991; teleost fishes: Amanze and Thorogood 1992).

Other attributes of the model are that it provides possible explanations for compositional change in the mesenchymal lineage of homologous elements and for the adaptive changes characterizing regulation after experimental perturbation. With regard to the former, the contribution from the two principal mesenchymal lineages to the component parts of the neurocranium can be changed experimentally (see Noden 1983) or phylogenetically during the course of evolution. An early specification of morphogenetic fate which is intrinsic to the mesenchymal cells is difficult to equate with such phenomena; yet if pattern is imposed upon a mesenchyme, irrespective of its source, by a second, reference tissue then such phenomena become explicable. In fact, the flypaper model does not distinguish where mesenchyme comes from. It assumes that both neural crest–derived and mesoderm-derived mesenchyme cells respond equally well to the same signals, a conclusion reached independently from analysis of heterospecific chimeras (Le Lièvre 1978) and from the osteogenic response of mixed-composition mesenchyme to epithelia (Tyler 1983). The (neuro)epithelium specifies, to a responsive mesenchyme, irrespective of source, when and where cartilage will form, by way of the spatial positioning of the appropriate interactions. Similarly, with regard to regulation, if only mesenchyme is lost and that mesenchymal defect is corrected by infilling migration, then the cells, assuming a certain level of potency, may have their fate altered by interaction with any reference tissues (i.e., epithelium) remaining at the site. They are therefore responding to the epigenetic factors, emanating from the epithelium, which would normally determine skeletal form and pattern. Furthermore, one can see that the effect of removing supporting tissues (see earlier discussion; and McKee and Ferguson 1984) will be not only to remove factors permitting migration but also to remove patterning (or reference) tissues. Thus, epigenesis can provide an explanation for regulation—a phenomenon which is difficult to reconcile with a supposed specification of morphogenetic fate prior to migration.

However, certain questions remain to be answered and apparent contradictions resolved. For instance, type II collagen cannot be a signal specific to chondrogenic interactions alone since it is also found at a number of other locations in the avian embryo where no chondrogenesis-promoting tissue interactions occur (in addition to the long-recognized ocular locations). Thus, it is found in the early limb bud (Fitch et al. 1989) and in the mesonephros and interface between epimyocardium and endocardium in the developing heart (Kosher and Solursh 1989). Given this widespread distribution, Kosher and Solursh suggest that type II at tissue interfaces might have a more general function unrelated to chondrogenesis, but involving other roles of the basement membrane at a particular site and developmental stage. It is unlikely, however, that the presence of a single matrix molecule would be the only signal or differentiation cue and more probable that particular combinations of matrix components are necessary, the combination perhaps differing in relation to the nature of the mesenchymal subpopulations at the interface in question. A cataloguing of these matrix molecule combinations is going to be necessary before we can assess their full significance. It will be necessary to plot not only spatiotemporal patterns of accumulated gene products, but also the spatiotemporal patterns of relevant gene transcription by in situ hybridization, as has been done for the developing limb bud (e.g., Mallein-Gerin et al. 1988; Swalla et al. 1988) and cornea (Hayashi et al. 1988). Currently, only limited progress is resulting from analysis of matrix composition. Two candidates for signal molecules which might possibly be coexpressed with type II are cartilage-specific proteoglycan and minor cartilage collagens. The lack of regular coexpression of cartilage-specific proteoglycan and type II collagen at tissue interfaces where matrix-mediated, chondrogenesis-promoting interactions occur, has been discussed earlier (Heath and Thorogood 1989) and it can tentatively be concluded that such proteoglycan might serve a signaling function only at some interfaces, if at all. The only minor cartilage collagen to have been investigated in any depth is type IX, which is normally considered to have a role cross-linking type II fibrils in mature cartilage matrix (Muller-Glauser et al. 1986). Two laboratories have independently reported that type IX does not codistribute with type II at early stages apart from in the cornea, vitreous, and perinotochordal sheath (Fitch et al. 1989; Kosher and Solursh 1989) and my personal observations confirm this. Thus, type IX does not seem to be involved in signaling. Its role at these early stages may be similar to its role in mature cartilage, i.e., a cross-linking function permitting the formation of multilayers of collagen fibrils in the matrix of the primary corneal stroma and perinotochordal sheath (Fitch et al. 1989). However, it is important to recognize also the correlation between transient type II collagen expression and the absence of type IX. Type II in the cornea and perinotochordal sheath persists from early stages, whereas at most of the interfaces listed in fig. 4.4 (and illustrated in fig. 8 in Thorogood et al. 1986) type II is present only temporarily and disappears long before the overt expression of a chondrogenic phenotype. This transience may reflect a turnover of type II in the absence of type IX which would otherwise cross-link and stabilize the type II collagenous matrix. Clearly we need to define more precisely the role of type II at all interfaces where it is found. It is possible that its "signaling" role is nonspecific and simply elicits a critical change in cell shape—from an irregular, locomotory phenotype, for example, to a rounded one—thereby promoting chondrogenesis in a responsive mesenchyme. (It has long been recognized that a rounded cell phenotype is a prerequisite for chondrogenic expression; for a recent account of the relationship between cell shape, the cytoskeleton, and chondrogenic expression, see Watt and Dudhia 1988.) Alternatively, or additionally, they might function to bind other molecules, such as growth factors, which in turn act as signals (reviewed Lyons et al. 1991; Rosen and Thies 1992), promoting or inhibiting skeletogenesis (e.g., Rosen et al. 1988; Wozney et al. 1990). For instance, TGFβ-related proteins are known to bind not only to the cell surface but also to extracellular molecules, including both proteoglycans and collagens (reviewed Messauge 1991), which is significant given the multiple influences that TGFβ has on skeletogenic differentiation (reviewed Rizzino 1988).

One apparent contradiction is that the flypaper model proposes epithelial determination of mesenchymal fate, whereas dogma generally argues for the converse, i.e., that mesenchyme normally determines the fate of associated ectodermal cells, at least postcephalically (for examples, see Wessells 1979). This is more difficult to resolve but may reflect the fact that the head mesenchyme cells, of both lineages, undergo dramatic rearrangements during craniofacial development of a magnitude simply not seen in the trunk. Given the inherent problems that might be posed in terms of controlling pattern formation and differentiation, a genetically economic and simple strategy would be to use another tissue as a stable frame of positional reference for subsequent differentiation of mesenchyme cells. The epithelia of the head, in spite of the various invaginations and evaginations, could provide such a planar reference, whereby a two-dimensional "prepattern" becomes translated into a three-dimensional form as a result of the mesenchymal cells' differentiative response. A justified criticism of the model is that it does not in itself constitute an answer; the establishment of the prepattern expressed in the epithelium (or at least its matrix) still has to be explained.

DIFFERENT INTERPRETATIONS OF A SINGLE MECHANISM, OR TWO MECHANISMS?

At this point we must ask ourselves whether "morphogenetic specification" and epigenetic determination of chondrocranial form are as mutually exclusive as they first appear. (See also discussion in Noden 1988; Thorogood 1988). Of undoubted relevance is that they are each based largely on the study of different parts of the embryonic chondrocranium. The interpretations of Wagner (1949; 1955), Andres (1949), and Noden (1983) emerged from experimental perturbation of branchial arch formation, i.e, the cartilaginous viscerocranium (and in Noden's case, some bony elements, too). In contrast, the epigenetic flypaper model emerges from investigation of the cartilaginous neurocranium. Superficially, at least, it would appear that the basic tenets upon which each interpretation is based are incompatible. However, two recently initiated lines of enquiry might enable us, in time, to resolve this issue.

First are the conclusions from the recent, detailed fate-mapping of the avian forebrain primordium prior to neural fold fusion. As a result of elegant isotopic and isochronic grafting experiments to create chick/quail chimeric neural plates and folds, Couly and Le Douarin (1987, 1990) have catalogued the derivatives of the entire prosencephalic neural primordium; furthermore, they have mapped the distribution of the progenitor cells for these derivatives to locations within the neural plate and folds (see fig. 4.8). It has been generally assumed that the apices of the neural folds are comprised largely, if not entirely, of neurectodermal cells, destined to de-epithelialize and form neural crest; but unexpectedly, Couly and Le Douarin found that the neural folds included groups of cells which will give rise to much facial and cranial ectoderm. Given, therefore, that the neural folds contain far more than just crest, and include tissues which may have a patterning role, it is not surprising that grafted neural folds can sometimes give rise to supernumary structures; possibly, the grafted cells do not always respond to novel patterning influences at the site of grafting but can respond to those transplanted alongside them within the graft. (Noden's observation that supernumerary egg teeth form from grafts, and the mapping of the egg tooth progenitor cells to the prosencephalic neural folds—see fig. 4.8—demonstrate clearly that more than just crest is transplanted in a neural fold graft. In other words, the supernumerary egg tooth may be not so much induced as grafted as presumptive tissue.) It is conceivable that, in this way, experimental observations which have been interpreted as evidence of morphogenetic specification might be reconciled with the concept of epigenetic control of chondrocranial form as mediated by local tissue interactions. Undoubtedly, further fate-mapping, with this degree of resolution, of the remaining mesencephalic and rhombencephalic primordia will reveal other unexpected and potentially interesting cell associations.

A second line of enquiry concerns the molecular biological analysis of regulatory genes within the developing head. A number of homeobox-containing regulatory genes, encoding for proteins with DNA binding domains and therefore with putative transcription factor roles, have been identified on the basis of sequence homology with their *Drosophila* counterparts (e.g., Wilkinson et al. 1989; see also chapter in this volume by Langille and Hall). Significantly, certain homeobox-containing genes of the

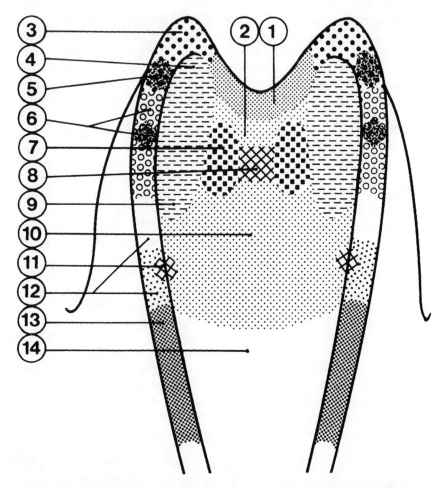

Fig. 4.8. Fate map of the anterior neural primordium at stage 8 in the avian embryo, derived from heterospecific chick/quail chimeras. Note that much facial ectoderm, including that of the olfactory placodes, that of the nasal cavity, and that covering the frontonasal area (including upper beak and egg tooth) are, at this stage, located with the neural fold. 1. Adenohypophysis. 2. Hypothalamus. 3. Ectoderm of nasal cavity. 4. Floor of telencephalon. 5. Olfactory placode. 6. Ectoderm of upper beak and egg tooth. 7. Optic vesicles. 8. Neurohypophysis. 9. Roof of telencephalon. 10. Diencephalon. 11. Hemiepiphysis. 12. Ectoderm of calvaria and caudal prosencephalic neural crest (light spotted area). 13. Rostral mesencephalic neural crest (dense spotted area). 14. Mesencephalon. (With permisssion, from Couly and Le Douarin 1987).

Antennapedia class are expressed in very precise spatial patterns within the embryonic hindbrain (rhombencephalon), and the anterior limits of the expression domains of particular genes coincide with the anterior limits of the hindbrain segments, or "rhombomeres" (reviewed by Hunt, Whiting, et al. 1991). Such expression patterns, initially expressed in the neuroepithelium of the neural tube, are maintained in an axial level–specific pattern by the migrating neural crest cells, which retain expression of the same *Hox* genes that characterize their axial level of origin in the neural tube (Hunt, Wilkinson, et al. 1991). Thus, at any one particular axial level in the hindbrain region of the embryonic head, neural tube and neural crest will express identical combinations of these regulatory *Hox* genes. This has led to the proposal that there is a combinatorial "*Hox* code" in which the array of *Hox* genes expressed not only correlates with a particular branchial region of the head but is causally involved in specifying the morphogenetic fate of the cells concerned (Hunt, Gulisano, et al. 1991). In this way, regional specification of morphogenetic fate at the level of the segmented hindbrain is extended into the corresponding branchial arches by the migrating crest cells (see fig. 2 in Hunt and Krumlauf 1991). The possibility of a combinatorial code is attractive given what appears to be a comparable system in the trunk whereby a trunk *Hox* code correlates with the phenotype of individual vertebrae along the antero-posterior axis of the embryo, and experimental transformation of vertebral phenotype correlates with a corresponding change in *Hox* code (Kessel and Gruss 1991). At this stage however, caution must be urged, on two grounds. First, the causal relationship between the head *Hox* code and the specification of morphogenetic fate remains to be experimentally demonstrated in a thorough and unequivocal fashion. At present the evidence is largely correlative; in the transgenic animals created to date, it has proved difficult to define the precise pedigree of causality between changed pattern of *Hox* gene expression and craniofacial abnormality (e.g., Balling et al. 1989; Chisaka and Cappecchi 1991). Second, the identity of the downstream genes, whose expression is controlled by the *Hox* gene products, remains to be established.

However, the rate of progress to date has been auspicious and this topic is currently the subject of intensive research. It should be noted that the proposed *Hox* code for the head does not correlate with differentiation of any particular cell or tissue type but rather with different regions of the embryo. In the segmental branchial arch region of the head this means an equivalent range of tissue types (e.g., cartilage, bone, and muscle), but in different and characteristic patterns in successive arches. Moreover, there is to date no demonstrated 1 : 1 relationship between expression of any particular *Hox* gene (or combination thereof) and the specification of any individual component parts of the head skeleton. Nevertheless, that the

Hox code is apparently expressed only in the rhombencephalic/branchial arch region of the head, in which the viscerocranium forms, is significant. A *Hox* code expressed in neural crest cells may constitute a genetic mechanism of specification of morphogenetic fate established before the crest cells begin to migrate. Such a possibility might be explored by experimental strategies which confront crest cells with new axial environments; monitoring whether their *Hox* code changes in relation to a new or unaltered morphogenetic fate will elucidate the role of these regulatory genes. (How such a code might be implemented in terms of three-dimensional anatomy can only be conjectured at this stage.)

Perhaps the single most significant point in the context of this discussion is that it may now be more accurate for us to think in terms of dual mechanisms underlying the specification of chondrocranial form. These two mechanisms, each of which is partly definable in molecular terms, appear to correlate precisely with the anatomists' rationalization of the chondrocranium into two main parts. Thus, we can envisage the cartilaginous neurocranium (for which there is as yet no evidence of any regulatory gene code operating) being specified epigenetically by the brain and sense organ primordia, via matrix-mediated tissue interactions in which type II collagen would appear to be the signaling molecule or would serve to bind another molecule with a signaling role. In contrast, the form of the cartilaginous viscerocranium (i.e., the branchial arches, including Meckel's cartilage) would be specified in certain crest cells before migration by means of a combinatorial code of expression of homeobox-containing genes, which specifies the morphogenesis of each branchial arch skeleton which will subsequently form. The compatability of a *Hox* code specification with the results of various experimental perturbations (such as default first arch morphogenesis in heterotopic grafts, and regulation) will need to be clarified. However, on the basis of available evidence it does appear that there are indeed two mechanisms operating. These different mechanisms probably reflect the evolution of the neurocranium and viscerocranium as independent events during early vertebrate ancestry (Thorogood and Hanken 1992), in which case, analyses such as those reviewed here are likely to clarify not only how the skull is specified developmentally but also how it evolved.

ACKNOWLEDGMENTS

It is a pleasure to acknowledge discussion held over a number of years with former graduate students and postdoctoral colleagues, in particular, Dee Amanze, Andy Wood, Lindsay Heath, and Paul Hunt. Barry Lockyer gave photographic assistance in the preparation of this paper. Masando Hayashi generously communicated unpublished results. Work from my own laboratory has been supported by grants from the Wellcome Trust and the Medical Research Council (U.K.).

REFERENCES

Alberch, P. 1982. Development constraints in evolutionary processes. In *Evolution and Development*, J. Bonner, ed., Berlin: Springer Verlag, pp. 313–331.

Amanze, D., and P. Thorogood. 1992. Neural crest cell behaviour studied *in vivo* during craniofacial morphogenesis. Manuscript.

Andres, G. 1949. Untersuchungen an Chimaeren von *Bombinator* und *Triton*. Genetica 24: 1–148.

Balling, R., G. Mutter, P. Gruss, and M. Kessel. 1989. Craniofacial abnormalities induced by ectopic expression of the homeobox gene *Hox 1.1* in transgenic mice. Cell 58: 337–347.

Baltzer, F. Von. 1952. Experimentelle Beiträge zur der Homologie. Experientia 8: 285–324.

Baroffio, A., E. Dupin, and N. M. Le Douarin. 1988. Clone-forming ability and differentiative potential of migratory neural crest cells. Proceedings of the National Academy of Science, U.S.A. 85: 5325–5329.

Baroffio, A., E. Dupin, and N. Le Douarin. 1991. Common precursors for neural and mesectodermal derivatives in the cephalic neural crest. Development 112: 301–306.

Bee, J. A., and P. Thorogood. 1980. The role of tissue interactions in the skeletogenic differentiation of avian neural crest cells. Developmental Biology 78: 47–66.

Bissell, M. J., and M. H. Barcellos-Hoff. 1987. The influence of extracellular matrix on gene expression: Is structure the message? Journal of Cell Science, 8 (suppl.): 327–343.

Bradamante, Z., and B. K. Hall. 1980. The role of epithelial collagen and proteoglycan in the initiation of osteogenesis by avian neural crest cells. Anatomical Records 197: 305–315.

Brigham, G., L. Scaletta, L. Johnson, Jr., and J. Occhino. 1977. Antigenic differences among condylar, epihyseal, and nasal septal cartilages. In *The Biology of Occlusal Development*, J. A. McNamara, ed. Ann Arbor: University of Michigan Press, pp. 313–331.

Bronner-Fraser, M., and S. E. Fraser. 1988. Cell lineage analysis reveals multipotency of some avian neural crest cells. Nature 335: 161–164.

Cheah, K. S. E., E. T. Lau, P. K. C. Au, and P. L. Tam. 1991. Expression of the mouse $\alpha1(II)$ collagen gene is not restricted to cartilage during development. Development 111: 945–954.

Chiakulas, J. J. 1957. The specificity and differential fusion of cartilage derived from mesoderm and mesectoderm. Journal of Experimental Zoology 136: 287–300.

Chibon, P. 1966. Analyse expérimentale de la régionalisation et des capacités morphogénétiques de la crête neurale chez l'Amphibien Urodele *Pleurodeles waltlii* Michah. Memoires de la Société zoologique de France 36: 4–107.

————. 1970. Capacité de régulation des excédents dans la crête neurale d'Amphibien. Journal of Embryology and Experimental Morphology 24: 479–496.

Chisaka, O., and M. R. Cappecchi. 1991. Regionally restricted developmental defects resulting from targeted disruption of the mouse homeobox gene *Hox 1.5*. Nature 350: 473–479.

Coulombre, A. J. 1965. The eye. In *Organogenesis*, R. L. Dehaan and H. Ursprung, eds. New York: Holt, Reinhart and Winston, pp. 219–251.

Coulombre, A. J., J. L. Coulombre, and H. Mehta. 1962. The skeleton of the eye. I. Conjunctival papillae and scleral ossicles. Developmental Biology 5: 382–401.

Couly, G., and N. M. Le Douarin. 1987. Mapping of the early neural primorium in quail-chick chimaeras. II. The prosencephalic neural plate and neural folds: Implications for the genesis of cephalic human congenital abnormalities. Developmental Biology 120: 198–214.

Couly, G., and N. M. Le Douarin. 1990. Head morphogenesis in embryonic avian chimaeras: Evidence for segmental pattern in the ectoderm corresponding to the neuromeres. Development 108: 543–558.

Croucher, S., and C. Tickle. 1989. Characterization of epithelial domains in the nasal passages of chick embryos: Spatial and temporal mapping of a range of extracellular matrix and cell surface molecules during development of the nasal placode. Development 106: 493–509.

Drews, U., U. Kocher-Becker, and U. Drews. 1972. Die Induktion von Klemenknorpel aus Kopfneuralleistenmaterial durch prasumptiven kiemendarm in der Gewebkultur un das Bewegungsverhalten der Zellen wahrend ihrer Entwicklung zu Knorpel. Roux' Archives of Developmental Biology 171: 17–37.

Epperlein, H. H., and R. Lehmann. 1975. Ectomesenchymal endodermal interaction system (EEIS) of *Triturus alpestris* in tissue culture. 2. Observations of the differentiation of visceral cartilage. Differentiation 4: 159–174.

Farley, J. R., J. E. Wergedal, and D. J. Baylink. 1983. Fluoride directly stimulates proliferation and alkaline phosphatase activity of bone forming cells. Science 222: 330–332.

Fitch, J. M., A. Mentzer, R. Mayne, and T. F. Linsenmayer. 1989. Independent deposition of collagen types II and IX at epithelial-mesenchymal interfaces. Development 105: 85–96.

Fyfe, D. M., and B. K. Hall. 1979. Lack of association between cartilages of different embryological origins when maintained *in vitro*. American Journal of Anatomy 154: 485–495.

Gans, C. 1989. Stages in the origin of vertebrates: Analysis by means of scenarios. Biological Reviews 64: 221–268.

Gans, C., and G. Northcutt. 1983. Neural crest and the origin of vertebrates. Science 220: 268–274.

Graveson, A. C., and J. B. Armstrong. 1987. Differentiation of cartilage from cranial neural crest in the Axolotl (*Ambystoma mexicanum*). Differentiation 35: 16–20.

Hall, B. K. 1968. *In vitro* studies on the mechanical evocation of adventitious cartilage in the chick. Journal of Experimental Zoology 168: 283–306.

————. 1978. Initiation of osteogenesis in mandibular mesenchyme in the embryonic chick in response to mandibular and non-mandibular epithelium. Archives of Oral Biology 23: 1157–1161.

————. 1981. 1981. Specificity in the differentiation and morphogenesis of neural crest–derived scleral ossicles and of epithelial scleral papillae in the eye of the embryonic chick. Journal of Embryology and Experimental Morphology 66: 175–190.

————. 1982a. Distribution of osteo- and chondrogenic cells and of osteogenically inductive epithelia in mandibular arches of embryonic chicks. Journal of Embryology and Experimental Morphology 68: 127–136.

————. 1982b. The role of tissue interactions in the growth of bone. In *Factors and Mechanisms Influencing Bone Growth,* A. S. Dixon and B. G. Sarnat, eds. New York: A. R. Liss, pp. 205–215.

————. 1984. Genetic and epigenetic control of connective tissues in the craniofacial structures. Birth Defects: Original Article Series 20 (3): 1–17.

————. 1987a. Earliest evidence of cartilage and bone development in embryonic life. Clinical Orthopaedics 225: 255–272.

————. 1987b. Initiation of chondrogenesis from somitic, limb, and craniofacial mesenchyme: Search for a common mechanism. In *Somites in Developing Embryos,* R. Bellairs, D. A. Ede, and J. W. Lash, eds. New York: Plenum, pp. 247–259.

————. 1987c. Sodium fluoride as an initiator of osteogenesis from embryonic mesenchyme *in vitro*. Bone 8: 111–116.

————. 1991. Cellular interactions during cartilage and bone development. Journal of Craniofacial Genetics and Developmental Biology 11: 238–250.

————. 1992. *Evolutionary Developmental Biology.* New York: Chapman & Hall.

Hall, B. K., and S. Hörstadius. 1988. *The Neural Crest.* 2d ed. Oxford: Oxford University Press.

Hall, B. K., R. J. Van Exan, and S. L. Brunt. 1983. Retention of epithelial basal lamina allows isolated mandibular mesenchyme to form bone. Journal of Craniofacial Genetics and Developmental Biology 3: 253–267.

Hammond, W. S., and C. L. Yntema. 1964. Depletions of pharyngeal arch cartilages following extirpation of cranial neural crest in chick embryos. Acta anatomica 56: 21–34.

Harrison, R. G. 1938. Die Neuralleiste. Anatomischer Anzeiger, Jena 85: 4–30.

Hayashi, M., Y. Ninomiya, K. Hayashi, T. F. Linsenmayer, B. R. Olsen, and R. L. Trelstad. 1988. Secretion of collagen types I and II by epithelial and endothelial cells in the developing chick cornea demonstrated by *in situ* hybridization and immunohistochemistry. Development 103: 27–36.

Heath, L. A., and P. Thorogood. 1989. Keratan sulfate expression during avian craniofacial morphogenesis. Roux' Archives of Developmental Biology 198: 103–113.

Heath, L. A., A. Wild, and P. Thorogood. 1992. Monoclonal antibodies raised against pre-migratory neural crest reveal population heterogeneity during crest development. Differentiation 49: 151–165.

Hörstadius, S. 1950. *The Neural Crest: Its Properties and Derivatives in the Light of Experimental Research.* Oxford: Oxford University Press.

Hörstadius, S., and S. Sellman. 1946. Experimentelle Untersuchungen uber die Determination des Knorpeligen Kopfskelettes bei Urodelen. Nova acta Regiae societatis scientiarum Upsaliensis, ser. 4, 13: 1–170.

Hunt, P., M. Gulisano, M. Cook, M.-H. Sham, A. Faiella, D. Wilkinson, E. Boncinelli, and R. Krumlauf. 1991. A distinct *Hox* code for the branchial region of the vertebrate head. Nature 353: 861–864.

Hunt, P., and R. Krumlauf. 1991. Deciphering the Hox code: Clues to patterning the branchial regions of the head. Cell 66: 1075–1078.

Hunt, P., J. Whiting, I. Muchamore, H. Marshall, and R. Krumlauf. 1991. Homeobox genes and models for patterning the hindbrain and branchial arches. Development 1 (suppl.): 187–196.

Hunt, P., D. Wilkinson, and R. Krumlauf. 1991. Patterning the vertebrate head: Murine *Hox 2* genes mark distinct subpopulations of premigratory and migrating cranial neural crest cells. Development 112: 43–50.

Johnston, M. C. 1964. Facial malformations in chick embryos resulting from removal of neural crest. Journal of Dental Research 43 (suppl. 5): 822.

———. 1966. A radioautographic study of the migration and fate of cranial neural crest cells in the chick embryo. Anatomical Records 156: 143–156.

Juriloff, D. M., and M. J. Harris. 1983. Abnormal facial development in the mouse mutant *First arch.* Journal of Craniofacial Genetics and Developmental Biology 3: 317–337.

Kessel, M., and P. Gruss. 1991. Homeotic transformation of murine vertebrae and concomitant alteration of *Hox* codes induced by retinoic acid. Cell 67: 89–104.

Klymkowsky, M. W., and J. Hanken. 1991. Whole-mount staining of *Xenopus* and other vertebrates. Methods in Cell Biology 36: 413–434.

Kosher, R. A., and R. L. Church. 1975. Stimulation of *in vitro* chondrogenesis by procollagen and collagen. Nature 258: 327–330.

Kosher, R. A., and M. Solursh. 1989. Widespread distribution of type II collagen during embryonic chick development. Developmental Biology 131: 558–566.

Kratochwil, K. 1983. Embryonic induction. In *Cell Interactions and Development,* K. M. Yamada, ed. New York: John Wiley & Sons, pp. 99–122.

Langille, R. M., and B. K. Hall. 1988a. Role of the neural crest in development of the cartilaginous cranial and visceral skeleton in the medaka, *Oryzias latipes* (Teleostei). Anatomy and Embryology 177: 297–305.

———. 1988b. Role of the neural crest in development of the trabeculae and branchial arches in the embryonic sea lamprey, *Petromyzon marinus.* Development 102: 301–310.

Lash, J. W., and N. S. Vasan. 1978. Somite chondrogenesis *in vitro:* stimulation by exogenous extracellular matrix components. Developmental Biology 66: 151–171.

Le Douarin, N. M. 1973. A biological cell labelling technique and its use in experimental embryology. Developmental Biology 30: 217–222.

Le Lièvre, C. 1974. Rôle des cellules mésectodermiques issues des crêtes neurales céphalique dans la formation des arcs branchiaux et du squelette viscéral. Journal of Embryology and Experimental Morphology 31: 453–477.

———. 1978. Participation of neural crest–derived cells in the genesis of the skull in birds. Journal of Embryology and Experimental Morphology 47: 17–37.

Linsenmayer, T. F., G. N. Smith, and E. D. Hay. 1977. Synthesis of two collagen types by chick embryonic corneal epithelium in vitro. Proceedings of the National Academy of Science, U.S.A. 74: 39–43.

Luder, H. U., C. P. Leblond, and K. Von Der Mark. 1988. Cellular stages in cartilage formation as revealed by morphometry, radioautography, and type II collagen immunostaining of the mandibular condyle from weaning rats. American Journal of Anatomy 182: 197–214.

Lumsden, A. G. S. 1987. The neural crest contribution to tooth development in the mammalian embryo. In Developmental and Evolutionary Aspects of the Neural Crest, P. F. A. Maderson, ed. New York: John Wiley and Sons, pp. 261–300.

Lyons, K. M., C. M. Jones, and B. L. M. Hogan. 1991. The DVR gene family in embryonic development. Trends in Genetics 7: 408–412.

Mallein-Gerin, S., R. A. Kosher, W. A. Upholt, and M. L. Tanser. 1988. Temporal and spatial analysis of cartilage proteoglycan core protein gene expression during limb development by in situ hybridization. Developmental Biology 126: 337–345.

Marks, S. C., and S. N. Popoff. 1988. Bone cell biology: Regulation of development, structure, and function in the skeleton. American Journal of Anatomy 183: 1–44.

Massague, J. 1991. A helping hand from proteoglycans. Current Biology 1: 117–119.

McKee, G. J., and M. W. J. Ferguson. 1984. The effects of mesencephalic neural crest cell extirpation on the development of chick embryos. Journal of Anatomy 139: 491–512.

Morriss, G. M., and P. V. Thorogood. 1979. An approach to cranial neural crest migration and differentiation in mammalian embryos. In Development of Mammals, M. H. Johnston, ed., vol. 3. Amsterdam: North Holland. pp. 363–412.

Moss, S. E., and M. J. Crumpton. 1990. The lipocortins and the EF hand proteins; Ca^{2+}-binding sites and evolution. Trends in Biochemistry 15: 11–12.

Muller-Glauser, W., B. Humbel, M. Glatt, P. Strauli, K. H. Winterhalter, and P. Bruckner. 1986. On the role of type IX collagen in the extracellular matrix of cartilage: Type IX collagen is localized to intersections of collage fibrils. Journal of Cell Biology 102: 1931–1939.

Murray, P. D. F., and M. Smiles. 1965. Factors in the evocation of adventitious (secondary) cartilage in the chick embryo. Australian Journal of Zoology 13: 351–381.

Nakamura, H., and C. Ayer-Le Lièvre. 1982. Mesectodermal capabilities of the trunk neural crest in birds. Journal of Embryology and Experimental Morphology 70: 1–18.

Noden, D. M. 1975. An analysis of the migratory behaviour of avian cephalic neural crest cells. Developmental Biology 42: 106–130.

————. 1978. The control of avian cephalic neural crest cytodifferentiation. I. Skeletal and connective tissues. Developmental Biology 67: 296–312.

————. 1983. The role of the neural crest in patterning of avian cranial skeletal, connective, and muscle tissue. Developmental Biology 96: 296–312.

————. 1984. Craniofacial development: New views on old problems. Anatomical Records 208: 1–13.

————. 1986. Origins and patterning of craniofacial mesenchymal tissues. Journal of Craniofacial Genetics and Developmental Biology 2: 15–31.

————. 1988. Interactions and fates of avian craniofacial mesenchyme. Development 103 (suppl.): 121–140.

Pinto, C. B., and B. K. Hall. 1991. Towards an understanding of the epithelial requirement for osteogenesis in scleral mesenchyme of the embryonic chick. Journal of Experimental Zoology 259: 92–108.

Rizzino, A. 1988. Transforming growth factor-β: Multiple effects on cell differentiation and extracellular matrices. Developmental Biology 130: 411–422.

Rosen, D. M., S. A. Stempien, A. Y. Thompson, and S. M. Seyedin. 1988. Transforming growth factor-β modulates the expression of osteoblast and chondroblast phenotypes in vitro. Journal of Cellular Physiology 134: 337–346.

Rosen, V., and R. S. Thies. 1992. The BMP proteins in bone formation and repair. Trends in Genetics 8: 97–102.

Schowing, J. 1968. Mise en évidence du rôle inducteur de l'encephale dans l'ostéogenèse du crâne embryonnaire du poulet. Journal of Embryology and Experimental Morphology 75: 165–188.

Sellman, S. 1946. Some experiments on the determination of larval teeth in Ambystoma mexicanum. Odontologisk Tidskrift 54: 7–128.

Serbedziga, G. N., M. Bronner-Fraser, and S. E. Fraser. 1989. A vital dye analysis of the timing and pathways of avian trunk neural crest cell migration. Development 106: 809–816.

Smith, G. N., T. F. Linsenmayer, and D. A. Newsome. 1976. Synthesis of type II collagen in vitro by embryonic chick neural retina tissue. Proceedings of the National Academy of Science, U.S.A. 73: 4420–4423.

Smith, L., and P. Thorogood. 1983. Transfilter studies on the mechanism of epithelio-mesenchymal interaction leading to chondrogenic differentiation of neural crest cells. Journal of Embryology and Experimental Morphology 75: 165–188.

Smith, M. M., and B. K. Hall. 1990. Development and evolutionary origins of vertebrate skeletogenic and odontogenic tissues. Biological Reviews 65: 277–373.

Stent, G. S. 1985. The role of cell lineage in development. Philosophical Transactions of the Royal Society of London, ser. B, 312: 3–19.

Stone, L. S. 1929. Experiments showing the role of migrating neural crest (mesectoderm) in the formation of the head skeleton and loose connective tissue in Rana palustris. Wilehlm Roux' Archiv für Entwicklungsmechanik der Organismen 118: 40–77.

————. 1932. Transplantation of hyobranchial mesentoderm, including the right lateral anlage of the second basibranchium, in *Ambylstoma punctatum*. Journal of Experimental Zoology 62: 109–123.

Swalla, B. J., W. A. Upholt, and M. Solursh. 1988. Analysis of type II collagen RNA localization in chick wing buds by *in situ* hybridization. Developmental Biology 125: 51–58.

Thompson, D'Arcy. 1942. *On Growth and Form*. 2d ed. Cambridge: Cambridge University Press.

Thorogood, P. 1979. *In vitro* studies on the skeletogenic potential of membrane bone periosteal cells. Journal of Embryology and Experimental Morphology 54: 185–207.

————. 1983. Morphogenesis of cartilage. In *Cartilage,* vol. 2, B. K. Hall, ed. New York: Academic Press, pp. 223–254.

————. 1987. Mechanisms of morphogenetic specification in skull development. In *Mesenchymal-Epithelial Interactions in Neural Development,* J. R. Wolff, J. Sievers, and M. Berry, eds. Berlin: Springer-Verlag, pp. 141–152.

————. 1988. The developmental specification of the vertebrate skull. Development 103 (suppl.): 141–153.

————. 1991. The development of the telost fin and implications for our understanding of tetrapod limb evolution. In *Developmental Patterning of the Vertebrate Limb,* J. R. Hinchliffe, J. M. Hurle, and D. Summerbell, eds. New York: Plenum Publishing Corporation, pp. 347–354.

Thorogood, P., J. Bee, and K. Von Der Mark. 1986. Transient expression of collagen type II at epitheliomesenchymal interfaces during morphogenesis of the cartilaginous neurocranium. Developmental Biology 116: 497–509.

Thorogood, P., and J. Hanken. 1992. Body building exercises. Current Biology 2: 83–85.

Thorogood, P., and L. Smith. 1984. Neural crest cells: The role of extracellular matrix in their differentiation and migration. In *Matrices and Cell Differentiation,* R. B. Kemp and J. R. Hinchliffe, eds. New York: A. R. Liss, pp. 171–185.

Thorogood, P., L. C. Smith, A. Nichol, R. McGinty, and D. Garrod. 1982. Effects of vitamin A on the behaviour of migratory neural crest cells *in vitro*. Journal of Cell Science 51: 331–350.

Tyler, M. 1983. Development of the frontal bone and cranial meninges in the embryo chick: An experimental study of tissue interactions. Anatomical Records 206: 61–70.

Tyler, M. S., and B. K. Hall. 1977. Epithelial influences on skeletogenesis in the mandible of the embryonic chick. Anatomical Records 188: 229–240.

Vasan, N. S. 1987. Somite chondrogenesis: The role of the microenvironment. Cell Differentiation 21: 147–159.

Von Der Mark, K., J. Mollenauer, M. Pfaffle, M. Van Menxel, and P. K. Muller. 1986. Role of Anchorin CII in the interaction of chondrocytes with extracellular collagen. In *Articular Cartilage Biochemistry,* K. Kuettner, ed. New York: Raven Press, pp. 125–141.

Wagner, G. 1949. Die Bedeutung der Neuralleiste für die kopfgestaltung der Amphibienlarven. Revue suisse de zoologie 56: 519–620.

————. 1955. Chimaerische Zahnlagen aus *Triton-Schmelzorgan* und *Bombina-tor*-Papille. Journal of Embryology and Experimental Morphology 3: 160–188.

Watt, F. M., and J. Dudhia. 1988. Prolonged expression of differentiated phenotype by chondrocytes cultured at low density on a composite substrate of collagen and agarose that restricts cell spreading. Differentiation 38: 140–147.

Weiss, P., and R. Amprino. 1940. The effect of mechanical stress on the differentiation of scleral cartilage *in vitro* and in the embryo. Growth 4: 245–258.

Wessells, N. K. 1979. *Tissue Interactions and Development.* Menlo Park, Calif.: W. A. Benjamin.

Wilde, C. E. 1955. The urodele neuroepithelium in the differentiation *in vitro* of the cranial neural crest. Journal of Experimental Zoology 130: 573–591.

Wilkinson, D., S. Bhatt, M. Cook, E. Boncinelli, and R. Krumlauf. 1989. Segmental expression of *Hox-2* homeobox-containing genes in the developing mouse hindbrain. Nature 341: 405–409.

Wood, A., D. E. Ashhurst, A. Corbett, and P. Thorogood. 1991. The transient expression of type II collagen at tissue interfaces during mammalian craniofacial development. Development 111: 955–968.

Wozney, J. M., V. Rosen, M. Bryne, A. J. Celeste, I. Moutsatos, and E. A. Wang. 1990. Growth factors influencing bone development. Journal of Cell Science 13 (suppl.): 149–156.

Zanetti, M., A. Ratcliffe, and F. Watt. 1985. Two subpopulations of differentiated chondrocytes identified with a monoclonal antibody to keratan sulfate. Journal of Cell Biology 101: 53–59.

5

Epigenetic and Functional Influences on Skull Growth

Susan W. Herring

POINTS OF VIEW

Definitions

THIS CHAPTER ADDRESSES the problem of how the various parts of the skull achieve their characteristic sizes and shapes. Although the story has a beginning, at the point where early events such as pattern formation and cytodifferentiation have been completed, it has no end other than death, because vertebrate skulls never cease to change during life (Behrents 1985). Skeletal growth can be influenced in many ways by many factors; mechanical factors are among the best documented and will be emphasized in this review. Because the terms "epigenesis" and "function" have had a variety of definitions and a history of acrimonious debate as applied to the skull, I will start by giving my versions of these terms.

Epigenesis. Classically, the term "epigenetic" referred to the transformation of a homogeneous primordium into a differentiated organism, and epigenesis was an alternative to preformation (Rieppel 1986, 1987). More recently the concept has been repopularized by Løvtrup (e.g., 1981) with a different connotation, leading to some confusion. Løvtrup restricts epigenetics to the study of the mechanisms responsible for transforming a single cell to a complex adult. Since genes are DNA sequences, not mechanisms, this view of epigenetics is strictly nongenetic. Moreover, Løvtrup argues that genes which affect morphogenesis (regulatory genes) are few and have evolved little. This general definition and attitude have been adopted by most developmental biologists, but with individual variations. While some authors consider any stimulus that elicits a developmental process to be epigenetic (e.g., Hall 1983), others have made a distinction between stimuli that are external to the organism (environmental) and those that are internal (epigenetic) (e.g., van Limborgh 1972). However, it seems fruitless to make such a distinction in many cases. For example, the

153

stimuli that influence musculoskeletal growth are frequently mechanical in nature (Horder 1981), yet similar mechanical loads can arise either internally (pressures within an artery) or externally (reaction forces from locomotion). Thus, this essay will follow Hall in considering any stimulus with an effect on skull growth to be epigenetic.

Function. This seemingly simple word becomes confusing when applied to movements made by embryos and fetuses. Postnatally, the functional role of movements such as jaw opening and closing is clearly to accomplish feeding and other oral behaviors, but what do we call essentially identical movements in unborn animals, which (with the exception of some caecilians [Wake 1977]) do not feed? In this chapter I will take the broad view that even fetal movements are functional in the sense that they serve to develop coordination (Bekoff 1981) or to promote differentiation and growth (Murray and Drachman 1969; Herring and Lakars 1981), and I will call all muscular activity functional regardless of developmental stage. Viewed in this way, functional activity provides a source of epigenetic stimuli.

Function and the Skull: A Short History

Evolutionary or Physiological Adaptations. It is a truism in biology that form is matched to function. However, a fundamental dichotomy among morphologists concerns the interpretation of the match. To oversimplify the matter somewhat, the dichotomy parallels the problem with the word "adaptation," which can be construed either in an evolutionary context, implying that an inherited trait has been selected in a species, or in a physiological context, implying that a trait (not necessarily inherited) has been elicited by external stimuli during the life of an individual. For morphology, the equivalent concepts are "genetic" for evolutionary and "epigenetic" for physiological.

For example, take the familiar contrast between the mandibles of a mammalian herbivore such as a horse and a carnivore such as a dog (fig. 5.1). The herbivore has a large angular process, small coronoid process, and high condyle, while the carnivore has the reverse. The genetic-evolutionary interpretation, exemplified by the classic paper by Maynard Smith and Savage (1959), explicitly assumes that jaw geometry is a product of natural selection, and seeks a functional explanation in terms of the mechanics of feeding. Genes for, say, a large coronoid process are assumed to exist and to have been selected in order to give the temporalis muscle increased mechanical advantage in carnivores. In contrast, an epigenetic-physiological interpretation would explain the differences in the size of the angular and coronoid processes as being due to differences in the forces delivered by the attaching musculature, and the difference in condyle height as related to loading from reaction forces on the jaw joint. The only

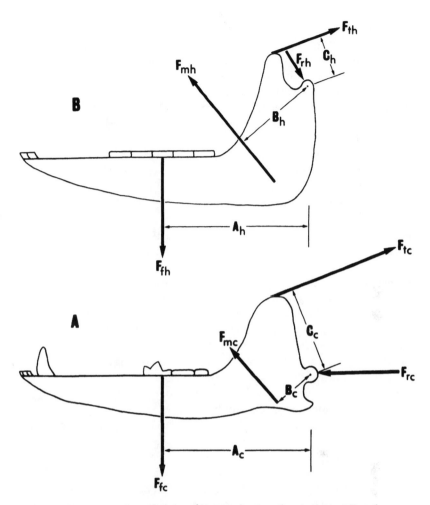

Fig. 5.1. Diagrammatic lateral views of jaw mechanics of a carnivore (A) and a herbivore (B). F_{mc} and F_{mh} represent the masseters in carnivore and herbivore, respectively, F_{tc} and F_{th} the temporalis muscles, and F_{fc} and F_{fh} the forces at the tooth row. A, B, and C are the moment arms for the bite force, masseter, and temporalis respectively. F_{rc} and F_{rh} show the reaction forces at the jaw joint. A genetic interpretation of the carnivore jaw is that natural selection produced the short condylar neck to provide mechanical advantage for the temporalis; an epigenetic interpretation would posit that the neck is short because large joint reaction forces reduced its growth. (From Scapino 1972, with permission)

"bone genes" involved would be those related to the response of osteoblasts to load, and these are presumed to have reached an evolutionarily
stable state somewhere at the base of vertebrate, or at least mammalian,
phylogeny; there would not have been any "bone evolution" when the
orders Carnivora or Perissodactyla arose. The question remains open as to
whether any nonbone genes (e.g., for relative muscle size) would be involved or whether the phenomenon could be purely epigenetic (e.g., differential muscle usage patterns stemming from a different diet).

Both the genetic and epigenetic interpretations are functional in the
sense that the mechanical functioning of the system dictates morphology,
but in the former function works indirectly through natural selection and
in the latter function is the immediate cause of morphology. Although the
alternatives are not mutually exclusive (indeed, Waddington's concept of
genetic assimilation [1962, 227] was intended as a fusion), in practice biologists tend to be either genetic or epigenetic in orientation.

Environmental, Genetic, and Epigenetic Views of the Skull. Historically,
the genetic and epigenetic interpretations have waxed and waned in popularity. As pointed out by Russell (1916), nineteenth-century American pa-
leontologists had a neo-Lamarckian orientation that was epigenetic in its
expression. For example, Cope (1888) explained the characteristic features
of rodent jaws as mechanical sequelae of the elongated incisors, which
were in turn attributed to continued use. Since the era of modern biology
began, however, no one has seriously considered that environmental influences alone could determine the final form of the skull—for one thing,
genetic information is required to synthesize collagen and other necessary
materials.

Although a broadened epigenetic view has remained current among
developmental biologists, morphologists abandoned it for a purely genetic
interpretation after the advent of the neo-Darwinian synthesis. A genetic
view assumes that all the necessary information is present in the genome
and thus is subject to evolutionary modification. Thus, studies on the vertebrate skull commonly assume explicitly or implicitly that each individual
feature is genetically determined (Bailey 1986) and the product of selection
(e.g., Nur and Hasson 1984; Thomason and Russell 1986).

Two recent developments have led to resurgence of interest in epigenetic regulation of skull morphology. First, heritability studies have shown
a substantial environmental component for variation in craniofacial characters (Atchley, this volume). Second, a wealth of experimental data has
demonstrated the ease of altering cranial form by such stimuli as colder
temperatures (Steegman and Platner 1968; Weaver and Ingram 1969;
Heath 1984), imposed loads (Smith 1981), experimental extirpations of
muscles (Pratt 1943; Avis 1959, 1961; Moore 1967, 1973; Schumacher et

al. 1979; but cf. Boyd et al. 1967), and dietary changes (Watt and Williams 1951; Moore 1965; Bouvier and Hylander 1981; Corruccini and Beecher 1982; Beecher et al. 1983). Thus, a completely genetic view appears to be untenable. Current opinion, although not uniform, stresses various combinations of genetic information and epigenetic instructions for determining skull growth. While these combinations are infinite, I will briefly discuss three theories that have attracted converts.

First, many workers believe that initial form of the skull is self-differentiating, that is, genetic, but that when function begins (usually assumed to occur after birth or hatching), epigenetic regulation takes over. Evidence for this view comes from experiments in which rat or mouse mandibular primordia are reported to develop normally as transplants or in organ culture (Baker 1941; Manson 1968; Glasstone 1971), as well as from the assumption that functional (here understood to mean mechanical) influences could not exist in early embryos. The evidence is weakened somewhat by an absence of quantification of the morphology of the transplants—experimental embryologists are notoriously tolerant of aberrant anatomical details as long as the specimen is alive and recognizable. Indeed, one report (Felts 1961) emphasizes the altered morphology of the transplants. Moreover, the absence of movement in young embryos does not imply a forceless environment—pressure, tension, and shear can result from differential tissue growth (Packard and Jacobson 1979; Tuckett and Morriss-Kay 1985), myoblast contractions (Grubić et al. 1983), and fibroblast activities (Harris et al. 1981, 1984; Stopak and Harris 1982). In older embryos and fetuses it is clear that movements analogous to postnatal movements occur with great frequency (reviewed by Hamburger 1973; Bekoff 1981; Herring 1985).

The second theory makes a distinction between tissues, rather than developmental stages. In a view popularized by Scott (1954), the growth of cranial cartilages is considered to be genetically determined, while that of the bones is epigenetically regulated by the cartilage, i.e., cartilage is the pacemaker for skeletal growth. Evidence for this view is supplied by the ability of some cranial cartilages to grow almost normally in vitro or as transplants (Dorenbos 1972; Rönning and Kylämarkula 1982; Copray 1986; but cf. Koski and Rönning 1969), implying an intrinsic regulation. Moreover, the servility of bone to external regulation is obvious (references above). In particular, in growth disorders that primarily affect cartilage, such as achondroplasia or acromegaly, bone growth closely matches that of cartilage, proving its lack of independence (Delaire and Precious 1987). The contrast of independent cartilage and subservient bone remains a valid one, but in the face of increasing evidence that the growth rate of cartilage can be altered by mechanical means (see below), this tissue can no longer be accepted as under simple genetic control.

The third theory of skull growth, the "functional matrix" hypothesis, is probably the best known, in part because of vigorous proselytism by Melvin Moss. As summarized by Moss in 1968, the hypothesis posits that, at least after their initial formation, the growth of skeletal units (whether cartilaginous or bony) is secondary to the growth of the functional matrix, or soft tissues and functioning spaces, in which the skeletal units are embedded. Two types of functional matrix are distinguished, a periosteal type in which soft tissues such as muscles act directly on skeletal units, and a capsular type in which a functioning space such as the pharyngeal cavity acts indirectly by causing a spatial translation of skeletal units. As a general statement, the functional matrix hypothesis has been well accepted, although there are continuing arguments over a few points, such as the role of cartilage growth and the mechanisms by which spaces can influence the skeleton (Johnston 1976; Behrents and Johnston 1984).

Caveats

It is logical to consider epigenetic mechanisms as initial hypotheses for explaining morphology. If the rules of development suffice to determine form, there is no need for recourse to more indirect explanations (although one still can investigate the genetic basis of the developmental rules). If, however, an epigenetic hypothesis can be rejected after experimental testing, then genetic hypotheses should be considered. In this chapter I will take the attitude that all the tissues in the skull can be epigenetically regulated, although the epigenetic rules may vary from one site to another and from time to time. I will give evidence for this view where it exists, but a few extrapolations and assumptions are unavoidable and will be mentioned here.

Species Differences. While there is an extensive literature on the regulation of skull growth in postnatal laboratory and domestic mammals, especially humans, and a moderate literature on chick embryos, few studies have dealt with fishes, amphibians, or reptiles, by far the majority of the vertebrate world. Thus, this review is necessarily biased toward mammals, although some differences among vertebrate groups clearly exist. For example, secondary cartilage, an epigenetically regulated tissue important for mandibular growth in mammals, is not found in heterothermic vertebrates (Hall and Hanken 1985; Irwin and Ferguson 1986). The acellular bone of many fishes can hardly be expected to remodel in response to various stimuli (Parenti 1986). Allometric changes in lizard limb bones differ from those in mammals (Peterson and Zernicke 1987). At the same time there are similarities. At least one teleost fish has a tissue analogous to secondary cartilage which contributes significantly to cranial growth (Huysseune and Verraes 1986; Huysseune et al. 1986). Correlations between ossification and developing muscles have been pointed out for a caecilian amphibian (Wake and Hanken 1982) and a lizard (Rieppel 1987) as well as for mammals (Spyropoulos 1977). Extirpation studies on the turtle *Chelydra* yield similar findings to those on chicks (Toerien 1965). Although the mechanisms of palate closure are different in alligators and mice, at least one (abnormal) response was common to both taxa in culture, the development of large cartilages (Ferguson et al. 1984). A high priority of future research should be to determine the generality of epigenetic relationships in the vertebrate skull.

Tissue Differences. In addition to the very different determinants of growth in bone and cartilage, each of these tissues has a number of subtypes. As will be reviewed below, secondary cartilages differ from primary cartilages under experimental conditions. Some reports have indicated that primary cartilages from different sites vary in their epigenetic responses (Koski and Rönning 1969). Transplants of osteoblasts from mouse calvaria result in bones structurally different from those induced by epiphyseal chondrocytes (Moskalewski et al. 1986). Embryonic regions are differentially sensitive to epigenetic regulation (Runner 1986). For purposes of this review, it is particularly important to ask whether there is anything special about cranial tissues. Much more work has been performed on long bones than on the skull, and it would be helpful to be able to extrapolate. I will assume that cranial tissues have at least qualitatively similar reactions to those of histologically identical postcranial tissues, but since cranial tissues often come from unusual sources (e.g., neural crest), this assumption may turn out to be false.

Age Changes. Tissues change with age. In the postnatal period alone, dramatic alterations in cellularity, extracellular matrix, and growth potential occur (condylar cartilage: Silbermann and Livne 1979; McNamara et al. 1982; Hinton and McNamara 1984a; temporal bone: Hinton and Mc Namara 1984b; periosteum: Chong et al. 1982). The changes during embryonic and fetal periods must be at least as large. Most in vitro studies have been carried out on fetal or neonatal material, and conclusions drawn from them may not be valid for other ages.

Epigenetic Conversion versus Modulation. Epigenetic regulation of morphology may take the form of conversion, in which an epigenetic cue activates an alternate genetic pathway and results in a qualitatively different morph. Alternatively, the regulation may be one of modulation, where different levels of epigenetic cues elicit different degrees of expression of some phenotype (Smith-Gill 1983). The epigenetic and functional influences discussed here are of the modulation category. However, instances of apparent conversion for vertebrate heads have been reported in fish, amphibians, and reptiles, although in no case is the mechanism clear. Greenwood's (1965) suggestion that differing morphology of the pharyngeal jaws in cichlid fish could be the epigenetic result of dietary differences has been supported and extended to other structures by more recent work (Witte 1984; Hoogerhoud 1986; Meyer 1987). In tiger salamanders, a cannibal morph with broadened head and enlarged vomerine teeth occurs as a response to population density (Collins and Cheek 1983; Collins and Holomuzki 1984). Among reptiles, Legler (1981) has reported a striking remodeling of the skull ("megacephaly") in individuals of the freshwater turtle *Emydura,* which he has hypothesized to be a response to the ingestion of mollusks by these individuals. Other vertebrate skull morphs appear to be genetic rather than environmentally induced, although epigenetic amplification magnifies the genetic differences (Sage and Selander 1975; Liem and Kaufman 1984).

Nature of the Stimulus. Innumerable factors are known to affect skeletal growth and are therefore epigenetic under the broad definition used here. These include factors with a general effect on the skeletal system as a whole (circulating hormones, metabolic rate) and factors with very local effects (blood supply, mechanical stress). In many cases the factors involved are unknown and may be general, local, or both. For example, bill length and other morphological characters in red-winged blackbirds show nongenetic location-specific differences, but how the environment accomplishes these modifications is unknown (James 1983). Similarly, cranial proportions are altered in mammals reared under cold conditions (Heath 1984) or under nutritional deficiencies (Pucciarelli 1981), but the factors involved are a matter of speculation only. At present these "black box" examples of epigenetic influences on skull growth remain obscure, and this review will concentrate on cases in which the epigenetic factors can be at least tentatively identified. Most attention will be given to mechanical factors, because (1) the biological role of the skeleton is largely a mechanical one, (2) growth changes in the skeleton are thought to be mechanically adaptive (e.g., Wolff's well-known law that the shape of bone is determined by function [Wolff 1892]), and (3) the literature on mechanical influences is more extensive than for other epigenetic factors.

PRIMARY CARTILAGE

Initial Formation and Growth

Primary cartilages important in skull growth are derived from the chondrocranium (cranial base, nasal septum) and from the splanchnocranium

(Meckel's cartilage). While comparatively little experimental work has been performed on the growth of cranial primary cartilages, most studies have indicated that the chondrocranial derivatives perform similarly to long bone cartilages in the sense that when explanted or transplanted they continue to grow at rates comparable to, although usually less than, in vivo rates (Charlier and Petrovic 1967; Dorenbos 1972; Rönning and Kylämarkula 1982; Copray 1986). Presumably, then, the regulatory factors are the same.

Primary cartilages grow interstitially by cell proliferation and the synthesis of extracellular matrix. Appositional growth also occurs as chondrogenesis by the perichondrium. This can be thought of as a differentiation event, since the cells of the perichondrium are also capable of differentiating into osteoblasts (Meikle 1975).

Because differentiation is part of cartilage growth, any agent that affects chondrogenesis also affects growth. Epigenetic factors involved in the differentiation of primary cartilages have been discussed by Hall (1978, 1984b), Archer et al. (1982), Hinchliffe and Johnson (1983), Hunter and Caplan (1983), and Thorogood (this volume), among others. Briefly, chondrogenesis is stimulated by low nicotinamide and high cAMP levels, low vascularity and oxygen tension, and any feature, chemical or mechanical, that leads to cell aggregation or rounding (Archer et al. 1982, 1985; Ede 1983; Hunter and Caplan 1983; Solursh 1983). Small alternating electrical currents have been found to inhibit chondrogenesis (Archer and Ratcliffe 1983). The mechanism of action of all these epigenetic factors may be the same; Hunter and Caplan (1983) have suggested that cellular NAD level is important in the final common pathway. These factors are all local in nature and could lead to differential growth of various cartilages.

Primary cartilage growth is stimulated postnatally by growth hormone, which may increase the number of cells producing local growth factors, thus stimulating clonal expansion of proliferating chondrocytes (Nilsson et al. 1986). Many other hormones influence cartilage growth, either directly or indirectly through metabolic effects (reviewed by Hinchliffe and Johnson 1983; Silbermann 1983; Hintz 1985). In theory, not all primary cartilages may be equally exposed to circulating hormones, because they have little or no direct blood supply and there may be local variation in diffusion. Cartilages may also differ in hormone receptivity. In practice, most workers assume that endocrine factors are systemic. Thus, hormones are considered unlikely to provide explanations for differential growth of cartilages (for examples see Hinchliffe and Johnson 1983, 273), although they may be very pertinent to intra- or interspecific differences in skull form (Hanken and Hall 1986, 1988).

On the basis of isolated blastemata forming normally in organ culture (Murray 1936), it has been claimed that the growth pattern of individual cartilages is "determined" by the time the prechondrogenic condensations are formed (Hinchliffe and Johnson 1983). Richman and Diewert (1988) found different fates for different portions of cultured rat Meckel's cartilage, for example. The "determination" refers to gross qualitative rather than quantitative aspects of form. As figured by Murray (1936, 15), chick long bones grafted onto the chorioallantoic membrane do indeed have heads despite the absence of articulations, but these heads are far from normal in either size or shape (see also Thorogood 1983). Additionally, the qualitative "determinations" might be epigenetic events that took place before the blastemata were removed. Archer et al. (1985) were able to alter cartilage morphogenesis in culture by varying cell density at innoculation and the relative amount of prechondrogenic mesenchyme. Moreover, even after removal the explants and grafts are not totally deprived of environmental features that might have an epigenetic effect. For example, in a number of studies (but not that of Richman and Diewert) the explants retained their perichondria; the periosteum is thought to have a major influence on growth rate of endochondral bones prenatally (Amprino 1985) and postnatally (Rodríguez et al. 1985), even when transplanted (Feik and Storey 1983).

Mechanical Effects

Numerous studies have addressed the growth of primary cartilage under various loading conditions. Normally, most cartilages appear to be under net compression. In vivo the sources of compressive force include the periosteum, muscle and ligament action, and body weight. Apparent exceptions to the general rule of compressive loading are the so-called traction epiphyses where muscles attach, for instance the femoral trochanters, and sesamoid cartilages within tendons (for a discussion of traction epiphyses in the skull, see Cave 1965). However, Oxnard's (1971) analysis of the patella (a sesamoid bone) suggests that these apparent exceptions may not be under net tension after all. In fact, efforts to place cartilages under net tension have resulted in cessation of growth and replacement of the cartilage by fibrous tissue (Heřt 1969; reviewed by Bonnel et al. 1984). A possible mechanism for this shift may relate to the positive electrical charge developed by stretched collagen fibrils; charge may control proteoglycan synthesis by adjacent cells (Gillard et al. 1979).

In contrast to its poor performance under tension, primary cartilage continues to grow well under a wide range of compressive loadings, although extremely high pressure causes destruction (Goodship et al. 1979; reviewed by Bonnel et al. 1984). However, a number of experimental approaches have suggested that longitudinal growth rate and the magnitude of the force are inversely related and that even normal compressive loads retard the intrinsic growth rate of the tissue. "Distracting" forces applied directly to long bone anlagen or growth plates either intermittently (Smith and Cunningham 1957) or continuously (Heřt 1969; Amprino 1985; Fjeld and Steen 1988; Wilson-MacDonald et al. 1990) resulted in at least temporary acceleration of growth at the adjacent growth plate. Similar findings have been reported for distraction of the callus in surgically injured bone (Kojimoto et al. 1988). At least part of the growth was due to enlargement of the cells, particularly along the axis of distraction (Smith and Cunningham 1957; Storey and Feik 1985), and Heřt (1969, 200) reported that the cartilages were "more active" as well. Similar results (acceleration, at least in the short term) have been achieved by circumferential sectioning of the periosteum. This procedure is thought to reduce the continuous compressive stress placed on bones by their stretched periosteal envelopes (Crilly 1972; Warrell and Taylor 1979; McLain and Vig 1983; Wilson-MacDonald et al. 1990). Extirpation of the upper beak, which removes one source of compression on the lower beak, results in elongation of Meckel's cartilage in chicks (Wouterlood and van Pelt 1979). One contrary report, suggesting that increased intermittent compression caused by bipedalism in rats leads to increased rather than decreased growth (Simon 1978), has recently been challenged (Kay and Condon 1987). Frost (1986, vol. 2) has suggested a more complex model, as yet unsupported by quantitative data, in which cartilage growth is increased either by higher or lower levels of compression, depending on the initial level.

In contrast to longitudinal growth, transverse growth of primary cartilages is increased by higher levels of long-axis compression (short of destructive levels, of course) and decreased by lower levels. Thus, transplants growing in the cerebral or other body cavities, freed from functional compressive loads, are often much thinner than normal even though their lengths are unaffected (Meikle 1975; Feik and Storey 1983). In Meikle's study the reduction in diameter was due to a decrease in proliferation as well as differentiation of perichondrial cells into osteoblasts rather than chondroblasts. Another possible example of unloading leading to cartilage thinning may be the reduction in the ridging of the elastic cartilage of the rat auricle after paralysis of the ear muscles (Chiu et al. 1979). Thickening of cartilage after increased compression has been shown by Amprino (1985), among others. In vitro intermittent compressive forces result in larger chondroblasts that secrete more matrix than unloaded controls (Veldhuijzen et al. 1987). Sah and Grodzinsky (1989) and Sah et al. (1989) have found that static compression tends to decrease matrix synthesis, while higher frequencies of compressive cycles increase synthesis. However, matrix production is not necessarily a good predictor of cartilage growth, which is primarily a function of cell proliferation and especially cell shape modeling (Hunziker and Schenk 1989).

Summarizing, primary cartilages do not survive under tensile loads or extreme compressive loads but will grow under varying degrees of pressure. Both intermittent and continuous loads are probably effective, although not to the same degree. In general, higher levels of compression lead to shorter, fatter cartilages and lower levels lead to longer, thinner cartilages. In vivo, most cartilages may be under intermediate loads, since experimental manipulation can produce changes in both directions. The transducer for mechanical signals is not known, although the monocilium of the chondrocyte has been proposed (Stockwell 1987).

Nasal Septum and Cranial Base. Growth at the nasal septum and cranial base is usually thought of in terms of primary cartilage, even though bony resorption and apposition are prominent phenomena on the endocranial and ectocranial surfaces of the base (Björk and Kuroda 1968).

Alterations in cranial base morphology as a result of achondroplasia (Delaire and Precious 1987), population variation (Kean and Houghton 1982), or surgical interference (DuBrul and Laskin 1961) are known to trigger many secondary changes in cranial form. Because primary cartilage growth was for so long believed to be immutably determined by genetic factors, functional effects on the cranial base itself were not looked for. However, continued research has yielded many examples of epigenetic changes in cranial base growth. Flattening of the base can be produced in humans by modifying head posture (Björk 1972), and alterations also occur in rats with amputated forelimbs (Fanghänel 1972). A causal connection between the descent of the hyolaryngeal apparatus and the development of cranial flexion in children has been suggested by Laitman et al. (1978).

Loading of the adult cranial base is probably mainly compression due to weight of the braincase and its contents (Demes 1985). Thus the situation is analogous to the compression of primary cartilages generally. However, the rapid expansion of the brain during growth may provide a tensile component that partially unloads the cartilaginous elements or, later in life, the synchondroses (Moss 1976). By exerting pressure on all of the endocranial surfaces (thus presumably causing net resorption; see below), the brain may be thought of as preserving the containerlike form. The brain does seem to be a major influence on the prenatal growth of the cranial base. Anencephalic human babies show such an increase in angulation that the cranial base presents a strongly convex, rather than slightly concave, surface to the braincase (Fields et al. 1978). The amount of cartilage is greater in both anencephalics and microcephalics than in normal babies (Melsen and Melsen 1980), possibly reflecting unloading. Ossification of the cranial base was reported by Melsen and Melsen to be retarded (1980) but by Fields et al. to be accelerated (1978 and literature cited). In a review of literature on changes produced experimentally by altering the neural contents, Moss (1976) associated reductions in brain size with decreases in synchondrosis length, and enlargements of the cranial contents with increases. These results support the concept of cranial base growth as a function of mechanical unloading from the growth of the brain in fetal and very young mammals (but for a jaundiced view, see Johnston 1976).

SECONDARY CARTILAGE AND THE MANDIBULAR CONDYLE

Evocation

Secondary cartilage is a tissue of particular interest to a consideration of functional influences on skull growth, since "[it] *only* differentiates in response to mechanical stimulation, and often from progenitor cells which would otherwise have differentiated into osteoblasts and formed bone" (Hall 1984a, 156; for another opinion see Beresford 1981, 33). Factors contributing to the differentiation of secondary cartilage have been reviewed by Hall (1978) and Beresford (1981); even though the tissue may not be homologous in birds and mammals (Hall 1984a), its properties are similar in the two classes.

Eight secondary cartilage sites in the developing chick skull were described by Murray (1963). All but one were articulations, and three were described as making substantial contributions to the prenatal growth of the skull. Posthatching, the cartilages are replaced by bone or fibrocartilage (Hall 1968). Absence of movement almost totally prevents the development of these cartilages (Murray and Smiles 1965). In Murray's view, pressure was the most likely mechanical evocator of secondary cartilage. The mechanism by which pressure would cause differentiation into secondary cartilage is unknown and could conceivably be the same as that responsible for primary cartilage differentiation.

In mammals secondary cartilages are associated with many cranial bones, sutures, and both upper and lower alveolar processes (for a list, see Beresford 1981, 26). The locations of secondary cartilage are for the most part either articulations or muscle attachments, suggesting that their differentiation is also due to mechanical stimulation. Only the mandibular condyle is considered a major growth site, although the cartilage of the mandibular angle probably is also important in prenatal rodent growth (Vilmann 1982). The vast majority of the literature addresses only the mandibular condyle.

Unlike the chick, immobilized mouse embryos and explants do develop secondary cartilage (Glasstone 1971; Herring and Lakars 1981). This evidence has been used to argue against the mechanical origin of secondary cartilage (Beresford 1981). However, such a conclusion is premature since, as mentioned above, the absence of gross movement does not imply an absence of force. Interestingly, a major difference between chick and rodent development is the timing of embryonic motility (Narayanan et al. 1971). In rats oral movements begin at day 16 (Angulo y Gonzalez 1932), while the condylar cartilage is well differentiated only one day later (Cunat et al. 1956). Chicks, which have a similar gestation period, show active oral movements by day 5 of incubation (Freeman and Vince 1974, 271), well before the secondary cartilages first appear at day 11 (Murray 1963).

Unlike primary cartilage, transplanted condylar cartilage is not maintained in the absence of functional loading. Young rat condyles transplanted intracerebrally reverted to osteogenesis (Meikle 1973). Transplantation to a functional environment preserves chondrogenesis, however (Engelsma et al. 1980).

Growth of Secondary Cartilage

Epigenetic controls on condylar cartilage growth are generally similar to those on primary cartilage growth, except that the condylar cartilage appears to be much more sensitive to both hormonal (Petrovic et al. 1975; Silbermann 1983, 337) and mechanical regulation. The growth pressure of rat condyles in culture is far less than that of primary cartilages (Copray et al. 1985d). In humans reduction of function is associated with diminished growth of the condyles (Larheim and Haanaes 1981), and absence of normal loading may lead to small abnormal condyles that are soon resorbed (Herring et al. 1979). Differences in masticatory behavior are thought to account for the spatial and temporal differences in condylar dimensions of various human populations (Hinton 1981; Hinton and Carlson 1979). Other secondary cartilages are similarly sensitive to functional changes (e.g., Hinton 1988).

Studies on experimental animals have yielded more specific information on the nature of the mechanical effects. Like primary cartilage, secondary cartilages are normally loaded under net compression. Procedures designed to increase compression reduce longitudinal growth and increase transverse growth; these procedures have included retractive forces on the mandible (Petrovic et al. 1975; Asano 1986) and surgical interference with protrusion, such as experimental microglossia (Simard-Savoie and Lamorlette 1976) and sectioning the lateral pterygoid muscle (Petrovic et al. 1975; but cf. Goret-Nicaise et al. 1983). A reduction in condylar cartilage thickness occurs in rats when incisor function is lost; Simon (1977) attributed this change to a decrease in compressive loads (contrary to the interpretation of compressive effects here), but a repeat of the study with an additional control by Hinton and Carlson (1986) suggests that this procedure actually increases compression because the animals protrude their jaws less.

Conversely, experiments designed to relieve compression at the temporomandibular joint by protruding or lowering the mandible result in increased longitudinal growth (McNamara and Bryan 1987; Buchner 1982; but cf. Tewson et al. 1988). In rats such treatments are effective even in adult animals (Lindsay 1977), whereas in monkeys the adaptive potential diminishes with age (Hinton and McNamara 1984a). Procedures that alter the position of the condyle in the fossa can change its shape, possibly by directing mesenchymal cells toward either chondrogenesis or osteogenesis (Kantomaa 1986b; Kantomaa and Hall 1988).

By analogy with primary cartilage growth, pressure-relieving conditions would be expected to result in more slender condyles. In cases where major masticatory muscles (the presumed source of normal compression) are paralyzed (Herring and Lakars 1981) or detached (Ghafari and Heeley 1982), the diameters of the condylar and angular cartilages are indeed greatly reduced (fig. 5.2).

A reasonable proportion of experiments intended to alter condylar or mandibular growth are uninterpretable mechanically. These include sectioning of the periosteum (Rönning and Koski 1974; McLain et al. 1982; Koski et al. 1985) and sectioning (Ghafari and Heeley 1982) or denervating (Sato et al. 1986) masticatory muscles. These studies altered the direction more than the magnitude of condylar growth. Moreover, short-term and long-term responses differ (Koski et al. 1985). The confusion probably arises from our ignorance of normal loads on the condyle and our very profound ignorance of how these loads are altered by experimental manipulation.

The complexity of the in vivo situation makes it unlikely that quantitative assessment of the epigenetic responses of the condylar cartilage will be accomplished in the near future. However, a series of elegant in vitro studies has been carried out by Copray and his colleagues (1985a, b, c, d). These workers devised a system allowing rat cartilages to be cultured under a variety of intermittent and continuous compressive loads. Under low continuous forces the condyle grew at the same rate as unloaded controls, but at forces over 3 g growth ceased. Intermittent compression slowed growth somewhat, but the condyles were able to continue growing until the force reached 8 g. All compressive regimes resulted in slight width increases and prevented the loose arrangement of prechondroblasts seen in the controls (Copray et al. 1985c). Proliferative and synthetic activity were not affected in parallel; low continuous force stimulated proliferation but depressed matrix synthesis, while low intermittent force had the opposite effect (Copray et al. 1985b). As in the case of primary cartilage, however, the relevance of proliferation and matrix synthesis to growth is moot, because cell enlargement accounts for most of condylar growth in vivo (Luder et al. 1988). Copray et al. (1985c) suggest that the continuous low

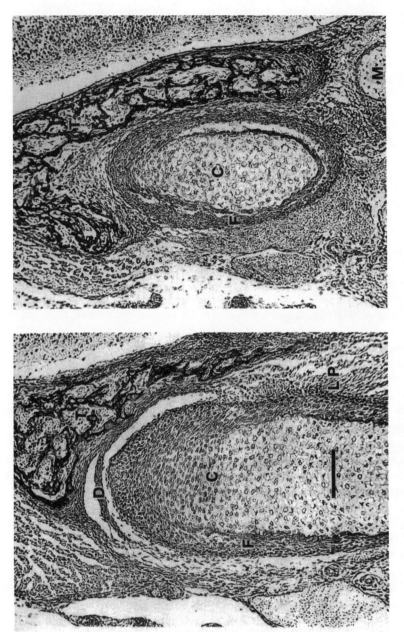

Fig. 5.2. Coronal sections through the jaw joints of normal (left) and paralyzed (*muscular dysgenesis*) 18-day mouse fetuses. In the paralyzed mutant, note the reduced width of the condylar cartilage and the absence of a joint space and intra-articular disc. C, condylar cartilage; D, disc (normal only); F, perichondrium; Lp, lateral pterygoid (visible in normal only); M, Meckel's cartilage (visible in mutant only); T, temporal bone. The bar represents 0.1 mm. (From Herring and Lakars 1981)

compression resembles the resting in vivo condition and establishes a basic growth rate, while intermittent forces during function regulate and reduce the growth rate. The fundamental similarity of these findings to in vivo observations provides a comforting validation of the latter.

Thus, in vitro and in vivo results are consistent in showing that mechanical loads affect the condylar cartilage in roughly the same ways they affect primary cartilage. More heavily loaded condyles become short and fat, less heavily loaded condyles are long and thin. As in the case of primary cartilage, however, the mechanisms by which the loads induce changes in cellular activity are not known. Suggestions include modifying the diffusion of nutrients (Copray et al. 1985b) or oxygen tension (Kantomaa 1986a), regulation of intracellular sodium ion concentration (Petrovic 1982), and stimulation of membrane-bound enzymes (Copray et al. 1985b).

BONE

A special problem with bone is whether the factors involved in evoking membranous and endochondral bone are the same. Hall (1970) has reviewed evidence that cartilage and bone arise from common germinal cells, suggesting that a general resemblance is to be expected. Nevertheless, the cells maturing in a limb bone have a different developmental history than those in the braincase, and this different history may be responsible for the somewhat different results when cells from the two regions are transplanted (Moskalewski et al. 1986). The majority of experimental work concerns long bones of endochondral origin, but the majority of the skull consists of membranously ossified elements. Moskalewski et al. (1989) have found that although transplanted scapular and calvarial osteoblasts formed differently shaped bones, the transplants responded similarly to mechanical support. In the absence of evidence to the contrary, this review will assume that all bone tissue behaves similarly in response to epigenetic stimuli.

Osteogenesis

The factors involved in triggering osteogenesis have been discussed by Hall (1970). They include increased vascularity and oxygen tension as well as mechanical stress. It was Murray's (1936) opinion that while mechanical loading might account for the magnitude and direction of bone growth, the initiation of bone formation was not under mechanical control. The matter still cannot be considered settled. Two examples have attracted recent attention, the formation of bone around the cartilaginous models of long bones and the initiation of centers of ossification in the bones of the braincase.

Using chick embryo long bones, Pechak et al. (1986a, b) have postulated that osteoprogenitor cells form as early as chondroprogenitor cells, so bone differentiation is not likely to be a response to mechanical loading, even though mineralization may be. Osdoby and Caplan (1979, 1981) reached the same conclusion on the basis of tissue culture studies. More recently, however, Caplan (1991) has pointed out that the differentiation of mesenchymal stem cells into either cartilage or bone can be manipulated by altering the seeding density of cell cultures. This is clearly an epigenetic, if not necessarily mechanical, effect. Further, Carter et al. (1987) have proposed that the appearance and extension of primary and secondary ossification sites are accelerated by shear stresses but can be prevented or inhibited by intermittent hydrostatic pressure, which maintains the cartilaginous anlagen instead.

A number of early workers, such as Thoma and Kokott (reviewed by Murray 1936) constructed elaborate theories relating the initiation of ossification centers to high stresses originating directly from growth of the brain or indirectly from stretching the fibrous tracts of the dura mater. A more recent version has been put forth by Blechschmidt (1976). Murray himself and most later workers have rejected this notion because some or all of the dermal elements can be found even in anencephalic fetuses (de Beer 1937; Garol et al. 1978). However, increased intracranial volume (e.g., in hydrocephaly) can lead to the formation of sutural bones, which represent extra, mechanically induced ossification centers (de Beer 1937). Sutural bones are also induced by cranial deformation in southwest Indians (Gottlieb 1978) and by neural tube abnormalities in both humans (Pryles and Khan 1979) and mice (Johnson 1976). Thus, brain growth and its mechanical consequences are not the proximate causes of ossification of the dermal bones, but abnormalities do lead to the formation of additional ossification centers.

Bone Growth

There seems to be general agreement that once bone is established, growth is epigenetically regulated. In addition to the mechanical environment, and not always independent of it, hormonal and metabolic factors are important, especially those concerned with calcium regulation (Wronski and Morey 1982; Hintz 1985; Soskolne et al. 1986; Bertram and Swartz 1991). Local factors include prostaglandin synthesis (Yeh and Rodan 1984) and electrical effects (Bassett 1972; Chakkalakal and Johnson 1981; Pollack 1984; Krukowski et al. 1990), both of which are in part associated with mechanical events. The orientation of newly laid-down bone is determined by the orientation of the blood vessels in both endochondral and membranous bones (Pechak et al. 1986b), but the orientation of the vessels is in turn a response to mechanical conditions (Murray 1936; Warrell and Taylor 1979).

Views on precisely how mechanical loads affect bone growth are divided into the belief that the matter is simple and straightforward and the belief that the matter is too complex to be resolved. A contributing cause of confusion is, as before, ignorance of normal and experimental loading patterns. Situations which are mechanically simple give simple results, but there are not very many of these. Three matters in particular need discussion: (1) whether growth and remodeling are the same phenomenon; (2) whether continuous loads can trigger a response or whether only intermittent loads are effective; and (3) the relationship of compressive, tensile, and shear forces to the magnitude and direction of the response.

Growth versus Remodeling. Frost (1983) has distinguished among *growth,* which is strictly size increase, *modeling,* which is the shaping of tissues during growth, and *remodeling,* which is tissue turnover. The process of interest here is modeling. Remodeling involves an obligatory but not always coordinated coupling between bone resorption and formation (Frost 1983). While related to mechanical usage (Frost 1987), remodeling is primarily important for mineral homeostasis (Currey 1984b) and is found only to a limited extent in heterothermic vertebrates (Enlow 1969; Ricqles 174; Throckmorton 1979). The formation aspect of remodeling is probably functionally similar to that of modeling in that it is mechanically adaptive (Lanyon et al. 1982; Currey 1984b; Burr et al. 1989).

Intermittent or Continuous Loading. Murray (1936) has summarized early debate on this issue. Initially, the notion that intermittent and continuous loads had different effects seems to have come from the observation that continuous pressure, for example from the contents of the cranial cavity or from blood vessels, is associated with resorption, so that these structures leave impressions or grooves on bony surfaces. On the contrary, intermittent compression from cyclic functions such as locomotion or mastication is associated with apposition of bone. Actually, this contrast is based on an inaccurate premise; the loads are not comparable. In the continuous-load models, simple compressive forces are applied directly to the periosteal surface of the bones. During cyclic activity bones are loaded in complex combinations of bending and torsion, not simple compression. Moreover, the cyclic compressive loads are delivered through the mediation of articular cartilage, and the compression is directed along the long axis of the bone. In the continuous model, resorption takes place along the lines of compression, whereas in the cyclic model apposition is observed along the shaft, perpendicular to the lines of compression.

More modern statements of the argument compare similar loads delivered either intermittently or continuously. A variety of experiments have suggested that although dynamic bending loads stimulate bone modeling, similar loads that are static have a much smaller effect (Chamay and Tschantz 1972) or no effect at all (Lanyon and Rubin 1984). These results have been thought to bear out the importance of electrokinetic signals in triggering osteogenesis, since these are necessarily dynamic in nature (Pollack 1984).

Opposed to this view are another group of workers who find that remodeling is readily elicited in bones continuously loaded under compression (Meade et al. 1984) or bending (Storey and Feik 1985). These authors also point to electrical phenomena as supporting their position, in this case the bioelectric currents from blood flow, cell membranes, and injured tissue (Rubinacci and Tessari 1983; Borgens 1984).

A reasonable compromise position at the moment is that continuous loads can produce bone remodeling, but not as effectively (in terms of both threshold and magnitude of response) as intermittent loads.

Compression, Tension, and Shear. Probably the one most striking need in the area of functional influences on bone growth is to characterize the real loading regimes of skeletal elements. Computer models have been invaluable in showing broad views of strain distribution (e.g., Carter et al. 1987), but of necessity they must ignore almost all local effects and make many assumptions about applied forces. In vivo studies of strain (e.g., Lanyon et al. 1979) remedy these deficiencies but give information only about very limited areas under a small range of functions. Given our ignorance about the real strain histories of bones, it is no wonder that there is no agreement about how specific loads correspond with specific responses.

An additional complicating factor is that, although all bone is thought to respond to strain, not all sites respond to the same strain levels. Rubin and Lanyon (1987) resort to the catchall notion that various locations have different genetic programming, a concept which is not helpful in the context of an organism whose cells all have the same genome. Frost (1987) has expressed roughly the same notion in a form which is operationally useful, by pointing out that both the "setpoint" and the response of the system will be modified by many mechanical and nonmechanical, systemic and local (i.e., epigenetic) effects.

The history of research on bone adaptation includes many attempts at simple mechanical explanations, most successfully by Frost (1964, 1973). Currey, however, has argued forcefully that no simple model can produce an adaptive response under all conditions of loading and therefore unknown factors such as the nervous system must somehow modify the response (1968, 1984a, b). Bertram and Swartz (1991) have even suggested that many examples of mechanical adaptation may in fact be due to non-mechanical factors such as trauma. Indeed, the premise that all bone remodeling is mechanically adaptive is not universally true; Matsuda et al. (1986) have described a case in which the bones of exercised animals actually became weaker than those of controls. The reader is referred to these authors for their detailed analyses. For the present purpose, the empirical literature will be surveyed for broad patterns that may be heuristically applicable to skull growth.

In brief, it will be argued that the direction of periosteal bone growth is generally well predicted by the orientation of tensile strain, while resorption corresponds to the orientation of compressive strain. This hypothesis is actually an ancient once based on empirical observations to be summarized below. Wolff (1892) opposed the hypothesis, as have many authors subsequently, on the basis of counterexamples, especially the case of bent long bones, in which apposition occurs on the "compressive" concave surface. As mentioned above, this counterexample is inappropriate in that it fails to take into account that the apposition does not occur along the lines of compressive strain but at right angles to them. When a compressive load is applied along the axis of a bone, as in this case, the radial and tangential strains are tensile, not compressive. The relative amount of tensile strain is known as Poisson's ratio, which for bone is 30–40% of the longitudinal compressive strain (data compiled by Currey 1984b). The compressive load is applied only to the ends of the bone, which are protected from resorption by the cushioning of articular cartilage (in fact, the attachment of cartilage fibrils to the bone ends [Broom and Marra 1986] may provide a tensile force). Thus, a re-examination of this famous counterexample suggests that the general notion of periosteal cells responding to tension by osteogenesis and to compression by resorption may still be viable. Most available data support this concept.

In experimental systems it has been possible to put limited areas of bone under either direct compression or tension. As mentioned earlier, periosteal surfaces that are in line with continuous compressive forces are always resorptive, possibly via occlusion of the blood vessels (Rygh et al. 1986). The case for surfaces in line with intermittent compressive forces is not clear. Arteries that groove bones, such as the middle meningeal and facial in humans, were one of the cases cited above as examples of resorption caused by continuous force, but their pulsating flow might actually cause intermittent compression. If intermittent compression against a bony surface also causes resorption, this would explain why osteoarthritic joint surfaces (no longer protected by articular cartilage) are resorptive. (The osteophytes which typically form near arthritic joint surfaces are oriented radially, i.e., along lines of tension.)

Direct continuous tension has the opposite effect of causing osteogenesis in line with the tensile force. Linden (1986, 62) has proposed that cartilage proliferation controls bone formation by putting connective tissue fibers under tension to trigger directed osteogenesis. The direct effect of tension has been seen at muscle attachments placed under artificial tension (Yeager 1985), in the mandibular fossa when the posterior attachment of the articular disc is tensed by forward displacement (Hinton and McNamara 1984b), and in alveolar bone when the periodontal ligament is tensed by orthodontic tooth movement (Reitan and Kvam 1971; Rygh et al. 1986). These situations have one feature in common, the periosteum being pulled away from the bony surface, possibly with an increase or reorientation of blood supply. Since the inner layer of the periosteum is osteogenic, this pulling away may be the means by which tension induces apposition.

The periosteum can also be pulled away from the bony surface under static loading conditions that are not predominantly tensile. An example is the compensatory bone formation on the outer surface of alveolar bone being resorbed on the inner surface. Reitan and Kvam (1971) have suggested that the entire bony wall is deflected outward during application of force to the tooth. After resorption has created a space on the inner side, the wall tends to return to its original position. The periosteum, being the trailing edge for this rebound, would be pulled away from the bone. Another example is the osteogenesis that occurs on the concave side of long bones held in static bending (Narbaitz et al. 1983; Amprino 1985; Storey and Feik 1985); histological examination of these cases reveals that the periosteum is separated from the concave bone surface and fronds of new bone stretch out to it perpendicular to the shaft (fig. 5.3).

Intermittent loading situations, including normal function, usually involve complex and variable shearing stresses. Most experimental studies have not characterized the details of the resulting strain patterns, but simply document that strains are elevated from the control condition. There are a few exceptions, however. Keller and Spengler (1989) verified with strain gages that their running exercise regimen in rats did not alter the orientation of the principal strain and that consistent strain magnitudes were maintained by bone modeling. Swimming, a nonweightbearing activity which is assumed to alter strain orientation, does result in appropriate changes in rat long bone morphology (Simkin et al. 1989). A roughly linear relation between strain magnitude and amount of new bone has been noted (Rubin and Lanyon 1985). The pattern of bone growth is essentially the same as on the concave sides of bent bones mentioned above, radially oriented fronds which later are consolidated into compact bone. In experiments where artificial compressive loading causes naturally curved bones to bend, the fronds form on only part of the cross section of the bone. Chamay and Tschantz (1972) report specifically that fronds

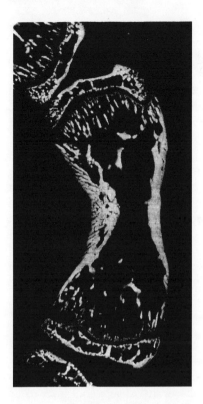

Fig. 5.3. Microradiograph of a caudal vertebra from a rat tail that had been bent into a sharp loop. Under the continuous compressive load on the concave side, trabeculae of new bone have formed at right angles to the shaft, along lines of tension. (From Storey and Feik 1985, with permission)

formed from the concave (compression) side, and this also seems likely in the studies of Rubin and Lanyon (1984) and Meade et al. (1984). This pattern is the same as that observed under continuous bending (fig. 5.3). Where natural (but increased) loading led to more uniform compression, fronds were formed all around the shaft of the bone (Goodship et al. 1979). As explained earlier, such apposition is along the lines of tension, perpendicular to the applied compressive load. It should be noted that these examples of periosteal apposition have been dismissed as pathological by Frost (1986, vol. 1); however, their consistency and predictability suggest a fundamental mechanism, although perhaps not the only one.

Although this discussion leaves in the dark the questions of how much strain suffices to start or stop bone formation and which processes are involved in later rearrangement of the bone, it does provide a crude guideline for where to expect apposition and resorption. A local area under tension, either directly from a pull on the periosteum or indirectly from a compressive load at right angles, should show apposition along the lines of tension. An area under direct compression should show resorption. These heuristic considerations are empirical correlations only, and do not address basic mechanisms such as electrical or metabolic effects.

The Braincase

De Beer (1937, 477) summarized evidence that the shape of the braincase was "to a large extent dependent on the volume of its contents." Thus, when growth in one dimension is constrained, compensatory increases are observed in other dimensions (Smit-Vis and Griffioen 1987).

At least in mammals, the initial growth of the neurocranial ossifications is radial, along the lines of tension created by the expanding brain. Murray pointed out (1936, 67) that it may be the blood vessels that are influenced by tension with the bony trabeculae merely following along. In anencephalic fetuses position and growth of the neurocranial bones are very abnormal; the radial arrangement is not found and growth is minimal (Garol et al. 1978). Thus tension seems to be required for normal growth. Until the bones meet to form sutures (see next section), tension from the brain and dural fiber tracts may be the dominant influence on neurocranial growth. Before adjacent bones make contact, in fact, compressive loading is physically difficult. The bones grow as simple sheets expanding at their edges.

Postnatally, while the brain is still growing rapidly, the neurocranial bones continue to grow primarily at their edges, now the sutural margins (Mednick and Washburn 1956; Duterloo and Enlow 1970). This has usually been interpreted as indicating that the brain capsule continues to be loaded in tension, especially because removal of the coronal suture in young rabbits actually accelerates separation of the bones (Babler et al. 1982; Alberius 1983). In fact, however, the loading of the braincase is debatable and has not been measured directly. The anatomy of the coronal suture area in rats has been used to buttress arguments of both tensile (Smith and McKeown 1974) and compressive (Prahl-Andersen 1968) stress environments. The apparent contradiction is unresolvable at present. The cited studies were inferential with regard to the actual loading on the skull and in any case refer only to static conditions along one axis. Actual loading could involve different strains anteroposteriorly and transversely along the skull and dynamic changes in direction and magnitude.

Later in development, sutural growth becomes negligible and apposition and resorption become the most important factors in skull growth and the final determination of cranial shape (Brash 1934). Compressive loads, including weight-bearing (reaction force from the occipital condyles) and bite force transmitted from the jaws, probably predominate in the walls of the braincase, except for the sagittal suture area where contraction of the temporalis causes tensile strain (Behrents et al. 1978). Compressive loads transmitted across the bones of the calvaria would be

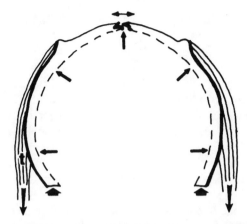

Fig. 5.4. Heuristic model of braincase loading and growth, shown on a diagrammatic coronal section. Except for the summit (around the sagittal suture), the braincase wall is presumed loaded in compression from the weight of the cranium and the pull of the temporalis muscles (t), resisted by the vertebral column. Compression along the axis of the bones would be expected to result in apposition on both endocranial and ectocranial surfaces (along the lines of tension). However, the endocranial surface is additionally subjected to radial compression from the expanding cranial contents. Thus, it shows net resorption. Axial tension at the sagittal suture leads to apposition at the sutural margins. Heavy lines: expected appositional surfaces; dashed lines: expected resorptive surfaces.

expected to lead to increased thickness of the neurocranium, with apposition occurring mainly on the outer surface of the skull, since intracranial pressure would discourage osteogenesis on the inner surface (fig. 5.4).

While not so well studied, it seems likely that the growth of other "volumetric" parts of the skull is similarly regulated by the enlargement of their contents (the capsular matrices of Moss, as mentioned above). For example, the studies of Tonneyck-Müller (e.g., 1976) show extensive disturbance of the orbits and related parts of the skull after enucleation of the eyes in chick embryos.

Cranial Sutures

The fibrous joints between the dermal bones of the skull have received a surprising amount of attention, perhaps because their accessibility makes them easy to study. In the context of this review, sutures are interesting in that both their morphology and their persistence are influenced by stress. While most studies have involved sutures of the braincase, those of the face presumably behave similarly.

Loading of Sutures. For the most part the loading environment of sutures is unknown, but the information available to date makes clear that tension

(Behrents et al. 1978), compression (Jaslow 1987), and bending with tension on one surface and compression on the other (Smith and Hylander 1985) can all occur during various activities at various sutures. Indeed, in the pig zygomatico-squamosal suture, compression and tension occur simultaneously in different parts of the suture, and the pattern reverses under certain loading conditions (Herring and Mucci 1991). The actual load on the bony margins of the sutures may not reflect skull loading; in particular, compressive loads may be borne by fibers, which transmit the load to bone as tension, just as compressive loads on teeth are resisted by tension in the periodontal ligament (Herring 1972). Age changes in the attachment and orientation of sutural fibers (Persson 1973) could thus have a major effect on stress transmission in the sutures. The occurrence of secondary cartilage in some sutures may indicate a true compressive load.

Kokich (1986) has reviewed evidence that experimental compression causes resorption at sutural edges, while tension enhances growth. For example, an orthodontic appliance putting retractive force on the maxilla of rhesus monkeys causes resorption at the zygomatico-frontal suture, which is normally an appositional surface; anterior displacement results in the development of bony spicules between the maxillary tuberosity and the palatine bone (Adams et al. 1972). The tensile stress is presumably delivered by suture-crossing fibers. Using a rat model, Koskinen (1977) noted a tendency for more apposition to occur at sutural sites with attaching fibers than in neighboring fiberless areas. In vitro work also indicates that tension stimulates the growth of sutural tissues, possibly by a general promotion of protein synthesis (Meikle et al. 1979, 1982). These findings appear to correspond with the general expectations for bone growth, apposition along lines of tension, and resorption along lines of direct compression. Although Meikle et al. (1982) suggested that growth of the suture under tension might be an indirect effect mediated by general metabolism, more recent work (Miyawaki and Forbes 1987; Southard and Forbes 1988; Wagemans et al. 1988) has shown a specific connective tissue response correlated to applied tension and related to osteogenesis.

Suture Morphology. Moss (1957) has classified sutures as butt-ended or beveled, straight or interdigitated. While the functional role of beveling may be to allow relative movement of skull bones (Moss 1957; Herring 1972; Oudhof and van Doorenmaalen 1983) or fast growth (Koskinen et al. 1976), compressive loads can transform butt-ended sutures into beveled sutures (Moss 1957) and increase the overlap of existing beveled sutures (Prahl-Andersen 1968); a possible natural example of the latter is the squamosal suture of *Australopithecus boisei* (Rak 1978). There seem to be no cases of beveled sutures becoming butt-ended.

Levels of interdigitation have been correlated with growth rates (Koskinen et al. 1976), the length of the growth period (Massler and Schour 1951), and cranial stress (Herring 1972). These factors are often difficult to separate. For example, when Washburn (1947) removed the temporalis of rats, he observed simpler sutures. Because this procedure reduces growth as well as stress, it is not clear which factor (if any of these) acted directly on sutural morphology. A few studies have suggested that stress alone suffices to increase interdigitation. For example, Gottlieb (1978) found the lambdoid sutures of cradleboard Indian skulls to be more complex than normal; cradleboarding should have little if any effect on braincase size (although the contribution of various bones might be altered) but probably creates unusual skull stresses.

The literature is devoid of experimental demonstrations that sutural complexity is epigenetically determined by skull loading. However, comparative studies have built a strong circumstantial case for the association of sutural complexity with patterns of loading. Jaslow (1989) studied sexual differences in sutural morphology in *Ovis orientalis,* a wild sheep species in which the males but not the females indulge in forceful horn clashing. Juvenile males and females did not differ. In adults, most facial sutures were similar, but most braincase sutures were more complex in males than in females, suggesting that complexity developed as a consequence of horn growth or usage. Intergeneric comparisons of pigs and peccaries (Herring 1972) indicated that generic differences in suture complexity were correlated with probable stress differences. For example, the sutures around the pterygoid bone were highly interdigitated in pigs, in which the bone forms part of the origin of the lateral pterygoid muscle. However, in peccaries the muscle does not impinge on the pterygoid bone and all of the pterygoid's sutures were simple. In addition, the pattern of interdigitation was found to reflect probable stress "trajectories." While some interdigitated sutures had complex spicule patterns capable of resisting forces from all directions, others were strongly oriented, often providing a mortise-and-tenon arrangement (fig. 5.5).

Synostosis. Finally, there has been debate on the factors responsible for fusion of the sutures. While the order of suture fusion is known for many mammals (the information is used for aging skulls), functional analyses are rare. Herring's (1972) comparison of pig and peccary genera implicated both growth patterns and differential stresses as determinants of suture closure. Almost everyone who has succeeded in inducing fusion experimentally has commented that immobility is a precondition (Hinrichson and Storey 1968; Engström et al. 1985, 1986), as is cessation of growth (Persson 1973; Smith and McKeown 1974); these phenomena are not necessarily independent, since mobility would be expected to stimulate growth by putting some or all of the suture under tension. Immobilization alone is

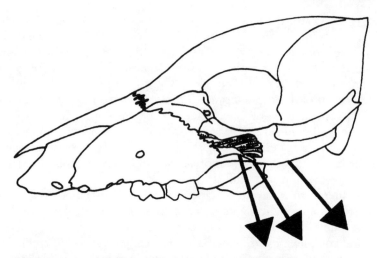

Fig. 5.5. Skull of a young domestic pig (*Sus scrofa*), showing some of the
interdigitations of the maxillary bone at the maxillo-jugal suture through a
transparent jugal bone. Ridges of the jugal surface sit in the valleys of the maxillary
surface. The masseter muscle (arrows) pulls inferiorly on the jugal, constituting a
compressive load which seats the ridges and valleys of the suture more firmly. The
load is presumably borne by intersutural fibers; the sutural borders themselves are
probably not under direct compression. (From Herring 1972)

apparently not sufficient to produce synostosis; experiments testing this
association have been confounded by an interaction between the periosteum and the glue used to hold the suture (Nappen and Kokich 1983).

Given that the suture must be relatively immobile, the factors involved
in synostosis are those which promote bony apposition. Within the suture
itself, fusion frequently begins as ossification along the transverse fibers
uniting the bones (Persson et al. 1978; Engström et al. 1985). Such fibers
are found (in humans and rats, at least) only after growth is essentially
complete (Persson 1973); this explains why synostosis requires cessation
of growth. Since fibers can transmit only tensile forces, the apposition is
along the lines of tension. Synostosis can also be initiated on the extracranial surface when the periosteum is distorted and pulled away from the
bone (Engström et al. 1985), just as in bent long bones (fig. 5.3). Moss
(1959) has argued that tension on the endocranial dural attachment surfaces, caused by abnormalities in the cranial base, can cause premature
synostosis in the human braincase.

Muscle Activity and the Jaws

Muscles are intimately associated with the skeleton, and muscle growth
and use are causally related to cranial growth even in invertebrates (Bernays 1986). Because the function of muscles is to produce force, it is easiest

to think about their effect on skeletal growth in mechanical terms. Nevertheless, it is important to point out the existence of other possible mechanisms. The vascular supply of bones is affected by muscle activity, directly because muscular arteries are a major source of that supply and indirectly because of volume and pressure changes during muscle contraction and movement. It is also conceivable that muscles might produce growth modulators for the skeleton, as local areas of the retina have been proposed to do for the sclera (Wallman et al. 1987).

Muscles as Forces. Muscles apply forces to skeletal elements in two ways. First, they pull directly on their attachment areas. Although this force is referred to as "tension," most muscles probably put complex loads on their attachment areas (Haskell et al. 1986; fig. 5.6A). While growth of the muscles seems intuitively to point to bone apposition, because of the tension applied and the teleological need for larger attachment surfaces, a muscle growing and functioning in an enclosed area such as the temporal fossa will actually result in compression and a resorptive surface (Hoyte 1971). A generalized version of this notion, called the "accommodational hypothesis," was suggested by Lanyon (1980) to account for the absence

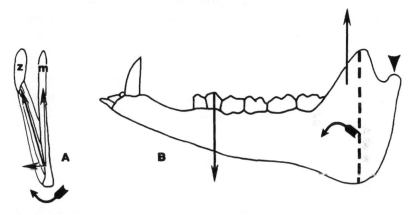

Fig. 5.6. A. Diagrammatic coronal section through the zygomatic arch (z), masseter muscle, and mandible (m) of a mammal at the level indicated by the dashed line in (B). The masseter's line of action is shown by the heavy arrow superimposed on the muscle; it runs from the insertion at the angular process of the mandible to the origin at the zygomatic arch. The line of action can be resolved (thin arrows) into a compressive load vertically up the ascending ramus of the mandible and a smaller, laterally directed tensile load. In addition, the muscle tends to evert the lower border of the mandible (curved arrow), compressing the lateral surface (left side) and tensing the medial surface (right side). B. Lateral view of a mandible, showing how the bite force, muscle pull, and reaction force apply three-point bending to the body of the bone. The upper surface will be under tension and the lower surface under compression. Because the muscles are lateral to the teeth, there will be torsion as well.

of normal tibial curvature after paralyzing the limb muscles. Muscles also pull on the periosteum, modifying the influence of the periosteum on growth plates (Dysart et al. 1989). The complexity of muscle loading on bone is presumably responsible for the lack of simple correspondence between muscle attachment and bone apposition. After a careful investigation of muscle attachment areas in rabbit skulls, Hoyte and Enlow (1966, 208) reported that areas of resorption and deposition could lie side by side, with "no seeming change in muscle relationships." Since as yet there are no measurements of bone strain at muscle attachments during function, the nature of loading at appositional or resorptive sites is unknown.

Second, during functional activities muscles cause bones to be loaded as beams or levers, with associated bending or torsion (fig. 5.6B). These overall loading patterns are better studied than the localized loads on inaccessible attachment areas. The literature abounds with theoretical treatments (e.g., Badoux 1968; Haskell et al. 1986), experimental analysis of models (e.g., Alexandridis et al. 1985; Demes 1985), and strain gauge recordings both in vitro (Endo 1966; Fisher et al. 1976) and in vivo (Weijs and de Jongh 1977; Hylander et al. 1987 and references therein).

Presumably, the influence of muscle action on skull growth is by the means of compressive and tensile strains as discussed above. Experimental studies have been necessarily indirect, and usually alterations in strain patterns are unknown. Various approaches, discussed below, have included comparing normal and paralyzed embryos, extirpating or denervating muscles, and changing the level of activity through altered diet or occlusion.

Developmental Studies. In mammals the ability of the palatal shelves to meet in the midline depends on the ability of the tongue to get out of their way, normally by flattening in the enlarging oral space (Wragg et al. 1972). Thus, paralysis, such as in the muscular dysgenetic mouse, is associated with clefting (Pai 1965; for a review see Carey et al. 1982). Even after closure of the shelves, the shape of the palate is molded by the tongue (Walker and Quarles 1976).

A general association between ossification of skull elements and their use in activities such as feeding and respiration has been noted in both fish (Weisel 1967) and mammals (Maier 1987). In particular for the muscles of mastication, a temporal correspondence between the appearance of muscle anlagen and their attachment areas has been noted in several groups. Wake and Hanken (1982) related the early ossification of the suspensorium in the caecilian *Dermophis* to the prenatal use of the jaws in feeding. In the lizard *Podarcis* Rieppel (1987) found that the coronoid bone ossified within the aponeurosis of the external adductor muscle. Most of the other cranial bones he studied ossified prior to the attachment of the jaw muscles, but the muscle anlagen were already present and probably exerting tissue forces. Similarly, in human fetuses the masseter and temporalis anlagen precede the ossification of their attachment areas, and the coronoid process differentiates within the temporalis, only later uniting with the mandible (Spyropoulos 1977).

There is also suggestive evidence that the rate of prenatal jaw growth is controlled in part by muscle activity. In mammals the jaw-opening musculature, which attaches to the lower but not the upper jaw, matures earlier than the jaw-closing musculature, which attaches to both lower and upper jaws (for a review, see Herring 1985). In both humans (Humphrey 1971) and hamsters (Lakars and Herring 1980) a growth spurt of the lower jaw accompanies the "quickening" of the openers and a later spurt of the upper jaw accompanies the "quickening" of the closers. Humphrey (1971) suggested that the mechanism was a vascular stimulation of bone growth, although of course other explanations are possible.

Paralysis and Dystrophies. Changes in cranial form have been reported after drug-induced paralysis in chick embryos (Murray and Drachman 1969) and in congenital paralysis of mice (Pai 1965; Herring and Lakars 1981). During the rapid growth in the embryonic period, the effects on the secondary cartilages are most marked; as mentioned above, in chicks the cartilages do not even form, and in mice their growth, particularly in width, is dramatically reduced. However, changes in osseous elements are also marked. Length of the bones is unaffected; in fact, the mandible of paralyzed chicks is actually longer than that of controls (Murray and Drachman 1969), presumably because of the overgrowth of the unloaded Meckel's cartilage (Wouterlood and Pelt 1979). However, like the cartilages, the bones are typically more slender than normal, reflecting the reduced loads.

The unchanging position of the paralyzed embryos causes distortions in the bones. An unusual curvature of the mandible in paralyzed mice was thought to be due to pressure from the shoulder (Herring and Lakars 1981), while in chicks the two sides of the jaw become asymmetrical (Hall and Herring 1990).

Movements mediated by embryonic and fetal muscles are necessary for the maturation of synovial joints. As is the case in the postcranial skeleton, cranial joints of paralyzed mice or chicks do not develop complete cavities or intra-articular discs (Murray and Drachman 1969; Herring and Lakars 1981; fig. 5.2). A particularly intriguing speculation is that embryonic movements cause the breakdown of Meckel's cartilage in mammalian ontogeny (Scott 1951), but no experimental evidence exists on this point.

Since paralysis of the jaw muscles does not allow survival, later changes cannot be studied. Interestingly, however, normal mice that are heterozygous for the gene causing paralysis (*muscular dysgenesis*) show asymmetry in mandibular muscle attachment areas, a developmental instability that may be related to variability in the muscles (Atchley et al. 1984). Another postnatal approach to a paralysis analogue is the investigation of mandibular growth in muscular dystrophies. A study by Vilmann et al. (1985) on various bones, including the mandible, of dystrophic mice showed that while absolute mandibular length was reduced compared to that in normal mice, mandibular length relative to the cube of body weight was greater than normal. Further, the dystrophic mandibles had disproportionately small condylar and angular processes. In humans myotonic muscular dystrophy is associated with narrowed jaws with anterior open bite and a high arched palate (Müller and Punt-van Manen 1982). In both mice and humans these changes are analogous, although not as severe, to those seen in paralyzed fetuses.

Alterations in Level of Function. Paralysis and muscular dystrophy presumably mimic disuse atrophy, producing overall reduction or even elimination of muscle forces. Reasoning that the most important loading of the mammalian skull occurs during mastication, a number of studies have attempted to reduce loading by feeding animals only soft food requiring minimal preparation. In rats such a diet leads to notable reductions in the size of the condylar surface (Bouvier and Zimny 1987) and the angular process (Watt and Williams 1951; Moore 1965) and decreases in the thickness of the mandible and breadth of the maxilla (Watt and Williams 1951), that is, essentially the same changes as in muscular dystrophy. Rhesus monkeys on a soft diet had relatively shallow mandibular bodies and low levels of remodeling in the mandible (Bouvier and Hylander 1981). Squirrel monkeys treated similarly had jaws comparable in length to hard-diet animals but greatly reduced breadths and a high arched palate (Beecher et al. 1983). Again, these findings are reminiscent of those in human muscular dystrophy.

Thus, reduction in muscle forces, whether due to defects in the muscles or to reduced use, has a consistent effect on skull morphology. The bones are little reduced in length, but they are slender and the viscerocranium as a whole is narrower than normal. Major muscle attachment areas are decreased in all dimensions. Since blood supply and innervation were intact in all of the examples cited, the mechanism would appear to be a direct muscular effect on bone growth.

The reverse experiment, stimulating cranial muscles to exert higher than usual forces on the skull, does not seem to have been performed. However, it is well known that hypertrophy of the masseter muscle in humans is associated with expansion and flaring of its attachment area, the angular process (Moss 1968). Moreover, a regimen of daily chewing of pine resin apparently changed the direction of facial growth in a group of children receiving orthodontic treatment (Ingervall and Bitsanis 1987).

Extirpations and Transpositions. A number of studies have attempted to elucidate the role of muscles in determining bone form by surgically removing them. Given the information presented above, it is clear that these studies are almost impossible to interpret. The removal of a jaw muscle not only deprives a bony surface of the mechanical and vascular inputs from the muscle, but also inevitably changes the masticatory stroke and thus the entire loading pattern on the skull. Since different species have different masticatory loadings, each will be changed in a different way. Thus it is no surprise that except for the direct effect on the attachment areas, there are few common features in the studies on muscle extirpations.

The temporalis has been partially removed in rats (Washburn 1947; Moss and Meehan 1970), guinea pigs (Boyd et al. 1967), cats (Avis 1959), and dogs and sheep (Schumacher et al. 1979). Except for the study of Boyd and coworkers, the results have included diminished size or loss of the coronoid process and the temporal ridges on the skull. The Boyd group attributed the absence of an effect to their maintenance of a good vascular supply and suggested that the reductions of growth were due less to the loss of muscle traction than to a damaged blood supply. This interpretation has in general not been accepted, and the study has been criticized, especially by Moss and Meehan (1970), for selecting an inappropriate animal (the guinea pig has a vanishingly small coronoid process). In several of the rat (Moss and Meehan 1970) and cat (Avis 1959) experiments the muscle was not completely severed; the diminished coronoid process was more vertically oriented than usual, a finding attributed to the vertical pull of the more intact deeper fibers of temporalis. These studies imply that the coronoid process grows in the direction of muscle pull, i.e., along the lines of tension applied by the temporalis.

Changes in more distant parts of the skull after temporalis removal have not been reported in detail. Schumacher et al. (1979) briefly discuss a dissertation from the Soviet Union (Nikitjuk 1961), in which unilateral resection of the temporalis of dogs resulted in decreased bone apposition but increased sutural growth on the "mechanically relieved side"; this suggests the typical long and thin development of an unloaded bone. Interestingly, the braincase is reported to be wider but shorter in rats after bilateral temporalectomy (Moore 1967). Such a phenomenon could result from decreased resorption in the temporal fossa in the absence of pressure from the contracting muscle, but without histological studies it is fruitless to speculate further, or even this far.

The masseter, with or without the medial pterygoid, has been removed in dogs and sheep (Schumacher et al. 1979), but most studies have involved rats (Pratt 1943; Avis 1961; Moore 1967, 1973). As expected, the greatest effect is on the angular process of the mandible; indeed when both muscles are removed unilaterally, there is no angular process (Avis

1961). Unlike the temporalis, these muscles should place their insertion area largely under compression, not tension (Herring and Lakars 1981; fig. 5.6). Therefore, the simplistic mechanical explanation propounded herein does not account for the failure of the angular process to enlarge. Epker and Frost (1966) have explained the changes in terms of their postulate that apposition occurs when surfaces are made more concave, as is the angle when the masseter and medial pterygoid contract.

Extirpation of the masseters has a far-reaching effect on the growing rat skull. One difficulty is that animals with bilateral surgery cannot eat standard rat pellets and must be fed soft diets, resulting in all of the changes reported above for reduction of function by a soft diet (Moore 1967, 1973). Beyond these changes, rats without masseters have buccally inclined teeth, lighter skulls that are especially reduced in their linear dimensions, and mandibles with reduced condylar processes (Moore 1967, 1973). Unilateral operations result in severe asymmetry and malocclusion, obscuring the specific effects of the myotomies (Pratt 1943; Avis 1961). In addition to the expected problems of interpretation, the concentration of these studies on rats makes them particularly difficult to extrapolate to other species because the rodent masticatory apparatus is highly specialized, particularly with regard to the morphology and function of the masseter.

Because of its putative importance in regulating growth of the condylar cartilage, several attempts have been made to sever the lateral pterygoid muscle, again using rats (Petrovic et al. 1975; Goret-Nicaise et al. 1983; Hinton 1990). Petrovic has argued that this muscle stimulates condylar growth by protruding, thereby unloading the condyle. Thus, traumatizing the muscle should reduce mandibular growth. His group has reported that sectioning the lateral pterygoid leads to reductions in cell division and cartilage differentiation, and that these effects can be reversed if appliances are used to protrude the jaw. However, Goret-Nicaise and colleagues (1983) have criticized the use of mitotic indices to assess growth, and suggest instead that the changes at the condyle following lateral pterygoid section are comparable to osteoarthritis. These workers found resorption at the anterior surface of the condylar process and increased growth at the posterior surface. This is an arrangement that might be expected to lead to increased, rather than decreased, elongation of the mandible as a whole. However, Hinton's results support the Petrovic group, and he has suggested that the findings of Goret-Nicaise et al. were related to their use of a unilateral surgical model. Since no study to date has examined changes in function or overall cranial growth, a full understanding of the role of the lateral pterygoid is not at hand.

A study on *Macaca nemestrina* (Hohl 1983) involved the transposition, rather than extirpation, of the masseter and temporalis. Both muscles

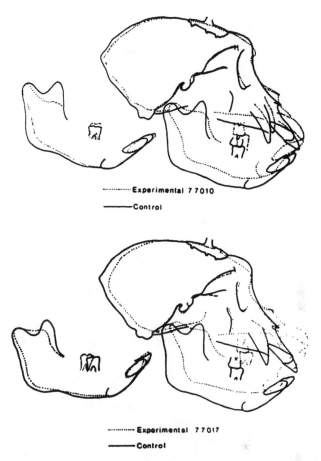

Fig. 5.7. Transpositions of masticatory muscles in rhesus macaques. Superimpositions of lateral cephalometric tracings of age- and sex-matched control and experimental animals. In the experimental monkeys the insertions of the masseters and temporalis muscles (with coronoid processes) had been moved postero-superiorly. Alteration of the muscle action lines was associated with more antero-superiorly directed facial growth than normal. As shown in the mandibular tracings to the left of each skull, the mandibles undergo minimal shape change other than the loss of the coronoid process. The notable difference in position of the mandible is secondary to the alteration in the shape of the middle face. (From Hohl 1983)

were moved to new locations that made their lines of action more anteriorly directed than before. Gross chewing patterns were found to be normal six weeks after surgery. While there were alterations in the attachment areas of the muscles, the most striking change was a reorientation of cranial growth such that the face became tilted up relative to the braincase (fig. 5.7). While still not mechanically interpretable in that neither the

changes in bone strain nor alterations in appositional or resorptive surfaces are known, this experiment is important in showing a major growth
effect as the result of an anatomical rather than functional muscle change.
That is, the reoriented muscles were used at levels and in patterns comparable to those of control monkeys, but their direction of pull was different. This situation may be a reasonable experimental approach to the
investigation of whether species-level variation in muscle anatomy can epigenetically lead to differences in cranial form.

SUMMARY AND PROSPECTUS

In the conflict between genetic and epigenetic interpretations of skull form,
this contribution has taken the side of epigenetics and attempted to show
how even major changes in morphology can be produced epigenetically by
mechanical loading. The rules governing the growth of cartilage and bone
in the skull appear to be the same as those which operate in the rest of the
skeleton.

Primary cartilages, including those of the cranial base and probably
Meckel's cartilage, require a compressive environment. Higher compressive loads result in shorter, wider cartilages, while reductions in load
produce long, thin elements. Secondary cartilages, represented by the mandibular condyle, respond similarly to mechanical stimuli but appear to be
more sensitive.

Although the responses of bone to mechanical stimuli have been long
debated, I argue that the direction of periosteal growth is well predicted
by the orientation of tensile stress, while resorption occurs at surfaces subjected to direct pressure. This heuristic model accounts for the thickening
of long bones under axial compression by noting that radial and tangential
strains under such conditions are tensile. Both the growth of primary cranial cartilages and the enlargement of capsular areas of the skull are regarded as possible tensile stimuli for the growth of the dermal bones of the
skull. Muscle function appears to have the general effect of causing compressive or bending loads, and thus decreased levels of muscle activity are
associated with skeletal elements that are of reasonably normal length but
reduced diameter. Unfortunately, many experimental studies attempting to
manipulate skull growth (e.g., myotomies and diet alterations) are not interpretable mechanically because neither the normal nor the altered strain
regime has been defined.

Although the epigenetic story of skull growth is reasonably coherent,
it is still very incomplete and some of the evidence is very sparse. Two areas
in particular need work urgently. First, the story is based almost entirely
on mammals, in fact mostly on laboratory rats with a smattering of other

domesticated species, notably humans. The scraps of information available for other vertebrates instill no confidence that the parameters of epigenetic response will be the same. The simple experiment of loading a long bone in a lizard to see where remodeling will take place has apparently never been performed. A primary need is to extend the range of species studied experimentally to include fishes, amphibians, and reptiles and birds other than the omnipresent chick embryo.

Second, an even more pressing problem is our ignorance of in vivo functioning of the skull. Almost all theories of skeletal modeling rely on mechanical loading, but in fact the normal loading of bones is unknown except for a very few systems which have been studied with in vivo strain gauges. Conjecture and untested computer models do not suffice; real data are necessary. Until the actual stresses in functioning bones are known, it will be impossible to evaluate the available hypotheses critically.

ACKNOWLEDGMENTS

I am grateful to Ken Gordon, Zane Muhl, Rick Sumner, and the editors for their helpful criticism of the manuscript, to Kurt Schwenk for telling me about the cannibalistic salamanders, and to F. Witte for introducing me to the cichlid literature.

REFERENCES

Adams, C. D., M. C. Meikle, K. W. Norwick, and D. L. Turpin. 1972. Dentofacial remodelling produced by intermaxillary forces in *Macaca mulatta*. Archives of Oral Biology 17: 1519–1535.

Alberius, P. 1983. Roentgen stereophotogrammetric analysis of cranial vault growth in rabbits. Ph.D. diss., University of Lund, Sweden.

Alexandridis, C., A. A. Caputo, and C. E. Thanos. 1985. Distribution of stresses in the human skull. Journal of Oral Rehabilitation 12: 499–507.

Amprino, R. 1985. The influence of stress and strain in the early development of shaft bones. Anatomy and Embryology 172: 49–60.

Angulo y Gonzalez, A. W. 1932. The prenatal development of behavior in the albino rat. Journal of Comparative Neurology 55: 395–442.

Archer, C. W., and N. A. Ratcliffe. 1983. The effects of pulsed magnetic fields on chick embryo cartilaginous skeletal rudiments in vitro. Journal of Experimental Zoology 225: 243–256.

Archer, C. W., N. A. Ratcliffe, and C. P. Cottrill. 1985. Cartilage morphogenesis in vitro. Journal of Embryology and Experimental Morphology 90: 33–48.

Archer, C. W., P. Rooney, and L. Wolpert. 1982. Cell shape and cartilage differentiation of early chick limb bud cells in culture. Cell Differentiation 11: 245–251.

Asano, T. 1986. The effects of mandibular retractive force on the growing rat mandible. *American Journal of Orthodontics and Dentofacial Orthopedics* 90: 464–474.

Atchley, W. R. 1993. Genetic and developmental aspects of variability in the mammalian mandible. In *The Skull*, vol. 1, J. Hanken and B. K. Hall, eds. Chicago: University of Chicago Press.

Atchley, W. R., S. W. Herring, B. Riska, and A. A. Plummer. 1984. Effects of the muscular dysgenesis gene on developmental stability in the mouse mandible. *Journal of Craniofacial Genetics and Developmental Biology* 4: 179–189.

Avis, V. 1959. The relation of the temporal muscle to the form of the coronoid process. *American Journal of Physical Anthropology* 17: 99–104.

———. 1961. The significance of the angle of the mandible: An experimental and comparative study. *American Journal of Physical Anthropology* 19: 55–61.

Babler, W. J., J. A. Persing, K. M. Persson, H. R. Winn, J. A. Jane, and G. T. Rodeheaver. 1982. Skull growth after coronal suturectomy, periostectomy, and dural transection. *Journal of Neurosurgery* 56: 529–535.

Badoux, D. M. 1968. Cremona diagrams of framed structures in the skull of *Canis familiaris* and *Sus scrofa scrofa*. *Proceedings Koninklijke Nederlandse Akadamie van Wetenschappen*, ser. C, 71: 229–244.

Bailey, D. W. 1986. Genes that affect morphogenesis of the murine mandible. *Journal of Heredity* 77: 17–25.

Baker, L. W. 1941. The influence of the formative dental organs on the growth of the bones of the face. *American Journal of Orthodontics* 27: 489–506.

Bassett, C. A. L. 1972. A biophysical approach to craniofacial morphogenesis. *Acta morphologica neerlando-scandinavica* 10: 71–86.

Beecher, R. M., R. S. Corruccini, and M. Freeman. 1983. Craniofacial correlates of dietary consistency in a nonhuman primate. *Journal of Craniofacial Genetics and Developmental Biology* 3: 193–202.

Behrents, R. G. 1985. *Growth in the Aging Craniofacial Skeleton*. Monograph 17, Craniofacial Growth Series. Ann Arbor: University of Michigan.

Behrents, R. G., D. S. Carlson, and T. Abdelnour. 1978. In vivo analysis of bone strain about the sagittal suture in *Macaca mulatta* during masticatory movements. *Journal of Dental Research* 57: 904–908.

Behrents, R. G., and L. E. Johnston, Jr. 1984. The influence of the trigeminal nerve on facial growth and development. *American Journal of Orthodontics* 85: 199–206.

Bekoff, A. 1981. Behavioral embryology of birds and mammals: Neuroembryological studies of the development of motor behavior. In *Behavioral Development*, K. Immelmann, G. W. Barlow, L. Petrinovich, and M. Main, eds. Cambridge: Cambridge University Press, pp. 152–163.

Beresford, W. A. 1981. *Chondroid Bone, Secondary Cartilage, and Metaplasia*. Baltimore: Urban and Schwarzenberg.

Bernays, E. A. 1986. Diet-induced head allometry among foliage-chewing insects and its importance for graminivores. *Science* 231: 495–497.

Bertram, J. E. A., and S. M. Swartz. 1991. The "law of bone transformation": A case of crying Wolff? *Biological Reviews* 66: 245–273.

Björk, A. 1972. The role of genetic and local environmental factors in normal and abnormal morphogenesis. Acta morphologica neerlando-scandinavica 10: 49–58.

Björk, A., and T. Kuroda. 1968. Congenital bilateral hypoplasia of the mandibular condyles associated with congenital bilateral palpebral ptosis. American Journal of Orthodontics 54: 584–600.

Blechschmidt, M. 1976. The biokinetics of the basicranium. In Development of the Basicranium, J. F. Bosma, ed. Bethesda, Md.: U.S. Department of Health, Education, and Welfare, pp. 44–53.

Bonnel, F., A. Dimeglio, P. Baldet, and P. Rabischong. 1984. Biomechanical activity of the growth plate. Anatomia clinica 6: 53–61.

Borgens, R. B. 1984. Endogenous ionic currents traverse intact and damaged bone. Science 225: 478–482.

Bouvier, M., and M. L. Zimny. 1987. Effects of mechanical loads on surface morphology of the condylar cartilage of the mandible in rats. Acta anatomica 129: 293–300.

Bouvier, M., and W. L. Hylander. 1981. Effect of bone strain on cortical bone structure in macaques (Macaca mulatta). Journal of Morphology 167: 1–12.

Boyd, T. G., W. A. Castelli, and D. F. Hvelke. 1967. Removal of the temporalis muscle from its origin: Effects on the size and shape of the coronoid process. Journal of Dental Research 46: 997–1001.

Brash, J. C. 1934. Some problems in the growth and developmental mechanics of bone. Edinburgh Medical Journal, 3d ser., 41: 305–387.

Broom, N. D., and D. L. Marra. 1986. Ultrastructural evidence for fibril-to-fibril associations in articular cartilage and their functional implication. Journal of Anatomy 146: 185–200.

Buchner, R. 1982. Induced growth of the mandibular condyle in the rat. Journal of Oral Rehabilitation 9: 7–22.

Burr, D. B., M. B. Schaffler, K. H. Yang, M. Lukoschek, N. Sivaneri, J. D. Blaha, and E. L. Radin. 1989. Skeletal change in response to altered strain environments: Is woven bone a response to elevated strain? Bone 10: 223–233.

Caplan, A. I. 1991. Mesenchymal stem cells. Journal of Orthopaedic Research 9: 641–650.

Carey, J. C., R. M. Fineman, and F. A. Ziter. 1982. The Robin sequence as a consequence of malformation, dysplasia, and neuromuscular syndromes. Journal of Pediatrics 101: 858–864.

Carter, D. R., T. E. Orr, D. P. Fyhrie, and D. J. Schurman. 1987. Influences of mechanical stress on prenatal and postnatal skeletal development. Clinical Orthopaedics 219: 237–250.

Cave, A. J. E. 1965. Traction epiphyses in the mammalian skull. Proceedings of the Zoological Society of London 145: 495–508.

Chakkalakal, D. A., and M. W. Johnson. 1981. Electrical properties of compact bone. Clinical Orthopaedics 161: 133–145.

Chamay, A., and P. Tschantz. 1972. Mechanical influences in bone remodeling: Experimental research on Wolff's law. Journal of Biomechanics 5: 173–180.

Charlier, J. P., and A. Petrovic. 1967. Recherches sur la mandibule de rat en culture d'organes: Le cartilage condylien a-t-il potential de croissance indépendant? L'orthodontie française 38: 165–175.

Chiu, D. T., G. F. Crikelair, and M. L. Moss. 1979. Epigenetic regulation of the shape and position of the auricle in the rat. Plastic and Reconstructive Surgery 63: 411–417.

Chong, D. A., C. A. Evans, and J. D. Heeley. 1982. Morphology and maturation of the periosteum of the rat mandible. Archives of Oral Biology 27: 777–785.

Collins, J. P., and J. E. Cheek. 1983. Effect of food and density on development of typical and cannibalistic salamander larvae in *Ambystoma tigrinum nebulosum*. American Zoologist 23: 77–84.

Collins, J. P., and J. R. Holomuzki. 1984. Intraspecific variation in diet within and between trophic morphs in larval tiger salamanders (*Ambystoma tigrinum nebulosum*). Canadian Journal of Zoology 62: 168–174.

Cope, E. D. 1888. The mechanical origin of the dentition of the Rodentia. American Naturalist 22: 3–11.

Copray, J. C. V. M. 1986. Growth of the nasal septal cartilage of the rat in vitro. Journal of Anatomy 144: 99–111.

Copray, J. C. V. M., H. W. B. Jansen, and H. S. Duterloo. 1985a. Effect of compressive forces on phosphatase activity in mandibular condylar cartilage of the rat in vitro. Journal of Anatomy 140: 479–489.

———. 1985b. Effects of compressive forces on proliferation and matrix synthesis in mandibular condylar cartilage of the rat in vitro. Archives of Oral Biology 30: 299–304.

———. 1985c. An in-vitro system for studying the effect of variable compressive forces on the mandibular condylar cartilage of the rat. Archives of Oral Biology 30: 305–311.

———. 1985d. The role of biomechanical factors in mandibular condylar cartilage growth and remodeling in vitro. In *Developmental Aspects of Temporomandibular Joint Disorders*, D. S. Carlson, J. A. McNamara, and K. A. Ribbens, eds. Monograph 16, Craniofacial Growth Series. Ann Arbor: University of Michigan.

Corruccini, R. S., and R. M. Beecher. 1982. Occlusal variation related to soft diet in a nonhuman primate. Science 218: 74–76.

Crilly, R. G. 1972. Longitudinal overgrowth of chicken radius. Journal of Anatomy 112: 11–18.

Cunat, J. J., S. N. Bhaskar, and J. P. Weinmann. 1956. Development of the squamosomandibular articulation in the rat. Journal of Dental Research 35: 533–546.

Currey, J. D. 1968. The adaptation of bones to stress. Journal of Theoretical Biology 20: 91–106.

———. 1984a. Can strains give adequate information for adaptive bone remodeling? Calcified Tissue International 36: S118–S122.

———. 1984b. *The Mechanical Adaptations of Bones*. Princeton, N.J.: Princeton University Press.

de Beer, G. R. 1937. *The Development of the Vertebrate Skull*. London: Oxford University Press. Reprint. Chicago: University of Chicago Press, 1985.

Delaire, J., and D. Precious. 1987. Interaction of the development of the nasal septum, the nasal pyramid, and the face. International Journal of Pediatric Otorhinolaryngology 12: 311–326.

Demes, B. 1985. Biomechanics of the primate skull base. Advances in Anatomy, Embryology, and Cell Biology 94: 1–59.

Dorenbos, J. 1972. In vivo cerebral implantation of the anterior and posterior halves of the spheno-occipital synchondrosis in rats. Archives of Oral Biology 17: 1067–1072.

DuBrul, E. L., and D. M. Laskin. 1961. Preadaptive potentialities of the mammalian skull. American Journal of Anatomy 109: 117–132.

Duterloo, H. S., and D. H. Enlow. 1970. A comparative study of cranial growth in *Homo* and *Macaca*. American Journal of Anatomy 127: 357–368.

Dysart, P. S., E. M. Harkness, and G. P. Herbison. 1989. Growth of the humerus after denervation: An experimental study in the rat. Journal of Anatomy 167: 147–159.

Ede, D. A. 1983. Cellular condensations and chondrogenesis. In *Cartilage*, vol. 2, B. K. Hall, ed. New York: Academic Press, pp. 143–185.

Endo, B. 1966. Experimental studies on the mechanical significance of the form of the human facial skeleton. Journal of the Faculty of Science, University of Tokyo, sec. 5(3): 1–106.

Engelsma, S. O., H. W. B. Jansen, and H. S. Duterloo. 1980. An in-vivo transplantation study of growth of the mandibular condyle in a functional position in the rat. Archives of Oral Biology 25: 305–311.

Engström, C., S. Kiliaridis, and B. Thilander. 1985. Facial suture synostosis related to altered craniofacial bone remodelling induced by biomechanical forces and metabolic factors. In *Normal and Abnormal Bone Growth: Basic and Clinical Research*, A. D. Dixon and B. G. Sarnat, eds. New York: Alan R. Liss, pp. 379–391.

———. 1986. The relationship between masticatory function and craniofacial morphology. II. A histological study in the growing rat fed a soft diet. European Journal of Orthodontics 8: 271–279.

Enlow, D. H. 1969. The bone of reptiles. In *Biology of the Reptilia*, vol. 1A, C. Gans and A. d'A. Bellairs, eds. London: Academic Press, pp. 45–80.

Epker, B. N., and H. M. Frost. 1966. Biomechanical control of bone growth and development: A histologic and tetracycline study. Journal of Dental Research 45: 364–371.

Fanghänel, J. 1972. The influence of statics on the maxillo-mandibular apparatus. In *Morphology of the Maxillo-Mandibular Apparatus*, G.-H. Schumacher, ed. Leipzig: Thieme, pp. 59–64.

Feik, S. A., and E. Storey. 1983. Remodelling of bone and bones: Growth of normal and transplanted caudal vertebrae. Journal of Anatomy 136: 1–14.

Felts, W. J. L. 1961. In vivo implantation as a technique in skeletal biology. International Review of Cytology 12: 243–302.

Ferguson, M. W. J., L. S. Honig, and H. C. Slavkin. 1984. Differentiation of cultured palatal shelves from alligator, chick, and mouse embryos. Anatomical Record 209: 231–249.

Fields, H. W., Jr., L. Metzner, J. D. Garol, and V. G. Kokich. 1978. The craniofacial skeleton in anencephalic human fetuses. I. Cranial floor. Teratology 17: 57–66.

Fisher, J. L., K. Godfrey, and R. I. Stephens. 1976. Experimental strain analysis of infant, adolescent, and adult miniature swine skulls subjected to simulated mastication forces. Journal of Biomechanics 9: 333–338.

Fjeld, T. O., and H. Steen. 1988. Limb lengthening by low rate epiphyseal distraction: An experimental study in the caprine tibia. Journal of Orthopaedic Research 6: 360–368.

Freeman, B. M., and M. A. Vince. 1974. *Development of the Avian Embryo.* London: Chapman and Hall.

Frost, H. M. 1964. *The Laws of Bone Structure.* Springfield, Ill.: Charles C Thomas.

———. 1973. *Bone Modeling and Skeletal Modeling Errors.* Springfield, Ill.: Charles C Thomas.

———. 1983. The skeletal intermediary organization. Metabolic Bone Diseases and Related Research 4: 281–290.

———. 1986. *Intermediary Organization of the Skeleton.* 2 vols. Boca Raton, Fla.: CRC Press.

———. 1987. The mechanostat: A proposed pathogenic mechanism of osteoporoses and the bone mass effects of mechanical and nonmechanical agents. Bone and Mineral 2: 73–85.

Garol, J. D., H. W. Fields, Jr., L. Metzner, and V. G. Kokich. 1978. The craniofacial skeleton in anencephalic human fetuses. II. Calvarium. Teratology 17: 67–74.

Ghafari, J., and J. D. Heeley. 1982. Condylar adaptation to muscle alteration in the rat. Angle Orthodontist 52: 26–37.

Gillard, G. C., H. C. Reilly, P. G. Bell Booth, and M. H. Flint. 1979. The influence of mechanical forces on the glycosaminoglycan content of the rabbit flexor digitorum profundus tendon. Connective Tissue Research 7: 37–46.

Glasstone, S. 1971. Differentiation of the mouse embryonic mandible and squamomandibular joint in organ culture. Archives of Oral Biology 16: 723–729.

Goodship, A. E., L. E. Lanyon, and H. McFie. 1979. Functional adaptation of bone to increased stress. Journal of Bone and Joint Surgery 61-A: 539–546.

Goret-Nicaise, M., M. Awn, and A. Dhem. 1983. The morphological effects on the rat mandibular condyle of section of the lateral pterygoid muscle. European Journal of Orthodontics 5: 315–321.

Gottlieb, K. 1978. Artificial cranial deformation and the increased complexity of the lambdoid suture. American Journal of Physical Anthropology 48: 213–214.

Greenwood, P. H. 1965. Environmental effects on the pharyngeal mill of a cichlid fish, *Astatoreochromis alluandi,* and their taxonomic implications. Proceedings of the Linnean Society of London 176: 1–10.

Grubić, Z., V. M. Tennyson, H. W. Chang, and A. S. Penn. 1983. Cholinergic receptors are present in the myotome prior to innervation. Anatomical Record 205: 70A.

Hall, B. K. 1968. The fate of adventitious and embryonic articular cartilage in the skull of the common fowl, *Gallus domesticus* (Aves: Phasianidae). Australian Journal of Zoology 16: 795–805.

———. 1970. Cellular differentiation in skeletal tissues. Biological Reviews 45: 455–484.

———. 1978. *Developmental and Cellular Skeletal Biology.* New York: Academic Press.

———. 1983. Epigenetic control in development and evolution. In *Development and Evolution,* B. C. Goodwin, N. Holder, and C. G. Wylie, eds. Cambridge: Cambridge University Press, pp. 353–379.

———. 1984a. Developmental processes underlying the evolution of cartilage and bone. Symposium, Zoological Society of London 52: 155–176.

———. 1984b. Genetic and epigenetic control of connective tissues in the craniofacial structures. Birth Defects: Original Article Series 20 (3): 1–17.

———. 1986. The role of movement and tissue interactions in the development and growth of bone and secondary cartilage in the clavicle of the embryonic chick. Journal of Embryology and Experimental Morphology 93: 133–152.

Hall, B. K., and J. Hanken. 1985. Repair of fractured lower jaws in the spotted salamander: Do amphibians form secondary cartilage? Journal of Experimental Zoology 233: 359–368.

Hall, B. K., and S. W. Herring. 1990. Paralysis and growth of the musculoskeletal system in the embryonic chick. Journal of Morphology 206: 45–56.

Hamburger, V. 1973. Anatomical and physiological basis of embryonic motility in birds and mammals. In *Studies in the Development of Behavior and the Nervous System,* G. Gottlieb, ed. New York: Academic Press, pp. 51–76.

Hanken, J., and B. K. Hall. 1986. Endocrine control of cranial ossification in amphibians analyzed using hormone implants. American Zoologist 26: 93A.

———. 1988. Skull development during anuran metamorphosis. II. Role of the thyroid hormone in osteogenesis. Anatomy and Embryology 178: 219–227.

Harris, A. K., D. Stopak, and P. Warner. 1984. Generation of spatially periodic patterns by a mechanical instability: A mechanical alternative to the Turing model. Journal of Embryology and Experimental Morphology 80: 1–20.

Harris, A. K., D. Stopak, and P. Wild. 1981. Fibroblast traction as a mechanism for collagen morphogenesis. Nature 290: 249–251.

Haskell, B., M. Day, and J. Tetz. 1986. Computer-aided modeling in the assessment of the biomechanical determinants of diverse skeletal patterns. American Journal of Orthodontics 89: 363–382.

Heath, M. E. 1984. The effects of rearing-temperature on body conformation and organ size in young pigs. Comparative Biochemistry and Physiology 77B: 63–72.

Herring, S. W. 1972. Sutures: A tool in functional cranial analysis. Acta anatomica 83: 222–247.

———. 1985. The ontogeny of mammalian mastication. American Zoologist 25: 339–349.

Herring, S. W., and T. C. Lakars. 1981. Craniofacial development in the absence of muscle contraction. Journal of Craniofacial Genetics and Developmental Biology 1: 341–357.

Herring, S. W., and R. J. Mucci. 1991. In vivo strain in cranial sutures: The zygomatic arch. Journal of Morphology 207: 225–239.

Herring, S. W., U. F. Rowlatt, and S. Pruzansky. 1979. Anatomical abnormalities in mandibulofacial dysostosis. American Journal of Medical Genetics 3: 225–259.

Heřt, J. 1969. Acceleration of the growth after decrease of load on epiphyseal plates by means of spring distractors. Folia morphologica (Prague) 17: 194–203.

Hinchliffe, J. R., and D. R. Johnson. 1983. Growth of cartilage. In Cartilage, vol. 2, B. K. Hall, ed. New York: Academic Press, pp. 255–295.

Hinrichsen, G. J., and E. Storey. 1968. The effect of force on bone and bones. Angle Orthodontist 38: 155–165.

Hinton, R. J. 1981. Form and function in the temporomandibular joint. In Craniofacial Biology, D. S. Carlson, ed. Monograph 10, Craniofacial Growth Series. Ann Arbor: University of Michigan, pp. 37–60.

———. 1988. Response of the intermaxillary suture cartilage to alterations in masticatory function. Anatomical Record 220: 376–387.

———. 1990. Myotomy of the lateral pterygoid muscle and condylar cartilage growth. European Journal of Orthodontics 12: 370–379.

Hinton, R. J., and D. S. Carlson. 1979. Temporal changes in human temporomandibular joint size and shape. American Journal of Physical Anthropology 50: 325–334.

———. 1986. Response of the mandibular joint to loss of incisal function in the rat. Acta anatomica 125: 145–151.

Hinton, R. J., and J. A. McNamara, Jr. 1984a. Effect of age on the adaptive response of the adult temporomandibular joint. Angle Orthodontist 54: 154–162.

———. 1984b. Temporal bone adaptations in response to protrusive function in juvenile and young adult rhesus monkeys (Macaca mulatta). European Journal of Orthodontics 6: 155–174.

Hintz, R. L. 1985. Control mechanisms of prenatal bone growth. In Normal and Abnormal Bone Growth: Basic and Clinical Research, A. D. Dixon and B. G. Sarnat, eds. New York: Alan R. Liss, pp. 25–34.

Hohl, T. H. 1983. Masticatory muscle transposition in primates: Effects on craniofacial growth. Journal of Maxillo-Facial Surgery 11: 149–156.

Hoogerhoud, R. J. C. 1986. Ecological Morphology of Some Cichlid Fishes. Thesis, Rijksuniversiteit Leiden, chap. 3, pp. 75–90.

Horder, T. J. 1981. On not throwing the baby out with the bath water. In Evolution Today, G. G. E. Scudder and J. L. Reveal, eds. Pittsburgh: Carnegie-Mellon University, pp. 163–180.

Hoyte, D. A. N. 1971. Mechanisms of growth in the cranial vault and base. Journal of Dental Research 50: 1447–1461.

Hoyte, D. A. N., and D. H. Enlow. 1966. Wolff's law and the problem of muscle attachment on resorptive surfaces of bone. American Journal of Physical Anthropology 24: 205–214.

Humphrey, T. 1971. Development of oral and facial motor mechanisms in human fetuses and their relation to craniofacial growth. Journal of Dental Research 50: 1428–1441.

Hunter, S. J., and A. I. Caplan. 1983. Control of cartilage differentiation. In Cartilage, vol. 2, B. K. Hall, ed. New York: Academic Press, pp. 87–119.

Hunziker, E. B., and R. K. Schenk. 1989. Physiological mechanisms adopted by chondrocytes in regulating longitudinal bone growth in rats. Journal of Physiology 414: 55–71.

Huysseune, A., W. Vanden Berghe, and W. Verraes. 1986. The contribution of chondroid bone in the growth of the parasphenoid bone of a cichlid fish as studied by oblique computer-aided reconstructions. Biologische Jahrbuch Dodonaea 54: 131–141.

Huysseune, A., and W. Verraes. 1986. Chondroid bone on the upper pharyngeal jaws and neurocranial base in the adult fish Astatotilapia elegans. American Journal of Anatomy 177: 527–535.

Hylander, W. L., K. R. Johnson, and A. W. Crompton. 1987. Loading patterns and jaw movements during mastication in Macaca fascicularis: A bone-strain, electromyographic, and cineradiographic analysis. American Journal of Physical Anthropology 72: 287–314.

Ingervall, B., and E. Bitsanis. 1987. A pilot study of the effect of masticatory muscle training on facial growth in long-face children. European Journal of Orthodontics 9: 15–23.

Irwin, C. R., and M. W. J. Ferguson. 1986. Fracture repair of reptilian dermal bones: Can reptiles form secondary cartilage? Journal of Anatomy 146: 53–64.

James, F. C. 1983. Environmental component of morphological differentiation in birds. Science 221: 184–186.

Jaslow, C. R. 1987. A functional analysis of skull design in the Caprini. Ph.D. diss., University of Chicago.

———. 1989. Sexual dimorphism of cranial suture complexity in wild sheep (Ovis orientalis). Zoological Journal of the Linnean Society 95: 273–284.

Johnson, D. R. 1976. The interfrontal bone and mutant genes in the mouse. Journal of Anatomy 121: 507–513.

Johnston, L. E., Jr. 1976. The functional matrix hypothesis: Reflections in a jaundiced eye. In Factors Affecting the Growth of the Midface, J. A. McNamara, Jr., ed. Monograph 6, Craniofacial Growth Series, Ann Arbor: University of Michigan, pp. 131–168.

Kantomaa, T. 1986a. The effect of increased oxygen tension on the growth of the mandibular condyle. Acta odontologica scandinavica 44: 307–312.

———. 1986b. New aspects of the histology of the mandibular condyle in the rat. Acta anatomica 126: 218–222.

Kantomaa, T., and B. K. Hall. 1988. Mechanism of adaptation in the mandibular condyle of the mouse. Acta anatomica 132: 114–119.

Kay, E. D., and K. Condon. 1987. Skeletal changes in the hindlimbs of bipedal rats. Anatomical Record 218: 1–4.

Kean, M. R., and P. Houghton. 1982. The Polynesian head: Growth and form. Journal of Anatomy 135: 423–435.

Keller, T. S., and D. M. Spengler. 1989. Regulation of bone stress and strain in the immature and mature rat femur. Journal of Biomechanics 22: 1115–1127.

Kojimoto, H., N. Yasui, T. Gato, S. Matsuda, and Y. Shimomura. 1988. Bone lengthening in rabbits by callus distraction. Journal of Bone and Joint Surgery [British] 70-B: 543–549.

Kokich, V. G. 1986. The biology of sutures. In Craniosynostosis: Diagnosis, Evaluation, and Management, M. M. Cohen, Jr., ed. New York: Raven Press, pp. 81–103.

Koski, K., and O. Rönning. 1969. Growth potential of subcutaneously transplanted cranial base synchondroses of the rat. Acta odontologica scandinavica 27: 343–357.

Koski, K., O. Rönning, and T. Nakamura. 1985. Periosteal control of mandibular condyle growth. In Normal and Abnormal Bone Growth: Basic and Clinical Research, A. D. Dixon and B. G. Sarnat, eds. New York: Alan R. Liss, pp. 413–423.

Koskinen, L. 1977. Adaptive sutures. Academic diss., University of Turku.

Koskinen, L., K. Isotupa, and K. Koski. 1976. A note on craniofacial suture growth. American Journal of Physical Anthropology 45: 511–516.

Krukowski, M., R. A. Shively, P. Osdoby, and B. L. Eppley. 1990. Stimulation of craniofacial and intramedullary bone formation by negatively charged beads. Journal of Oral and Maxillofacial Surgery 48: 468–475.

Laitman, J. T., R. C. Heimbuch, and E. S. Crelin. 1978. Developmental change in a basicranial line and its relationship to the upper respiratory system in living primates. American Journal of Anatomy 152: 467–482.

Lakars, T. C., and S. W. Herring. 1980. Ontogeny of oral function in hamsters (Mesocricetus auratus). Journal of Morphology 165: 237–254.

Lanyon, L. E. 1980. The influence of function on the development of bone curvature: An experimental study on the rat tibia. Journal of Zoology 192: 457–466.

Lanyon, L. E., A. E. Goodship, C. J. Pye, and J. H. MacFie. 1982. Mechanically adaptive bone remodelling. Journal of Biomechanics 15: 141–154.

Lanyon, L. E., P. T. Magee, and D. G. Baggott. 1979. The relationship of functional stress and strain to the processes of bone remodelling: An experimental study on the sheep radius. Journal of Biomechanics 12: 593–600.

Lanyon, L. E., and C. T. Rubin. 1984. Static vs dynamic loads as an influence on bone remodelling. Journal of Biomechanics 17: 897–905.

Larheim, T. A., and H. R. Haanaes. 1981. Micrognathia, temporomandibular joint changes and dental occlusion in juvenile rheumatoid arthritis of adolescents and adults. Scandinavian Journal of Dental Research 89: 329–338.

Legler, J. M. 1981. The taxonomy, distribution, and ecology of Australian freshwater turtles (Testudines: Pleurodira: Chelidae). National Geographic Society Research Reports 13: 329–404.

Liem, K. F., and L. S. Kaufman. 1984. Intraspecific macroevolution: Functional biology of the polymorphic cichlid species Cichlasoma minckleyi. In Evolution of Fish Species Flocks, A. A. Echelle and I. Kornfeld, eds. Orono: University of Maine at Orono Press, pp. 203–215.

van der Linden, F. P. G. M. 1986. *Facial Growth and Facial Orthopedics*. Chicago: Quintessence Publishing Co.

van Limborgh, J. 1972. The role of genetic and local environmental factors in the control of postnatal craniofacial morphogenesis. Acta morphologica neer-lando-scandinavica 10: 37–47.

Lindsay, K. N. 1977. An autoradiographic study of cellular proliferation of the mandibular condyle after induced dental malocclusion in the mature rat. Archives of Oral Biology 22: 711–714.

Løvtrup, S. 1981. Introduction to evolutionary epigenetics. In *Evolution Today*, G. G. E. Scudder and J. L. Reveal, eds. Pittsburgh: Carnegie-Mellon University, pp. 139–144.

Luder, H. U., C. P. Leblond, and K. von der Mark. 1988. Cellular stages in cartilage formation as revealed by morphometry, radioautography and type II collagen immunostaining of the mandibular condyle from weanling rats. American Journal of Anatomy 182: 197–214.

Maier, W. 1987. The ontogenetic development of the orbitotemporal region in the skull of *Monodelphis domestica* (Didelphidae, Marsupialia) and the problem of the mammalian alisphenoid. In *Morphogenesis of the Mammalian Skull*, H.-J. Kuhn and U. Zeller, eds. Hamburg: Paul Parey, pp. 71–90.

Manson, J. D. 1968. *A Comparative Study of the Postnatal Growth of the Mandible*. London: Henry Kempton.

Massler, M., and I. Schour. 1951. The growth pattern of the cranial vault in the albino rat as measured by vital staining with alizarine red "S." Anatomical Record 110: 83–101.

Matsuda, J. J., R. F. Zernicke, A. C. Vailas, V. A. Pedrini, A. Pedrini-Mille, and J. A. Maynard. 1986. Structural and mechanical adaptation of immature bone to strenuous exercise. Journal of Applied Physiology 60: 2028–2034.

Maynard Smith, J., and R. J. G. Savage. 1959. The mechanics of mammalian jaws. School Science Review 40: 289–301.

McLain, J. B., and P. S. Vig. 1983. Transverse periosteal sectioning and femur growth in the rat. Anatomical Record 207: 339–348.

McLain, J. B., P. S. Vig, and D. C. Hamilton. 1982. The influence of circumferential periosteal section on mandibular morphology and growth in the rat. In *Factors and Mechanisms Influencing Bone Growth*, A. D. Dixon and B. G. Sarnat, eds. New York: Alan R. Liss, pp. 581–596.

McNamara, J. A., Jr., and F. A. Bryan. 1987. Long-term mandibular adaptations to protrusive function: An experimental study in *Macaca mulatta*. American Journal of Orthodontics and Dentofacial Orthopedics 92: 98–108.

McNamara, J. A., Jr., R. J. Hinton, and D. L. Hoffman. 1982. Histologic analysis of temporomandibular joint adaptation to protrusive function in young adult rhesus monkeys (*Macaca mulatta*). American Journal of Orthodontics 82: 288–298.

Meade, J. B., S. C. Cowin, J. J. Klawitter, W. C. Van Buskirk, and H. B. Skinner. 1984. Bone remodeling due to continuously applied loads. Calcified Tissue International 36: S25–S30.

Mednick, L. W., and S. L. Washburn. 1956. The role of the sutures in the growth of the braincase of the infant pig. American Journal of Physical Anthropology 14: 175–191.

Meikle, M. C. 1973. In vivo transplantation of the mandibular joint of the rat: An autoradiographic investigation into cellular changes at the condyle. Archives of Oral Biology 18: 1011–1020.

———. 1975. The influence of function on chondrogenesis at the epiphyseal cartilage of a growing long bone. Anatomical Record 182: 387–400.

Meikle, M. C., J. K. Heath, R. M. Hembry, and J. J. Reynolds. 1982. Rabbit cranial suture fibroblasts under tension express a different collagen phenotype. Archives of Oral Biology 27: 609–613.

Meikle, M. C., J. J. Reynolds, A. Sellers, and J. T. Dingle. 1979. Rabbit cranial sutures in vitro: A new experimental model for studying the response of fibrous joints to mechanical stress. Calcified Tissue International 28: 137–144.

Melsen, B., and F. Melsen. 1980. The cranial base in anencephaly and microcephaly studied histologically. Teratology 22: 271–277.

Meyer, A. 1987. Phenotypic plasticity and heterochrony in Cichlosoma managuense (Pisces, Cichlidae) and their implications for speciation in cichlid fishes. Evolution 41: 1357–1369.

Miyawaki, S., and D. P. Forbes. 1987. The morphologic and biochemical effects of tensile force application to the interparietal suture of the Sprague-Dawley rat. American Journal of Orthodontics and Dentofacial Orthopedics 92: 123–133.

Moore, W. J. 1965. Masticatory function and skull growth. Journal of Zoology 146: 123–131.

———. 1967. Muscular function and skull growth in the laboratory rat (Rattus norvegicus). Journal of Zoology 152: 287–296.

———. 1973. An experimental study of the functional components of growth in the rat mandible. Acta anatomica 85: 378–385.

Moskalewski, S., J. Malejczyk, and A. Osiecka. 1986. Structural differences between bone formed intramuscularly following the transplantation of isolated calvarial bone cells or chondrocytes. Anatomy and Embryology 175: 271–277.

Moskalewski, S., A. Osiecka, A. Hyc, and J. Malejczyk. 1989. Difference in shape of bone formed by isolated calvarial and scapular osteoblasts transplanted under various conditions. Folia histochemica et cytobiologica 27: 25–34.

Moss, M. L. 1957. Experimental alteration of sutural area morphology. Anatomical Record 127: 569–590.

———. 1959. The pathogenesis of premature cranial synostosis in man. Acta anatomica 37: 351–370.

———. 1968. The primacy of functional matrices in orofacial growth. Dental Practitioner 19: 65–73.

———. 1976. Experimental alteration of basi-synchondrosal cartilage growth in rat and mouse. In Development of the Basicranium, J. F. Bosma, ed. Bethesda, Md.: U.S. Department of Health, Education, and Welfare, pp. 541–575.

Moss, M. L., and M. Meehan. 1970. Functional cranial analysis of the coronoid process in the rat. Acta anatomica 77: 11–24.

Müller, H., and J. A. Punt-van Manen. 1982. Maxillo-facial deformities in patients with dystrophic myotonica and the anaesthetic implications. Journal of Maxillo-Facial Surgery 10: 224–228.

Murray, P. D. F. 1936. *Bones*. Cambridge: Cambridge University Press, Reprint. 1985.

———. 1963. Adventitious (secondary) cartilage in the chick embryo, and the development of certain bones and articulations in the chick skull. Australian Journal of Zoology 11: 368–430.

Murray, P. D. F., and D. B. Drachman. 1969. The role of movement in the development of joints and related structures: The head and neck in the chick embryo. Journal of Embryology and Experimental Morphology 22: 349–371.

Murray, P. D. F., and M. Smiles. 1965. Factors in the evocation of adventitious (secondary) cartilage in the chick embryo. Australian Journal of Zoology 13: 351–381.

Nappen, D. L., and V. G. Kokich. 1983. Experimental craniosynostosis in growing rabbits. Journal of Neurosurgery 58: 101–108.

Narayanan, C. H., M. W. Fox, and V. Hamburger. 1971. Prenatal development of spontaneous and evoked activity in the rat (*Rattus norvegicus albinus*). Behaviour 40: 100–134.

Narbaitz, R., K. Sarkar, and B. Fragiskos. 1983. Differentiation of bones and skeletal muscles in chick embryos cultured on albumin. Revue canadienne de biologie expérimentale 42: 271–277.

Nikitjuk, B. A. 1961. Eksperimentalno morfologiceskoje issledovanija y formoobrazovanii cerepa mlekopitajuscich. Medical diss., Moscow.

Nilsson, A., J. Isgaard, A. Lindahl, A. Dahlström, A. Skottner, and O. G. P. Isaksson. 1986. Regulation by growth hormone of number of chondrocytes containing IGF-1 in rat growth plate. Science 233: 571–574.

Nur, N., and O. Hasson. 1984. Phenotypic plasticity and the handicap principle. Journal of Theoretical Biology 110: 275–297.

Osdoby, P., and A. I. Caplan. 1979. Osteogenesis in cultures of limb mesenchymal cells. Developmental Biology 73: 84–102.

———. 1981. First bone formation in the developing chick limb. Developmental Biology 86: 147–156.

Oudhof, H. A. J., and W. J. van Doorenmaalen. 1983. Skull morphogenesis and growth: Hemodynamic influence. Acta anatomica 117: 181–186.

Oxnard, C. E. 1971. Tensile forces in skeletal structures. Journal of Morphology 134: 425–436.

Packard, D. S., Jr. and A. G. Jacobson. 1979. Analysis of the physical forces that influence the shape of chick somites. Journal of Experimental Zoology 207: 81–92.

Pai, A. C. 1965. Developmental genetics of a lethal mutation, muscular dysgenesis (*mdg*), in the mouse. I. Genetic analysis and gross morphology. Developmental Biology 11: 82–92.

Parenti, L. R. 1986. The phylogenetic significance of bone types in euteleost fishes. Zoological Journal of the Linnean Society 87: 37–51.

Pechak, D. G., M. J. Kujawa, and A. I. Caplan. 1986a. Morphological and histo-chemical events during first bone formation in embryonic chick limbs. Bone 7: 441–458.

———. 1986b. Morphology of bone development and bone remodeling in embryonic chick limbs. Bone 7: 459–472.

Persson, M. 1973. Structure and growth of facial sutures. Odontologisk revy 24 (suppl. 26): 1–146.

Persson, M., B. C. Magnusson, and B. Thilander. 1978. Sutural closure in rabbit and man: A morphological and histochemical study. Journal of Anatomy 125: 313–321.

Peterson, J. A., and R. F. Zernicke. 1987. The geometric and mechanical properties of limb bones in the lizard, Dipsosaurus dorsalis. Journal of Biomechanics 20: 902.

Petrovic, A. G. 1982. Postnatal growth of bone: A perspective of current trends, new approaches, and innovations. In Factors and Mechanisms Influencing Bone Growth, A. D. Dixon and B. G. Sarnat, eds. New York: Alan R. Liss, pp. 297–331.

Petrovic, A. G., J. J. Stutzmann, and C. L. Oudet. 1975. Control processes in the postnatal growth of the condylar cartilage of the mandible. In Determinants of Mandibular Form and Growth, J. A. McNamara, Jr., ed. Monograph 4, Craniofacial Growth Series. Ann Arbor: University of Michigan, pp. 101–153.

Pollack, S. R. 1984. Bioelectrical properties of bone. Orthopedic Clinics of North America 15: 3–14.

Prahl-Andersen, B. 1968. Sutural growth. Ph.D. diss., University of Nijmegen.

Pratt, L .W. 1943. Experimental masseterectomy in the laboratory rat. Journal of Mammalogy 24: 204–211.

Pryles, C. V., and A. J. Khan. 1979. Wormian bones. American Journal of Diseases of Children 133: 380–382.

Pucciarelli, H. M. 1981. Growth of the functional components of the rat skull and its alteration by nutritional effects: A multivariate analysis. American Journal of Physical Anthropology 56: 33–41.

Rak, Y. 1978. The functional significance of the squamosal suture in Australopithecus boisei. American Journal of Physical Anthropology 49: 71–78.

Reitan, K., and E. Kvam. 1971. Comparative behavior of human and animal tissue during experimental tooth movement. Angle Orthodontist 41: 1–14.

Richman, J. M., and V. M. Diewert. 1988. The fate of Meckel's cartilage chondrocytes in ocular culture. Developmental Biology 129: 48–60.

de Ricqles, A. J. 1974. Evolution of endothermy: Histological evidence. Evolutionary Theory 1: 51–80.

Rieppel, O. 1986. Atomism, epigenesis, preformation, and pre-existence: A clarification of terms and consequences. Biological Journal of the Linnean Society 28: 331–341.

———. 1987. The development of the trigeminal jaw adductor musculature and associated skull elements in the lizard Podarcis sicula. Journal of Zoology 212: 131–150.

Rodríguez, J. I., E. Delgado, and R. Paniagua. 1985. Changes in young rat radius following excision of the perichondrial ring. Calcified Tissue International 37: 677–683.

Rönning, O., and K. Koski. 1974. The effect of periostomy on the growth of the condylar process in the rat. Proceedings of the Finnish Dental Society 70: 28–29.

Rönning, O., and S. Kylämarkula. 1982. Morphogenetic potential of rat growth cartilages as isogeneic transplants in the interparietal suture area. Archives of Oral Biology 27: 581–588.

Rubin, C. T., and L. E. Lanyon. 1984. Regulation of bone formation by applied dynamic loads. Journal of Bone and Joint Surgery 66-A: 397–402.

———. 1985. Regulation of bone mass by mechanical strain magnitude. Calcified Tissue International 37: 411–417.

———. 1987. Osteoregulatory nature of mechanical stimuli: Function as a determinant for adaptive remodeling in bone. Journal of Orthopaedic Research 5: 300–310.

Rubinacci, A., and L. Tessari. 1983. A correlation analysis between bone formation rate and bioelectric potentials in rabbit tibia. Calcified Tissue International 35: 728–731.

Runner, M. N. 1986. Epigenetically regulated genomic expressions for shortened stature and cleft palate are regionally specific in the 11-day mouse embryo. Journal of Craniofacial Genetics and Developmental Biology 2 (suppl.): 137–168.

Russell, E. S. 1916. Form and Function. London: John Murray. Reprint. Chicago: University of Chicago Press, 1982.

Rygh, P., K. Bowling, L. Hovlandsdal, and S. Williams. 1986. Activation of the vascular system: A main mediator of periodontal fiber remodeling in orthodontic tooth movement. American Journal of Orthodontics 89: 453–468.

Sage, R. D., and R. K. Selander. 1975. Trophic radiation through polymorphism in cichlid fishes. Proceedings of the National Academy of Sciences, U.S.A. 72: 4669–4673.

Sah, R. L.-Y., and A. J. Grodzinsky. 1989. Biosynthetic response to mechanical and electrical forces. In The Biology of Tooth Movement, L. A. Norton and C. J. Burstone, eds. Boca Raton, Fla.: CRC Press, pp. 335–347.

Sah, R. L.-Y., Y.-J. Kim, J.-Y. H. Doong, A. J. Grodzinsky, A. H. K. Plaas, and J. D. Sandy. 1989. Biosynthetic response of cartilage explants to dynamic compression. Journal of Orthopaedic Research 7: 619–636.

Sato, Y., H. Ohmae, T. Takano, M. Sakuda, and H. Nakagawa. 1986. Influence of unilateral masseteric denervation on the growth of mandibular condylar cartilage: An autoradiographic study. Journal of Osaka University Dental School 26: 177–186.

Scapino, R. P. 1972. Adaptive radiation of mammalian jaws. In Morphology of the Maxillo-Mandibular Apparatus, G.-H. Schumacher, ed. Leipzig: Thieme, pp. 33–39.

Schumacher, G.-H., D. Ivánkievicz, and J. Fanghänel. 1979. The role of function in the formation of the skull. Acta morphologica Academiae scientiarum hungaricae 27: 53–56.

Scott, J. H. 1951. The development of joints concerned with early jaw movements in the sheep. Journal of Anatomy 85: 36–43.

———. 1954. The growth of the human face. Proceedings of the Royal Society of Medicine 47: 91–100.

Silbermann, M. 1983. Hormones and cartilage. In *Cartilage,* vol. 2, B. K. Hall, ed. New York: Academic Press, pp. 327–368.

Silbermann, M., and E. Livne. 1979. Skeletal changes in the condylar cartilage of the neonate mouse mandible. Biology of the Neonate 35: 95–105.

Simard-Savoie, S., and D. Lamorlette. 1976. Effect of experimental microglossia on craniofacial growth. American Journal of Orthodontics 70: 304–315.

Simkin, A., I. Leichter, A. Swissa, and S. Samueloff. 1989. The effect of swimming activity on bone architecture in growing rats. Journal of Biomechanics 22: 845–851.

Simon, M. R. 1977. The role of compressive forces in the normal maturation of the condylar cartilage in the rat. Acta anatomica 97: 351–360.

———. 1978. The effect of dynamic loading on the growth of epiphyseal cartilage in the rat. Acta anatomica 102: 176–183.

Smith, D. W. 1981. Mechanical forces and patterns of deformation. In *Morphogenesis and Pattern Formation,* T. G. Connelly, L. L. Brinkley, and B. M. Carlson, eds. New York: Raven Press, pp. 215–223.

Smith, H. G., and M. McKeown. 1974. Experimental alteration of the coronal sutural area: A histological and quantitative microscopic assessment. Journal of Anatomy 118: 543–559.

Smith, K. K., and W. L. Hylander. 1985. Strain gauge measurement of mesokinetic movement in the lizard *Varanus exanthematicus.* Journal of Experimental Biology 114: 53–70.

Smith, W. S., and J. B. Cunningham. 1957. The effect of alternating distracting forces on the epiphyseal plates of calves: A preliminary report. Clinical Orthopaedics and Related Research 10: 125–130.

Smith-Gill, S. J. 1983. Developmental plasticity: Developmental conversion versus phenotypic modulation. American Zoologist 23: 47–55.

Smit-Vis, J. H., and F. M. M. Griffioen. 1987. Growth control of neurocranial height of the rat skull. Anatomische Anzeiger 163: 401–406.

Solursh M. 1983. Cell-cell interactions and chondrogenesis. In *Cartilage,* vol. 2, B. K. Hall, ed. New York: Academic Press, pp. 121–141.

Soskolne, W. A., Z. Schwartz, and A. Ornoy. 1986. The development of fetal mice long bones in vitro: An assay of bone modeling. Bone 7: 41–48.

Southard, K. A., and D. P. Forbes. 1988. The effects of force magnitude on a sutural model: A quantitative approach. American Journal of Orthodontics and Dentofacial Orthopedics 93: 460–466.

Spyropoulos, M. N. 1977. The morphogenetic relationship of the temporal muscle to the coronoid process in human embryos and fetuses. American Journal of Anatomy 150: 395–410.

Steegman, A. T., Jr., and W. S. Platner. 1968. Experimental cold modification of craniofacial morphology. American Journal of Physical Anthropology 28: 17–30.

Stockwell, R. A. 1987. Structure and function of the chondrocyte under mechanical stress. In *Joint Loading*, H. J. Helminen, I. Kiviranta, A.-M. Smnen, M. Tammi, K. Paukkonen, and J. Jurvelin, eds. Bristol: Wright, pp. 126–148.

Stopak, D., and A. K. Harris. 1982. Connective tissue morphogenesis by fibroblast traction. I. Tissue culture observations. Developmental Biology 90: 383–398.

Storey, E., and S. A. Feik. 1985. Remodelling of bone and bones: Effects of altered mechanical stress on caudal vertebrae. Journal of Anatomy 140: 37–48.

Tewson, D. H. T. K., J. K. Heath, and M. C. Meikle. 1988. Biochemical and autoradiographical evidence that anterior mandibular displacement in the young growing rat does not stimulate cell proliferation or matrix formation at the mandibular condyle. Archives of Oral Biology 33: 99–107.

Thomason, J. J., and A. P. Russell. 1986. Mechanical factors in the evolution of the mammalian secondary palate: A theoretical analysis. Journal of Morphology 189: 199–213.

Thorogood, P. 1983. Morphogenesis of cartilage. In *Cartilage,* vol. 2, B. K. Hall, ed. New York: Academic Press, pp. 223–254.

Throckmorton, G. S. 1979. The effect of wear on the cheek teeth and associated dental tissues of the lizard *Uromastix aegyptius* (Agamidae). Journal of Morphology 160: 195–208.

Toerien, M. J. 1965. Experimental studies on the columella-capsular interrelationship in the turtle, *Chelydra serpentina.* Journal of Embryology and Experimental Morphology 14: 265–272.

Tonneyck-Müller, I. 1976. Das Wachstum von Augen und Augenhöhlen beim Hühnerembryo. IX. Die Entwichklung der Augen- und Schädelanlage bei Embryonen von 3-9 Tagen mit künstlich erzeugter doppelseitiger Mikrophthalmie. Acta morphologica neerlando-scandinavica 14: 139–164.

Tuckett, F., and G. M. Morriss-Kay. 1985. The ontogenesis of cranial neuromeres in the rat embryo. II. A transmission electron microscopy study. Journal of Embryology and Experimental Morphology 88: 231–247.

Veldhuijzen, J. P., A. H. Huisman, J. P. W. Vermeiden, and B. Prahl-Andersen. 1987. The growth of cartilage cells in vitro and the effect of intermittent compressive force. A histological evaluation. Connective Tissue Research 16: 187–196.

Vilmann, H. 1982. The mandibular angular cartilage in the rat. Acta anatomica 113: 61–68.

Vilmann, H., M. Juhl, and S. Kirkeby. 1985. Bone-muscle interactions in the muscular dystrophic mouse. European Journal of Orthodontics 7: 185–192.

Waddington, C. H. 1962. *New Patterns in Genetics and Development*. New York: Columbia University Press.

Wagemans, P. A. H. M., J.-P. van de Velde, and A. M. Kuijpers-Jagtman. 1988. Sutures and forces: A review. American Journal of Orthodontics and Dentofacial Orthopedics 94: 129–141.

Wake, M. H. 1977. Fetal maintenance and its evolutionary significance in the Amphibia: Gymnophiona. Journal of Herpetology 11: 379–386.

Wake, M. H., and J. Hanken. 1982. Development of the skull of *Dermophis mexi-*

canus (Amphibia: Gymnophiona), with comments on skull kinesis and amphibian relationships. Journal of Morphology 173: 203–223.

Walker, B. E., and J. Quarles. 1976. Palate development in mouse foetuses after
tongue removal. Archives of Oral Biology 21: 405–412.

Wallman, J., M. D. Gottlieb, V. Rajaram, and L. A. Fugate-Wentzek. 1987. Local
retinal regions control local eye growth and myopia. Science 237: 73–76.

Warrell, E., and J. F. Taylor. 1979. The role of periosteal tension in the growth of
long bones. Journal of Anatomy 128: 179–184.

Washburn, S. L. 1947. The relation of the temporal muscle to the form of the skull.
Anatomical Record 99: 239–248.

Watt, D. G., and C. H. Williams. 1951. The effects of the physical consistency of
food on the growth and development of the mandible and maxilla of the rat.
American Journal of Orthodontics 37: 895–928.

Weaver, M. E., and D. L. Ingram. 1969. Morphological changes in swine associated with environmental temperature. Ecology 50: 710–713.

Weijs, W. A., and H. J. de Jongh. 1977. Strain in mandibular alveolar bone during
mastication in the rabbit. Archives of Oral Biology 22: 667–675.

Weisel, G. F. 1967. Early ossification in the skeleton of the sucker (*Catostomus
macrocheilus*) and the guppy (*Poecilia reticulata*). Journal of Morphology
121: 1–18.

Wilson-MacDonald, J., G. R. Houghton, J. Bradley, and E. Morscher. 1990. The
relation between periosteal division and compression or distraction of the
growth plate. Journal of Bone and Joint Surgery [British] 72-B: 303–308.

Witte, F. 1984. Consistency and functional significance of morphological differences between wild-caught and domestic *Haplochromis squamipinnis* (Pisces,
Cichlidae). Netherlands Journal of Zoology 34: 596–612.

Wolff, J. 1892. *The Law of Bone Remodelling.* Berlin. Translated by P. Maquet
and R. Furlong. Berlin: Springer-Verlag, 1986.

Wouterlood, F. G., and W. van Pelt. 1979. The influence of the lower beak on the
interorbital septum-prenasal process complex in the chick embryo. Journal of
Embryology and Experimental Morphology 49: 61–72.

Wragg, L. E., V. M. Diewert, and M. Klein. 1972. Spatial relations in the oral
cavity and the mechanism of secondary palate closure in the rat. Archives of
Oral Biology 17: 683–690.

Wronski, T. J., and E. R. Morey. 1982. Skeletal abnormalities in rats induced by
simulated weightlessness. Metabolic Bone Diseases and Related Research 4:
69–75.

Yeager, V. L. 1985. Periosteal stimulation by artificial tension. Journal of Experimental Pathology 2: 37–40.

Yeh, C.-K., and G. A. Rodan. 1984. Tensile forces enhance prostaglandin E synthesis in osteoblastic cells grown on collagen ribbons. Calcified Tissue International 36: S67–S71.

6

Genetic and Developmental Aspects of Variability in the Mammalian Mandible

WILLIAM R. ATCHLEY

INTRODUCTION

THE VERTEBRATE CRANIOMANDIBULAR REGION is a complex morphogenetic structure whose origin and patterns of evolutionary diversification are of interest to a broad spectrum of biologists and clinicians (reviews in Crompton 1963; Wood 1965; Hall 1978; Moore 1981; Moore and Lavelle 1974; Thorogood and Tickle 1988; Atchley and Hall 1991). Studies on the craniomandibular region have focused on broad questions in genetics, development, systematics, evolution, human biology, and clinical sciences.

An eventual understanding of the origin and evolution of complex structures like those of the craniomandibular region requires resolution of a series of complicated questions which must be examined at different hierarchical levels of organization. At one level, concerns about developmental and genetical architecture of a given complex morphological trait are generally dealt with at the level of the individual organism. Questions about developmental architecture focus upon defining the component parts of a complex structure, determining how these parts are produced and how they are assembled into a complex morphological structure during ontogeny. Questions about genetic architecture include ascertaining which genes control the synthesis of the developmental parts and how many genes are involved, and determining their gene products and how these genes regulate the assembly of the developmental components.

Once we have ascertained how a complex morphological structure is assembled, we must ask about how variability in morphology among a group of organisms is generated and what the evolutionary fate of this variability potentially will be. Resolution of evolutionary questions about the origin and evolution of craniomandibular diversity requires that we focus our attention on analyses at the level of the biological population. The evolution of morphology is, in fact, the evolution of those underlying developmental processes which produced the morphology (Atchley 1987; Atchley and Hall 1991).

Evolutionary diversity in the form of a complex morphological structure has been hypothesized to have arisen from selection acting upon genetic diversity in the ontogenies of its component morphogenetic parts
(Atchley 1984, 1987, 1990; Atchley et al. 1990; Atchley and Hall 1991).
The importance of this hypothesis is that it defines evolutionary change in
complex traits to be the result of changes in heritable patterns of variability
of the various component developmental parts and their interactions during ontogeny. Thus, to understand the evolution of complex morphological structures, we need to ascertain which developmental components
exhibit heritable variability among individuals or populations, how the
variability is regulated, and whether this variability responds to selection.

To achieve this goal requires a robust genetic theory which integrates
information from development and morphology using a metric common
to models of evolutionary change by selection. This ingredient has been
missing from most evolutionary studies of development. Indeed, Sewall
Wright (1960) indicated that "evolution is something that happens in populations and without a mathematical theory connecting the phenomena in
populations with those in individuals, there can be no very clear thinking
on the subject."

In this essay, I will summarize some of the recent work on the genetics
and development of morphological change in complex structures using the
rodent mandible as a paradigm. This discussion includes comments on
three major topics: (1) the developmental composition of complex morphological traits, (2) a genetic model for complex traits, and (3) some genetic and developmental aspects of morphological variability in mandible
form within and between rodent populations.

DEVELOPMENTAL ORIGIN OF THE MAMMALIAN MANDIBLE

Understanding how a complex structure like the mandible is assembled
from its component parts during ontogeny is necessary to understanding
the origin and control of mandibular variability. What follows is a brief
summary of some of the major aspects of development in the rodent mandible. A more detailed summary is found in Atchley and Hall (1991) and
other chapters in the present volume.

The mammalian mandible is a complex skeletal structure which is developmentally and functionally divisible into a number of major skeletal
regions, including the horizontal ramus, the molar and incisor alveolar
components (those parts of the ramus associated with the teeth), and the
coronoid, condyloid, and angular processes (fig. 6.1). These morphogenetic components, together with other skeletal, dental, muscular, and connective tissues in the embryonic craniofacial region, originate from cells

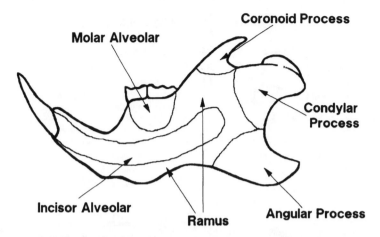

Fig. 6.1. A drawing showing the four morphogenetic components comprising the rodent mandible. These components include the ramus and three processes. Six morphogenetic units (one ramal, two alveolar, and three processes) produce the four morphogenetic regions.

which arise in the embryonic neural crest (Hall and Hörstadius 1988). Neural crest cells, which arise from the folds of the neural tube, migrate to the area of the first mandibular arch along pathways provided by extracellular molecules, and there they provide the embryonic mesenchyme of the mandibular skeletal, dental, and connective tissues (fig. 6.2). Individual neural crest cells undergo cell division during migration to produce a larger population of cells at their final destination. Following migration, these neural crest–derived cells aggregate into mesenchymal condensation(s) which then differentiate into bone or cartilage. These mesenchymal aggregations must occur prior to differentiation since chondrogenesis or oesteogenesis is initiated within individual mesenchymal condensations. Growth, differentiation, and morphogenesis of the cells derived from these mesenchymal condensations produce a series of skeletal elements which collectively comprise the mammalian mandible (Atchley and Hall 1991). Figure 6.3 describes the hypothesized derivation of the various skeletal components of the mandible from these differentiated mesenchymal tissues and their assembly into a functional mandible.

The cellular characteristics of these mesenchymal condensations are hypothesized to be fundamentally important in the early determination of adult skeletal form in the mandible (Atchley and Hall 1991). For example, activities occurring during cell migration but before the formation of mesenchymal condensations can exert control over normal development and growth of tissues derived from the neural crest cells (fig. 6.2). These controls include: (1) the number of cells leaving the neural tube, (2) the rate

Origin of Rodent Mandible

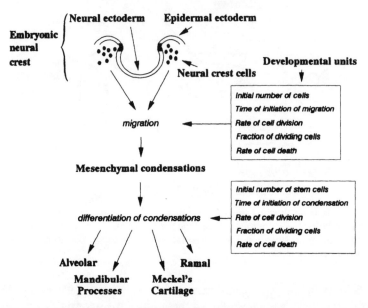

Fig. 6.2. Embryological origins of the rodent mandible. This figure summarizes the neural crest origin of Meckel's cartilage and the six major morphogenetic units of the mandible, i.e., the two alveolar, one ramal, and three processes. During migration of the neural crest cells, and during differentiation of the mesenchymal condensations, there are several developmental units which are important in the production of mandibular form.

at which they migrate, (3) the proportion of these migrating cells that divide, (4) the minimal period of time between successive divisions, and (5) the number of cells that die along the way. Variation in any of the developmental processes involved with migration of the neural crest cells can cause variation in the size of the entire mandibular structure. Thus, mutations at those loci regulating the number of neural crest cells, their migration, or their rates of division may produce mandibles which are larger or smaller overall than normal.

Condensation size is very important to the initiation of skeletogenesis since this process will not start if condensations are too small (Grüneberg 1963, 1975; Hall 1982a, b; Solursh 1983; Johnson 1986; Cottrill et al. 1987). Correspondingly, abnormally large bones develop if condensations are abnormally large.

Atchley and Hall (1991) designated as fundamental "developmental units" specific events or processes that can potentially exercise important levels of control over development and variability in mandibular form.

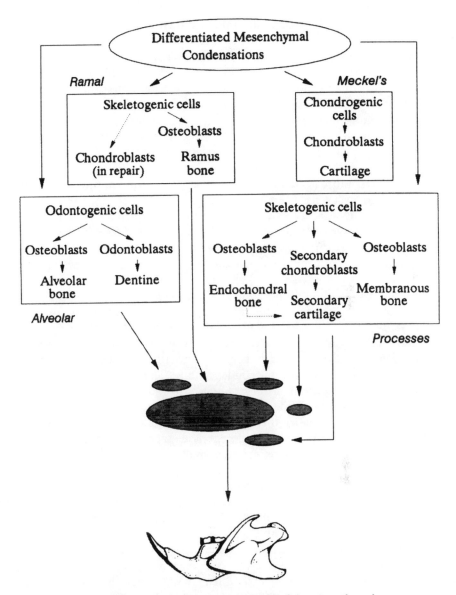

Fig. 6.3. A developmental map of the differentiation of the mesenchymal condensations into Meckel's cartilage and the various morphogenetic units of the mandible. These various units are then assembled into a consolidated and functioning skeletal structure.

This designation was made to dramatize their importance in growth and morphogenesis of skeletal structures, and to facilitate thinking about them in an evolutionary genetic sense. Developmental units are defined as those basic structural entities or regulatory phenomena necessary to assemble a complex morphological structure and whose alteration brings about morphological evolution. In early skeletal development, relevant developmental units include various cellularity parameters, such as those described above for migrating neural crest cells. Later in morphogenesis, other important developmental parameters come into operation (Atchley and Hall 1991).

Above, I discussed important activities occurring during migration of the neural crest cells. There are equivalent activities or processes occurring after the migrating cells have formed into mesenchymal condensations. These latter activities and processes can be expected to exhibit important regulating effects at a later point in the ontogeny of the mandible (fig. 6.2). Thus, within each mesenchymal condensation, important developmental units include (1) the number of preskeletal stem cells in each condensation; (2) the relative time of initiation of the condensation; (3) the rate of cell division in the condensation; (4) the fraction of the total cell population that is mitotically active; and (5) the rate of cell death. Variation in the developmental process characterizing each individual mesenchymal condensation can potentially generate variation in those skeletal tissues derived from the individual condensations. Thus, variation in these developmental units prior to differentiation could affect the overall size of the entire mandible, while variation in these equivalent processes after differentiation may change the shape of the mandible. There are equivalent developmental units in many different tissue types (Atchley and Hall 1991) and these units are often reiterated at multiple levels in the developmental hierarchy.

Complex morphological structures arise from a collection of component parts, and the assembly of these components into the final structure involves the coordination of activities occurring at different levels of hierarchical organization. (The temporal and spatial patterns of morphogenetic integration of these mesenchymal derivatives have been described as a "developmental choreography"; Atchley et al. 1990). As a consequence, variation in the form of the mandible may arise not only from variation in the primary characteristics of the mesenchymal condensations but also from variation in the regulation of the patterns of integration of the derivatives of mesenchymal condensations. That is, variation in morphological form can arise from changes in the patterns and timing of integration of embryologically separate component parts. Superimposed upon these hierarchically arranged events and processes are heritable epigenetic effects which arise from interactions with embryologically distinct tissues. For the mandible, these epigenetic interactions include those arising from the effects of variation in muscle development, development of the teeth, and related activities (Atchley and Hall 1991; Herring 1993). Thus, in addition to heritable ontogenetic variability in the components of bone tissue, there are also extrinsic components arising from the interactions with nonskeletal tissues.

This brief picture of mandible development together with figures 6.1–6.3 shows that this morphogenetically complex structure arises from the integration of a number of embryologically distinct parts whose integration is necessary to generate the final skeletal structure. In addition to summarizing the developmental origin of the mandible, this brief discussion of the multipartite nature of development of the rodent mandible dictates the type of genetic model we must embrace if we are to understand the evolution of morphological diversity in the craniomandibular region.

A GENETIC MODEL FOR EVOLUTIONARY CHANGE IN CRANIOMANDIBULAR TRAITS

What is an appropriate genetic model to describe evolutionary changes in patterns of growth and morphogenesis of skeletal structures? This is often a point of confusion among biologists attempting to understand the evolution of developmental processes. An appropriate genetic model for understanding evolutionary change in complex morphological structures is one that effectively describes the relevant genetical biology of the organism, but yet is simple enough in its parameters so that deductions can be made and relevant hypotheses tested (Atchley and Newman 1989). Genetic analyses of craniofacial features have often focused on major malformations within individuals (e.g., Grüneberg 1963; Neuberg and Merker 1975; Johnson 1986). Genetic control of these malformations is often quite simple. Single gene mutations occur which affect some critical step during development. The result is a significant disruption of the normal sequence of events, leading to a conspicuous and malformed phenotype. While such major gene mutations are valuable for studying the sequence of developmental events, they are generally of limited utility in studies about the evolution of morphological diversity. Evolutionary studies deal with genetic variation in normal phenotypes. Most major mutations have a significant negative impact upon reproductive fitness and, as a result, they are of little value in evolutionary analyses.

Many of the morphological, developmental, physiological, and metabolic aspects of normal development of greatest importance to evolutionary analyses generally do not exhibit discrete phenotypes; rather, these traits vary continuously over a range of phenotypic values. Such continuous variability—the hallmark of quantitative traits—arises because of complex patterns of actions and interactions among a large number of independently segregating genetic factors. These factors may be expressed differentially during ontogeny, and their expression is often modulated significantly by heritable epigenetic effects as well as by nonheritable environmental factors. Description of the underlying genetic elements controlling continuously varying traits has always been very difficult because of the absence of a simple correspondence between expression of a craniomandibular trait and segregation at one or a few loci. As a consequence, quantitative genetic models have traditionally been used to deal with evolutionary problems in continuously varying traits.

An appropriate genetic model of development must be one that can deal with a complex array of interacting developmental processes, whose variability arises from heritable intrinsic and epigenetic sources as well as from nonheritable environmental effects. In addition to accounting for continuous variability, an optimal genetic model of development must account for the developmental and genetic complexity of the traits involved, and permit experiments to test important biological hypotheses.

Simple Quantitative Genetic Models

The most widely used genetic models for describing and predicting evolutionary change in morphological traits are direct-effects models which have been derived from classical population genetics theory. In these simple models, the phenotypic variance (V_P) for a morphological trait is simply the sum of additive genetic (G) and nonadditive genetic and environmental variances (E); that is,

$$V_P = V_G + V_E.$$

Under this genetic model, the covariance between genotype and phenotype is the additive genetic variance, and the regression of genotype onto phenotype is the narrow-sense heritability. The rate of response to directional selection is determined by the narrow-sense heritability and the selection differential (Falconer 1989).

Direct-effects genetic models have often been used in both experimental and theoretical discussions and, in some cases, they provide an adequate description of the phenotype for some traits. Many of the recent theoretical expositions in evolutionary quantitative genetics have stressed this direct-effects model (e.g., Bulmer 1980; Lande 1979, 1980, 1982, 1988; Lande and Arnold 1983; Arnold and Wade 1984a, b; Thompson and Thoday 1979; and Barton and Turelli 1989).

Developmental Quantitative Genetic Models

While this direct-effects model is very simple in terms of its parameters, is it the appropriate genetic model for studying evolutionary change in mam-

Genetic Model of Mandible Development

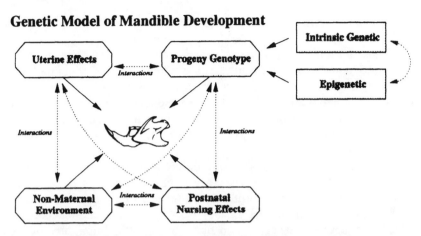

Fig. 6.4. A quantitative genetic model of mandible development which includes the individual's own genome as well as the prenatal and postnatal contributions made by the mother. The progeny genotype includes both intrinsic genetic and heritable epigenetic effects. Solid lines with single-headed arrows represent the actions of causal factors, dashed lines with double-headed arrows represent interactions between causal factors.

malian traits? Consider the underlying biological assumptions of a simple direct-effects quantitative genetics model. It assumes that (1) genetic factors are inherited in a Mendelian fashion; (2) only one generation of organisms is involved in expression of the trait; (3) all relevant evolutionary information is contained in the direct genetic components; (4) high correlation exists between genotype and phenotype; (5) epigenetic factors such as maternal effects are absent; (6) genotype × environment interactions and covariances have zero expectation; and (7) correlation between sexes for a given trait is unity.

As stated earlier, systematic evolutionary change in morphological traits results from evolutionary changes in those underlying heritable developmental processes or components which produce the traits (Atchley 1987; Atchley and Hall 1991). Thus, genetic models for understanding and predicting the magnitude and direction of evolutionary change in morphological traits must incorporate information from development. First, a genetic model of mammalian development must account for the fact that the control of most traits involves two genomes (the individual's own genome and that of its mother) and three different environments (uterine, nursing, and postweaning) (fig. 6.4). Second, the model must incorporate information from the four major categories of controlling factors which regulate development, growth, and morphogenesis. These include (1) intrinsic genetic factors, (2) heritable epigenetic phenomena, (3) maternal genetic factors, and (4) nonheritable environmental effects (Atchley and Newman 1989; Atchley and Hall 1991; Cowley and Atchley, 1992).

Thus, a simple direct-effects genetic model as described above ignores too many real-life complexities inherent to even the simplest of developmental systems—not to mention the development systems of organisms like mammals. Specifically, these models are inadequate because they ignore two developmental aspects which are important to understanding evolutionary change, i.e., maternal (or paternal) and epigenetic effects.

Why is it so important to use a model which is complicated by inclusion of all these factors? The answer lies in the need to be able to predict accurately the magnitude and direction of response to selection in evolutionary studies. The efficacy of selection is determined by the correlation between genotype and phenotype. With simple direct-effects models, it is assumed that the correlation between phenotype and genotype is an accurate prediction of the proportion of phenotypic variation that will respond to selection. However, there is an extensive literature on mammals showing that maternal effects and epigenetic phenomena can affect the expression of genes controlling development of many morphological traits. One important consequence of these phenomena is that there may be a significant decrease in the correlation between genotype of an individual and its phenotype (Atchley and Newman 1989; Kirkpatrick and Lande 1989; Cowley and Atchley, 1992). Obviously, any phenomena affecting the correlation between genotype and phenotype can have a significant impact on the rate of evolutionary change by directional selection.

Three classes of biological phenomena participate in determining the final morphological phenotype in a developing organism and for accurately ascertaining the correlation between genotype and phenotype.

Intrinsic Genetic Effects. The intrinsic genetic component represents genes which act locally (intrinsically) by coding for structural or regulatory elements that either confer characteristic properties on cells or regulate their expression, activities, and developmental program. Locally acting genes affecting skeletal development include those specifying the makeup of the proteins and polysaccharides forming the skeleton, enzymes governing their metabolism, and their selective expression in skeletogenic cells (Atchley and Hall 1991).

Epigenetic Effects. Epigenetic factors refer to locally or globally acting heritable processes which extrinsically regulate the expression and the interaction of genetic materials. Epigenetic factors may be indirect in action and are often inductive in their effects. "Epigenetic control" is the influence genes regulating one cell or group of cells have on a different cell or group of cells (Atchley and Hall 1991). For example, locally acting epigenetic effects can originate from embryonic inductions involving adjacent cells or tissues. A well-documented example of a heritable inductive epigenetic effect is the ability of muscle to determine the shape of bone (e.g., Herring and Lakars 1981; Atchley et al. 1984; Herring 1993). Similarly, epigenetic factors may act globally where the source of the epigenetic effect is distant to the target cell and, as a result, the epigenetic factor can simultaneously affect many different populations of developing cells. The classic example of a globally acting epigenetic factor is a hormone.

Clearly, nonheritable processes are involved in gene expression; however, these nonheritable processes must be included as nonheritable environmental factors in quantitative genetic models of development (Atchley and Hall 1991; Cowley and Atchley, 1992).

Waddington (1939, 1940) is credited with originating the concept of epigenetic factors which arise from interactive activities during development. Epigenetic interactions are fundamental to understanding the mechanics of development and their relationship to evolutionary change. As shown by Atchley and Hall (1991), contrasting intrinsic and heritable epigenetic effects can greatly clarify the concept of pleiotropy and the origins of genetic associations among different traits.

Maternal Effects. In mammalian species, prenatal (uterine) and postnatal (nursing) interactions that occur between the mother and her developing progeny may affect the developing progeny's phenotype. These interactions, termed "maternal effects," stem from heritable processes arising in the genome of the mother which condition the expression of genes in the developing progeny. The term "maternal inheritance" has been coined for the influence the mother has on the phenotype of her progeny over and above the direct transmission of her nuclear genes (Kirkpatrick and Lande 1989) which arises from this maternal conditioning.

Maternal effects fit all the attributes of an epigenetic factor, i.e., they represent heritable phenomena, they extrinsically regulate the expression of a cell's DNA, they are indirect in their action. However, maternal effects are a special class of epigenetic factors, because the effect is interorganismal in origin, since two separate genomes are involved (maternal and progeny), and, as a result, it involves organisms from two generations. Therefore, it is important to make the distinction between "intraorganismal" epigenetic effects arising from interactions among the progeny's own genes, and maternal effects where another genome is involved.

In an evolutionary sense, maternal-fetal interactions may have a potentially significant impact on the phenotype of the progeny with a resultant change in the way that this phenotype is "seen" by selection. First, the covariance between genotype and phenotype now includes more than simple intrinsic additive genetic effects. For example, some authors have described the existence of "maternal constraints" where maternal factors expressed in utero prevent the fetus from completely expressing its genetically determined potential for growth (Gluckman and Liggins 1984). These constraints arise from the maternal "conditioning" of the progeny genome. Experimental evidence for the occurrence of significant maternal constraints in utero and the persistence of their effects into adult organisms is found by Cowley et al. (1989) and Atchley et al. (1991). Thus, maternal effects alter the correlation between genotype and phenotype and thereby affect evolutionary change by selection.

Second, the fitness of the offspring depends in part on the offspring phenotype and in part on the mother's phenotype. Thus, the response to selection depends in part on the change due to selection in the previous generation, and it can also involve transitory environmental effects through the maternal inheritance (Kirkpatrick and Lande 1989; Cowley and Atchley, 1992). Cheverud (1984) demonstrated that selection response with maternal effects can be delayed or can temporarily occur in a direction opposite to the direction of selection. Kirkpatrick and Lande (1989) have shown that maternal effects can cause selection response to continue after selection ceases, and that in general, the initial rate of evolutionary response differs from the asymptotic rate. Perhaps the most important point to be emphasized regarding maternal effects is that without a good understanding of the developmental system, it is impossible to generalize about the expected outcome of selection.

Thus, maternal-fetal interactions not only make important contributions to offspring development, they can potentially complicate predictions about the rate and direction of evolution.

Nonheritable Environmental Influences. This category refers to the myriad of nonheritable influences which may act locally or globally and have a significant impact upon development. While these latter influences may have a significant impact on the phenotype during any particular generation, their impact over evolutionary time is minimal.

Summary of Causal Factors. An evolutionary genetic model for partitioning the phenotypic variability (V_P) in a given trait into its relevant developmental components is thus written as

$$V_P = V_A + V_E + V_M + V_R,$$

where V_A is the additive intrinsic genetic variance, V_E is the genetic variance due to epigenetic effects, V_M is the prenatal and postnatal maternal effects, and V_R is the residual nonheritable environmental effects. For the sake of simplicity, covariance terms have been excluded from the above formulation of this genetic model. A detailed discussion of evolutionary change by selection which incorporates intrinsic, maternal, and epigenetic effects is given in Cowley and Atchley (1992).

To date, few if any studies have experimentally partitioned out intrinsic and epigenetic effects in such a way as to provide robust quantitative estimates of their relative contribution to phenotypic variability. Published studies to date have simply estimated the additive and nonadditive genetic variances for a given morphological trait and those variances which include both intrinsic and extrinsic effects. Emphasis in the future must be focused upon generating experimental designs which permit the relative contributions of intrinsic and epigenetic factors to be estimated.

GENETIC ASPECTS OF VARIABILITY IN MANDIBLE FORM WITHIN POPULATIONS

What is the extent of heritable variation in mandible form? This question is fundamental to understanding the evolution of morphological form, since the rate and direction of response to selection is a function of the extent of additive genetic variability and covariability in relevant traits. Quantitative genetic analyses of mandible form in rodents, which are necessary to provide an answer to this question, have been reasonably common (Atchley 1983; Atchley et al. 1985a, b, 1990, 1992; Bailey 1956, 1985, 1986; Festing 1973; Lavelle 1983; Lovell and Johnson 1983; Lovell et al. 1984; and Nonaka and Nakata 1984). In this section, I will review some of the experimental evidence relating to (1) the causal basis for variability in morphological form of the mandible; (2) the patterns of genetic and environmental correlation among mandible components; (3) the effects of variation in body size on mandibular form; and (4) briefly comment on the number of genes involved in mandibular variability.

Causal Basis of Variability

What are the relative contributions made by the underlying causal factors to variability in the rodent mandible? I will report first on a conventional set of morphometric measures representing nine linear dimensions of the rodent mandible. Then I will discuss a set of six area traits which represent the skeletal derivatives of the mesenchymal condensations described ear-

TABLE 6.1. Mandible traits included in various analyses, together with a short descriptive code

Code	Linear dimension	Code	Linear dimension
a	Posterior mandible length	f	Condyloid width
b	Anterior mandible length	g	Condyloid length
c	Height at incisor region	h	Coronoid height
d	Height at mandibular notch	j	Angular process length
e	Height of ascending ramus		

Area definitions
Anterior alveolar area: Polygon defined by points 4, 5, 6, 8
Posterior alveolar area: Polygon defined by points 3, 4, 8, 9, 11
Coronoid area: Triangle (11, 12, 14) minus the area of (12, 13, 14)
Masseter area: Polygon defined by points 3, 11, 14, 19
Condylar area: Polygon defined by points 14, 15, 18, 19
Angular area: Polygon defined by points 1, 2, 3, 19

Note: Refer to figure 6.5 for further information about landmarks and the origins of the measurements.

lier. These linear dimensions and areas are described in table 6.1 and figure 6.5.

Causal Basis of Variability in Linear Dimensions. Table 6.2 describes the relative contributions of additive genetic variability (= narrow-sense heritability, h^2), dominance genetic variance (d^2), and the variability due to postnatal maternal effects (m^2) for nine linear dimensions of the mandible in adult (70-year-old) random-bred ICR mice (Atchley et al. 1985a, b). Within this large random-bred population, the narrow-sense heritability ranges from 9% for condylar width to 44% for notch height. The geometric mean of the heritability averaged over all nine traits is 21%; that is, an average of about 21% of the variability in linear dimensions of mandible within this population arises from the additive effects of genes.

Deviations from additivity due to dominance effects contribute to the phenotypic manifestation of a trait in every generation; however, dominance effects are not of much impact in evolutionary change because organisms transmit genes rather than genotypes to their progeny. The contribution to the phenotypic variance by dominance effects ranges from zero for incisor height and ramus height to 15% for condyloid width. The average contribution of dominance effects over these traits is 8%.

How much of the observed morphological variability in a population arises from variability in the mothers by way of postnatal nursing effects? In these 70-day-old ICR random-bred mice, postnatal maternal effects range from zero for ramus height, incisor height, condyloid width, and angular process length to 26% for notch height. Mandible traits with a

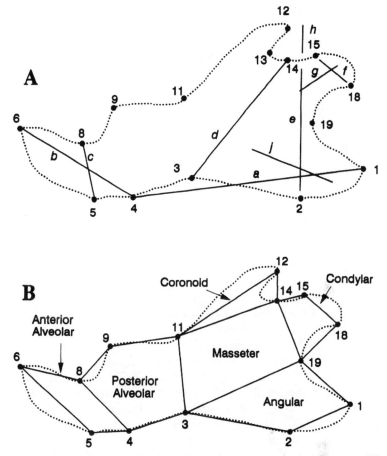

Fig. 6.5. A drawing of the rodent mandible showing a series of landmarks. (A) defines nine linear dimensions while (B) depicts a series of area traits representing skeletal derivatives of the mesenchymal condensations. Both sets of traits are subjected to quantitative genetic analyses.

reasonably large postnatal effect at 70 days of age include posterior mandible length (13%) and coronoid height (11%). Thus, at 70 days of age, 26% of the phenotypic variability in notch height arose from postnatal maternal effects which the mouse was exposed to during the first 21 days of postnatal life.

Atchley et al. (1981) examined 17 craniomandibular traits in 189-day-old rats and found that postnatal maternal effects had an impact on phenotypic variability even at this late age. They found that postnatal maternal effects accounted for 14% of the total variability in skull length,

TABLE 6.2.   Estimates of additive (h^2), dominance (d^2), and postnatal maternal variance (m^2) for linear dimensions in ICR random-bred mice

	h^2	d^2	m^2
Posterior mandible length	0.21	0.07	0.13
Anterior mandible length	0.24	0.10	0.07
Notch height	0.44	0.08	0.26
Incisor height	0.25	0.00	0.00
Ramus height	0.27	0.00	0.00
Condyloid process width	0.09	0.15	0.00
Condyloid process length	0.26	0.07	0.01
Coronoid process height	0.26	0.05	0.11
Length of angular process	0.10	0.06	0.00

12% in skull width, and 18% in zygomatic length. In other traits, e.g., width of the palate, postnatal maternal effects did not contribute to observed phenotypic variability at 189 days.

What is the impact of uterine maternal effects? That is, what is the effect of the genotype of the female providing the uterine environment during prenatal ontogeny? Quantifying the impact of prenatal maternal effects is difficult with random-bred organisms and has only been done to date using techniques such as embryo transplantation in homozygous inbred strains. Using reciprocal transfer procedures among three isogenic strains of mice, Atchley et al. (1991) demonstrated a significant uterine maternal effect on the major dimensions of the mandible. These authors found that the genotype of the female in which gestation occurred had a statistically significant impact upon anterior and posterior mandible length and notch height. Mothers from the isogenic strain having larger body size produced mice with larger mandible dimensions. When the effect of body size was removed, anterior mandible length still showed a statistically significant effect due to maternal uterine genotype.

Uterine litter size can be experimentally manipulated as a nonheritable environmental variable in embryo transfer studies. Atchley et al. (1991) found that uterine litter size had a statistically significant negative impact upon seven dimensions of the mouse mandible, including angular process length, condyloid length, height of the coronoid process, notch height, posterior mandible length, ramus height, and molar tooth area. For these traits, mothers developing larger litters gave birth to pups with significantly smaller mandibles.

Causal Basis of Variability in Area Traits. To understand the evolution of the rodent mandible, we must be able to relate alternations in the underlying developmental components to changes in their derivative skeletal components. Table 6.3 summarizes the relative contributions to phenotypic variability of additive genetic effects, postnatal maternal effects, and random environmental variability in six areas of the mandible for both mice and rats (Atchley 1992; Atchley et al. 1992). These areas correspond to the skeletal derivatives of mesenchymal condensations described earlier in this paper and discussed in considerable detail by Atchley and Hall (1991). Further, they correspond to important sites of muscle insertion and tooth development.

There is a statistically significant portion of the phenotypic variability which arises from additive genetic variability in all the area traits in both species. The narrow-sense heritabilities of these mandibular areas in mice range from 21% to 41% in mice and from 43% to 62% in rats. All of the skeletal derivatives of these mesenchymal condensations exhibit significant genetic variability in both mice and rats.

The higher heritabilities in rats may stem from fitting a more detailed statistical model. The rats described here arose from a large selection experiment (Atchley and Rutledge 1980) and the data include control and selected lines and their replicates derived from a selection experiment. The effects of the selected lines and their replicates were removed statistically from these analyses (Atchley and Rutledge 1980; Atchley et al. 1981, 1982). However, fitting the additional terms for selection and replicate lines in the model may have removed a greater portion of the environmental variance than occurred with the analyses of the mice. This could have resulted in a higher estimate of heritability in rats compared to mice.

There are statistically significant postnatal maternal effects for poste-

TABLE 6.3. Estimates of the relative proportions of phenotypic variability due to additive genetic variance (h^2), postnatal maternal variance (m^2), and residual environmental variance (e^2) for six area traits in the adult mandible for mice and rats.

Trait	Mice			Rats		
	h^2	m^2	e^2	h^2	m^2	e^2
Anterior alveolar area	0.30	0.01	0.69	0.52	0.13	0.29
	±.06	±.02	±.05	±.13	±.05	±.09
Posterior alveolar area	0.41	0.14	0.46	0.62	0.06	0.40
	±.06	±.03	±.05	±.16	±.04	±.12
Masseter area	0.39	0.13	0.51	0.60	0.15	0.31
	±.07	±.03	±.05	±.15	±.05	±.11
Coronoid area	0.21	0.03	0.76	0.43	0.11	0.52
	±.06	±.03	±.05	±.13	±.05	±.10
Condyloid area	0.23	0.06	0.71	0.43	0.11	0.52
	±.06	±.03	±.71	±.13	±.05	±.10
Angular area	0.23	0.09	0.67	0.44	0.01	0.48
	±.06	±.03	±.05	±.13	±.03	±.10

Notes: Standard errors are provided for each estimate. See figure 6.5 for further information about the traits.

TABLE 6.4. Genetic and environmental correlations among nine linear dimensions of the mandible for ICR random-bred mice

	Pm1	Am1	Nh	Ih	Rh	Cpw	Cp1	Cph	Lap
Posterior mandible length	—	0.19	0.25	0.18	0.46	0.05	0.20	-0.16	0.55
Anterior mandible length	0.06	—	0.20	0.33	0.30	0.22	-0.01	0.14	0.40
Notch height	0.40	0.35	—	0.32	0.26	0.08	-0.39	0.09	0.32
Incisor height	0.18	0.45	0.33	—	0.16	0.14	-0.24	0.19	0.28
Ramus height	0.26	0.54	0.50	0.12	—	0.28	0.33	-0.15	0.31
Condyloid process width	0.41	0.65	0.41	0.62	0.54	—	0.12	-0.03	-0.05
Condyloid process length	0.15	-0.09	-0.30	-0.19	0.23	0.01	—	-0.25	0.13
Coronoid process height	0.10	-0.13	0.01	-0.50	-0.13	-0.24	-0.21	—	-0.01
Length of angular process	0.58	0.65	0.39	0.06	0.12	0.48	0.01	-0.04	—

Note: The lower half of the matrix gives the genetic correlations while the upper half gives the environmental correlations.

rior alveolar, masseter, and angular areas in mice, and anterior alveolar, masseter, coronoid, and condyloid areas in rats. Postnatal maternal effects range from 1% to 15% in these animals. Dominance deviations were not estimated for these area traits.

Causes of Covariability among Linear Mandible Dimensions. The next important question is to ascertain the underlying origins of the phenotypic associations among the different dimensions and components of the mandible. The various developmental and skeletal components of the mandible do not exist in isolation, but rather during development they become integrated into a single functioning skeletal structure. Many of these developmental components and skeletal dimensions share genetic determinants as a result of common developmental pathways, pleiotropic gene action, and heritable epigenetic interactions. Further, just as genetic factors can generate correlations among traits, nongenetic factors can likewise produce phenotypic associations between traits. The cellular environment, nutrition, and related factors interact among each other as well as with the developing organism's genome to produce associations between traits. These nonheritable associations are important in generating the observed phenotype at any point in ontogeny; however, they are of little consequence for evolutionary change.

A matrix of additive genetic correlations among nine linear dimensions of the random-bred ICR mice is given in table 6.4. Additive genetic correlations estimate the common genetic component between a pair of traits. Genetic correlations are an integral part of understanding correlated response to selection and the overall magnitude of evolutionary changes due to selection (Falconer 1989).

The elements of this genetic correlation matrix range from −0.50 between coronoid height and incisor height to 0.65 between anterior mandible length and both condyloid width and angular process length. The average correlation is only 0.19 for these 36 values, which is not a high value for a number of measurements from what appears to be a single skeletal unit. The low average correlation is apparently the result of the morphogenetic heterogeneity of the mandible as discussed by Atchley et al. (1985b) and Atchley and Hall (1991) and apparently stems from the embryological heterogeneity of the mandible.

The extent of correlation arising from nonheritable environmental effects among these nine linear dimensions is given in table 6.4. Overall, these correlations are lower in magnitude than the genetic correlations. They range from −0.39 between notch height and condyloid process length to 0.55 between posterior mandible length and the length of the angular process.

It is usually difficult to discern whether patterns exist among a group

TABLE 6.5. Principal components analysis for genetic and environmental correlations among nine mandible traits in ICR random-bred mice

	Genetic correlations				Environmental correlations			
	I	II	III	IV	I	II	III	IV
Posterior mandible length	54	−51	−26	43	69	−32	37	−10
Anterior mandible length	79	8	9	−21	63	14	−28	36
Notch height	67	−27	31	−20	56	45	12	−51
Incisor height	61	58	29	25	54	46	−16	1
Ramus height	64	−1	−32	−66	68	−42	−16	−15
Condyloid process width	87	14	−4	2	29	−15	−84	−16
Condyloid process length	−4	9	−96	1	8	−84	−5	35
Coronoid process height	−27	−78	22	−24	5	60	−9	58
Angular process length	67	−43	−8	38	74	−1	40	29
Variance explained	38.1	16.7	14.8	10.8	28.7	19.8	12.8	11.0

Vector correlations

		Environmental			
		I	II	III	IV
Genetic	I	92	−1	−29	−17
	II	−23	−14	−43	−29
	III	−7	93	−4	−24
	IV	1	−2	39	5

Note: Decimal points have been omitted.

of correlation coefficients by simply inspecting a matrix. Therefore, two statistical techniques were used to describe the patterns of covariation among these nine linear dimensions. First, a principal components analysis was carried out on each correlation matrix to identify the major independent (orthogonal) patterns of covariability and the relative contribution of each individual linear dimension to these major patterns. Table 6.5 gives the first four principal components for each matrix.

For the genetic correlations, the first multivariate pattern is one of general pleiotropic effects where all but two traits have large and positive contributions. Only the length of the condyloid process and the height of the coronoid process did not show a high correlation with this multivariate pattern of variation. The second pattern describes an inverse genetic relationship between incisor height and coronoid process height, posterior mandible length, and angular process length. The third pattern relates primarily to genetic variation in condyloid process length, while the fourth pattern describes an inverse genetic relationship between ramus height on the one hand, and posterior mandible length and angular process length on the other.

For the environmental correlations, the first pattern is a "general environmental effect" where all dimensions except condyloid process length and coronoid process height contribute significantly. The second environmental pattern is an inverse relationship between condyloid process length, ramus height, and posterior mandible length on the one hand, and coronoid process height, incisor height, and notch height on the other. The third pattern refers to an inverse environmental relationship between condyloid process width and angular process length and posterior mandible length. The fourth environmental pattern is an inverse relationship between notch height and several other dimensions, including coronoid process height, anterior mandible length, condyloid process length, and angular process length.

The patterns of genetic and environmental correlation structure among these various mandible traits can also be assessed in a hierarchical fashion by cluster analysis procedures. Figure 6.6 describes the results of a UPGMA cluster analysis of the genetic and environmental correlation structure for the nine linear dimensions in ICR mice. The clustering of the genetic correlations shows the heritable associations between posterior mandible length and angular process length. This high level of genetic association is not unexpected, given the overlapping nature of these measurements. Another genetic cluster comprises anterior mandible length, condyloid width, ramus height, notch height, and incisor height. Finally, condyloid length and coronoid height appear as genetically independent traits. These latter results reinforce the findings of the principal components analyses.

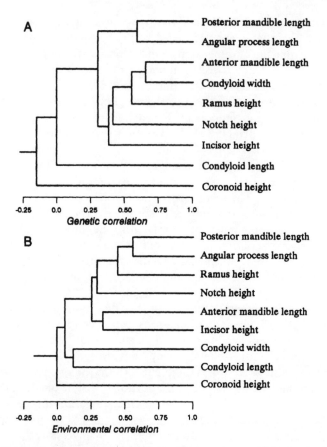

Fig. 6.6. Phenograms arising from UPGMA cluster analyses of the genetic (A) and environmental (B) correlation matrices for the nine linear dimensions described in figure 6.5A. The original correlation matrices are described in table 6.4.

The clustering of the environmental correlations shows a somewhat different pattern (fig. 6.6). There is a cluster comprising posterior mandible length, angular process length, ramus height, and notch height; another related cluster of anterior mandible length and incisor height; a rather loose cluster of condyloid width and length; and finally, coronoid height appears as an environmentally independent trait.

Since genetic and environmental processes are acting on the same set of developmental processes, one can inquire whether the genetic and environmental patterns of covariability are themselves correlated. There are several ways to answer this question. First, a matrix congruence procedure based on a permutation test was used (Dietz 1983). This test indicates that the patterns of elements in the genetic and environmental correlation matrices are highly significantly associated (P < .001). Thus, the magnitude and sign of the genetic and environmental correlation coefficients for these 11 mandible traits are very similar.

Since the elements of the genetic and environmental correlation matrices are significantly correlated, one might ask which elements or patterns of variability are interrelated. This question is answered by computing a correlation coefficient between the actual eigenvectors or principal components (Reyment et al. 1984). Table 6.5 provides a matrix of vector correlations which describes the extent of correlation between the major genetic and environmental patterns of covariability. There is a large and significant correlation between the first genetic and the first environmental vectors (r = 0.92) as well as the third genetic and second environmental vectors (0.93). The remaining patterns show very little association.

Are the genetic and environmental correlations correlated in morphological traits in other species? This question has been examined in detail in only a few other species. Atchley (1983), for example, examined the correspondence between genetic and environmental correlations for eight mandibular and maxillary traits in rats. The traits included mandible length, mandible height, mandible width, mandibular tooth row length, maxillary tooth row length, palatal length, width of the anterior portion of the palate, and width of the posterior portion of the palate. The permutation test indicates that there is no significant association between genetic and environmental correlation structure (P = 0.55) in these data.

Causes of Covariability in Area Traits. Table 6.6 gives the genetic correlations for the six area traits described in table 6.1 and figure 6.5 for both mice and rats. For mice, the genetic correlations range from values which are not significantly different from zero (condylar area and anterior alveo-

TABLE 6.6.   Genetic correlations among the six area traits for mice and rats

	Anterior alveolar area	Posterior alveolar area	Masseter area	Coronoid area	Condyloid area	Angular area
Anterior alveolar area	1.00	.45	.32	−.01	.25	.23
Posterior alveolar area	.54	1.00	.67	.31	.57	.10
Masseter area	.69	.78	1.00	.66	.66	.34
Coronoid area	.58	.70	.99	1.00	.56	.18
Condylar area	−.05	.46	.13	.47	1.00	.01
Angular area	.37	.41	.39	.32	−.02	1.00

Note: Matrix has the genetic correlations for mice in the lower triangular half and those for rats in the upper half.

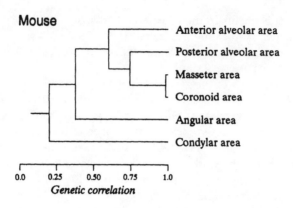

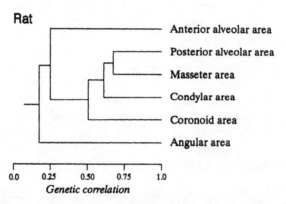

Fig. 6.7. Phenograms arising from UPGMA cluster analyses of the genetic correlation matrices from mice and rats for the six area traits described in figure 6.5B. The original correlation matrices are given in table 6.6.

lar area, angular area and condyloid area, and condylar area and masseter area) to statistically significant correlations among all other pairs of traits. In rats, there is no significant genetic correlation between anterior alveolar area and coronoid area, condylar area and angular area, and posterior alveolar area and angular area.

Figure 6.7 gives the hierarchical patterns among genetic correlations for both mice and rats as shown by a UPGMA cluster analysis. In mice, the masseter and coronoid areas form a tight cluster. Anterior and posterior alveolar areas are added to this cluster at a lower level of genetic correlation. Angular area and condylar areas appear as genetically more or less independent traits. In rats, there is a cluster comprised of posterior alveolar, masseter, condylar, and coronoid areas. Anterior alveolar area and angular area appear as genetically independent traits in this species.

Table 6.7 gives the principal components solutions for the genetic correlation matrices of the area traits in these two species. In mice, the first genetic vector has high positive values for anterior alveolar, posterior alveolar, masseter, and coronoid areas. Condylar and angular areas do not contribute significantly to this vector. Thus, the first principal component reflects the relationships shown in the UPGMA cluster analysis. The second principal component relates to condylar area and, to a lesser extent, to posterior alveolar and coronoid areas. The third vector reflects the genetic variation in angular area.

For the rats, the first principal component reflects genetic covariation in posterior alveolar, masseter, coronoid, and condylar areas. Anterior alveolar and angular areas do not contribute significantly to this principal component. Thus, as with the mice, the genetic relationships shown by first principal component vector are the same as those depicted in the UPGMA cluster analysis. The second vector reflects genetic covariation in anterior and posterior alveolar areas with a much smaller contribution made by masseter and condylar areas. The third vector describes genetic variation in angular area.

Are the genetic correlation matrices similar between mice and rats for these six area traits? Again, there are two ways to examine this question. First, a permutation test of the matrix elements (Dietz 1983) indicates that there is no significant correlation between the elements of these two genetic

TABLE 6.7. Principal components analysis of the additive genetic correlation matrices and partial additive genetic correlation matrices

| | Genetic correlations | | | | | |
| | Mice | | | Rats | | |
Trait	I	II	III	I	II	III
Anterior alveolar area	0.83	−0.21	0.22	0.01	0.90	0.18
Posterior alveolar area	0.68	0.47	0.34	0.57	0.67	−0.07
Masseter area	0.97	0.14	0.17	0.83	0.33	0.27
Coronoid area	0.89	0.40	0.09	0.88	−0.19	0.18
Condylar area	0.08	0.97	−0.03	0.82	0.29	0.16
Angular area	0.22	−0.01	−0.97	0.09	0.12	0.97
Eigenvalue	2.93	1.39	1.13	2.46	1.51	1.10

| | | Vector correlations | | |
| | | | Rats | |
		I	II	III
	I	0.77	0.67	0.40
Mice	II	0.83	0.26	−0.10
	III	0.26	0.43	0.91

Note: The concordance of the eigenvectors is determined by a vector correlation coefficient and the cosine of the angle.

correlation matrices. Second, the vector correlation procedure associated with the principal components analyses (table 6.7) shows that significant vector correlations exist between several vectors. For example, there is a significant correlation between the first principal components of each genetic matrix; however, inspection of these vectors shows that some relationships between traits are the same between species but other relationships are quite different (e.g., inclusion of anterior alveolar area in mice but not in rats, and inclusion of condylar area in rats but not in mice). There is also a significant vector correlation between mouse genetic vector II and rat vector I; however, this arises from the high coefficients on anterior and posterior alveolar area and masseter area. The coefficients for other traits are quite different. The only vector where there is real similarity between the species is genetic vector III, which relates to variation in angular area in both species. This procedure is not a very robust procedure in this particular instance because of the small number of traits being compared.

Atchley et al. (1992) have compared the genetic correlation structures for mandible traits in mice and rats and found importance differences between these two species in their genetic correlation structures.

Effect of Body Size Variability on Mandible Form

Interrelationships of morphological dimensions within a complex trait are important for ascertaining morphological form. However, important relationships also usually exist between skeletal traits and the overall body size of an organism. These latter associations are fundamental to studies of the ontogeny of size scaling and shape of morphological traits. Genetically based allometric relationships are also important in attempts to ascertain the genetic architecture of traits. Genetic correlations among traits present problems because a significant number of loci affecting mandible growth and morphogenesis may be systematically acting loci which have general pleiotropic effects over the entire skeletal system rather than simply loci specifically affecting only the mandible. This would be a complicating factor in attempts to ascertain the genetic architecture of a craniomandibular trait.

Atchley et al. (1985a) and Bailey (1985) examined genes affecting body size variability and their impact on mandible dimensions. Among the traits discussed here, Atchley et al. (1985a) found that anterior mandible length, notch height, incisor height, ramus height, condylar length, coronoid area, and posterior alveolar area had statistically significant genetic correlations with body weight at 70 days of age. This indicates significant patterns of pleiotropic gene activity between these mandible traits and body size.

However, the phenomenon of pleiotropic gene activity between body size and mandible dimensions is more complex than simple genetic correlations between adult body weight and adult mandible form. The patterns of genetic correlation change significantly during postnatal ontogeny. Indeed, in mice three ontogenetic patterns of genetic correlation were found (Atchley et al. 1985a). In one pattern (exemplified by condylar length), the genetic correlation between adult mandible dimensions and body weight during ontogeny was rather stable. That is, condylar length in mice had a significant positive genetic correlation with body weight at 14 days of age and this significant correlation persisted through skeletal maturity at 70 days of age. A second pattern occurred where there was a genetic correlation not different from zero between body weight at 14 days and mature mandible dimensions. However, there followed an increase in the genetic correlation during ontogeny to a very high value for mature body weight and mandible dimensions. This pattern is exhibited by anterior mandible length and incisor height. The third pattern was one where there was a low genetic correlation between mature mandible dimensions an early body weight: the correlation increased significantly at about 35 days of age and then decreased to near zero at 70 days of age. This pattern is exhibited by posterior alveolar area, condylar width, and posterior mandible length. Complex changes in genetic correlation structure also occur between mandible dimensions and weight gain.

Bailey (1985) approached the problem of size scaling in a slightly different way. He focused upon the correlation between mandible dimensions and various long bones. His results suggest that genes affecting long bone dimensions are not necessarily the same as those affecting mandible shape.

Atchley et al. (1992) examined the problem of genetic scaling effects arising from body size on mandibular form in a different way. Recall from previous discussion that the genetic correlation structure for mice for the six area traits shows no statistical similarity to the genetic correlation structure in rats. Based upon this observation and the marked size differences between mice and rats, Atchley et al. (1992) asked whether the differences in genetic correlation structure for the six mandibular area traits described in this paper were due to a genetic scaling effect arising from the great differences in body size. To test this hypothesis, we computed genetic correlations among mandibular dimensions, holding body weight constant. That is, we computed a partial genetic correlation between mandibular areas after the genetic correlation with adult body weight had been removed.

We rejected the hypothesis that the different genetic correlation structures arose from genetic scaling to great differences in body weight. Using a matrix permutation test on the two partial genetic correlations, we showed that the elements of the matrices were uncorrelated. Further, a principal components analysis of these matrices in each species showed that the orthogonal genetic patterns of covariation were quite different.

Number of Genes

Questions about genetic complexity of a trait usually lead to queries about genetic architecture (e.g., Atchley and Newman 1989; Sing et al. 1985, 1988). Few critical experimental data exist about the genetic architecture of the mandible, that is, which genes control the synthesis of the developmental components, the nature of their gene products, and how these genes regulate the assembly of these developmental components. There are several schools of thought about the genetic complexity of the rodent mandible. Bailey (1985), for example, suggested that divergence in the form of the mandible among several inbred mouse strains involves variation in over 100 genetic factors. Johnson (1986), on the other hand, suggests that there are very few actual skeletal genes in the restricted sense. He argues that only those loci specifying the composition of the proteins and polysaccharides forming the skeleton and the enzymes specifying them and governing their metabolism might be considered as skeletal genes *sensu stricto*. Johnson argues that the skeleton is a secondary structure produced as a result of interactions during development and therefore is the result of secondary, tertiary, and quaternary effects. Thus, many genes may affect the skeleton en passant as a result of activity elsewhere.

Much of this seeming disparity is semantic in origin; however, it contains an important lesson in how one approaches problems dealing with genetic control of biological processes. Johnson is concerned with the numbers of loci involved in the development of a structure within an individual. In the terminology of Atchley and Hall (1991), he is contrasting intrinsic genetic versus heritable epigenetic factors in his estimates about genetic architecture. Bailey, on the other hand, is concerned with the number of loci involved in the divergence of mandibular form among taxa. Thus, his question is a populational one (in spite of the fact that he is working with inbred strains of mice). Further, his estimates about genetic architecture lump together intrinsic genetic and heritable epigenetic factors.

GENETIC ASPECTS OF VARIABILITY IN MANDIBLE FORM BETWEEN TAXA

While quantitative genetic variability *within* populations for mandible traits has been relatively well studied, the genetic composition of the morphological variability *among* taxa has been poorly studied. In this section,

I will briefly review some of the experimental evidence bearing upon four questions: (1) How much of the observed variation in mandible morphology between taxa is genetic in origin? (2) Are the patterns of genetic divergence in mandibular morphology concordant with estimates of genetic divergence at the level of major gene loci? (3) Does divergence between taxa in mandibular traits occur through changes in the skeletal derivatives of the mesenchymal condensations as proposed by Atchley and Hall (1991)? (4) Are changes in the "developmental choreographies" of complex morphological structure responsible for intertaxa differentiation?

Questions about how much genetic variability occurs between taxa can be examined at several different levels of biological organization. For example, Atchley and Fitch (1991) described the genetic divergence among 24 inbred strains of mice at 144 so-called major gene loci, i.e., loci coding for specific proteins, enzymes, and immune factors. These authors have shown that this approach gives a highly accurate picture of divergence among taxa because the genetic basis of each of these traits is very simple, the traits closely adhere to a simple direct-effects genetic model, the phenotype associated with each allele is usually a discrete entity which is easily scored, and the patterns of genetic divergence over all loci adhere very closely to the patterns of known genealogical divergence among these inbred strains (Fitch and Atchley 1985; Atchley and Fitch 1991).

It would be valuable to have robust estimates of the number of genes involved in producing a given amount of morphological change. However, accurate estimates of the extent of genetic divergence among taxa based upon morphological data are much more difficult to obtain because of the complex nature of the genetic control of complex morphological structures. As noted previously, the underlying genetic model is much more complex and morphological traits are often strongly affected by nonheritable environmental factors. As a consequence, variability in most morphological traits is usually continuous, making assessment of the effects of allelic substitutions very difficult. With morphological phenotypes, many loci make indirect contributions through pleiotropic and epigenetic interactions. For example, Bailey (1985, 1986a, b) suggested that the form of the mandible is determined by the actions of literally hundreds of genes whose effect is transient and localized in both time and space. However, Atchley and Hall (1991) criticized Bailey's estimate since it ignores a number of important epigenetic processes known to affect mandibular form. Finally, morphological traits are usually developmentally complex and represent a compilation of several embryologically distinct parts.

It is possible to circumvent some of these problems associated with estimating genetic divergence in morphological traits (although certainly not all of them) through the use of special breeding systems. Inbred strains are a good example. Inbred strains are produced by many generations of brother × sister matings so that individuals within each inbred strain are assumed to be isogenic (except for mutations). The morphological variability observed *within* groups arises from nongenetic or environmental causes while variability *between* groups arises from genetic causes. Thus, the among-groups component of variability in an analysis of variance is a measure of the extent of genetic variability among taxa. An appropriate statistic for assessing the extent of among-groups variability in individual traits in this instance is the intraclass correlation (Sokal and Rohlf 1979). The intraclass correlation for each trait in completely inbred strains in this case is an estimate of the broad-sense heritability of normal variability among the strains for the trait in question. Further, the Mahalanobis pair-wise distance among these inbred lines is a multivariate genetic distance estimate for quantitatively controlled traits (Atchley et al. 1988).

Genetic Basis of Differences between Taxa

Atchley et al. (1988) provided intraclass correlation coefficients for 11 mandible traits from a study of nine inbred strains of mice (table 6.8). These coefficients estimate the proportion of the morphological divergence between strains that is of genetic origin. The intraclass correlation coefficients range from 44% (condyloid width) to 80% (height at the incisor region). Thus, between 44% and 80% of the divergence between these nine inbred strains of mice is due to differentiation in the genes controlling the development and expression of mandibular form. The geometric mean of intraclass correlation coefficients over the 11 mandible traits was 0.64.

TABLE 6.8.   Intraclass correlation coefficients, t, among nine inbred mouse strains for several mandible traits

Mandible trait	t
Posterior mandible length	0.72
Anterior mandible length	0.72
Height at mandibular notch	0.62
Height at incisor region	0.80
Height of ascending ramus	0.72
Condyloid width	0.44
Condyloid height	0.67
Coronoid height	0.67
Angular process length	0.73
Posterior alveolar area	0.50
Coronoid area	0.52

Note: Standard errors for the intraclass correlation range from 0.020 to 0.030.

Table 6.9 gives two estimates of the amount of genetic divergence which has occurred among these nine inbred mouse strains. One estimate is based upon the 144 so-called major gene loci as described above. These pair-wise genetic distance values between strains represent the proportion of the 144 loci at which different alleles have become fixed during the inbreeding process (Atchley and Fitch 1991). Some of these loci may be involved in morphological divergence of the mandible and others are not. The second matrix is composed of genetic distance estimates based upon 11 linear dimensions of the mandible. Each element of this latter matrix is the square root of the Mahalanobis distance. These elements provide a multivariate distance which estimates the genetic distance between pairs of strains based upon simultaneous variation in 11 mandible dimensions.

Concordance in Measures of Genetic Divergence

Table 6.9 provides two estimates of genetic divergence among these strains, one based on a large number of major gene loci from throughout the genome, the other specific to the dimensions of the mandible. Are these two estimates concordant?

Figure 6.8 gives a bivariate plot of these two estimates of genetic divergence and it is clear that there is a significant linear relationship between the two distance measures. The Kendall's tau correlation coefficient from a matrix permutation test (Dietz 1983) indicates that there is a statistically significant association between these genetic distance estimates ($P = 0.05$). However, is the extent of association between these two estimates of genetic divergence sufficient to provide the same estimates of phylogenetic relationships among the various taxa?

Inspection of figure 6.8 shows that several of the pair-wise genetic distance estimates for strains exhibiting the most morphological divergence do not show the greatest genetic divergence. Likewise, some of the comparisons showing the most divergence in major gene loci are not exhibiting the most morphological differentiation in mandible dimensions. Figure 6.9 gives the results of UPGMA cluster analyses of these two genetic distance matrices. Extensive previous analyses of divergence in the major gene loci indicate that they recapitulate the genealogical relationships among these mouse strains almost exactly (Atchley and Fitch 1991). Figure 6.9 shows that the two estimates of genetic divergence are not very concordant.

Such discordance in different genetic distance estimates is a complicating factor when one is trying to resolve questions about phylogeny. However, such discordancies are to be expected when genetic distances are estimated using traits that differ considerably in the underlying genetic and developmental complexity. Indeed, major gene loci fit closely to the direct-

TABLE 6.9. Matrices of genetic distances among nine inbred strains of mice

	A/J	BALB	CBA	C57BL	C3H	DBA	SEA	SEC	SWR
A/J	—	43.8	48.8	45.4	45.0	37.7	39.0	41.9	40.3
BALB	6.83	—	44.4	47.1	37.0	41.9	23.4	9.6	47.6
CBA	5.57	6.22	—	59.3	20.1	40.7	44.2	43.6	45.6
C57BL	7.04	7.84	4.87	—	54.8	57.4	42.9	41.5	50.0
C3H	6.27	6.13	4.98	6.24	—	41.5	35.5	38.7	46.4
DBA	5.55	6.66	3.38	6.76	6.77	—	45.5	39.4	39.7
SEA	6.04	4.99	4.80	7.29	5.33	5.80	—	26.8	57.3
SEC	7.21	2.92	6.10	8.72	6.07	5.91	5.38	—	39.1
SWR	7.27	8.60	5.06	5.97	5.44	6.02	6.81	7.82	—

Note: The lower half of the matrix relates to a polygenic distance based upon mandible dimensions. The upper half of the matrix refers to a genetic distance based upon 144 major gene loci.

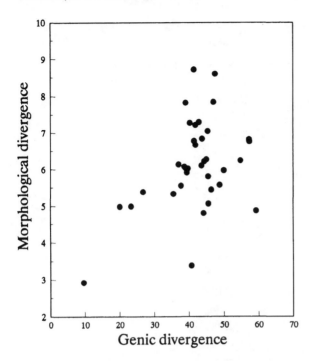

Fig. 6.8. A bivariate plot of the elements of two genetic distance matrices describing divergence among nine inbred strains of mice. One distance estimate (genic) represents the percentage out of 144 fixed alleles that differ between strains. The other genetic distance is the square root of the Mahalanobis pairwise distance statistic which measures genetic divergence among taxa in completely inbred strains.

effects genetic model described earlier while the genetic model describing the control of morphological structures in mammalian species is much more complex (Atchley 1987; Atchley and Newman 1989; Atchley and Hall 1991). Further, it has recently been shown that genetic distance estimates using large numbers of gene loci at the same levels of organization (i.e., protein-coding versus immune system loci) can produce highly discordant estimates of phylogenetic relationships (Atchley and Fitch 1991).

Morphogenetic Components of Mandibular Divergence

Does divergence between taxa in mandibular traits occur through changes in the skeletal derivatives of the mesenchymal condensations? In the developmental model proposed by Atchley and Hall (1991), it was suggested that the adult mandible is produced by the assembly of a number of morphogenetically separate components. Does evolutionary divergence in mandible form occur by means of changes among the skeletal derivatives of these various mesenchymal condensations?

Experimentally, this question can be answered most effectively by histological analyses of the various developmental and cellular parameters involved in mandibular differentiation and morphogenesis. However, such histological data is not yet available. As a consequence, we will have to depend upon analyses of the skeletal derivatives of these condensations.

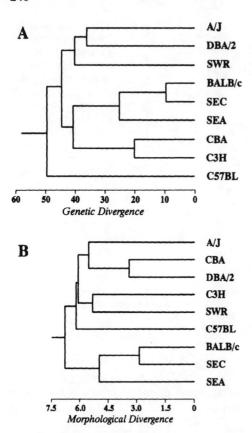

Fig. 6.9. Phenograms arising from UPGMA cluster analyses of the genic and morphological distance statistics given in table 6.9 and plotted in figure 6.8.

Several recent studies involving various rodent taxa have been carried out on divergence in area of the mandible corresponding to the skeletal derivative of these mesenchymal condensations as described in table 6.1. Several studies have used both parametrical statistical analyses and finite element scaling to examine the divergence among inbred strains of mice (Cheverud et al. 1991), between selected lines of mice (Atchley 1992), and the extent divergence between mice and rats (Atchley et al. 1992).

These various studies indicate that significant divergence in mandible form among rodent taxa occurs in the skeletal derivatives of these condensations. For example, significant amounts of divergence occur among various inbred strains of mice in the angular, condyloid, and coronoid processes. Ranking the areas as to their contribution to the divergence in mandibular form among these inbred strains indicates that angular process area and condylar process area showed the greatest divergence, while posterior alveolar area contributed the least.

Atchley et al. (1990) and Atchley (1992) examined mandibular differ-

entiation in five strains of mice which had been selected over 13 generations for percentage fatness and leanness. Two strains of mice were
selected for high and low fat percentage and two strains for high and low
lean percentage, and a fifth was randomly selected as a control strain.
Morphometric analyses of these showed that significant divergence in the
mandible occurred in all of the skeletal areas described in figure 6.5.

Atchley et al. (1992) examined the differentiation in mandibular form
between rats and mice and asked whether morphological differentiation
between these species had occurred in the skeletal derivatives from the
mesenchymal condensations. The mice and rats were adjusted to a common size by removing the effects of differences in overall body size. After
this adjustment, significant differences were found in the size of anterior
and posterior alveolar areas, masseter area, and condylar area. Further, it
was found that the genetic correlation structure among these six skeletal
areas was significantly different between species.

Thus, the findings from several different studies indicate that significant divergence in the form of the mandible in rodents occurs through
changes in the skeletal derivatives of those mesenchymal condensations
described in figures 6.2–6.3. Studies to date have not elucidated the underlying developmental processes which have been changed in order to
produce these skeletal changes. Resolution of questions about the underlying developmental mechanisms awaits critical studies at the cellular level.

Changes in Developmental Choreographies

"Developmental choreography" is a term that refers to the spatial and
temporal coordination of the various component parts of a complex structure and the patterns of integration of these various parts into the final
composite structure (Atchley et al. 1990). "Choreography" is a particularly appropriate term for this dynamic process because it brings to mind
an organized program of events exquisitely coordinated in time and space
(Atchley 1992).

This concept is quite useful in understanding how evolutionary
changes in morphology come about. As described earlier, the evolution of
complex morphological structures is, in fact, the evolution of their underlying developmental processes. Thus, do the different embryologically derived skeletal areas exhibit different temporal patterns of postnatal
growth? Further, how are these patterns and choreographies and their integration altered by selection? Does the amount of relative divergence
among these skeletal areas change during ontogeny?

The various components of the rodent mandible exhibit different patterns of growth and morphogenesis. For example, significant growth in the
anterior alveolar area is completed by 6 weeks postnatal age while significant ontogenetic changes in the size of angular process may continue until

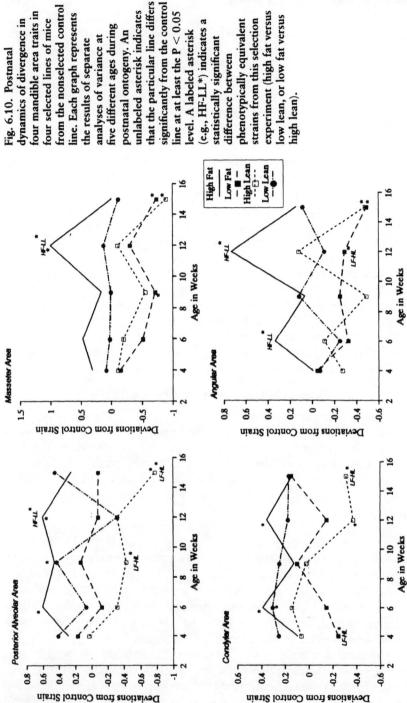

Fig. 6.10. Postnatal dynamics of divergence in four mandible area traits in four selected lines of mice from the nonselected control line. Each graph represents the results of separate analyses of variance at five different ages during postnatal ontogeny. An unlabeled asterisk indicates that the particular line differs significantly from the control line at at least the P < 0.05 level. A labeled asterisk (e.g., HF-LL*) indicates a statistically significant difference between phenotypically equivalent strains from this selection experiment (high fat versus low lean, or low fat versus high lean).

15 weeks of age (Atchley 1992). Does morphological evolution occur through the alternation of the timing of such growth patterns? Figure 6.10 summarizes the effects of changes in the components of body weight (fatness and leanness) on the patterns of postnatal growth for posterior alveolar area, masseter area, condylar area, and angular area as deviations of the selection lines form the randomly selected control strain. These five lines include mice selected over 13 generations for high and low lean percentage, high and low fat percentage, and a randomly selected control line (Eisen 1987). The effects are shown at 4, 6, 9, 12, and 15 weeks postnatal age. Further, this figure demonstrates the points of time during postnatal ontogeny where there are significant differences in mandible morphology between phenotypically similar lines (i.e., high fat and low lean, low fat and high lean). Studies on these particular selected lines show selection has systematically altered the times during postnatal ontogeny during which significant growth begins and ends. Further, selection has altered the age-specific covariance structure among areas and linear dimensions in these mice.

SUMMARY

In this paper, I have provided a brief review of some of the developmental and genetic aspects of variability in the form of the rodent mandible. A developmental model was discussed which considers the mandible to be a complex morphogenetic entity comprised of the skeletal derivatives originating from a series of mesenchymal condensations of neural crest origins. It is suggested that variation in the form of the mature mandible arises from variability underlying the development of the individual skeletal components and variability in the patterns of their integration into a functioning complex structure. A developmental quantitative genetic model is described which would account for genetic variability in mammalian mandibular form. This model includes causal factors representing intrinsic genetic, heritable epigenetic, prenatal and postnatal maternal effects, and random environmental effects.

Quantitative genetic analyses show that considerable genetic variation exists within and between rodent taxa in these various skeletal components. This heritable variation occurs in both linear dimensions as well as in a series of area traits representing skeletal derivatives of the various mesenchymal condensations. Additionally, there is significant variability which arises from prenatal and postnatal maternal effects.

Artificial selection studies show that evolutionary changes in mandibular form involve changes in those mandibular areas which represent the skeletal derivatives of these condensations. The morphological changes are achieved, in part, by alternations in the underlying patterns of growth in the skeletal components, including changes in the initiation and termination of significant periods of postnatal growth. Further, significant changes have occurred between taxa in the genetic correlation structure among the various linear dimensions and areas of mandible.

Considerable further research on the genetic control of mandibular growth and morphogenesis is needed to clarify the genetic architecture of the mandible, to quantify the relative contributions of intrinsic and heritable epigenetic factors during development, and to further ascertain the genetic mechanisms underlying evolutionary divergence in this complex morphological structure.

ACKNOWLEDGMENTS

The research reported in this paper has been very generously supported by a series of grants from the National Science Foundation and the National Institutes of Health. I gratefully acknowledge my current grant support (NIH GM-45344 and NSF BSR-9107108).

REFERENCES

Arnold, S. J., and M. J. Wade. 1984a. On the measurement of natural and sexual selection: Applications. Evolution 38: 720–734.

———. 1984b. On the measurement of natural and sexual selection: Theory. Evolution 38: 709–719.

Atchley, W. R. 1983. A genetic analysis of the mandible and maxilla in the rat. Journal of Craniofacial Genetics and Developmental Biology 3: 409–422.

———. 1984. Ontogeny, timing of development, and genetic variance-covariance structure. American Naturalist 123: 519–540.

———. 1987. Developmental quantitative genetics and the evolution of ontogenies. Evolution 41: 316–330.

———. 1990. Heterochrony and morphological change: A quantitative genetic approach. Seminars in Developmental Biology 1: 289–297.

———. 1992. Selection, developmental choreographies, and heterochronic change in craniofacial development of the mouse. Manuscript.

Atchley, W. R., D. E. Cowley, E. J. Eisen, H. Prasetyo, and D. Hawkins-Brown. 1990. Correlated response in the developmental choreographies of the mouse mandible to selection for body composition. Evolution 44: 669–688.

Atchley, W. R., D. E. Cowley, C. Vogl, and T. McLellan. 1992. Shape change and genetic correlation structure in the rodent mandible. Systematic Biology 41: 196–221.

Atchley, W. R., and W. M. Fitch. 1991. Gene trees and the origins of inbred strains of mice. Science 254: 554–558.

Atchley, W. R., and B. K. Hall. 1991. A model for development and evolution of complex morphological structures. Biological Reviews 66: 101–157.

Atchley, W. R., S. W. Herring, B. Riska, and A. A. Plummer. 1984. Effects of the muscular dysgenesis gene on developmental stability in the mouse mandible. Journal of Craniofacial Genetics and Developmental Biology 4: 179–189.

Atchley, W. R., T. Logsdon, D. E. Cowley, and E. J. Eisen. 1991. Uterine effects, epigenetics, and postnatal skeletal development in the mouse. Evolution 45: 891–909.

Atchley, W. R., and S. Newman. 1989. Developmental quantitive genetic aspects of evolutionary change. American Naturalist 134: 468–512.

Atchley, W. R., S. Newman, and D. E. Cowley. 1988. Genetic divergence in mandible form in relation to molecular divergence in inbred mouse strains. Genetics 120: 239–253.

Atchley, W. R., A. A. Plummer, and B. Riska. 1985a. Genetic analysis of size-scaling patterns in the mouse mandible. Genetics 111: 579–595.

———. 1985b. Genetics of mandible form in the mouse. Genetics 111: 555–577.

Atchley, W. R., and J. J. Rutledge. 1980. Genetic components of size and shape variation. I. Dynamics of components of phenotypic variability and covariability during ontogeny in the laboratory rat. Evolution 34: 1161–1174.

Atchley, W. R., J. J. Rutledge, and D. E. Cowley. 1981. Genetics components of size and shape variation. II. Multivariate covariance patterns in the rat and mouse skull. Evolution 35: 1037–1055.

———. 1982. A multivariate statistical analysis of direct and correlated response to selection in the rat. Evolution 36: 677–698.

Bailey, D. W. 1956. A comparison of genetic and environmental principal components of morphogenesis in mice. Growth 20: 63–74.

———. 1985. Genes that affect the shape of the murine mandible. Journal of Heredity 76: 107–114.

———. 1986a. Genes that affect morphogenesis of the murine mandible. Journal of Heredity 77: 17–25.

———. 1986b. Genetic programming of development: A model. Differentiation 33: 89–100.

Barton, N., and M. Turelli. 1989. Evolutionary quantitative genetics: How little do we know? Annual Review of Genetics 23: 337–370.

Bulmer, M. 1980. The Mathematical Theory of Quantitative Genetics. Oxford: Clarendon Press.

Cheverud, J. M. 1984. Evolution by kin selection: A quantitative genetic model illustrated by maternal performance in mice. Evolution 38: 766–777.

Cheverud, J. M., S. E. Hartman, J. T. Richtsmeier, and W. R. Atchley. 1991. A quantitative genetic analysis of localized morphology in mandibles of inbred mice using finite element scaling analysis. Journal of Craniofacial Genetics and Developmental Biology 11: 122–137.

Cottrill, C. P., C. W. Archer, and L. Wolpert. 1987. Cell sorting and chondrogenic aggregate formation in micromass culture. Developmental Biology 122: 503–515.

Cowley, D. E., and W. R. Atchley. 1992. Quantitative genetic models for development, epigenetic selection, and phenotypic evolution. Evolution 46: 495–518.

Cowley, D. E., D. Pomp, W. R. Atchley, E. J. Eisen, and D. Hawkins-Brown. 1989.

The impact of maternal uterine genotype on postnatal growth and adult body size in mice. Genetics 122: 193–203.

Crompton, A. W. 1963. The evolution of the mammalian jaw. Evolution 17: 431–439.

Dietz, E. J. 1983. Permutation tests for association between two distance matrices. Systematic Zoology 32: 21–26.

Eisen, E. J. 1987. Selection for components related to body composition in mice: Direct responses. Theoretical and Applied Genetics 74: 793–801.

Falconer, D. S. 1989. *Introduction to Quantitative Genetics.* New York: Longman.

Festing, M. F. W. 1973. A multivariate analysis of subline divergence in the shape of the mandible in C57BL/Gr mice. Genetical Research 21: 121–132.

Fitch, W. M., and W. R. Atchley. 1985. Evolution in inbred strains of mice appears rapid. Science 228: 1169–1175.

Gluckman, P. D., and G. C. Liggins. 1984. Regulation of fetal growth. In *Fetal Physiology and Medicine,* R. W. Beard and P. W. Nathaniels, eds. New York: Marcel Dekker, pp. 511–557.

Grüneberg, H. 1963. *The Pathology of Development.* Oxford: Blackwell Scientific.

———. 1975. How do genes affect the skeleton? *New Approaches to the Evolution of Abnormal Embryonic Development,* D. Neuberg and H. J. Merker, eds. Stuttgart: Georg Thieme, pp. 354–359.

Hall, B. K. 1978. *Developmental and Cellular Skeletal Biology.* New York: Academic Press.

———. 1982a. How is mandibular growth controlled during development and evolution? Journal of Craniofacial Genetics and Developmental Biology 2: 45–49.

———. 1982b. Mandibular morphogenesis and craniofacial malformations. Journal of Craniofacial Genetics and Developmental Biology 2: 309–322.

Hall, B. K., and S. Hörstadius. 1988. *The Neural Crest.* London: Oxford University Press.

Herring, S. W. 1993. Epigenetic and functional influences on skull growth. In *The Skull,* J. Hanken and B. K. Hall, eds. Chicago: University of Chicago Press.

Herring, S. W., and T. C. Lakars. 1981. Craniofacial development in the absence of muscle contraction. Journal of Craniofacial Genetics and Developmental Biology 1: 341–357.

Johnson, D. R. 1986. *The Genetics of the Skeleton.* Oxford: Clarendon Press.

Kirkpatrick, M., and R. Lande. 1989. Selection, inheritance, and evolution of maternal characters. Evolution 43: 485–503.

Lande, R. 1979. Quantitative genetic analysis of multivariate evolution, applied to brain: body size allometry. Evolution 33: 402–416.

———. 1980. Sexual dimorphism, sexual selection, and adaptation in polygenic characters. Evolution 34: 292–305.

———. 1982. A quantitative genetic theory of life history evolution. Ecology 63: 607–615.

———. 1988. Quantitative genetics and evolutionary theory. In *Proceedings of the Second International Conference on Quantitative Genetics,* B. S. Weir, E. J.

Eisen, M. M. Goodman, and G. Namkoong, eds. Sunderland, Mass.: Sinauer, pp. 71–84.

Lande, R., and S. J. Arnold. 1983. The measurement of selection on correlated characters. Evolution 37: 1210–1226.

Lavelle, C. L. B. 1983. Study of mandibular shape in the mouse. Acta anatomica 117: 314–320.

Lovell, D. P., and F. M. Johnson. 1983. Quantitative genetic variation in the skeleton of the mouse. I. Variation between inbred strains. Genetical Research 42: 169–182.

Lovell, D. P., P. Totman, and F. M. Johnson. 1984. Variation in the shape of the mouse mandible. 1. Effect of age and sex on the results obtained from the discriminant functions used for genetic monitoring. Genetical Research 43: 65–73.

Moore, W. J. 1981. *The Mammalian Skull.* Cambridge: Cambridge University Press.

Moore, W. J., and C. B. Lavelle. 1974. *Growth of the Facial Skeleton in the Hominoidea.* London: Academic Press.

Neuberg, D., and H. J. Merker. 1975. *New Approaches to the Evolution of Abnormal Embryonic Development.* Stuttgart: Georg Thieme.

Nonaka, K., and M. Nakata. 1984. Genetic variation and craniofacial growth in inbred rats. Journal of Craniofacial Genetics and Developmental Biology 4: 271–302.

Reyment, R. A., R. E. Blackith, and N. A. Campbell. 1984. *Multivariate Morphometrics.* 2d ed. New York: Academic Press.

Sing, C. F., E. Boerwinkle, and P. P. Moll. 1985. Strategies for elucidating the phenotypic and genetic heterogeneity of a chronic disease with a complex etiology. In *Diseases of Complex Etiology in Small Populations,* R. Chakraborty and E. J. E. Szathmary, eds. New York: Alan R. Liss, pp. 39–66.

Sing, C. F., E. Boerwinkle, P. P. Moll, and A. R. Templeton. 1988. Characterization of genes affecting quantitative traits in humans. In *Proceedings of the Second International Conference on Quantitative Genetics,* B. S. Weir, E. J. Eisen, M. M. Goodman, and G. Namkoong, eds. Sunderland, Mass.: Sinauer.

Sokal, R. R., and F. J. Rohlf. 1979. *Biometry.* San Francisco: W. H. Freeman and Co.

Solursh, M. (1983). Cell-cell interactions and chondrogenesis. In *Cartilage,* vol. 2, B. K. Hall, ed., New York: Academic Press.

Thompson, J. N., Jr., and J. M. Thoday. 1979. *Quantitative Genetic Variation.* New York: Academic Press.

Thorogood, P., and C. A. Tickle, eds. 1988. *Craniofacial Development.* Cambridge: Company of Biologists.

Waddington, C. H. 1939. *An Introduction to Modern Genetics.* London: Allan and Unwin.

———. 1940. *Organisers and Genes.* Cambridge: Cambridge University Press.

Wood, A. E. 1965. Grades and clades among rodents. Evolution 19: 115–130.

Wright, S. 1960. Genetics and twentieth century Darwinism: A review and discussion. American Journal of Human Genetics 12: 365–372.

7

Developmental-Genetic Analysis
of Skeletal Mutants

DAVID R. JOHNSON

INTRODUCTION

THE VERTEBRATE SKULL is a complex integrated structure made up of a large number of bones and cartilages. Although there is a tendency toward reduction in this number as we proceed from fishes through amphibians and reptiles to mammals, it is still difficult to decide how to approach the problem of skull design. Form is based on function, but how is form determined and regulated in accord with the demands of function? Should we regard the finished object, the adult skull, as the end product of a large number of small clones of cells, all subjected to fine-grain genetical control, as suggested by Bailey (1985, 1986); or should we regard it as a total object, or perhaps more realistically as a series of coterminous objects, a brain case, a set of masticatory apparatus, a collection of cased sense organs each adapted to its particular function?

Developmental genetics looks at this problem by means of mutations which are random, naturally occurring or induced changes in DNA sequences, some of which do little enough damage to be viable, and some of which affect the skeleton. We can then see which areas of the skeleton (or in this context the skull) are tolerant of reorganization or disorganization, and the effects of this on other areas. We may then hope to extrapolate from these examples the course of normal development. This approach is, of course, fraught with difficulties. Grüneberg (1975), toward the end of a long and successful career, became disillusioned and suggested that the whole area of skeletal genetics was a lottery, and furthermore a "lottery in which people without tickets often win." This followed the realization that the skeleton is, in fact, largely a secondary structure built around other anatomical components. The so-called skeletal genes which Grüneberg pursued for half a lifetime are thus usually no such thing—they frequently change the skeleton en passant as a result of an often distant primary effect. In the strict sense there might, therefore, be relatively few major skeletal genes—limited to those specifying the makeup of the proteins and polysaccharides forming the skeleton and the enzymes governing their metabolism. But a neural tube gene which affects the skeleton only at fourth or fifth hand still gives us information about the skeleton, and this is potentially useful. It is hard to subscribe to Grüneberg's disillusionment and to follow his "spanner in the works" theory (Grüneberg 1975) which suggests that a nonskeletal gene tells us no more of the structure of the skeleton than does the study of broken glass about the structure of a window.

With this caveat—that the skeleton is in many respects secondary to other structures—firmly in mind we may begin to consider the skeletal gene in its best-studied context, the laboratory mouse. I shall also refer, as appropriate, to mutations in other animals, most notably the chick (table 7.1). Skeletal genes have been conventionally divided into three categories: major skeletal genes, modifiers, and the rest, known collectively as the genetic background.

The Major Skeletal Gene

The major skeletal gene is a unit of convenience produced by the skeletal geneticist. Major skeletal genes, by definition, (a) have a regular set of effects on the skeleton and (b) behave in general accord with Mendel's laws, allowing themselves to be classified as dominant, semidominant, or recessive and producing consistent constellations of defects. Animals carrying major skeletal genes form the main armory of the developmental geneticist.

Genetic Modifiers

Major skeletal genes are acted upon by genetic modifiers, which may be enhancing (positive) or suppressive (negative). Suppose we take a litter of mice, segregating for a gene for achondroplasia, which shortens the antero-posterior measurement of the skull. We could select for greater or lesser shortening by choosing individuals from which to breed. After a few generations the process of selection would result in two lines of achondroplastic mice, one with shorter skulls than before and one with longer skulls. The skull dimensions of normal littermates would be unaffected: selection was for modifiers of the original achondroplasia gene, which may often be located by appropriate linkage tests.

The Genetic Background

Mice carrying the same gene for achondroplasia may have different appearances when repeatedly outcrossed to different normal mouse strains.

TABLE 7.1. A representative sample of mutations affecting the blastema, cartilaginous, or osseous stages of skull development, listed in the order in which they are first mentioned in the text

Mutant	Symbol	Species
talpid	ta	chick
amputated	am	mouse
congenital hydrocephalus	ch	mouse
short ear	se	mouse
phocomelia	pc	mouse
shorthead	sho	mouse
nanomelia	nm	chick
cartilage matrix deficiency	cmd	mouse
Disproportionate micromelia	Dmm	mouse
spondylo-metaphyseal chondrodysplasia	smc	mouse
cartilage anomaly	—	rat
brachymorphic	bm	mouse
achondroplasia	ac	rabbit
stumpy	stm	mouse
achondroplasia	cn	mouse
Gyro	Gy	mouse
Hypophosphataemia	Hyp	mouse
Extra toes	Xt	mouse
Scott's polydactylous monster	Px	guinea pig
Patch	Ph	mouse
Tail short	Ts	mouse
first arch malformation	far	mouse
otocephaly	oto	mouse
shorthead	sho	mouse
Small eyes	Sey	mouse
Dancer	Dc	mouse
Twirler	Tw	mouse
chondrodysplasia	cho	mouse
brain hernia	bh	mouse
cerebral degeneration	cb	mouse
obstructive hydrocephalus	oh	mouse
dreher	dr	mouse
Sightless	Sig	mouse
visceral inversion	vi	mouse
hydrocephalus	hy^1, hy^2, hy^3	mouse
Looptail	Lp	mouse
muscular dysgenesis	mdg	mouse
Repeated epilation	Er	mouse

Source: Johnson 1986.

This could, of course, be considered to be the effect of specific genetic modifiers present in different strains: in practice these are usually thought of en masse as the genetic background.

Inbred Strains

The mouse is tolerant of a large degree of inbreeding. Because of this it is possible to brother/sister mate repeatedly and to achieve almost total homozygosity (barring mutation). There is, of course, no choice as to which alleles are fixed within such an inbred strain, but each strain serves as a different genetic background which may modify the effect of a particular major gene. A major gene can be introduced into an inbred strain of choice by repeated backcrossing. If more than one major gene is introduced into the same inbred strain in this way, we can be sure that we are comparing like with like, all potential modifiers being common to both genes.

Pleiotropism

Because skeletal genes are often a long way from the primary gene effect, they are often pleiotropic: that is, the same genes act in many tissues and changes in such genes tend to produce a suite of changes, often expressed as a syndrome. The origin of these syndromes is, of course, of interest to skeletal geneticists.

Grüneberg (1938) distinguished between genuine and spurious pleiotropism. Genuine pleiotropism was held to be the result of multiple primary gene effects, spurious pleiotropism to be based on a single primary gene effect which triggered off a series of secondary "symptoms" or developmental effects, often in different systems of the developing embryo. An analysis of these symptoms and their relationships, a "pedigree of causes" is a useful tool in sorting out the complicated schemes of interaction which are frequently encountered.

Genuine pleiotropism, as defined above, is now thought to be unlikely; the maxim "one gene, one enzyme" which came with the advances in cell biology of the 1960s rules it out. On the other hand painstaking linkage experiments and the newer techniques of chromosome analysis have shown us that some "genes" are in fact small deletions of genetic material. If such a deletion overlaps two codons, then both gene products may be damaged, and our single gene may produce a pedigree of causes which cannot be resolved to a single first cause. Spurious pleiotropism is now seen to occur from the enzyme level upward: cartilage, as we shall see, seems to be especially vulnerable to the level of certain metabolites. Mutations affecting any of these will affect cartilage growth and produce a chondrodysplasia which may be linked with a multitude of other symptoms, depending upon the pathways in which the mutant enzyme is involved.

THE SKULL AND FACIAL SKELETON

Skeletal genes act upon skeletal tissue either directly or indirectly. Many of the mutations listed below and in table 7.1, and others omitted for the sake of brevity, therefore affect the skull merely because it is part of the skeleton.

Ørvig (1967) listed the mineralized (or mineralizable) skeletal tissues as follows: bone, cartilage, enamel, dentine, and the inevitable residue which cannot be easily classified. Moss (1964) suggested that all skeletal tissues were produced by one basic cell type, the scleroblast, and thus implied that all skeletal tissues are closely related. This view, however, changes our preconceptions, for the scleroblast can be mesodermal (chondro-, osteoblast), ectodermal (ameloblast), or derived from the neural crest. The action of the same gene on different scleroblastlike cells would clearly raise the possibility of pleiotropy. For current views the reader should refer to the chapter by Beresford in volume 2 of this work.

The first sign of skeletogenesis is the formation of concentrations of skeletoblasts, usually referred to as condensations. These arise in areas where a bone is to form by intramembraneous ossification or where a cartilage is to appear (irrespective of whether or not this is later to ossify). This phenomenon is not unique to the skeletal system: mesenchymal condensations also precede muscle masses, ligaments, and tendons. The position of a skeletal condensation defines the location of the skeletal element of which it is a precursor, and its shape defines the basic (but not the detailed) shape of the element. Condensations are formed from cells which are either of local origin (as in the limb buds or parts of the skull, Hall 1971) or migrate from elsewhere (mesodermal cells migrate into the chick jaw and ectomesenchymal cells from the neural crest enter the skull, mandible, and pharynx (Jacobson and Fell 1941; Johnston and Listgaren 1972).

Johnson (1986) has reviewed some of the factors governing the formation of condensations (blastemata) and their subsequent fate. Blastemata formed from cells which have migrated from elsewhere will chondrify only if preblastemal cells come into contact with epithelia during their migration (Bee and Thorogood 1980). The bones of the lower jaw, for example, form after blastemal cells have contacted the epithelia of the mandibular arch (Tyler and Hall 1977). Scleral ossicles are formed only after neural crest blastemal cells have interacted with epidermal scleral papillae (Coulombre et al. 1962; Pinto and Hall 1991). Hall (1981) showed that the morphology of the induced bone depended on the blastemal cell type rather than on the type of epithelium with which it came into contact. In blastemata where migration is not seen, Newman (1977) concluded that the induction of cartilage was dependent upon cell density. Increase in cell density is, of course, a way of redefining the process of blastema formation.

Although an increase in mitotic rate in blastemata has been reported in some skeletal elements, including skull bones and the mandible (Hale 1956; Jacobson and Fell 1941; Fyfe and Hall 1983), autoradiography has failed to demonstrate it in others, such as limb cartilage (Janners and Searls 1970; Thorogood 1972), where the cell division rate tends to fall with time as more and more cells become specialized (Abbott and Holtzer 1966; Flickinger 1974). The increased cell density within such blastemata seems to reflect a progressive increase in adhesiveness between blastemal cells: intercellular spaces become smaller and matrix components are secreted in increasing amounts.

Mutations Affecting Blastemata

The Talpid Chick. Any mutant that affects blastemal formation might be expected to have a widespread effect on cartilage, cartilage replacement bone, and muscle. The talpid (ta) series of mutations in the chick (talpid[1], Cole 1942; talpid[2], Abbott et al. 1959; talpid[3], Hunton 1960) are so called because of their short, spadelike wings, which resemble the forelimbs of the mole, *Talpa*. Ede and Kelly (1964) described the defects in the head region (fig. 7.1). The eyes are drawn together in the midline and may partially fuse. There is no upper beak, or at best a small, peglike protrusion, and the nasal process forms a plaque above or between the eyes. The lower beak is often represented only as a midline protrusion. All these abnormalities are interpreted by Ede and Kelly as consequent upon the failure of the prechordal mesoderm to separate into lateral strips and a central prechordal plate. In the trunk and limbs we see similar defects, also consequent upon blastemal condensations which are aberrant in number, position, and size. Ede and Agerback (1968) and Ede and Flint (1975) demonstrated that talpid cells are more adhesive than normal, and suggested that this may be the reason for abnormal condensations.

The Amputated Mouse. Cell culture studies show that the amputated gene in the mouse (am, Flint 1977, Flint and Ede 1978) resembles talpid in affecting cell adhesion (Flint and Ede 1982). Facial development is abnormal and a cleft palate is invariably present (fig. 7.2).

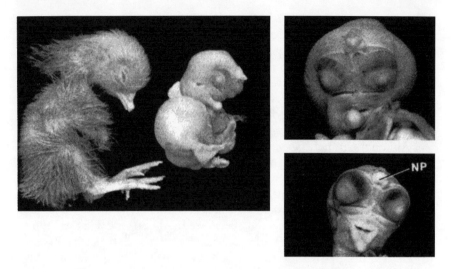

Fig. 7.1. *Left:* Normal and talpid³ embryos aged 14 days. *Right:* Frontal views of talpid³ embryos aged 14 days (above) and 11 days (below). (From Ede and Kelly 1964)

Other Conditions with Abnormal Blastemata. Using talpid and amputated as examples we can make educated guesses about other mutants which affect condensations, where no experimental work has been done. In congenital hydrocephalus in the mouse (ch, Grüneberg 1963, 1975) there is a whole series of abnormalities which suggest that chondrogenic blastemata are small or absent, together with other abnormalities where blastemata forming membrane bone are large and premature. The zygomatic blastema, for instance, is present a whole day earlier than normal in ch, and the large mandibular and maxillary blastemata undergo osseous fusion (fig. 7.3). It is obvious that this ability to "time shift" the appearance of blastemata, and hence their relative sizes at a given point in development, is a potentially important evolutionary mechanism, likely to upset the integrated timing necessary for the construction of a skeletal complex such as the skull (Hall 1984, 1992).

Several genes mimic ch in having reduced cartilaginous blastemata, though without concomitant size increase in those producing membrane bone. Short ear (se, Green 1951) has a whole series of smaller than normal bones and missing or reduced bony processes: membrane bones such as the nasal are also affected, but it is not known whether this is primary or due to the adjacent abnormal cartilage bones. Phocomelia (pc, Glueck-sohn-Waelsh et al. 1956) also affects both cartilaginous and membrane bones; nasals are absent, premaxillae reduced, part of the maxilla usually missing, and the mandible reduced in size. On each side of the nasal capsule an aberrant bar of cartilage forms near the palatal processes (Fitch

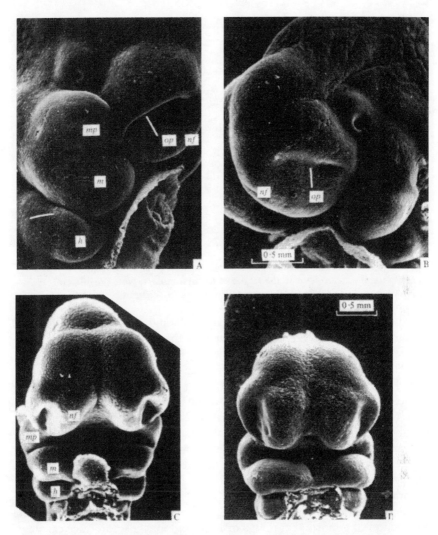

Fig. 7.2. 10.5-day normal (A, C) and amputated (am/am) heads (B, D). Note the shallow olfactory pit (op) is amputated. h, hyoid arch; mp, maxillary process; nf, nasal fold. (From Flint and Ede 1978)

1957) and probably interferes with closure of the secondary palate. Short-head (sho, Fitch 1961a, b), as the name suggests, has a broad, short head associated with a median cleft palate: the skull disproportion is present before cartilage matrix can be demonstrated.

These mutants demonstrate that the skeleton can often be seen to be abnormal at a very early stage in its development, at the time when blas-

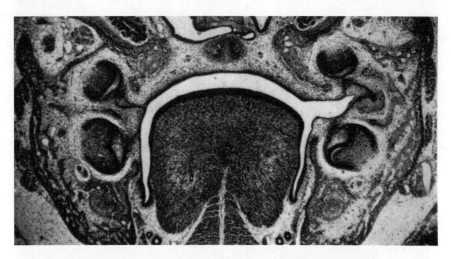

Fig. 7.3. Transverse section through the head of an 18-day-old congenital
hydrocephalus (ch/ch) fetus in the region of the first molars. Note the bilateral
fusion of maxilla and mandible. (From Grüneberg and Wickramaratne 1974)

temal and nonblastemal cells can first be distinguished. Using talpid and
amputated as guides we may suggest that the factor which seems to be
affected in this group of mutants is the degree of cell adhesion.

The blastema often gives us only post hoc notification of an abnormality, seen as a disturbance in bone or cartilage. Grüneberg (1963)
pointed out the consequences of blastematal disruption. Blastemal size is
usually reduced: different genes tend to reduce blastema according to a
specific pattern. Small or retarded blastemata will chondrify or ossify late
and may so retard an area that "developmental appointments" may be
missed. If a blastema is too small (though by what criteria we do not yet
know, see Hinchliffe and Johnson 1983; Thorogood 1983) it may not
chondrify or ossify at all.

It is clear that any mutant which produces blastemata may lead to the
production of abnormal cartilage or bone and may also produce cartilaginous or bony elements which are abnormal in shape or size. It is thus
rather difficult to define our next two categories of mutants, those which
primarily affect cartilage and bone, respectively, with any degree of accuracy: we always run the risk that the first lesion may, in fact, be an undiscovered abnormality of the blastema.

Mutations Affecting Cartilage: Chondrodystrophies

Since cartilage matrix is complex and composed of many components, we
may expect a priori to find mutations which disrupt any or all of them.

Abnormal matrix may be formed from unusual components: collagen, the matrix mucopolysaccharides, and the protein forming the mucopolysaccharide backbone are all suspect. Alternatively the overall balance of the tissue may be upset by over- or underproduction of one component, or all components may be normally balanced but underproduced, or degradation may be absent. Such matrix defects may occur in morphologically abnormal cells, or apparently morphologically normal cells may produce a morphologically normal matrix at a reduced rate, owing to a reduction in metabolic rate or even in the rate of cell division. The most easily recognized cartilage mutant is the classical chondrodystrophy, usually recognized by its effects in the limbs but affecting all cartilages in the body, characteristically shortening the cartilaginous skull base and leading to frontal bossing in the membranous skull vault and frequent cleft palate and abnormalities of the jaw.

Chondrodystrophy or disproportionate dwarfing is typified by human achondroplasia. However these conditions are best referred to as chondrodystrophies, of which achondroplasia is but one example. In humans this imprecision of terminology has led to confusion: in laboratory animals the first chondrodystrophy described in a species is usually termed "achondroplasia": these conditions may or may not correspond to achondroplasia in humans, and it is best to assume that they do not. All chondrodystrophies act rather late in development and affect the epiphyseal growth plates of cartilage replacement bones. Many such conditions of varying severity have been described: at the level of the light microscope we often see only deranged cartilage cell columns: more information comes from metabolic studies or ultrastructure. Johnson (1986) gives a full review of these conditions in various laboratory animals. Here it is sufficient to quote brief examples to show that many different kinds of defect can affect cartilage and thus produce chondrodystrophy.

The Nanomelic Chick, Cartilage Matrix Deficiency Mouse, and Disproportionate Micromelia Mouse: Specific Loss of Cartilage Components. The abnormal cartilage matrix of the nanomelic (nm) chick has been well documented, from Mathews (1967), who noticed that it contained only 10% of the normal mucopolysaccharide but normal levels of collagen, through a series of ever more sophisticated studies (Fraser and Goetinck 1971; Palmoski and Goetinck 1972; Stearns and Goetinck 1979; McKeown-Longo 1981), to the definitive work of Argraves et al. (1981), who showed that the proteoglycan core protein was defective. We also have a good ultrastructural description of nanomelic cartilage (Pennypacker and Goetinck 1976) and know that neural crest–derived cartilage is also affected (McKeown and Goetinck 1979).

Coincidentally a mutation in mouse (cartilage matrix deficiency, cmd) has a very similar first cause. Rittenhouse et al. (1978) described the morphology of the cmd mouse and the ultrastructure of its cartilage, and Kimata et al. (1981) its biochemistry. The latter authors were able to demonstrate the absence of specific core protein. Spondylo-metaphyseal chondrodysplasia (smc) in the mouse (Johnson 1984) and the cartilage anomaly rat (Fell and Grüneberg 1939) are microscopically similar in appearance to cmd, and this might be taken to indicate a similar underlying defect. But we must be careful when making such comparisons even within a species: the ultrastructure of nanomelic cartilage is markedly different from that of cmd.

In disproportionate micromelia (Dmm) in the mouse (Brown et al. 1981) another matrix component is disrupted. This gene preferentially affects the secretion of type II collagen into the extracellular matrix in both the developing appendicular skeleton (Brown et al. 1981) and the inner ear (Van der Water and Galinovic-Schwartz 1987).

The Brachymorphic Mouse and the Achondroplastic Rabbit: Generalized Metabolic Defects Reflected in Cartilage. The main defect in brachymorphic (bm) mice is undersulphation of the mucopolysaccharides in the cartilaginous matrix (Orkin et al. 1976) due to deficient conversion of adenosine 5′-phosphate (APS) to 3′-phosphoadenosine 5′-phosphate (PAPS), a sulphate donor (Sugahara and Schwartz 1979). This naturally implicates the enzyme which catalizes this step, APS kinase, but Schwartz et al. (1982) have also reported the involvement of ATP kinase.

The achondroplastic rabbit (ac) has a mitochondrial defect which results in the virtual absence of oxidative phosphorylation in the cytochrome oxidase region (site III, Bargman et al. 1972).

In both these mutants we see a nonspecific defect present in almost every cell in the body reflected as an achondroplasia. This suggests that cartilage is a tissue particularly vulnerable to metabolic defects.

Stumpy and the Achondroplastic Mouse: Defects in Cell Division. The cell kinetics of stumpy (stm, Ferguson et al. 1978) and achondroplasia (cn, Lane and Dickie 1968) in the mouse have been studied by Thurston et al. (1983, 1985), who showed clear differences from normal littermates. In stumpy, hypertropic cell height is reduced from 10 days; from 16 days onward the growth plate is very irregular with much cell debris present. This can be seen to originate from pairs of dead cells (Johnson 1983). Many lacunae contain large numbers of cells with complicated interdigitation of the membranes. One is forced to conclude that stumpy cells do not part readily after mitosis and that this is often fatal to the cell.

In achondroplasia (cn) there is much inconclusive biochemical evidence (reviewed by Johnson 1986), with a reduced proliferation zone size, mean labeling index, and hypertrophic cell height (Sannasgala and Johnson 1990).

These two mutations serve as examples of defects in cell division, presumably restricted to cartilage, which affect cell proliferation and hence growth.

Mutations Affecting Bone

Defects in bone are usually concerned with its deposition and resorption. There is a clear cascade effect in such genes as talpid[2], where Hinchliffe and Ede (1968) noted a failure of ossification confined to cartilage replacement bones, presumably due to defects at earlier stages. In some genes, however, bone is the first defective tissue seen.

Gyro and Hypophosphataemia: Defects in Bone Deposition. In the sex-linked Gyro (Gy/-, Sela et al. 1982) mouse male there is osteomalacia in the maxilla and inner ear with broad bands of osteoid and unmineralized foci in mineralized areas, and irregular ossification of cartilage. Hypophosphataemia in the mouse (Hyp, also sex-linked, Meyer et al. 1979) has many similarities with the human condition, with low plasma phosphate, low bone ash weight, and widened bands of osteoid.

The Osteopetroses. Many conditions in laboratory animals produce osteopetrosis with reduced bone resorption, failure of teeth to erupt, and occlusion of bony foramina. Dense, poorly mineralized bone is characteristic of all of them (Johnson 1986). As in the chondrodystrophy group of mutations the first causes may be very different in different mutations. All seem to concern specific defects in the numbers of osteoclasts or their biochemistry: no generalized metabolic defect manifesting as bone disease has yet been described. Presumably bone, with its excellent blood supply, is less vulnerable than avascular cartilage.

Mutations Specifically Affecting the Craniofacial Skeleton

We have already noted that some genes affect the skull en passant because they affect all skeletal tissue. Another group of mutations comprises those whose effects are wholly or chiefly limited to the head region and thus affect the skull because it is part of the head. These two facts, taken together, serve to emphasize the differences in the developmental process in these areas.

Conditions of this kind may be subdivided into several subgroups. The first of these affects the visceral arches, chiefly the maxillary arch. This often results in the development of split-faced individuals (when the maxillary arches fail to meet in the midline) or animals with grossly abnormal facial regions due to reduction (or indeed the overgrowth) of the facial processes. Secondly, there are major genes which cause regular cleft lip and palate. Third comes a series of inbred lines in which there is a regular low incidence of cleft lip and palate in the absence of any single major gene. The frequency of such clefts is often susceptible to teratogens and face shape is subtly altered. Fourth is a heterogeneous group with cleft palate alone, with a tendency to altered skull proportions. Lastly comes a group where skull proportions are changed, primarily affecting the braincase, but which may or may not involve palatal clefting.

Major Abnormalities of the Visceral Arches. *Extra-Toes.* This semidominant gene in the mouse (Xt, Johnson 1967) has multiple defects involving many regions. The homozygote is first recognized at nine days of gestation by a wavy neural tube and the large size of the first pharyngeal arch. By 10 days the arch has divided into a large maxillary portion and a mandibular part of normal size. By 13 days the enlarged maxillary arch partly or completely covers the eyes (fig. 7.4); later it carries more mystacial vibrissae than normal. Some Xt/Xt individuals are exencephalic, with a failure of the closure of the cranial neural tube and consequent failure of the vault of the skull to form. The increased size of the maxillary part of the first arch leads to multiple abnormalities in the facial skeleton and skull base, but the palate is closed (although the nasal chamber is grossly misshapen) and the mandible is not described as abnormal. In an allele of Xt, brachyphalangy (Xt^{bph}, Johnson 1969), the nasal processes are widely separated with unilateral or bilateral cleft lip. A similar phenotype was described in the guinea pig (Px, Scott 1937, 1938).

It seems clear that the facial defects in this group of mutants are due to initial overgrowth of the maxillary portion of the first arch, which then interferes mechanically with the eye and nose. The overgrowth may be ascribed to a defective ectodermal-mesodermal interaction (all these mutants are extravagantly pre- and postaxially polydactylous). Alternatively the cns defects also seen in these mutants may extend to the neural crest, which supplies ectomesenchyme to the pharyngeal arches. Both extra-toes and brachyphalangy produce belly spots in the viable heterozygote—an indication of possible neural crest involvement, given that pigment cells are neural crest derivatives.

Patch. Patch (Ph, Grüneberg and Truslove 1960) is another semidominant mouse gene producing a belly spot when heterozygous and lethal when homozygous. Again it is recognizable at nine days by a wavy neural tube.

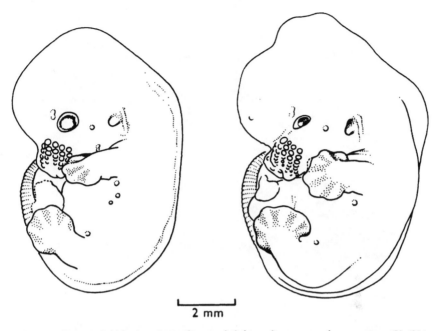

Fig. 7.4. Camera lucida drawings of normal (left) and extra-toes homozygous (Xt/Xt) mouse embryos aged 13 days. (From Johnson 1967)

The Ph/Ph embryo is also more or less waterlogged. Grüneberg and Trus-love describe a face bleb developing in the concavity between the nasal pits in a sectioned 10–11 day embryo: "Once formed, the bleb becomes a mechanical hinderance to the movement of the two halves of the nose to-wards the midline." In their opinion this bleb led to the later occurrence of a cleft-face phenotype (fig. 7.5), which often has the two halves of the face separated by a bleb. Erickson and Weston (1983) noted that fluid-filled blebs also occurred alongside the open patch neural tube at nine days, and that neural crest cells migrate early into these spaces. A face bleb is also seen in some putative Ph/+ individuals: a similar bleb was reported by Johnson (1969) in $Xt^{bph}/+$. The intracellular matrix is reported to be ab-normal within patch blebs (Morrison-Graham and Bork, in Morrison-Graham and Weston 1989). In ruthenium red–stained ultrathin sections, glycoseaminoglycan-like clusters are seen which are two to three times larger than those seen in normal littermates. It is suggested that these ab-normal matrix constituents may affect the migration or differentiation of neural crest–derived cells.

Tail Short. A very similar split-face phenotype was seen in the Tail short mouse (Ts, Morgan 1950) by Matta (1981), who placed the original Ts

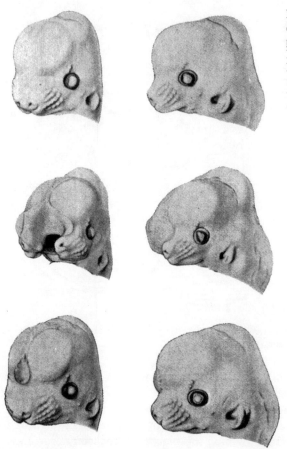

Fig. 7.5. Heads of 13-day embryos from the patch stock. *Top row:* Normal. *Middle row:* Ph/Ph with cleft face. *Bottom row:* ?Ph/ + with face bleb. (From Grüneberg and Truslove 1960)

gene on differing genetic backgrounds (fig. 7.6). Split face was not correlated with exencephaly or hare lip (both present on some backgrounds). Interestingly, Matta mentions oedema only in connection with Ts placed on the patch genetic background. She certainly saw no central face bleb separating the maxillary processes.

First Arch Malformation. The recessive mouse mutation (far, McLoed et al. 1980) affects the secondary palate along with many cranial bones originating chiefly from the first branchial arch. The defects can be traced back to day 12 of gestation. Palatal shelves are deficient and later develop into bizarre polypoid structures. The trigeminal nerve seems to be abnormal where it passes through the maxillary region and the maxillary vibrissal pads and lower eyelid are clearly defective. By day 16 cartilage/bone prep-

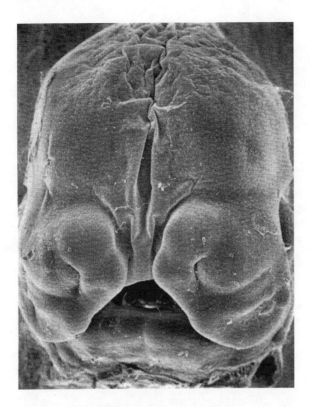

Fig. 7.6. Scanning
electron micrograph
of a 15-day-old Ts/ +
splitface embryo.

arations show clear skeletal abnormalities (fig. 7.7). The zygomatic arch is
thickened and flattened against the side of the head and centers of ossification for the squamosal and alisphenoid are absent. The mandible lacks
most of the coronoid process. By the time of birth the premaxilla is misshapen, and connections between it and the maxilla and between the maxilla and frontal are absent. The zygomatic bone is by now about five times
its normal thickness and the squamosal is virtually absent. There are
smaller defects in the ear ossicles and the styloid apparatus. The secondary
palate is cleft, but the primary palate and lip are intact. Most of these
defects, except the involvement of the styloid apparatus, suggest a defect
of the maxillary part of the first arch, with secondary involvement of the
mandible.

Juriloff and Harris (1983) found that far/far differed from normal
mice in face shape (fig. 7.8), being flattened and deficient in the maxillary
region. Palatal development was disrupted, with palatal shelves reduced in
size lying above the tongue and containing ossifications of abnormal shape.
In some embryos an abnormal rod of cartilage lies lateral to the palate

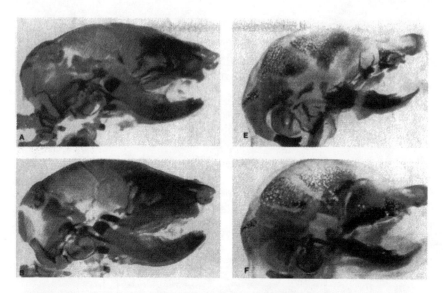

Fig. 7.7. Normal (A) and far/far (B) newborns. Normal (E) and far/far (F) 16-day embryos stained for cartilage and bone and cleared. (From McLoed et al. 1980)

(cf. pc, Fitch 1957). Meckel's cartilage and the lower jaw appear normal. Later, palatal shelves were lobed irregularly anteriorly and deficient posteriorly.

Amputated. Flint and Ede (1978) described facial development in the amputated (am) mouse, which we have already discussed as a blastematal mutant. Here the nasal pit fails to invaginate as deeply as usual (fig. 7.2). This region is largely of neural crest origin, but since amputated mice cannot be recognized (on the basis of a shortened body axis) until after the neural crest has migrated, a direct test of neural crest malfunction is not possible. However dorsal root ganglia are of normal size, the dermal skeleton of the head is not deficient, and mandibular, maxillary, and nasal portions of the skeleton are present, though shortened. Cell density at 9.5 to 10.5 days is normal in nasofacial mesenchyme, and Flint and Ede do not regard shortage of mesenchyme as a basis for the facial defects. Flint (1980) extended these studies to the palate (invariably cleft in amputated) and found no decrease in mitotic rate, but an increase in contact area between cells, suggesting once again increased cell adhesion as the basis of the amputated syndrome.

Otocephaly. The ultimate result of reduction in facial processes is otocephaly, a drastic reduction in the anterior part of the head. Juriloff et al.

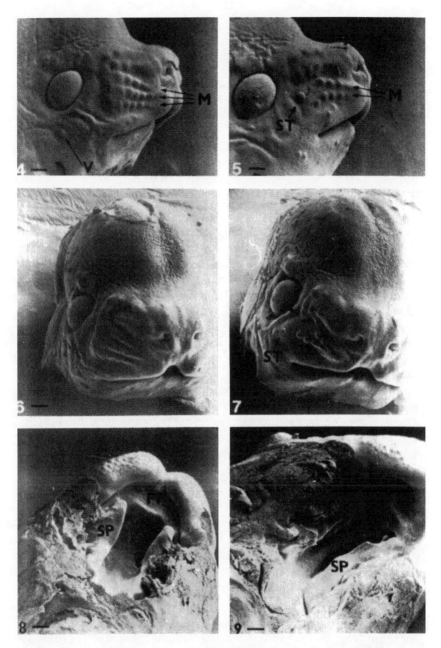

Fig. 7.8. Scanning electron micrograph of 13-day-old normal (4, 6) and far/far (5, 7) embryos, and 14-day-old normal (8) and far/far (9) palates. PP, primary palate; SP, secondary palate; ST, skin tag; M, mystacial vibrissae. (From Juriloff and Harris 1983)

(1985) have recently described such a defect due to a single gene (oto) in the mouse, which seems to be based upon a deficiency of certain mesodermal cell populations in the anterior part of the embryonic disc. At 16 days oto/oto mice may have only a single nostril, agnathia, a reduced tongue, and a univentricular telencephalon. The secondary palate is usually present but distorted, and the nasal septum is usually absent. Earlier stages (12–14 days) show a range of defects involving a progressive reduction of the structures of the head. At 10 days the head is narrow and the mandibular processes small and closely applied in the midline, although the maxillary processes appear relatively normal. At nine days the prosencephalic part of the neural tube can be seen to be defective.

Phocomelia In phocomelia (pc) Siskin and Glueksohn-Waelsch (1959) reported smallness of the head region, especially the mandible in 13.5-day-old embryos. Fitch (1957) had already described a reduction in the size of the condensations which are destined to become the mandible and maxilla, and by day 15 reported that the maxilla, premaxilla, and mandible are reduced and that the head is smaller and narrower than usual. The chondrocranium is not proportionately reduced, although abnormal in many areas. At birth (Glueksohn-Waelsch et al. 1956) the head is narrow and pointed with a wide palatal cleft, the nasal bones absent, the premaxilla reduced, the maxilla partially absent, and the mandible reduced in width and length.

Taken with the disproportionate dwarfing of the rest of the phocomelic skeleton and the incidence of poly- or syndactyly, the late-appearing abnormalities of the tissues of the pharyngeal arches suggest that arch tissue as such is not necessarily abnormal in this mutant, but that general misallocation of tissue at the blastemal stage has perhaps occurred.

Shorthead. The defects in shorthead (sho, Fitch 1961a, b) also seem to be based on defective facial processes. Abnormals can be identified at 12 days by their foreshortened heads; at 13 days the groove separating the left and right sides of the face is shallow and wide and the lower jaw flatter than normal. Shorthead mice go on to develop a wide median palatal cleft: premaxillae, maxillae, and sphenoids are small and of abnormal shape.

Small Eyes. The semidominant Small eyes (Sey, Roberts 1967) was named for the microphthalmia seen in the heterozygote. Hogan et al. (1986) identified the homozygous abnormal in litters from Sey/+ − Sey/+. Sey/Sey at 10.5 days has no nasal pits and no lens to the eye and later develops only small frontonasal protuberances (fig. 7.9). These embryos are viable at 18.5 days post coitus but are eaten by the mother at or after birth. Hogan et al. (1986) note that the maxillae are normal with the normal compliment of whisker follicles: Hogan et al. consider that the defect in Sey lies in the nasal placode (cf. Hill et al. 1991). Small eyes is allelic to a radiation-induced mutation (Small eyes Harwell, Sey^H) and to Dickie's Small eye (Sey^{Sey}).

Skull Proportions and Visceral Arch Abnormalities. Many mouse genes which affect the pharyngeal arches (the heterozygotes of Ph, Ts, Xt, sho/sho) have an increased incidence of the interfrontal bone, and pc has widely parted frontals. This suggests that the presence of an interfrontal bone may be used as an indicator of changed skull proportions. Johnson (1976) calculated a simple index of skull proportions in the presence or absence of an interfrontal bone. In those mice with no interfrontal the width/length index varied widely, but its size when present was positively correlated with relative increase in skull width.

Cleft Lip and Cleft Palate. The formation of the secondary palate in those reptiles where it is present in birds and in mammals is complex, relying as it does on the uniting in the midline of the palatine processes (themselves part of the maxillary processes of the first pharyngeal arch). This is complicated by the original caudal direction of growth of these processes, which must therefore rotate medially before fusion. Anteriorly the fused palatine processes must also make contact with the primitive palate in the premaxillary region and superiorly with the developing nasal septum. Failure of union of the palatine processes (palatal shelves) is conventionally described as cleft palate. Defects at the margins of the premaxilla are usually described as cleft (or hare) lips.

Dancer and Twirler. Dancer (Dc, Deol and Lane 1966; Trasler 1969) and twirler (Tw, Lyon 1958; Juriloff 1978) are rather similar in combining cleft lip and palate (of incomplete penetrance) with a constellation of behavioral defects. The cleft lip in dancer is thought to be due to a decrease in the mesenchyme of the nasal processes (Trasler and Leong 1976). It is not clear whether these mutants form a separate subgroup or should be regarded as an extension of the group affecting the pharyngeal arches.

Cleft Lip and Palate in Inbred Strains. Spontaneous cleft lip and palate has a low incidence in most strains of mice (Kalter 1978; Loevy 1968) but is much commoner (c. 10%) in certain derivatives of the A strain (Staats 1972). Outcrossing A strains to other mice produces offspring without

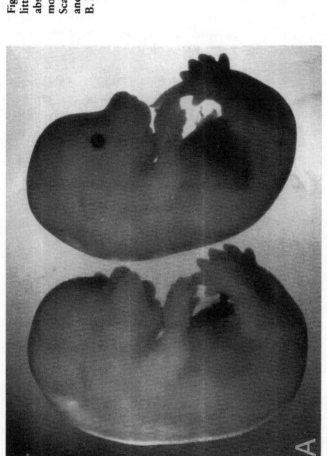

Fig. 7.9. A. Sey/Sey^H (left) and normal littermate aged 13.5 days. Sey/Sey^H shows absence of eyes and nose and retarded facial morphogenesis. (From Hogan et al. 1986). B, C. Scanning electron micrographs of Sey/Sey (left) and Sey/? (right) aged 11.5 days. (Courtesy of B. Hogan)

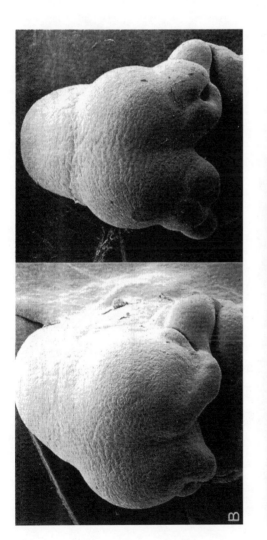
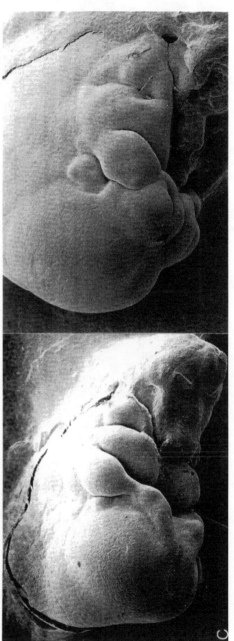

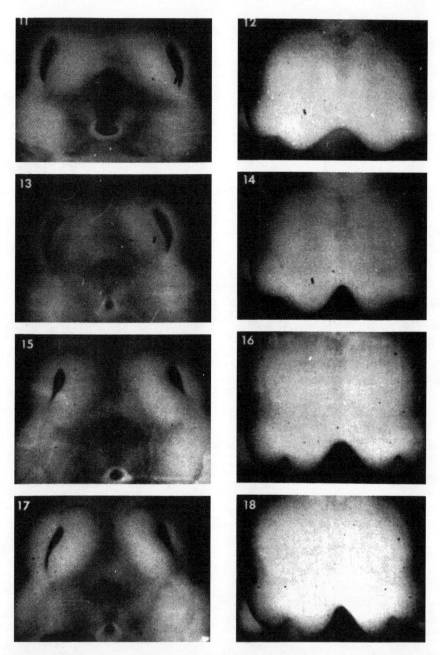

Fig. 7.10. Differences in face shape between C57BL (11, 12, 15, 16) and A/J (13, 14, 17, 18) mice. (From Trasler 1968)

clefts (Loevy 1968), thus ruling out a pure maternal effect and the presence of dominant genes. Backcrossing to A reintroduces the cleft at a lower frequency. The difference between backcross and parental strains suggests that no more than three or four genes are involved. There is often a maternal component in backcrosses (Francis 1973, Loevy 1968). The marked abnormalities of the face in such genes as Patch (Ph), Tail short (Ts), and Extra-toes (Xt) together with the altered skull proportions suggest that a less marked change in facial shape may be seen in A. Trasler (1968) compared A and C57BL fetuses and found differences in size and proportion (fig. 7.10) and frequent asymmetries in A which could be the forerunners of facial clefts. Millikovsky et al. (1982) looked at the areas of difference identified by Trasler, mainly the borders of lateral and medial nasal processes, using the scanning electron microscope (fig. 7.11) and found changes in the behavior of epithelial cells in this area (fig. 7.12)

Cleft Palate without Cleft Lip. *Major Genes.* Many mutant genes produce cleft palate alone or as part of a wider syndrome of abnormalities. This is obviously a heterogeneous group, but many of its members share with previously described abnormalities of the pharyngeal arches a tendency towards abnormal skull proportions, based on failure of the skull to elongate normally. Interruption of skull growth (as in the chondrodystrophies) may predispose to a palatal cleft. However many genes are known which produce a broad, short skull with a normal palate. Cleft palate is thus a regular feature of chondrodysplasia (cho, Seegmiller and Fraser 1977; fig. 7.13) and cartilage matrix deficiency (cmd, Rittenhouse et al. 1978), in both of which cartilage growth is affected, and of hypophosphataemia (Hyp, Iorio 1980), where bone growth is abnormal, but not in the short, wide skulls of brain hernia (bh, Bennett 1959), brachymorphic (bm, Lane and Dickie 1968), or achondroplasia (cn, Jolly and Moore 1975).

Inbred Strains. Once again we find a low incidence of cleft palate without cleft lip in some strains, and a higher incidence in others. And once again the A strain is most susceptible to the condition (Fraser and Faintstat 1951). Since cleft lip and palate and simple cleft palate have high incidences in the same strains and respond to the same teratogens, it seems likely that they are based on similar defects in development. For cleft lip and palate Biddle and Fraser (1977) suggested two or three loci, one of which was linked to the H-2 histocompatibility locus. This locus accounted for about 80% of the difference in susceptibility between strains, but since CBA/J and C3H/HeJ share the same H-2 haplotype but differ in susceptibility (Goldman et al. 1977), another locus or loci must be involved.

What exactly do these genes do? Leong et al. (1973) looked at the

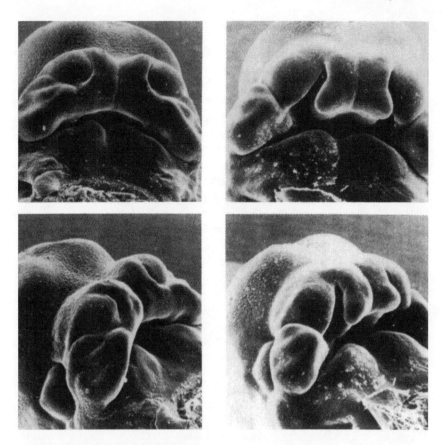

Fig. 7.11. Scanning electron micrographs of C57BL/6J (left) and CL/Fr mice (right) at the 18-tail somite stage. (From Millikovsky et al. 1982)

growth of the cranial base in A strain mice. They thought, following Harris (1964, 1967), that growth of the cranial base might be important in palatal closure. Harris suggested that the upward extension of the cranial base would raise the nasal septum and primary palate so that the anterior extremities of the palatal shelves could be brought above the tongue and that the increased size of the oral cavity so produced would allow forward growth or movement of the tongue and lower jaw. Harris noted strain-dependent differences in this extension and a decrease in cortisone-treated fetuses. Smiley (1967), Barbula et al. (1970), Wragg et al. (1970) and Leong et al. (1973) all made measurements of cranial growth. Leong et al. additionally extended the work by looking for areas of high mitotic rate in the cranial base cartilage. Vertical, unrotated palatal shelves are associated with a curved sphenoid; embryos whose shelves had rotated but not

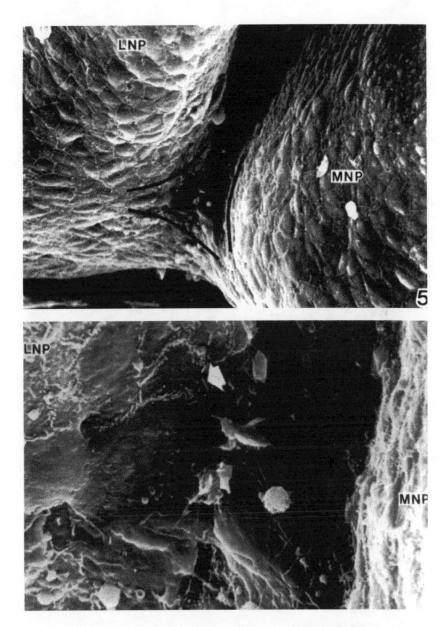

Fig. 7.12. Fusion of median nasal processes (MNP) and lateral nasal processes (LNP) in C57BL (above) and CL/Fr (below) mice. In CL/Fr the median and lateral nasal processes are widely separated. (From Millikovsky et al. 1982)

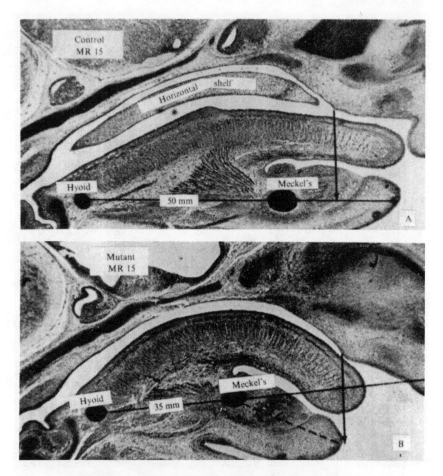

Fig. 7.13. Midsagittal sections through the head of (A) normal and (B) cho/cho mouse fetuses aged 15 days. (From Seegmiller and Fraser 1977)

yet fused had less curved sphenoids, and straight sphenoids were associated with complete palatal fusion. Areas of rapid cartilaginous growth were seen in craniopharyngeal, presphenoid, and mesethmoid regions. 6-aminonicatinomide (a teratogen increasing the number of cleft palates seen) led to the reduction of mitotic rate in the presphenoid and craniopharyngeal regions.

Miller et al. (1978) used chimeras between a susceptible strain (T1Wh) and the resistant C57BL to show that the more T1Wh cells present in the palatal region, the greater the chance of a palatal cleft.

The relationship between cleft lip and palate is now a little clearer. If the rotation of the palatal shelves depends upon sufficient growth of the basicranium allied to straightening of the basicranial axis, we must allow that in some cases the basicranium would straighten and the shelves try to unite but be impeded, perhaps by the tongue. This would produce a subgroup with straight basicranial axis and incomplete palate. The A strain cleft lip and palate are of this type. Trasler and Fraser (1963) suggested a series of possible mechanisms for palatal clefting in A-strain mice where the sphenoid has straightened. They were: (1) intrinsic shelf force was impaired (affected by cortisone), (2) resistance of tongue increased (as following amniotic puncture), (3) head was too wide to allow palatal shelves to meet in the midline (see Smiley et al. 1971), (4) shelves were too narrow to meet in the midline, and (5) fusion was inhibited.

Trasler and Fraser found that in A strain mice with cleft lip and palate the median nasal processes are larger than normal (leading to cleft lip) and that the tongue is also enlarged. The tip of the enlarged tongue is closely applied to the tip of the enlarged nasal processes. In normal embryos the tongue starts to move forward as the palatal processes start to unite above it posteriorly; in individuals with cleft lip and palate the tongue remains applied to and indented by the medial nasal processes. The tongue therefore arches craniad as seen in longitudinal section and obstructs further palatal closure, or at least delays it until the shelves, on becoming horizontal, can no longer meet in the midline.

Diewert (1982) compared craniofacial growth in four strains of mice (A/J, SWV, C3H, and C57BL/6J; fig. 7.14) and found the same developmental processes present in all, with C57BL the most advanced and A/J the most retarded at any given chronological age. One key relationship in palatal closure seems to be that between the lengths of the mandible and the primary palate, which allows the change in position of the tongue in the oronasal cavity. The relative position of the head and thorax is also critical: lifting the head increases the vertical dimension of the oronasal cavity and tends to decrease the effective length of the nasomaxilary region by rotating the upper face.

The Braincase. Several mutations interfere with the neurocranium in ways other than the restriction of the cranial base seen in chondrodysplasias. These are usually due to increases in the size of the brain, which are, in turn, usually due to hydrocephalus or disruption of the vault, such as that produced by anencephaly.

Hydrocephalus. Hydrocephalus is a fairly common feature of skeletal mutations. In brain hernia (already mentioned for its effect on skull proportions; Bennett 1959), for instance, hydrocephaly and microphthalmia allied to a cerebral herniation between frontal and parietal bones reshape the braincase. Similar secondary rearrangement of the vault by an abnor-

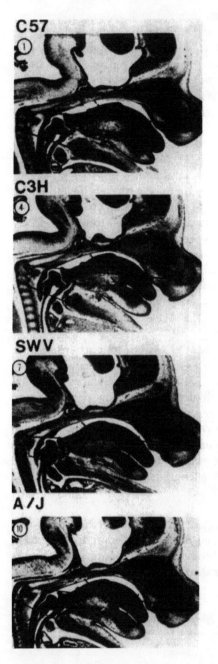

Fig. 7.14. Midsagittal sections through the heads of four strains of mouse fetus at a bodyweight of approx. 200 mg showing variation in head shape. (From Diewert 1982)

mal brain is seen in cerebral degeneration (cb, Deol and Truslove 1963), congenital hydrocephalus (ch, Grüneberg 1953; Green 1970), obstructive hydrocephalus (oh, Borit and Sidman 1972), dreher (dr, Fischer 1956), sightless (Sig, Searle 1965), and visceral inversion (vi, Tihen et al. 1948). Besides these conditions, often associated with eye or ear defects, three other genes have been named for hydrocephalus, which is the major presenting symptom. Hydrocephalus-1 (hy-1, Clark 1932) and hydrocephalus-2 (hy-2, Zimmerman 1933) are not allelic; hydrocephalus-3 (hy-3, Grüneberg 1943) has not been tested for allelism with the others. In all cases a classic dome-shaped head is present at birth or develops in the early weeks of life. The condition may be lethal or prevent breeding. In all cases it seems reasonable to assume that the effects on the skull vault are secondary to the increased size of the brain.

Anencephaly. The above remarks on hydrocephalus may apply even more strongly to anencephaly. In conditions such as Xt^{bph} (Johnson 1969) where the neural tube fails to close it may be thought that there is no possibility of the development of a normal brain, and hence no possibility of development of a normal skull. We must, however, beware of an oversimplistic view of anencephaly. In many cases (Xt^{bph}, Bn, Johnson 1976; Looptail, Lp, Strong and Hollander 1949; Smith and Stein 1962) there are indications of early, profound defects of axial elongation or the early development of the neural tube to which anencephaly may be secondary; some defects in the skulls of such mice may therefore be due to neural tube or neural crest defects.

Extraneous Factors Interfering with Skull Development

In addition to defects of the neural tube other systems may affect the development of the face. Two are mentioned here as examples. Pai (1965) noted the effects on the cranium of the gene muscular dysgenesis (mdg) in the mouse. The crania of homozygous abnormals (which die perinatally) are domelike, with slender zygomatic arches displaced dorsally. Cleft palate is common. The posterior part of the mandible is distorted and compressed dorso-ventrally and condylar and angular cartilages are reduced in width. Herring and Lakars (1981) suggest that the defects seen in the skull are a result of development in the absence of muscular contraction. Atchley et al. (1984) found an increase in fluctuating asymmetry (again suggestive of a secondary effect) but no statistically significant size or shape differences in the + /mdg mandible.

The epithelium covering the head may also be defective and upset normal development of the cranium. Tassin et al. (1983) describe the development of the cranial region in the mutant Repeated epilation (Er). Heterozygote mice have a defective coat, while homozygotes die at birth with severe malformations of the face, limbs, and tail. Holbrook et al. (1982) demonstrated abnormal epidermal keratinization, hyperplastic epidermis, and certain biochemical defects in this mutant. Homozygotes have small heads from 13 days onward. At 13.5 days their lips fuse from their lateral edges. The palatal shelves remain vertical or become horizontal but do not fuse, since the medio-palatal epithelium persists (as, interestingly, it does in normal development outside the mammalia). The defects seen here are once again put down to the effects of systems outside the skeleton, in this case the skin.

MUTATION AND NORMAL DEVELOPMENT

I have demonstrated that the effects of mutant genes upon the developing skull are of several kinds. First there are the purely trivial: an increase in brain size occurring late in fetal development or after birth is accommodated by an increase in the size of its container, the neurocranium. At some unspecified limit the skeleton becomes unable to cope with the increase in size demanded from it (perhaps running out of suitable raw material, i.e., skeletogenic cells) and the skull is left incomplete. Secondly there are the systemic defects in the three phases of skeletogenesis—membranous blastemata, cartilage, and bone—which lead inexorably to generalized reduced growth, defective cartilage formation, or defective ossification. The skull is no more and no less prone to show these defects than the rest of the skeleton. Thirdly, and most interesting, are defects in the skull caused by defects in the formation of the head, chiefly the pharyngeal arches. Here early developmental abnormalities are seen to result in a whole spectrum of defects of the facial region and palate, often confirming what we already knew of the embryological origins of various regions and offering the possibility of our knowing more.

When the first draft of this paper was prepared it was possible to consider skeletal mutations which affected pattern without reference to a rather esoteric group of genes containing ancient, conserved regions known as homeoboxes which seemed to specify positional information, notably in insects. Since then our knowledge of homeoboxes has spread, conserved sequences have been identified in vertebrates, and the time of appearance and spatial location of their gene products have been mapped. The findings of Frohman et al. (1990) will serve as an example of the way in which these genes add to our knowledge and as an entree into the homeobox literature.

The basic vertebrate body plan develops by a series of coordinated movements of ectoderm, mesoderm, and endoderm during gastrulation. This, and the specification of the neural tube and of regional identities along the antero-posterior axis is fairly well understood in amphibian and avian embryos, which are susceptible to experimental manipulation, but less well understood in mammals (see Beddington 1982, 1986). However it seems reasonable to infer that positional information in all classes lies in the mesoderm and is disseminated late in gastrulation or early in neurulation (the time of formation of the neural tube).

One group of *Drosophila* genes, the Antp-like *Hox* gene family, are sequentially expressed along the A-P axis and determine segmental identity (Akam 1989; Lewis 1989). In *Xenopus* the same sequence (X1HBox-1) is expressed in mesoderm and ectoderm with the same anterior and posterior boundaries (Oliver et al. 1988), suggesting that the transfer of position-specifying information across germ layers. Frohman et al. (1990) point out that such coterminous expression is hard to demonstrate at midgestation in mice (when most studies have been carried out, since the gene products are most easily visualized at these later stages), since the germ layers have undergone relative movement. *Hox* 2.9 in the mouse, however, is expressed earlier, and the expression in ectoderm and mesoderm is consistent with the hypothesis that mesoderm gives positional clues to apposed neurectoderm during neurulation. Interestingly the expression of this gene wanes after neurulation in the mesoderm associated with rhombomere four of the prospective hindbrain. This is consistent with findings in the chick (Kieny et al. 1972; Noden 1988) that the A-P identities of hindbrain paraxial mesoderm do not become irreversibly determined at this stage, but can be respecified by, for example, neural crest cells. The expression of *Hox* 2.9 may therefore also shed light on the later development of the branchial arches. Trunk mesoderm, in contrast, seems to retain its original positional specification.

Hox 2.9 as used by Frohman et al. (1990) is a normal gene: it takes little imagination to see that a nonlethal mutation within this ancient conserved DNA could produce changes in pattern formation corresponding to one or another of the genes described in this chapter, and it seems likely to be only a matter of time before one or another of the entities which we now know as skeletal genes is mapped into a homeobox. In fact, the Small eyes mutant has now been shown to be a mutation of a pairedlike homeobox gene (Hill et al. 1991).

The gradation through normal variation to gross abnormality reminds us that mutation in the skeleton need not be major to be of interest. The complicated final shape of the normal vertebrate skull must be the end product of many subtle genetic control mechanisms, each contributing to change in shape. The abnormalities produced by major skeletal genes are unsubtle and produce massive, often crude changes in skull morphology. These are naturally of interest, since similar massive crude changes in humans produce unfortunate individuals needing medical or surgical intervention. In this context, however, we must proceed from major to minor: when we understand the causes of normal variation in morphology we shall begin to understand how a skull is made.

REFERENCES

Abbott, U. K., and H. Holtzer. 1966. The loss of phenotypic traits by differentiated cells. III. The reversible behaviour of chondrocytes in primary cultures. Journal of Cell Biology 28: 473–478.

Abbott, U. K., L. W. Taylor, and H. Abplanalp. 1959. A second talpid like mutation in the fowl. Poultry Science 38: 1185.

Akam, M. 1989. Hox and HOM: Homologous gene clusters in insects and vertebrates. Cell 57: 347–349.

Argraves, W. S., P. J. McKeown-Longo, and P. F. Goetinck. 1981. Absence of glycoprotein core protein in the cartilage mutant nanomelia. FEBS Letters 132: 265–268.

Atchley, W. R., S. W. Herring, B. Riska, G. G. Plummer. 1984. Effects of the muscular dysgenesis gene on developmental stability in the mouse mandible. Journal of Craniofacial Genetics and Developmental Biology 4: 179–189.

Bailey, D. W. 1985. Genes that affect the shape of the murine mandible: Cogenic strain analysis. Journal of Heredity 76: 107–114.

———. 1986. Genes that affect the morphogenesis of the murine mandible. Journal of Heredity 77: 17–25.

Barbula, W. J., G. R. Smiley, and A. D. Dixon. 1970. The role of the cartilaginous nasal septum in midfacial growth. American Journal of Orthodontics 58: 250–263.

Bargman, G. J., B. Mackler, and T. H. Shepard. 1972. Studies of oxidative energy deficiency. I. Achondroplasia in the rabbit. Archives of Biochemistry and Biophysics 150: 137–146.

Beddington, R. S. P. 1982. An autoradiographic analysis of tissue potency in different regions of the embryonic ectoderm during gastrulation in the mouse. Journal of Embryology and Experimental Morphology 69: 265–285.

———. 1986. Analysis of tissue fate and prospective potency in the egg cylinder. In *Experimental Approaches to Mammalian Development,* J. Rossant and R. A. Pederson, eds. Cambridge: Cambridge University Press.

Bee, J., and P. V. Thorogood. 1980. The role of tissue interactions in the skeletogenic differentiation of avian neural crest cells. Developmental Biology 78: 47–60.

Bennett, D. 1959. Brain hernia, a new recessive mutation in the mouse. Journal of Heredity 50: 264–268.

Biddle, G. G., and F. C. Fraser. 1977. Cortisone induced cleft palate in the mouse: A search for the genetic control of the embryonic response trait. Genetics 85: 289–302.

Borit, A., and R. L. Sidman. 1972. New mutant mouse with communicating hydrocephalus and secondary aqueductal stenosis. Acta neuropathologica, Berlin 21: 316–311.

Brown, K. S., R. E. Cranley, R. Greene, H. K. Kleinman, J. P. Pennypaker. 1981. Disproportionate micromelia (Dmm): An incomplete dominant mouse dwarfism with abnormal cartilage matrix. Journal of Embryology and Experimental Morphology 62: 165–182.

Clark, F. H. 1932. Hydrocephalus: A hereditary character in the house mouse. Proceedings of the National Academy of Science, U.S.A. 18: 654–656.

Cole, R. K. 1942. The "talpid" lethal in the domestic fowl. Journal of Heredity 33: 82–86.

Coulombre, A. J., J. L. Coulombre, and H. Mehta. 1962. The skeleton of the eye. I. Conjunctival papillae and scleral ossicles. Developmental Biology 5: 382–401.

Deol, M. S., and P. W. Lane. 1966. A new gene affecting the morphogenesis of the vestibular part of the inner ear in the mouse. Journal of Embryology and Experimental Morphology 16: 543–558.

Deol, M. S., and G. M. Truslove. 1963. A new gene causing cerebral degeneration in the mouse. In *Proceedings of the Eleventh International Congress of Genetics*, vol. 1, J. Geerts, ed. New York: Pergamon Press, pp. 183–184.

Diewert, V. M. 1982. A comparative study of craniofacial growth during secondary palate development in four strains of mice. Journal of Craniofacial Genetics and Developmental Biology 2: 247–263.

Ede, D. A., G. S. Agerback. 1968. Cell adhesion and movement in relation to the developing limb pattern in normal and talpid[3] mutant chick embryos. Journal of Embryology and Experimental Morphology 20: 81–100.

Ede, D. A., and O. P. Flint. 1975. Intercellular adhesion and the formation of aggregates in normal and talpid[3] mutant chick limb mesenchyme. Journal of Cell Science 18: 97–111.

Ede, D. A., and W. A. Kelly. 1964. Developmental abnormalities in the head region of the talpid[3] mutant of the fowl. Journal of Embryology and Experimental Morphology 12: 161–182.

Erickson, C. A., and J. A. Weston. 1983. An SEM analysis of neural crest migration in the mouse. Journal of Embryology and Experimental Morphology 74: 97–118.

Fell, H. B., and H. Grüneberg. 1939. The histology and self differentiating capacity of the abnormal cartilage in a new lethal mutation in the rat (Rattus norvegicus). Proceedings of the Royal Society B127: 257–277.

Ferguson, J. M., M. E. Wallace, and D. R. Johnson. 1978. A new type of chondrodystrophic mutation in the mouse. Journal of Medical Genetics 15: 128–131.

Fischer, H. 1956. Morphologische und mikroskopisch-anatomische Untersuchungen am Innenohr eines Stammes spontanmutierter Hausmäuse (dreher). Zeitschrift für microscopisch-anatomische Forschung 62: 348–406.

Fitch, N. 1957. An embryological analysis of two mutants in the mouse, both producing cleft palates. Journal of Experimental Zoology 136: 329–357.

———. 1961a. Development of cleft palate in mice homozygous for the shorthead mutation. Journal of Morphology 109: 151–157.

————. 1961b. A mutation in mice producing dwarfism, brachycephaly, and micromelia. Journal of Morphology 109: 141–149.

Flickinger, R. A. 1974. Muscle and cartilage differentiation in small and large explants from chick embryo limb bud. Developmental Biology 41: 202–208.

Flint, O. P. 1977. Cell interactions in the developing axial skeleton in normal and mutant mouse embryos. In Vertebrate Limb and Somite Morphogenesis, D. A. Ede, J. R. Hinchliffe, and M. Balls, eds. Cambridge: Cambridge University Press, pp. 465–484.

————. 1980. Cell behaviour and cleft palate in the mutant mouse amputated. Journal of Embryology and Experimental Morphology 58: 131–142,

Flint, O. P., and D. A. Ede. 1978. Facial development in the mouse: A comparison between normal and mutant (amputated) mouse embryos. Journal of Embryology and Experimental Morphology 48: 249–267.

————. 1982. Cell interactions in the developing somite: In vitro comparison between amputated (am/am) and normal mouse embryos. Journal of Embryology and Experimental Morphology 67: 113–125.

Francis, B. M. 1973. Influence of sex linked genes on embryonic sensitivity to cortisone in three strains of mice. Teratology 7: 119–126.

Fraser, F. C., and T. D. Fainstat. 1951. Production of congenital defects in the offspring of pregnant mice treated with cortisone. Pediatrics 8: 527–533.

Fraser, R. A., and P. F. Goetinck. 1971. Reduced synthesis of chondroitin sulphate by cartilage from the mutant nanomelia. Biochemical and Biophysical Research Communications 43: 494–503.

Frohman, M. A., M. Boyle, and G. R. Martin. 1990. Isolation of the mouse Hox-2.9 gene: Analysis of embryonic expression suggests that positional information along the anterior-posterior axis is specified by mesoderm. Development 110: 589–607.

Fyfe, D. M., and B. K. Hall. 1983. The origin of the ectomesenchymal condensations which precede the development of the bony scleral ossicles in the eyes of embryonic chicks. Journal of Embryology and Experimental Morphology 73: 69–86.

Gluecksohn-Waelsch, S., S. D. Hagedora, and B. F. Sisken. 1956. Genetics and morphology of a recessive mutation in the house mouse affecting head and limb skeleton. Journal of Morphology 99: 465–479.

Goldman, A. S., M. Katsumata, S. J. Yaffe, and D. L. Gasser. 1977. Palatal cytosol cortisol binding protein associated with cleft palate susceptibility and H-2 genotype. Nature 265: 643–645.

Green, M. C. 1951. Further morphological effects of the short ear gene in the house mouse. Journal of Morphology 88: 1–21.

————. 1970. The developmental effects of congenital hydrocephalus (ch) in the mouse. Developmental Biology 23: 585–608.

Grüneberg, H. 1938. An analysis of the "pleiotropic" effects of a new lethal mutation in the rat. Proceedings of the Royal Society B 125: 123–144.

————. 1943. Congenital hydrocephalus in the mouse: a case of spurious pleiotropism. Journal of Genetics 45: 1–21.

————. 1953. Genetical studies on the skeleton of the mouse. VII. Congenital hydrocephalus. Journal of Genetics 51: 327–38.

————. 1963. *The Pathology of Development.* Oxford: Blackwell.

————. 1975. How do genes affect the skeleton? In *New Approaches to the Evaluation of Abnormal Embryonic Development,* D. Neuberg and H. J. Merker, eds., Stuttgart: Georg Thieme, pp. 354–359.

Grüneberg, H., and G. M. Truslove. 1960. Two closely linked genes in the mouse. Genetical research 1: 69–90.

Grüneberg, H., and G. A. de S. Wickramaratne. 1974. A re-examination of two skeletal mutants of the mouse vestigial tail (vt) and congenital hydrocephalus (ch). Journal of Embryology and Experimental Morphology 31: 207–222.

Hale, L. J. 1956. Mitotic activity during early skeletal differentiation of the scleral bones of the chick. Quarterly Journal of the Microscopical Society 97: 333–353.

Hall, B. K. 1971. Histogenesis and morphogenesis of bone. Clinical Orthopaedics and Related Research 74: 249–268.

————. 1981. The induction of neural crest derived cartilage and bone by embryonic epithelia: An analysis of the mode of action of an epithelial-mesenchymal interaction. Journal of Embryology and Experimental Morphology 64: 305–320.

————. 1984. Developmental processes and heterochrony as an evolutionary mechanism. Canadian Journal of Zoology 62: 1–7.

————. 1992. *Evolutionary Developmental Biology.* London: Chapman and Hall.

Harirs, J. W. S. 1964. Oligohydramnios and cortisone induced cleft palate. Nature 203: 533–534.

————. 1967. Experimental studies on closure and cleft palate formation in the secondary palate. Scientific Basis of Medicine Annual Review: 354–370.

Herring, S. W., and T. C. Lakars. 1981. Craniofacial development in the absence of muscle contraction. Journal of Craniofacial Genetics and Developmental Biology 1: 341–357.

Hill, R. E., J. Favor, B. L. M. Hogan, C. C. T. Tom, G. F. Saunders, I. M. Hanson, J. Prosser, T. Jordan, N. D. Hastie, and V. van Heynngen. 1991. Mouse Small eye results from mutations in a paired-like homeobox-containing gene. Nature 354: 522–525.

Hinchliffe, J. R., and D. A. Ede. 1968. Abnormalities in bone and cartilage development in the talpid[3] mutant of the fowl. Journal of Embryology and Experimental Morphology 19: 327–339.

Hinchliffe, J. R., and D. R. Johnson. 1983. Growth of cartilage. In *Cartilage,* vol. 2, *Development, Differentiation, and Growth,* B. K. Hall, ed. New York: Academic Press, pp. 255–295.

Hogan, B. L. M., G. Horsburgh, J. Cohen, C. M. Hetherington, G. Fisher, and M. F. Lyon. 1986. Small eyes (Sey): A homozygous lethal mutation on chromosome 2 which affects the differentiation of both lens and nasal placodes in the mouse. Journal of Embryology and Experimental Morphology 97: 95–110.

Hogan, B. L. M., R. Krumlauf, and C. M. Hetherington. 1987. Allelism of small eyes (Sey) with Dickie's small eye (Dey) on chromosome 2. Mouse News Letter 77: 135–138.

Holbrook, K. A., B. A. Dale, K. S. Brown. 1982. Abnormal epidermal keratinisation in the repeated epilation mutant mouse. Journal of Cell Biology 92: 387–398.

Hunton, P. 1960. A study of some factors affecting hatchability of chicken eggs with special reference to genetic control. Master's thesis, Wye College, University of London.

Iorio, R. J., G. Murray, and R. A. Meyer. 1980. Craniometric measurements of craniofacial malformations in mice with X linked dominant hypophosphataemia. Teratology 22: 291–298.

Jacobson, W., and H. B. Fell. 1941. The developmental mechanics and potencies of the undifferentiated mesenchyme of the mandible. Quarterly Journal of Microscopical Science 82: 563–586.

Janners, M. T., and R. L. Searls. 1970. Changes in the rate of cellular proliferation during the differentiation of cartilage and muscle in the mesenchyme of the embryonic chick wing. Developmental Biology 23: 136–165.

Johnson, D. R. 1967. Extra toes: A new mutant gene causing multiple abnormalities in the mouse. Journal of Embryology and Experimental Morphology 17: 543–581.

———. 1969. Brachyphalangy, an allele of extra toes in the mouse. Genetical Research 13: 257–280.

———. 1976. The interfrontal bones and mutant genes in the mouse. Journal of Anatomy 121: 507–513.

———. 1983. Abnormal cartilage from the mandibular condyle of stumpy (stm) mutant mice. Journal of Anatomy 137: 715–728.

———. 1984. The ultrastructure of the condylar cartilage from mice carrying the spondylo-metaphyseal chondrodysplasia (smc) gene. Journal of Anatomy 138: 463–470.

———. 1986. The Genetics of the Skeleton. Oxford: Clarendon Press.

Johnston, M. C., and M. A. Listgaren. 1972. Observations on the migration interaction and early differentiation of the orofacial tissues. In Developmental Aspects of Oral Biology, H. K. Slavkin and L. A. Bavetta, eds. New York: Academic Press, pp. 56–80.

Jolly, R. J., and W. J. Moore. 1975. Skull growth in achondroplastic (cn) mice: A craniometric study. Journal of Embryology and Experimental Morphology 33: 1013–1022.

Juriloff, D. M. 1978. The genetics of clefting in the mouse. In Etiology of Cleft Lip and Palate, M. Melnick, D. Bixler, and E. D. Shields, eds. New York: Alan J. Liss, pp. 39–71.

Juriloff, D. M., and M. J. Harris. 1983. Abnormal facial development in the mouse mutant first arch. Journal of Craniofacial Genetics and Developmental Biology 3: 317–337.

Juriloff, D. M., K. K. Sulik, T. H. Roderick, B. K. Hogan. 1985. Genetic and developmental studies of a new mouse mutation that produces otocephaly. Journal of Craniofacial Genetics and Developmental Biology 5: 121–145.

Kalter, H. 1978. The structure and uses of genetically homogeneous lines of animals. In *Handbook of Teratology,* vol. 4, J. G. Wilson and F. C. Fraser, eds. New York: Plenum, pp. 155–190.

Kieny, M., A. Mauger, and P. Sengel. 1972. Early regionalisation of the somitic mesoderm as studied by the development of the axial skeleton of the chick embryo. Developmental Biology 28: 142–161.

Kimata, K., H. J. Barrach, K. S. Brown, and J. P. Pennypacker. 1981. Absence of proteoglycan core protein in cartilage from cmd/cmd (cartilage matrix deficiency) mouse. Journal of Biological Chemistry 256: 6961–6968.

Lane, P. W., and M. M. Dickie. 1968. Three recessive mutations producing disproportionate dwarfing in mice. Journal of Heredity 59: 300–308.

Leong, S. Y., K. S. Larsson, and S. Lohmander. 1973. Cell proliferation in the cranial base of A/J mice with 6-AN induced cleft palate. Teratology 8: 127–138.

Lewis, J. 1989. Genes and segmentation. Nature 341: 382–383.

Loevy, H. 1968. Cortisone induced teratogenic effects in mice. Proceedings of the Society for Experimental Biology and Medicine 128: 841–844.

Lyon, M. F. 1958. Twirler: A mutant affecting the inner ear of the house mouse. Journal of Embryology and Experimental Morphology 6: 105–116.

Mathews, M. B. 1967. Chondroitin sulphate and collagen in inherited skeletal defects of chickens. Nature 213: 1255–1256.

Matta, C. A. 1981. Genetic background and the effects of the gene Tail short in the mouse. Ph. D. diss., University of London.

McKeown, P. J., and P. F. Goetinck. 1979. A comparison of the proteoglycans synthesised in Meckel's and sternal cartilage from normal and nanomelic cell embryos. Developmental Biology 71: 203–215.

McKeown-Longo, P. F. 1981. Proteoglycan link protein synthesis by cartilage from normal and nanomelic chick embryos. Federated Proceedings of the American Society of Experimental Biologists 40: 1840.

McLoed, M. J., and M. J. Harris, G. F. Chernoff, and J. R. Miller. 1980. First arch malformation: A new craniofacial mutant in the mouse. Journal of Heredity 71: 331–335.

Meyer, R. A., J. Jowsey, and M. H. Meyer. 1979. Osteomalacia and altered magnesium metabolism in the X linked hypophosphataemic mice. Calcified Tissue International 27: 19–26.

Miller, J. R., K. Sulik, and R. L. Atnip. 1978. Allophenic mice in cleft palate investigations. Journal of Embryology and Experimental Morphology 47: 169–177.

Millikovsky G., L. J. H. Ambrose, and M. C. Johnson. 1982. Developmental alterations associated with spontaneous cleft lip and palate in CL/Fr mice. American Journal of Anatomy 164: 29–44.

Morgan, W. C. 1950. A new short tail mutation in the mouse whose lethal effects are conditioned by the residual genotypes. Journal of Heredity 41: 208–215.

Morrison-Graham, K., and J. A. Weston. 1989. Mouse mutants provide new insights into the role of extracellular matrix in cell migration and differentiation. Trends in Genetics 5: 116–121.

Moss, M. L. 1964. The phylogeny of mineralised tissues. International Review of General and Experimental Zoology 1: 297–331.

Newman, S. 1977. Lineage and pattern in the developing wing bud. In *Vertebrate Limb and Somite Morphogenesis,* D. A. Ede, J. R. Hinchliffe, and M. Balls, eds., Cambridge: Cambridge University Press, pp. 181–197.

Noden, D. M. 1988. Interactions and fates of avian craniofacial mesenchyme. Development 103: 121–140.

Oliver, G., C. V. E. Wright, J. Hardwicke, and E. M. De Robers. 1988. Differential antero-posterior expression of two proteins encoded by a homeobox gene in Xenopus and mouse embryos. EMBO J 7: 3199–3209.

Orkin, R. W., R. M. Pratt, and G. M. Martin. 1976. Undersulphated chondroitin sulphate in cartilage matrix of brachymorphic mice. Developmental Biology 50: 82–94.

Ørvig, T. 1967. Phylogeny of tooth tissues: Evolution of some calcified tissues in early vertebrates. In *Structural and Chemical Organization of Teeth,* A. E. W. Miles, ed. New York: Academic Press, pp. 45–110.

Pai, A. C. 1965. Developmental genetics of a lethal mutation, muscular dysgenesis (mdg) in the mouse. 1. Genetic analysis and gross morphology. Developmental Biology 11: 82–92.

Palmoski, M. J., and P. F. Goetinck. 1972. Synthesis of proteochondroitin sulphate by normal nanomelic and 5-bromodeoxyuridine treated chondrocytes in cell culture. Proceedings of the National Academy of Sciences, U.S.A. 69: 3385–3388.

Pennypacker, J. P., and P. F. Goetinck. 1976. Biochemical and ultrastructural studies of collagen and proteochondroitin sulphate in normal and nanomelic cartilage. Developmental Biology 50: 35–47.

Pinto, C. B., and B. K. Hall. 1991. Toward an understanding of the epithelial requirement for osteogenesis in scleral mesenchyme of the embryonic chick. Journal of Experimental Zoology 259: 92–108.

Rittenhouse, E., L. C. Dunn, J. Cookingham, C. Calo, M. Spiegelmann, G. B. Dooker, and D. Bennett. 1978. Cartilage matrix deficiency (cmd): A new autosomal recessive lethal mutation in the mouse. Journal of Embryology and Experimental Morphology 43: 71–84.

Roberts, R. C. 1967. Small eyes: A new dominant mutation in the mouse. Genetic Research, Cambridge 9: 121–122.

Sannasgala, S. S. M. M. K., and D. R. Johnson. 1990. Kinetic parameters in the growth plate of normal and achondroplastic (cn/cn) mice. Journal of Anatomy 172: 245–258.

Schwartz, N. B., J. Belch, J. Henry, J. Hupert, and K. Sugahara. 1982. Enzyme defect in PAPA synthesis of brachymorphic mice. Federated Proceedings of the American Society for Experimental Biology 41: 852.

Scott, J. P. 1937. The embryology of the guinea pig. III. The development of the polydactylous monster. Journal of Experimental Zoology 77: 123–157.

———. 1938. The embryology of the guinea pig. II. The polydactylous monster. Journal of Morphology 62: 299–311.

Searle, A. G. 1965. Mouse News Letter 33: 29.

Seegmiller, R. E., and F. C. Fraser. 1977. Mandibular growth retardation as a cause for cleft palate in mice homozygous for the chondrodysplasia gene. Journal of Embryology and Experimental Morphology 38: 227–238.

Sela, J., I. Bab, and M. S. Deol. 1982. Patterns of matrix vesicle calcification in osteomalacia of gyro mice. Metabolic Bone Disease and Related Research 4: 129–134.

Sisken, B. F., and S. Gluecksohn-Waelsch. 1959. A developmental study of the mutation "phocomelia" in the mouse. Journal of Experimental Zoology 142: 623–642.

Smiley, G. R. 1967. A profile of cephalometric appraisal of normal growth parameters in embryonic mice. Anatomical Record 157: 323.

Smiley, G. R., R. J. Vanek, and A. D. Dixon. 1971. Width of the craniofacial complex during formation of the secondary palate. Cleft Palate Journal 8: 371–378.

Smith, L. J., and K. F. Stein. 1962. Axial elongation in the mouse and its retardation in mice homozygous for looped-tail. Journal of Embryology and Experimental Morphology 10: 73–87.

Staats, J. 1972. Standardised nomenclature for inbred strains of mice. 5th listing. Cancer Research 32: 1609–1646.

Stearns, K., and P. F. Goetinck. 1979. Stimulation of chondroitin sulphate synthesis by beta D xyloside in chondrocytes of the proteoglycan deficient mutant nanomelia. Journal of Cell Physiology 100: 33–38.

Strong, L. C., and W. F. Hollander. 1949. Hereditary loop-tail in the house mouse accompanied by imperforate vagina and with craniorachischisis when homozygous. Journal of Heredity 40: 329–334.

Sugahara, K., and N. B. Schwartz. 1979. Defect in 3′ phosphadenosine 5′ phosphosulphate formation in brachymorphic mice. Proceedings of the National Academy of Sciences, U.S.A. 76: 6615–6681.

Tassin, M. T., B. Salzgeber, and Guénet, J.-P. 1983. Studies of "repeated epilation" mouse mutant embryos. I. Development of facial malformations. Journal of Craniofacial Genetics and Developmental Biology 3: 289–307.

Thorogood, P. V. 1972. Patterns of chondrogenesis and myogenesis in the limb buds of normal and talpid[3] chick embryos. Ph.D. diss., University of College of Wales, Aberystwyth.

———. 1983. Morphogenesis of cartilage. In Cartilage, vol. 2, Development, Differentiation, and Growth. B. K. Hall, ed. New York: Academic Press, pp. 223–254.

Thurston, M. N., D. R. Johnson, and N. F. Kember. 1985. Cell kinetics of growth cartilage of achondroplastic (cn) mice. Journal of Anatomy 140: 425–434.

Thurston, M. N., D. R. Johnson, N. F. Kember, and W. J. Moore. 1983. Cell kinetics of growth cartilage in stumpy: A new chondrodystrophic mutant in the mouse. Journal of Anatomy 136: 407–415.

Tihen, J. A., D. R. Charles, and T. O. Sippel. 1948. Inherited visceral inversion in mice. Journal of Heredity 39: 29–31.

Trasler, D. G. 1968. Pathogenesis of cleft lip and its relation to embryonic face shape in A/J and C57BL mice. Teratology 1: 33–50.

————. 1969. Differences in face shape of mouse with and without the gene dancer predisposing to cleft lip. Teratology 2: 271.

Trasler, D. G., and F. C. Fraser. 1963. Role of the tongue in producing cleft palate in mice with spontaneous cleft lip. Developmental Biology 6: 45–50.

Trasler, D. G., and S. Leong. 1976. Face shape and mitotic index in mice with 6-aminonicotinamide induced and inherited cleft lip. Teratology 9: A39–40.

Van der Water, T. R., and V. Galinovic-Schwartz. 1987. Collagen type II in the otic extracellular matrix: Effect on inner ear development. Hearing Research 30: 39–48.

Verrusio, A. C. 1970. A mechanism for closure of the secondary palate. Teratology 3: 17–20.

Tyler, M. S., and B. K. Hall. 1977. Epithelial influences on skeletogenesis in the mandible of the embryonic chick. Anatomical Record 188: 229–240.

Wragg, L. E., M. Klein, G. Steinvorth, and R. Warpeha. 1970. Facial growth accommodating secondary palate closure in rat and man. Archives of Oral Biology 15: 705–719.

Zimmermann, K. 1933. Eine neue Mutation der Hausmaus: **hydrocephalus**. Zeitschrift für induktive Abstammungs- und Vererbungslehre 64: 176–180.

8

Metamorphosis and the Vertebrate Skull: Ontogenetic Patterns and Developmental Mechanisms

CHRISTOPHER S. ROSE AND JOHN O. REISS

IN THIS CHAPTER we summarize present knowledge regarding the role of developmental mechanisms, hormonal and otherwise, in metamorphic remodeling of the vertebrate skull. The focus of developmental research into metamorphosis has traditionally been the neuroendocrine axis; this approach has been forged on the assumption that the endocrinological features of vertebrate metamorphosis justify its treatment as a mechanistically distinct aspect of vertebrate development. In contrast, our focus is directed primarily at the remodeling of the peripheral morphology; we address the cellular pathways involved in the transformation of cranial structures and the developmental mechanisms by which cranial and primarily skeletal tissues may regulate their own remodeling, i.e., epigenetic interactions and peripheral regulation of thyroid hormone.

Our review of this material is derived primarily from studies on anurans (frogs), urodeles (salamanders), lampreys, and flatfishes. Experimental investigations of these systems do not support the contention that cranial remodeling at metamorphosis is mechanistically distinct from development in nonmetamorphic systems. We emphasize that similar developmental interactions and cellular pathways seem to be utilized by both types of developmental system, although they are invoked at different scales and rates. Furthermore, within the developmental context of a metamorphic ontogeny, these same developmental factors may exercise a much greater influence upon the ontogenetic and hence evolutionary diversification of the peripheral morphology.

DEFINING METAMORPHOSIS

Discussion of the developmental structure of metamorphosis demands first a methodology for recognizing when a set of developmental events constitutes a metamorphosis. In reviewing the phylogenetic distribution of metamorphosis, we have come to the conclusion that the phenomenon is not easily defined and that the term "metamorphosis" does not carry a precise empirical meaning. Usage of the term has proceeded mainly at the discretion or whim of individual authors.

Among vertebrate morphologists and developmental biologists, metamorphosis has historically been considered as a discrete and mechanistically distinct phase of development. Vertebrate metamorphoses are often united under the theoretical standpoint that they share similar rules of onset, e.g., activation by thyroid hormone, and similar sorts of morphological change, e.g., loss of external gills. But such similarities cannot constitute a definition, since there appears to be no single cue employed by all metamorphic vertebrates, nor do all metamorphic vertebrates share common metamorphic events. Anurans and lampreys have equally dramatic metamorphoses, but the two sets of events bear no resemblance, nor do they appear to be activated in the same way. Even among closely related groups, structures may express a distinctly metamorphic response in one group yet develop independently of metamorphic cues in another, for example, the limb and tail in anurans and urodeles.

Ecologists, on the other hand, have consistently described metamorphosis in terms of ecological shifts, i.e., ontogenetic changes in habitat and/or feeding mode. However, defining metamorphosis as morphological changes coincident with an ecological shift is not sufficient, since abrupt and profound changes in morphology do not always correlate with an ecological shift. For example, the frog *Hymenochirus boettgeri* shows little appreciable change in habitat, feeding behavior, or food choice despite undergoing a pronounced morphological transformation (Sokol 1962, 1969). Moreover, abrupt ecological shifts, especially in habitat utilization, are typical of ontogenetic development in many vertebrates, yet these shifts are often unaccompanied by major morphological changes (see review by Werner and Gilliam 1984).

Many authors have been explicit in their usage of metamorphosis for transitions between larval and juvenile life history stages. However, there are numerous cases of dramatic changes in morphology at other points in ontogeny. The return of adults to a spawning habitat is marked by the extensive growth of caudal and dorsal fins in newts, the appearance of premaxillary hooks in salmon, and changes in the body proportions, fins, eyes, and dentition of parasitic lampreys. Embryonic and early larval events have even been regarded as a metamorphosis: Szarski (1957) describes coiling of the intestine and development of the operculum as a first metamorphosis in anurans.

We can find no tenable rationale for restricting the term "metamorphosis" to changes concurrent with one specific life-history event. We agree with Cohen (1985) that metamorphosis is really a metaphorical concept, rather than a specific and discrete process. Alberch (1989) elaborates upon this view by recognizing metamorphosis as a particular pattern in the temporal distribution of developmental events comprising the life cycle of the organism. A metamorphic ontogeny is one exhibiting a temporal concentration of postembryonic developmental events, this concentration being delimited at both ends by periods of growth and developmental quiescence (Alberch 1989).

According to Alberch's view, metamorphosis is not a specific process or phase of development, but rather an emergent property of the relative spacing of developmental events in ontogeny. This definition implies that metamorphosis is an arbitrarily determined and primarily quantitative phenomenon. A sufficient number of events must occur within a sufficiently short period of the postembryonic lifespan for one to be able to distinguish a period of concentrated development. Although inherently subjective, we find this definition conceptually valuable because it utilizes only temporal developmental criteria; it sets no a priori limits upon either the type of morphological changes or the nature of mechanistic factors involved, and thus provides a sound basis for addressing the diversity of these qualities within vertebrates.

THE DIVERSITY OF CRANIAL METAMORPHOSIS

A comparative discussion of any aspect of vertebrate metamorphosis is handicapped by the lack of an internally consistent assessment of the phylogenetic distribution of metamorphosis among vertebrates. This dilemma has led us to undertake such a survey, one which soon grew far beyond the scope of this chapter (Reiss and Rose, in preparation). Employing Alberch's (1989) definition, we reached the not surprising conclusion that metamorphosis has a phylogenetically disjunct occurrence in Vertebrata. Profoundly metamorphic ontogenies are found in lampreys, numerous teleost groups, and all three groups of lissamphibians; there is conversely no evidence for a metamorphosis in hagfish, chondrichthyans, many teleost groups, coelacanths, and lungfish (cf. Evans and Fernald 1990). This distribution, combined with the lack of homology among metamorphic events in different groups, makes it indisputable that metamorphosis has evolved many times within this subphylum.

The morphological literature on vertebrate metamorphosis is widely scattered, and inaccessible to anyone wanting a comparative treatment of skull development at a purely descriptive level. Yet only by considering a diversity of metamorphic ontogenies can one hope to gain a perspective upon what metamorphosis means as a developmental phenomenon. Detailed morphological observations, wherein each metamorphic change is described in its temporal and spatial relations to other events, are prerequisite for inferring the nature of underlying developmental interactions. Furthermore, a comparison of such observations for similar and disparate taxa provides one with a methodology for addressing the role of these mechanisms in morphological diversification. Therefore, as a starting point toward these goals, we provide the following brief overview of cranial skeletal changes characterizing the various vertebrate groups for which we recognize a metamorphosis (for a more thorough treatment see Reiss and Rose, in preparation). Although unable to give full references here, we attempt to provide an entry into the literature on skull development for each group. We adopt the terms "primary metamorphosis" to refer to developmental events occurring between larval and juvenile periods, and "secondary metamorphosis" to refer to events at sexual maturation.

Petromyzontiformes

The life history of all lampreys involves a freshwater microphagous larva, the ammocoete, which metamorphoses after a prolonged period of growth into a "macrophthalmic" juvenile. The juvenile migrates downstream and usually assumes a parasitic habit, either in the ocean or, in the case of landlocked forms, in fresh water. The maturing adult makes one return trip upstream to spawn and die. Although the evolution of a nonparasitic life history has been a recurring trend in lampreys (Vladykov and Kott 1979), the group as a whole remains morphologically conservative, and there has been little, if any, diversification of larval and adult cranial morphologies. Nonetheless, the primary metamorphosis in this group is perhaps the most profound within vertebrates, being remarkable for the scope of both its histological and morphological restructuring.

The main cranial changes (fig. 8.1) involve the transformation of the oral hood of the larva into a rasping disk, development of the tonguelike piston, maturation of the eyes, and extensive remodeling of the branchial region (Johnels 1948; Hardisty 1981). The skeletal support for the oral hood, which is composed of a histologically and developmentally unique tissue called mucocartilage (see Wright and Youson 1982; Langille and Hall 1988), is lost at metamorphosis, and many new cartilaginous elements develop to support the newly forming suctorial disk and piston; cartilages are also added to the neurocranium and branchial arches. Most of these changes correlate with the transition from microphagous to parasitic feeding.

Actinopterygii

Within the actinopterygians there is a complete spectrum of life history patterns from gradual development through profound metamorphosis (see

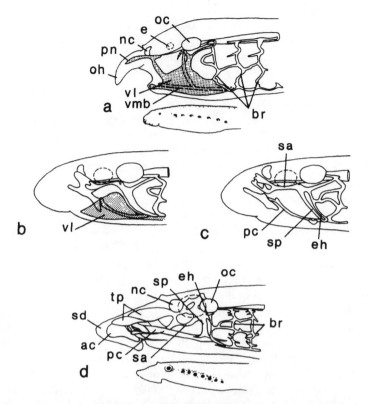

Fig. 8.1. Metamorphic changes in the skull of the lamprey *Lampetra planeri*. a. Larva. b, c. Midmetamorphic stages. d. Immature adult (size range of metamorphic individuals is 110 to 170 mm total length; Hardisty and Potter 1971a). Stippled elements are mucocartilage; all others are cartilage. The mucocartilage elements, which support the oral hood of the larva, are completely resorbed and replaced by a cartilaginous ring and dorso-lateral plates which support the suctorial disk of the adult. A cartilaginous support for the tonguelike piston develops in the floor of the mouth, a subocular arch develops lateral and parallel to the trabecula, and the styliform process forms in the wall of the pharynx at the opening of the velar valve. The branchial arches gain additional processes, as well as a new arch, the extrahyal, derived from the same blastema as the styliform process (b). ac, annular cartilage; br, branchial arch; e, eye; eh, extrahyal; nc, nasal capsule; oh, oral hood; oc, otic capsule; pc, piston cartilage; pn, prenasal plate; sa, subocular arch; sd, suctorial disk; sp, styliform process; tp, tectal plates; vl, ventro-lateral plate; vmb, ventro-median bar. Redrawn from Hardisty (1981), after Johnels (1948).

Bertin 1957; Moser et al. 1984; Youson 1988; Evans and Fernald 1990). Although the taxonomic distribution of these patterns is complicated, it is clear that gradual development is typical of freshwater and coastal fishes, while metamorphosis is usually associated with the settlement of marine fishes having planktonic larvae and benthic adults, with the vertical descent of the epipelagic larvae of marine meso- or bathypelagic fishes, and with the transition between freshwater and saltwater habitats in anadromous or catadromous fishes. As one might expect from their freshwater habit, none of the nonteleost or "lower" actinopterygians exhibits a metamorphic ontogeny, although gars, sturgeon, and paddlefish undergo a period of pronounced cranial development in early larval stages to produce the elongate rostra characteristic of the adults (Ryder 1890; Aumonier 1941; Ballard and Needham 1964; Jollie 1980). Teleosts, on the other hand, display a wide range of metamorphic patterns, only a few of which will be mentioned here.

In the elopomorphs (tarpons, bonefishes, halosaurs, and eels), the larvae are transparent, laterally compressed pelagic forms known as leptocephali (Castle 1984; Böhlke 1989). These larvae often undergo extensive shrinkage during metamorphosis to the juvenile, which may be freshwater, coastal, reef-dwelling, or bathypelagic. Metamorphic changes in the cranium are best known for the eels, in which there is extensive ossification of both dermal and endochondral elements and resorption of much of the larval chondrocranium (Norman 1926; Leiby 1979a, b). The entire branchial apparatus shifts caudally in relation to the neurocranium, and the elongate larval dentition is lost. Many eels also undergo a secondary metamorphosis, which can involve a pronounced reduction of the jaws and dentition (Nielsen and Smith 1978; Nielsen and Bertelsen 1985).

In the salmonids, anadromous forms undergo a primary metamorphosis (smoltification) during the downstream migration and a dramatic secondary metamorphosis, more pronounced in males, during the upstream spawning migration. Smoltification involves mainly physiological changes, although in *Oncorhynchus* teeth erupt on the jaws and tongue at this time (Gorbman et al. 1982). Secondary metamorphosis (fig. 8.2) involves extensive remodeling of the skull to produce an enlarged rostral region and a hook on the mandibular symphysis (Davidson 1935; Tchernavin 1937, 1938a, b). Also, the feeding teeth are completely replaced by a specialized breeding dentition. In *Oncorhynchus* these changes are terminal, but in *Salmo* and some other genera at least some individuals apparently undergo a regressive metamorphosis while migrating back downstream (Tchernavin 1938b), and they can repeat this cycle in subsequent seasons (Saunders and Schom 1985).

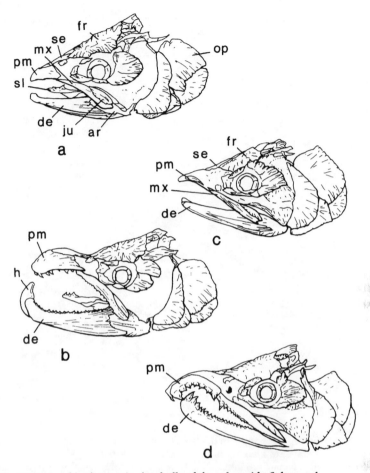

Fig. 8.2. Metamorphic changes in the skulls of the salmonids *Salmo* and *Oncorhynchus*. a, b. *S. salar* (56 mm and 66 mm skull widths, respectively), c, d. *O. keta* (sizes not available). a, c are coastal migrants; b, d are upstream migrants at the peak of the breeding season; all are male. The coastal migrant stage is marked in both genera by the loss of all feeding teeth, and the upstream migrant stage by pronounced lengthening of bones and cartilages in the rostral region, especially in the jaws. In male *Salmo* a connective tissue hook develops at the tip of the lower jaw; this is received by a hollow in the roof of the mouth. In male *Oncorhynchus* the premaxilla and dentary are enlarged by the fusion of additional tooth bases, producing a hooked upper jaw and a toothy knob at the tip of the lower jaw. Although females of both genera undergo some rostral enlargement, they do not develop the hook or toothy knob on the lower jaw. *Salmo* later undergoes regressive changes including loss of the hook; conversely, breeding development in *Oncorhynchus* is terminal. ar, articular; de, dentary; fr, frontal; h, connective tissue hook; ju, jugal; mx, maxilla; op, opercular; pm, premaxilla; se, supraethmoid; sl, supralingual (not shown are hyoid elements and branchiostegals). Redrawn from Tchernavin (1938b).

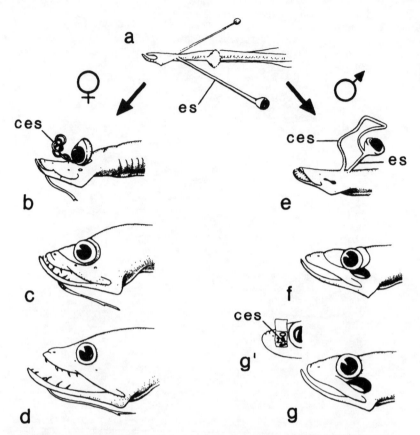

Fig. 8.3. Metamorphic changes in the head of the stomiiform *Idiacanthus fasciola*. a. Larva (16 mm Standard Length). b. Early metamorphic female (45 mm SL). c. Midmetamorphic female (48 mm SL). d. Late metamorphic female (43 mm SL). e. Early metamorphic male (40 mm SL). f. Midmetamorphic male (35 mm SL). g. Juvenile male (35 mm SL). g′. Same with flap of skin removed in front of eye. An extension of the lamina orbitonasalis provides support for the long eyestalk of the larva. At metamorphosis and as the eyestalk shortens, the cartilaginous support for the eyestalk begins to soften and bend (b, e); it subsequently bursts through its dermal sheath and coils in front of the eye (g′). The gape simultaneously enlarges as the suspensorium swings caudally; in the male this process ends at a stage (g) which is most comparable with the midmetamorphic stage c of the female—note the position of the jaw joint relative to the eye. ces, cartilaginous eyestalk support; es, eyestalk. Redrawn from Beebe (1934).

Another salmoniform, *Plecoglossus altivelis,* exhibits a gradual ontogenetic transition from an estuarine to fluviatile habitat, with an associated shift from planktivory to algal grazing or straining. Although there are no apparent external changes, the cranial changes associated with this transition are extensive, involving the jaws, dentition, and many soft tissues (Fukuhara and Fushimi 1986; Howes and Sanford 1987). However, the gradual nature of these changes distinguishes this as a very marginal case of metamorphosis.

The stomiiforms, which include the lightfishes, marine hatchetfishes, and viperfishes, exhibit a fascinating array of metamorphic patterns (Kawaguchi and Moser 1984; Ahlstrom, Richards et al. 1984). In general, metamorphosis is associated with a shift from epipelagic larvae to meso- or bathypelagic juveniles, and is marked by the appearance of numerous photophores. The basic pattern of cranial change involves enlargement of the gape via a caudal rotation of the suspensorium, increased ossification of the neurocranium, and the development of fanglike teeth (Belyanina 1977). This pattern has been markedly elaborated upon in some genera, the most extreme being *Idiacanthus* (fig. 8.3), which not only loses its incredibly long larval eyestalks, but shows sexual dimorphism in the extent of ossification and gape enlargement, with adult males closely resembling midmetamorphic females (Beebe 1934).

In the myctophids, or lanternfishes, metamorphosis is also associated with the shift from epipelagic larvae to mesopelagic juveniles, and is marked by completion of the adult count of photophores (Moser, Ahlstrom et al. 1984). Larval teeth are replaced by juvenile teeth, but unlike stomiiforms almost all cranial bones are present prior to metamorphosis (Moser and Ahlstrom 1970). However, the profound changes in head shape displayed by some species suggest that extensive remodeling may occur at this time.

In the ceratioids, or deep-sea anglerfishes, metamorphosis is again associated with the shift from epipelagic larvae to bathypelagic juveniles (Bertelsen 1951, 1984). Like the stomiiform *Idiacanthus,* ceratioids develop a remarkable sexual dimorphism at metamorphosis (fig. 8.4), here correlated with the parasitic habit of adult males. The most notable cranial event, exhibited by the males of some species, is the development of a unique secondary jaw-closing mechanism involving rostral denticles and the illicial pterygiophore (Bertelsen 1951). This is accompanied by resorption of the primary jaw bones and loss of the larval dentition, as the male uses its new jaws to attach itself to the female. Metamorphosis in females involves the progressive development of the illicial pterygiophore, the replacement of the larval dentition by long fangs, and in many species a notable enlargement of the gape. In females of the family Gigantactinidae,

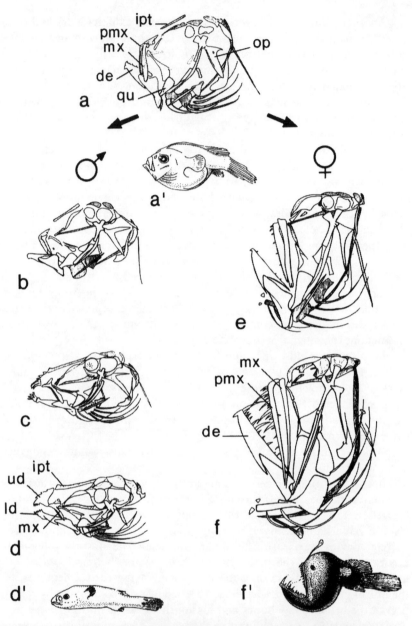

Fig. 8.4. Metamorphic changes in the skull of the ceratioid anglerfish *Melanocetus*.
All specimens except d are *M. johnsoni*; d is *M. murrayi*. a. Larval male (13 mm Total
Length). a'. Larval male (8.5 mm TL). b. Early metamorphic male (22 mm TL).
c. Midmetamorphic male (35 mm TL). d. Adult male (23.5 mm TL). d'. Adult male
(36 mm TL). e. Late metamorphic female (21 mm TL). f. Juvenile female (31 mm TL).

the osteocranium undergoes pronounced reduction, with several bones being completely resorbed (Bertelsen et al. 1981).

The pleuronectiforms, or flatfishes, are well known for their transformation from pelagic larvae to benthic juveniles (Norman 1934; Ahlstrom, Amaoka et al. 1984; Hensley and Ahlstrom 1984). The main event of this metamorphosis, the migration of one eye across the midline to the opposite side of the head, has understandably profound effects on the adult skull morphology, producing a pronounced asymmetry in the ethmoid, orbital, and, to a lesser extent, otico-occipital regions. During metamorphosis the supraorbital bars (orbital cartilages of de Beer 1937) and the overlying frontal bones are either bowed toward the future ocular side or resorbed to make way for the migrating eye (Williams 1901; Mayhoff 1914). Complex asymmetries can arise in the ethmoid region, apparently owing to differential growth of the ethmoidal cartilages. The palatoquadrate undergoes partial resorption, being functionally replaced by dermal bones of the palate. Larval teeth are replaced by juvenile teeth and many endochondral bones begin to ossify. Late in metamorphosis a novel structure, the pseudomesial bar, forms by the sutural fusion of extensions from the blind side frontal and lateral ethmoid bones; it supports the rostral end of the dorsal fin. In spite of similarities in the resulting morphology, the events and timing of eye migration vary widely among species, suggesting that the mechanisms involved also vary.

Dipnoi

The extant dipnoans, or lungfishes, are survivors of an extensive Paleozoic radiation. Although both the classical (Kerr 1899, 1909; Budgett 1901) and recent (e.g., Just et al. 1981) literature has described two of the three living genera as having a metamorphosis, we do not consider any living species to be metamorphic. Like urodele amphibians, lepidosirenids hatch with external gills that are subsequently resorbed, but unlike urodeles (and like the actinopterygian *Polypterus*), this resorption does not occur in synchrony with any notable internal remodeling or other external changes (see Agar

---

f'. Juvenile female (22 mm TL). Note the divergent transformation of males and females. The skull of the male elongates and rostral denticles appear (c), eventually fusing to form upper and lower denticles (d). The articulation of the upper denticle with the illicial pterygiophore creates a secondary jaw-closing mechanism which is used for attachment to the female. In contrast, the jaws and suspensorium of the female lengthen substantially and the dentary and premaxilla acquire long fangs (f). de, dentary; ipt, illicial pterigiophore; ld, lower denticle; mx, maxilla; op, opercular; pmx, premaxilla; qu, quadrate; ud, upper denticle. Figures a, a', d', and f' redrawn from Bertelsen (1951); b, c, e, and f from Regan and Trewavas (1932); and d from Parr (1930).

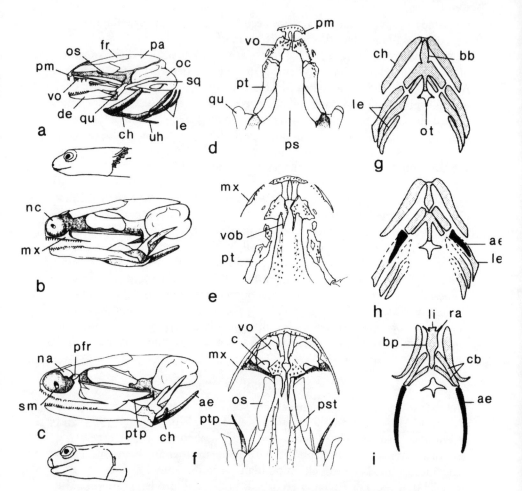

Fig. 8.5. Metamorphic changes in the skull of the plethodontid urodele *Eurycea bislineata*. a, d, and g are late larval specimens (approximately 20 to 22 mm Snout-Vent Length); b, e, and h are midmetamorphic (approximately 24 mm SVL); c, f, and i are recently metamorphosed (approximately 24 mm SVL). Chondrification of the nasal capsule (a, b) is followed by ossification of the maxilla and septomaxilla (b), and prefrontal and nasal (c). The ringlike scleral cartilage around the larval eye (not shown in a) is resorbed at stage b. In the palate (c-e), the pterygoid is resorbed and the vomer expands anteriorly to become indented by the choana. Posteriorly the vomer develops a long median bar which carries teeth caudally to form the parasphenoid tooth patch. Unlike salamandrids the vomerine bar is resorbed soon after its formation, so at no stage is it completely intact. In the hyobranchium (g-i), the ceratohyal, ceratobranchials, and os thyroideum (not yet ossified in a) separate from the basibranchial element; the ceratohyal develops a posterior hook to secure itself, via a ligament, to the quadrate (c); and the ceratobranchials converge posteriorly to articulate with the newly forming adult epibranchial. The long adult epibranchial

1906; Kerr 1909; Fox 1965; Bertmar 1966; Kemp 1987). This single event is not sufficient to constitute a metamorphosis under our definition.

Lissamphibia

Of the Lissamphibia, the urodeles, or salamanders, present the most generalized life history pattern, in which aquatic larvae with external gills, open gill slits, and a tail fin metamorphose into terrestrial juveniles lacking these structures (Duellman and Trueb 1986). Initial ossification of most bones is usually completed during the larval period, with the main cranial events at metamorphosis (fig. 8.5) being confined to the palate and hyobranchium (Smith 1920; Wintrebert 1922; Wilder 1925; Erdmann 1933; Keller 1946; Eyal-Giladi and Zinberg 1964; Corsin 1966; Bonebrake and Brandon 1971; Reilly 1986, 1987; Alberch et al. 1986). In general, metamorphic urodeles are consistent in their loss of elements but they show significant variation in the morphogenesis of new adult elements in the palate and hyobranchium. In the palate the palatopterygoid bone undergoes partial or complete resorption. The vomer is extensively remodeled, and in salamandrids and plethodontids it develops a tooth-bearing process which extends back along the parasphenoid to generate the parasphenoid tooth patch. In the hyobranchium most larval epibranchials are lost. The single adult epibranchial is derived either by retention of the anterior part of the larval first epibranchial (hynobiids, salamandrids, and ambystomatids) or from an outgrowth of this cartilage (at least some plethodontids); the latter pathway results in a longer and more slender cartilage used in tongue projection. A variable combination of radial and lingual cartilages forms anteriorly to support the tongue pad. Other metamorphic changes usually include loss of the splenial bone in the lower jaw, posterior elongation of the maxilla in the upper jaw, and reduction or resorption of the scleral cartilage of the eye.

Most anurans, or frogs and toads, undergo a profound metamorphosis associated with the transition from an aquatic, filter-feeding larva (tadpole) to a terrestrial, carnivorous juvenile (Duellman and Trueb 1986).

---

develops as an outgrowth from the anterior perichondrium of the larval first epibranchial. All larval epibranchial cartilages are eventually resorbed, and new cartilages are developed anteriorly to support the tongue pad. ae, adult epibranchial; bb, first basibranchial; bp, basibranchial plate; c, choana; cb, ceratobranchial; ch, ceratohyal; de, dentary; fr, frontal; le, larval epibranchial; li, lingual; mx, maxilla; na, nasal; nc, nasal capsule; oc, otic capsule; os, orbitosphenoid; ot, os thyroideum; pa, parietal; pfr, prefrontal; pm, premaxilla; pt, pterygoid; ptp, pterygoid process; ps, parasphenoid; pst, parasphenoid tooth patch; qu, quadrate; ra, radial; sm, septomaxilla; sq, squamosal; uh, urohyal; vo, vomer; vob, vomerine bar. Figures a-f and sketches of head redrawn from Wilder (1925).

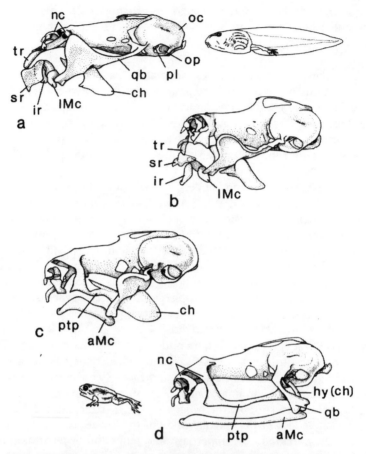

Fig. 8.6. Metamorphic changes in the chondrocranium of the anuran *Rana temporaria*. a. Early metamorphic (13 mm Body Length, 36 mm Total Length). b. Midmetamorphic (12 mm BL, 32 mm TL). c. Midmetamorphic (9 mm BL, 22 mm TL). d. Early juvenile (14 mm BL and TL). Note the elaboration of nasal cartilages, loss of the trabecular horns and suprarostral cartilages of the tadpole mouth, and the transformation of the broad ceratohyal into the slender hyale. The change in head shape is accomplished primarily by the posterior rotation and shortening of the quadrate bar, coupled with substantial lengthening of the pterygoid process and adult Meckel's cartilage. Not shown are the cup-shaped sclerotic cartilage on the medial side of the eye, and the tympanic annulus of the ear, both of which form at or soon after metamorphosis. aMc, adult Meckel's cartilage; ch, ceratohyal; hy, hyale; ir, infrarostral; lMc, larval Meckel's cartilage; oc, otic capsule; op, operculum; nc, nasal cartilages; pl, plectrum; ptp, pterygoid process; qb, quadrate bar; sr, suprarostral; tr, trabecular horn. Skulls redrawn from de Beer (1937), sketches from de Jong (1968).

Cranial changes are extensive, involving a fundamental restructuring of the entire chondrocranium (fig. 8.6) and the appearance of most bones (e.g., for *Ascaphus truei,* van Eeden 1951; for *Xenopus laevis,* Sedra and Michael 1957; for *Rana temporaria,* de Jongh 1968; for *Pelobates syriacus,* Rocek 1981; a nice review of the earlier literature on chondrocranial development is provided by Swanepoel 1970, while Trueb 1985 reviews ossification patterns). During metamorphosis the nasal cartilages develop in association with an increase in complexity of the olfactory organ, while the trabecular horns and the suprarostral cartilages, which support the upper lip of the tadpole, are resorbed. The quadrate bar supporting the jaw joint rotates posteriorly as the pterygoid process undergoes its pronounced elongation. At the same time the infrarostral and larval Meckel's cartilages fuse to form the adult Meckel's cartilage, which also lengthens greatly, thus increasing the gape. The sclerotic cartilage of the eyeball appears, as do the plectrum (columella), operculum, and tympanic annulus of the middle ear. The branchial basket, which supports the gills and filter apparatus in the larva, is remodeled into the hyobranchial plate and its associated processes, which function in tongue protrusion in the juvenile.

The third living amphibian group, the limbless caecilians or gymnophionans, primitively has a metamorphosis from an aquatic larva, characterized by a tail fin and at least one open gill slit, to a burrowing juvenile with a fully differentiated cephalic tentacle and no tail fin or gill slits (Breckenridge et al. 1987). However, the majority of living species are direct-developing or viviparous. Internally, caecilian metamorphosis involves a pronounced increase in the area of dermal bones in the skull roof, as well as changes in the palate and a rearrangement of the hyobranchial apparatus (compare the "juveniles" and adults of Visser 1963; see also Ramaswami 1947). The squamosal extends anteriorly, the maxilla grows posteriorly, and the orbital ("postfrontal") appears; together these processes complete the orbital rim and the lateral border of the subtemporal fenestra. The maxilla and palatine fuse to form a compound maxillopalatine, and in some species the parasphenoid and neurocranium fuse into a compound "basal" bone (in others this fusion occurs prior to metamorphosis). In *Ichthyophis* the cartilaginous larval hyobranchium undergoes minor remodeling, while in *Epicrionops* the extensively ossified elements of the larval hyobranchium are resorbed and replaced by newly formed cartilaginous elements (Wake 1989).

PATHWAYS OF DIVERSIFICATION IN METAMORPHIC ONTOGENIES

Metamorphic taxa express an enormous diversity in patterns of skull development. The evolutionary processes that have shaped this diversity can be broadly dissected into components of heterochrony, caenogenesis, and terminal addition (cf. Alberch 1989). Caenogenesis, the evolutionary appearance of larval specializations, and terminal addition, the evolution of adult specializations, play rather obvious roles in numerous groups. Striking examples of larval specializations include the mucocartilage skeleton of lamprey ammocoetes and the jaw cartilages of anuran tadpoles. Striking examples of terminal addition are the asymmetric skull of adult flatfishes and the secondary jaw-closing mechanism of adult male ceratioids.

Heterochrony, on the other hand, has numerous and often subtle manifestations. Within groups, there can be notable variation in the timing of events which characterize metamorphosis. For example, ossification of the maxilla, formation of the pterygoid process and nasal capsule, and the concomitant change in snout shape have a metamorphic occurrence in plethodontid urodeles; however, these events are typical of embryonic or larval development in other families. In anurans, the lamina orbitonasalis and sclerotic cartilage typically form well before metamorphosis, but they also form at metamorphosis in some species. Similarly, the plectrum of the middle ear and antero-lateral process of the hyobranchial plate, which typically develop at metamorphosis, can also form much later (Hetherington 1987). In addition, a few groups bear evidence of an evolutionary shift in the timing of a developmental event from primary to secondary metamorphic periods. Lampreys typically undergo oral disk enlargement as a late event in the primary metamorphic period. There are, however, a few parasitic forms which retain a small oral disk during the juvenile period and initiate disk enlargement only during the sexual maturation (Hardisty and Potter 1971b). Similarly, the caudal displacement of the branchial apparatus and pectoral girdle that is characteristic of the primary metamorphosis in eels does not occur in the primary metamorphosis of nemichthyids, although it does occur during secondary metamorphosis in males (Nielsen and Smith 1978).

Heterochrony can also generate recurring evolutionary trends within certain groups that are primitively metamorphic. Paedomorphosis modifies metamorphic ontogenies by delaying and eventually eliminating metamorphic events, thereby creating adult morphologies ranging from a mosaic of larval and metamorphic characters to a completely larval condition. Anurans and urodeles both exhibit numerous cases of a specific skeletal event being lost by particular taxa; these events often occur during late metamorphosis or adulthood in related species (Larsen 1963; Trueb and Alberch 1985; Wake and Larson 1987). As noted above, the stomiiform teleost *Idiacanthus* presents the case of a sexually dimorphic partial metamorphosis, in which numerous skeletal elements in the male develop only to a stage comparable with midmetamorphic stages of the female

(Beebe 1934). Within urodeles, some families (Cryptobranchidae, Sirenidae, Proteidae, and Amphiumidae) are exclusively paedomorphic and display taxonomically specific patterns of partial metamorphosis (Duellman and Trueb 1986). For example, within the Cryptobranchidae, *Andrias,* but not *Cryptobranchus,* exhibits branchial arch reduction at metamorphosis (Edgeworth 1923), and cryptobranchids and sirenids both retain some degree of palatal remodeling during larval life (Noble 1929; Aoyama 1930; Jarvik 1942). Other families (e.g., Ambystomatidae, Salamandridae, and Plethodontidae) contain both paedomorphic and metamorphic species, some of the latter being facultatively neotenic. Neotenic ambystomatids and plethodontids tend to eliminate all or almost all metamorphic changes in the cranial skeleton (Wake 1966; Reilly 1987). Conversely, neotenic salamandrids tend to complete most changes in the skull but only a variable subset of the events in the hyobranchium and palate (Reilly 1987; Marconi and Simonetta 1988); larval hyobranchial cartilages may be retained and even ossified (Reilly 1987).

Direct development represents an alternative means of escape from a metamorphic ontogeny. Direct development in primitively metamorphic groups involves the loss of a free-living larva, with variable suppression of larval characters. This suppression may entail metamorphic and embryogenic events becoming condensed, overlapped, temporally dissociated, or lost altogether; such changes are collectively referred to as differential metamorphosis or dissociation (Wake 1966; Roth and Wake 1985). Direct development may also be coupled with either paedomorphic or peramorphic modifications to cranial morphology as demonstrated by various plethodontid urodeles (Alberch and Alberch 1981; Wake et al. 1983; Wake and Larson 1987); the occurrence of this phenomenon in other groups has not received adequate attention.

Direct-developing anurans vary widely in their suppression of larval chondrocranial characters. For example, the quadrate bar may form in a typical larval position but without its typical neurocranial attachments (e.g., *Arthroleptella,* de Villiers 1929); it may form with a position and attachments typical of midmetamorphic stages (e.g., *Breviceps,* Swanepoel 1970); or it may form directly in the adult position (e.g., *Eleutherodactylus,* Lynn 1942). Suprarostral cartilages may form in the typical larval position or not at all. Likewise, the trabecular horns may be resorbed and replaced as in typical larvae, or they may be converted directly into the inferior prenasal cartilages. Relatively little is known about skull development in direct-developing urodeles and caecilians. Some members of the former group recapitulate larval development in the hyobranchium (e.g., *Plethodon cinereus,* Dent 1942; *Desmognathus wrighti,* Alberch 1989), while others have completely eliminated these events (e.g., *Bolitoglossa subpalmata,* Wake 1966; Alberch 1989). One viviparous caecilian, *Dermophis mexicanus,* shows no sign of recapitulating any metamorphic events (Wake and Hanken 1982).

This diversity of ontogenetic patterns within metamorphic groups well illustrates the evolutionary lability of metamorphosis, as well as the fallacy of defining metamorphosis on the basis of character-specific criteria alone. All patterns of cranial remodeling are relative in their scope and intensity, and how one defines the set of events constituting a "complete" or "true" metamorphosis is essentially a taxonomic or cladistic issue. The evolutionary tendency of metamorphic systems to undergo a heterochronic restructuring of their metamorphoses implies that metamorphosis is more than the sum of numerous morphological changes being triggered by one global cue. That heterochronic changes may occur at both local and global scales, i.e., with events becoming delayed or accelerated independently of other events, and with contrasting sets of changes becoming superimposed upon one another, would strongly suggest that the underlying developmental regulation operates at several levels.

DEVELOPMENTAL MECHANISMS OF CRANIAL REMODELING IN METAMORPHOSIS

Dating back to Gudernatsch (1912), who first noted the activating potential of thyroid tissue upon frog metamorphosis, endocrinologists have given exhaustive attention to the role of the neuroendocrine system in triggering and integrating metamorphic events (Etkin 1963, 1968; see recent reviews by White and Nicoll 1981; Norris 1983; Fox 1983; Matsuda 1987). However, this research has focused mainly on anuran metamorphosis, and more specifically, on the internal and environmental controls of hormone production and the role of hormones in tissue activation. The endocrinological perspective consequently fails to provide insight into the diversification of the peripheral morphology in different metamorphic systems. To understand the evolutionary origin of differences in skull remodeling, one must first elucidate the developmental mechanisms governing the morphogenetic specificity of tissue responses in cartilage and bone. We are referring in particular to the synergism between hormonal and nonhormonal regulatory mechanisms, and to the cellular pathways that have been coopted for packaging and unfolding the morphological duality of metamorphic tissues.

In surveying the experimental literature on metamorphosis and cranial remodeling, it becomes apparent that a comparative framework for discussing these phenomena is lacking. We recognize four aspects of developmental mechanism which collectively define the developmental structure of metamorphic systems and which have, in one way or another, contributed to cranial diversification. These aspects are (1) the hormonal agent for activating tissue responses, (2) the development of tissue sensitivity or response capacity, (3) the development of tissue specificity, i.e., how different tissue and cell types acquire their specific instructions for morphogenesis and differentiation, and (4) the choice of cellular pathway for transforming larval organ systems into adult ones. While many mechanistic relationships have been elucidated by research on nonskeletal tissues only, we address what is known concerning their actual role in skull development at metamorphosis and offer some speculative comments regarding their potential role in the evolutionary diversification of pathways of skeletal morphogenesis. We conclude with the observation that metamorphic systems utilize developmental mechanisms that are not qualitatively distinct from those characterizing nonmetamorphic development. However, within the context of a metamorphic system, i.e., an ontogeny incorporating a midontogenetic period of concentrated and morphologically pervasive development, these developmental interactions may have a far greater potential for promoting morphogenetic diversification.

Hormonal Agents of Activation

The role of various hormones as global activators of metamorphic tissue responses has been tested using two techniques: (1) the effective removal of endogenous hormone, via gland or hypophysis removal or gland-inhibiting drugs (in the case of the thyroid, goitrogens), to cause the suppression of metamorphic events, and (2) exogenous hormone application to precociously induce metamorphic events, this being the more rigorous method when done in conjunction with gland removal.

Thyroid hormones (TH) have received indisputable confirmation as the principal activating agent for primary metamorphosis in frogs (see Gudernatsch 1912; Etkin 1955; Kollros 1961 and references therein for exogenous induction; Allen 1916 for thyroid gland and hypophysis removal; Gordon et al. 1943; Hughes and Astwood 1944; Lynn and Peadon 1955; and Lynn 1948 for thyroid inhibitors), urodeles (see Gudernatsch 1914 for exogenous induction; Lynn 1947 for thyroid inhibitors), and flatfish (see Inui and Miwa 1985 and Miwa and Inui 1987 for exogenous induction and thyroid inhibitors). There are some preliminary experiments which implicate the thyroid gland in eel metamorphosis (Vilter 1946; Kitajima et al. 1967), as well as more circumstantial histological evidence supporting its role in the primary metamorphoses of caecilians (Klumpp and Eggert 1934) and other actinopterygians, including bonefish (see reviews by Pickford and Atz 1957; Eales 1979; Youson 1988).

However, the exact role of TH in activating skeletal tissue responses has received little direct investigation in metamorphic systems. Even for amniote systems there have been very few attempts to demonstrate TH-specific binding capacity in skeletal tissues (e.g., Kan and Cruess 1987). On the other hand, there is substantial evidence from anuran research to indicate peripheral interplay among multiple hormones. In particular, TH is thought to interact antagonistically with prolactin and gonadal steroids, and synergistically with corticosteroids to activate various aspects of tissue remodeling (e.g., Kaltenbach 1958; Kikuyama et al. 1983; Galton 1990; Gray and Janssens 1990), including chondrogenesis and osteogenesis in hind limbs (Tata et al. 1991). While certain of these interactions (TH-prolactin and TH-corticosterone, but not TH-testosterone—see Gray and Janssens 1990 and Tata et al. 1991) have been conclusively demonstrated to occur peripherally, i.e., at the hormone-cell interface, the exact mechanisms involved are not well understood (see Dent 1988; Dickhoff et al. 1990 for review).

In contrast to other metamorphic systems, lampreys have eluded all efforts to identify a key hormone for activating primary metamorphosis. Measured decreases in plasma TH at the onset of metamorphosis and repeated failures to initiate metamorphosis with exogenous TH rule against a primary endostyle or thyroid role (see reviews by Just et al. 1981; Hardisty and Baker 1982; Youson 1988). Interestingly, the only successful attempts at inducing metamorphosis in ammocoetes have been with goitrogens (Suzuki 1986, 1987a; see also Youson 1980), which suggests that the drop in plasma TH that is observed immediately after the onset of natural metamorphosis (Wright and Youson 1977; Lintlop and Youson 1983) may be a factor in metamorphic activation. There is histological and experimental evidence for both pineal and hypophysial involvement in lamprey metamorphosis (Eddy 1969; Cole and Youson 1981; Joss 1985; Wright 1989), and most accounts concede that several primary agents are probably involved. Lampreys, however, may not be unique in this regard, as there is a general consensus emerging that nonamphibian metamorphoses are typified by a weaker role of TH and a greater synergism among hormones and other factors than are amphibian metamorphoses (Eales 1979; Matsuda 1987).

Regarding the secondary metamorphoses of various groups, gonadal steroids have been widely confirmed as the primary inducing agent for secondary sexual characters (see Larsen 1974, 1980 for lampreys; Sassoon and Kelley 1986; Sassoon et al. 1986 for anurans; Noble and Davis 1928 for urodeles).

The Development of Response Capacity

In anurans there seems to be no doubt that most, if not all, metamorphic tissues respond directly to TH (see reviews by Kaltenbach 1968; White and Nicoll 1981; Dent 1988; Galton 1988). That many tissue responses, including those of skeletal elements, can occur independently has been demonstrated by the experimental uncoupling of localized remodeling events from systemic events (Hartwig 1940; Kaltenbach 1953a, b, c; Kaltenbach and Hobbs 1972) and of different classes of systemic events, for example, cranial chondrogenesis and osteogenesis (Hanken and Summers 1988b; Hanken and Hall 1988b), cranial muscle formation and muscle breakdown (Takisawa et al. 1976), and the global occurrences of programmed cell death and cell proliferation (Puckett 1937). In particular, Summers and Hanken's (1988) work with the jaw cartilages of the anuran *Bombina orientalis* demonstrates that all normal shape changes in these elements are inducible in vitro, which provides strong support for the direct and independent nature of TH responses in at least some cranial skeletal tissues. Yet in spite of these insights, we still do not know precisely how skeletal tissues acquire their response capacity, i.e., how they derive a meaningful signal from ontogenetic changes in the concentration of endogenous hormone, and in particular how they are instructed to initiate a response at the appropriate stage and maintain it at the appropriate rate thereafter.

The temporal sequence of metamorphic events is generally attributed to tissues having differential sensitivities and responding at different concentrations during a steady increase in plasma TH (see Hanken and Summers 1988b for a recent discussion). This model, however, receives somewhat equivocal support from empirical studies of endogenous hormone levels. Although radioimmunoassays have usually found plasma levels pooled from many individuals to undergo a surge in TH concentration at or slightly before metamorphic climax (see Miwa et al. 1988 for flatfish; Leloup and Buscaglia 1977; Regard et al. 1978; Schultheiss 1980 for anurans; Eagleson and McKeown 1978; Suzuki 1987b for urodeles; White and Nicoll 1981 and Dent 1988 for reviews), nonpooled sampling (Miyauchi et al. 1977; Mondou and Kaltenbach 1979; Suzuki and Suzuki 1981; Weil 1986 for anurans; Larras-Regard et al. 1981; Alberch et al. 1986; Norman et al. 1987 for urodeles) has commonly indicated substantial variation in this pattern. Individuals of some species may not even experience a conspicuous surge in plasma TH: a significant percentage of *Eurycea bislineata* individuals were found to have undetectably low TH levels at all midmetamorphic stages (Alberch et al. 1986). These discrepancies suggest that the metamorphic surge in plasma TH may provide at best a coarse-grained pulsatile signal to activate tissues (Rosenkilde 1979; White and Nicoll 1981), implying that the finer-grained specification of their responses is intrinsically determined prior to this signal. This conclusion is further supported by the finding that tadpoles thyroidectomized just prior to the climactic stages of metamorphosis are still able to complete all metamorphic changes (Kawamura et al. 1986).

The second shortcoming of this model is its failure to provide a developmental basis for differential tissue sensitivity. The original suggestion of an early, rapid, and full acquisition of response capacity (Etkin 1935, 1950, 1955) soon gave way to the consensus that most tissues acquire their response capacities slowly and continuously, over a range of larval stages and TH concentrations (Allen 1938; Geigy 1941; Kollros 1961; Etkin 1964; Chou and Kollros 1974; Miwa et al. 1988). It has also long been realized that anuran tissues can bind to TH at very early larval stages, and that this binding may be a prerequisite in the development of response capacity (Tata 1968, 1970; Knutson and Prahlad 1971). However, the most significant insight into this problem has come with the recent findings that larval and metamorphic tissues actively regulate the amount and type of hormone with which they interact, as well as their physiological sensitivity to that hormone (Galton 1983, 1988; Liegro et al. 1987).

Thyroid hormone is secreted by the thyroid gland in two forms, tetraiodothyronine (T_4) and triiodothyronine (T_3). The former is produced in greater abundance but is generally regarded as a prohormone or precursor to the more active latter form; both appear to bind to the same set of nuclear receptors (Galton 1986, 1988; Miwa and Inui 1987 and references therein; Evans 1988). Recent work on anurans has shown that tissues do in fact process plasma-bound thyroid hormone as it arrives at the cell interface: cytoplasmic enzyme systems can be activated to convert T_4 into active and inactive forms of T_3 which can then be converted into inactive T_2. Moreover, the activity of these deiodinating systems appears to be tissue-specific and to be regulated by ontogenetic changes in TH (Galton and Munck 1981; Galton and Hiebert 1987, 1988).

Tissues also regulate the expression of their thyroid hormone receptors throughout larval and metamorphic development. As in other vertebrates, two families of TH receptor gene, TRα and TRβ, have been recognized in the genome of the frog *Xenopus laevis* (Yaoita et al. 1990). Expression of these genes has been found to be both tissue- and stage-specific (Yaoita and Brown 1990; Kawahara et al. 1991). Moreover, there appears to be differential up-regulation of these genes by TH, with TRβ mRNA abundance being increased at a much greater rate in tadpoles exposed to exogenous hormone (Yaoita and Brown 1990; Kawahara et al. 1991). The converse situation, down-regulation of receptor density, has been demonstrated to occur in prolactin receptor induction (White et al. 1981). In addition to establishing tissue competence, receptor recruitment may also play a key role in specifying tissue fate at metamorphosis (Galton 1984, 1988; Kawahara et al. 1991). However, the full significance of this phenomenon will not be realized until the questions of translational regulation and pretranscription events, e.g., receptor-receptor interactions, are addressed as well (see Hoskins 1990 for review).

Current research on the cellular regulation of thyroid hormone abundance and receptor expression has been limited for experimental reasons mainly to whole animal assays and assays of nonskeletal tissue. However, one study (Kan and Cruess 1987) on the fetal bovine epiphysis provides circumstantial evidence for TH-induced receptor recruitment in growth-plate chondrocytes. Regarding metamorphic systems, although radioimmunoassays commonly do not detect plasma TH at larval stages, its presence in frogs has been confirmed by immunohistochemistry throughout the entire larval period (Kaltenbach 1982). In addition, the larval thyroid gland generally undergoes an increase in activity, as measured by iodine uptake (see Galton 1988 for review). There is also substantial evidence for TH having an active role in promoting the differentiation of bone and cartilage during this period. Kollros (1961) found that the stage to which hypophysectomized tadpoles could develop was directly proportional to the concentration of exogenous thyroid hormone applied, which indicates that larval development (or at least development of the hind limb staging criteria) relies upon endogenous hormone. This is supported by Kemp and Hoyt (1965, 1969), who used exogenous TH to induce periosteum formation in the tadpole femur well in advance of control animals. In addition, endocranial bones that normally ossify midway through the larval period in the plethodontid urodele *Eurycea bislineata* (the os thyroideum, orbitosphenoid, and the footplate and columella of the middle ear) can be induced to form precociously in larvae exposed to thyroid hormone (Rose, work in progress). These results suggest that the larval period entails some TH-dependent development in skeletal tissues. Furthermore, Hanken and Hall (1988a) report that bones of *Bombina orientalis* which are not visible until prometamorphosis in cleared and stained whole mounts derive from weakly differentiated blastemata that are actually formed at much earlier larval stages. It is tempting to speculate that this early differentiation is mediated by TH at very low levels, in anticipation of the later surge in TH which accelerates proliferation and differentiation to form the adult bone (Hanken and Hall 1988b).

To summarize, in re-evaluating the importance of thyroid hormone to metamorphic skeletogenesis, it is suggested that the specific cellular processes that are either activated or accelerated in metamorphic remodeling may in fact derive from a much longer term interaction with TH than was previously appreciated. Moreover, the possibility that different cellular responses at metamorphosis are precipitated by different mechanisms of peripheral TH regulation opens up the possibility that evolutionary changes in skeletal morphogenesis may result simply from temporal modulation of the endogenous TH signal during the larval period. However, the exact relationships between cell type (osteoblast or chondroblast), cell response (differentiation, division, apposition, death, etc.), and means of hormone regulation (deiodination, receptor recruitment, differential expression of receptor types) need to be elucidated before we can access the overall importance of peripheral TH regulation to skull morphogenesis.

The Development of Response Specificity

Cellular Responses to Metamorphic Hormones. Cranial skeletal tissues in TH-activated metamorphosis undergo a wide range of morphogenetic responses, including the complete resorption of larval elements, changes in the shape, size and/or position of elements, the de novo condensation and differentiation of adult elements, and the loss and gain of articulations. At a cellular level, these changes are accomplished via a combination of localized cell death, cell proliferation, cell migration, cell apposition, mineralization, matrix secretion and/or matrix resorption. All of these cell behaviors are presumably TH-induced, although outside Summers and Hanken's (1988) in vitro work on *Bombino orientalis* (see above), it remains unknown whether this induction is direct or indirect. In the parallel situation of secondary metamorphosis, gonadal steroids induce various cellular responses within skeletal tissues to accomplish similar types of morphogenesis. For example, testosterone promotes the proliferation of chondrocytes and perichondrial cells (as well as laryngeal myoblasts) in the larynx of male juvenile frogs (Sassoon and Kelley 1986; Sassoon et al. 1986); again, the nature of the induction is not known.

As one might expect, the role of these hormones in skeletogenesis in nonmetamorphic systems appears to be more limited, both in scope and spatial extent. In vivo studies of anamniote systems have revealed that TH stimulates sulphate uptake in the chondrocytes of salmon branchial cartilages (Barber and Barrington 1972), and that TH is essential for normal differentiation and matrix secretion in chondrocytes of the branchial and Meckel's cartilages of sharks (Alluchon-Gérard 1982); these effects are differentially expressed within different regions of the cartilages. In vitro studies of amniote growth-plate cartilage have revealed that TH directly accelerates the differentiation of chondrocytes from proliferative to hypertrophic states and also enhances the effects of somatomedins in promoting matrix deposition (Burch and Lebowitz 1982a, b; Burch and Van Wyk 1987); nongrowth-plate cartilage shows neither of these effects (Burch and Lebowitz 1982a; see also Silbermann 1983 for review). In mammalian bone, TH directly stimulates osteoclast activity in the degradation of collagen (Halme et al. 1972) and mineral resorption (Mundy et al. 1976), but it has no direct effect upon bone formation (see reviews by Canalis 1983; Mosekilde et al. 1990). Somatomedins, a family of insulin-like growth factors, are also important stimulators of collagen formation and osteoblast proliferation in bone, and this effect may again be enhanced by thyroid hormone (Canalis 1983; Mosekilde et al. 1990). With regard to gonadal steroids, early research had suggested an absence of estrogen receptors in mammalian bone, and the lack of a direct role for gonadal steroids in bone and cartilage development (Nutik and Cruess 1974; Chen and Feldman 1978; Silbermann 1983). However, more recent work has indicated estradiol receptors in osteoblastlike cells and androgen receptors in osteoblastlike cells and chondrocytes, and has demonstrated that both types of hormone exert direct anabolic effects on bone and cartilage cells (see Schwartz et al. 1991 and references therein). Moreover, the effects of these hormone appear to be sex-specific (Schwartz et al. 1991).

The majority of in vitro observations on TH and steroid effects are derived from studies of amniote growth-plate cartilage and long bones, in which the skeletal development proceeds through a stereotypic program of cell stages that are regionally distinct within skeletal elements. Anamniote cranial elements, on the other hand, do not necessarily exhibit a conspicuous regional differentiation in either cell size, cell packing, or distribution of matrix. For example, the larval Meckel's cartilage of *Xenopus laevis* is characterized by evenly distributed cells with large lacunae and little interlacunar matrix, and a thin perichondrium except in the immediate region of the articular surface (Thomson 1986). Similarly, the larval first epibranchial in the plethodontid urodele *Eurycea bislineata* is composed of chondrocytes that exhibit a typical morphology and uniform arrangement throughout the cartilage (Alberch and Gale 1986). These larval cartilages do not appear to be invested with any predefined structure that would dictate their program of morphogenesis at metamorphosis. One interpretation of this is that their cellular responses to metamorphic hormones are more localized and that their morphogenesis may require a more complex mediation than in growth-plate cartilage. The role of local growth regulators, i.e., locally released growth factors (Reddi 1982; Canalis 1983; Marks and Popoff 1988), deserves future attention in this regard.

It is also pertinent that the two major classes of hormone involved in activating metamorphic tissue responses, steroid and thyroid hormones, have nuclear receptors with similar DNA-binding regions, and presumably similar gene-regulating properties (Liegro et al. 1987; Evans 1988); these receptors are now considered to be evolutionarily derived from the same gene family (Weinberger et al. 1986). These observations suggest that the types of cellular response that are available for metamorphic remodeling are a function of the regulatory capacities shared by members of this family of hormone receptor. Furthermore, it appears that metamorphic systems have coopted certain regulatory mechanisms that are engaged in skeletal growth and differentiation in nonmetamorphic systems, but they have expanded the repertoire of cellular responses as well as the heterogeneity of cellular environments in which they occur.

The Nonhormonal Regulation of Cellular Responses. Granted that numerous cellular responses can be TH-activated in metamorphic systems, it remains to be seen how localized differences in cell response are established, especially when considering cells within the same larval tissue. Prior to the discovery of peripheral TH regulation, it was generally accepted that thyroxine had no role in conferring morphogenetic specificity. In Paul Weiss's words, "the morphogenetic action of hormone is not too unlike the action of the photographic developer in bringing out the latent picture on an exposed plate" (Weiss and Rosetti 1951). This long-standing view of metamorphic tissue responses as relying primarily upon predetermined or intrinsic specification has been reinforced by the many experiments on anurans showing that (1) heterotopically transplanted tissues adhere to origin-specific remodeling (see Schwind 1933 for cranial skeletal tissue; Schubert 1926 and Geigy 1941 for other tissues), and (2) TH pellet implants induce localized site-specific remodeling (see Kaltenbach 1953a for cranial skeletal tissue; Hartwig 1940; Kaltenbach 1953b, c; Kaltenbach and Hobbs 1972 for other tissues).

Most of these experiments were not sufficiently refined to detect the influence of small-scale tissue interactions, and many researchers have continued to perceive epigenesis to be a relatively unimportant source of regulation in metamorphic systems. In the absence of evidence for nonhormonal mediation of hormone processing and receptor induction during the larval period, the assumption persists that response specificity, including whatever mechanisms of peripheral TH regulation that may entail, is largely determined by early larval stages (Geigy 1941; Weiss and Rosetti 1951; Kaltenbach 1968; Tata 1970; Fox 1983; Matsuda 1987). However, an entirely mosaic and deterministic model for metamorphic remodeling runs contrary to our general impression of vertebrate development as a highly regulated process involving many epigenetic factors (Devillers 1965; Maderson 1975; Alberch 1980, 1982; Hall 1983a). Three amphibian researchers, O. M. Helff, Günter Clemen, and Irene Medvedeva, have invalidated the assumption of whole-scale determinism with demonstrations of inductive tissue interactions at metamorphosis that introduce qualitative changes in the cranial morphology.

Helff's (1927, 1928, 1931, 1934, 1940) classical work on anuran ear formation demonstrates that the tympanic annulus and pars externa plectri cartilages induce the dedifferentiation of adjacent larval integument and its subsequent differentiation into the thin fibrous epithelium and thickened lamina propria that comprise the adult tympanum. Heterotopic transplants reveal that the portion of larval integument adjacent to the middle ear is not predetermined to this fate, and that both aspects of tympanum formation can be induced in integument in other body regions. The membrane induction is essentially a contact phenomenon brought about by these two cartilages. It was very surprising though to find that the pala-toquadrate, which appears to give rise to the tympanic annulus at meta-morphosis, and, to a lesser extent, the suprascapular cartilage also display an inducing capacity when transplanted beneath skin. This led Helff (1934) to infer that "all hyaline cartilages may possess such potential influences to a greater or lesser degree." However, their remoteness from integument presumably precludes these other cartilages from exercising any inductive role.

Using transplants between post- and premetamorphic stages, Helff and Clemen both have demonstrated that the differentiation states of larval and adult integument are epigenetically determined. In salamandrid urodeles, for example, homotopic transplantation of adult oral epithelium to a larval palate causes it to revert to a larval state of differentiation with a renewed capacity to undergo metamorphosis (Clemen 1987). In anurans, the dermal plicae or dorsal ridges that form in the adult integument will regress when transplanted to larval integument; the same tissue can subsequently be induced to differentiate into a tympanic membrane (Helff 1933, 1937). These results may reflect inductive interactions with either adjacent skin or underlying mesenchyme. A more striking example of this phenomenon is the failure of tadpole tail muscle to resorb when exposed to TH, unless accompanied by tail epidermis or cultured in a medium containing epidermal factors (Niki et al. 1982, 1984).

Clemen's (1978, 1988a, b) experimental investigation of dentitional metamorphosis in ambystomatid and salamandrid urodeles has demonstrated that tooth replacement and changes in tooth pattern are contingent upon a nonspecific interaction between dental laminae and their associated dentigerous jaw and palatal bones. The connective tissue lining these bones is the main source of odontoblasts for tooth buds arising in the dental laminae. While a heterotopically transplanted dental lamina can recruit cells from the connective tissue associated with a foreign dentigerous bone, it cannot recruit cells when placed next to a foreign nondentigerous bone and instead undergoes resorption (see Clemen 1988a). The type of teeth (mono- or bicuspid) arising in a transplanted dental lamina is specific to the lamina and not to the bone providing the odontoblasts. Unlike the oral epithelium, metamorphic changes in dental laminae are irreversible (Clemen 1988a).

In salamandrids and plethodontids, the posterior expansion of the palatal dental lamina to form the parasphenoid tooth patch is correlated with the growth of an underlying vomerine bar (fig. 8.5d–f). This bar grows posteriorly from the medial (plethodontids) or lateral (salamandrids) edge of the vomer along the length of the cultriform process. Its growth is marked by the coalescence and multiplication of numerous tooth buds along its length, the most posterior ones going to form the parasphenoid tooth patch. Clemen's (1978, 1979b) transplant experiments on *Salamandra salamandra* demonstrate that development of the vomerine bar is dependent upon normal development of the tooth patch and vice versa. Clemen (1979a) further demonstrates that development of the bar requires the presence of an intact bordering nerve, the palatine branch of the facial nerve, although this observation may have been confounded by experimental disruption of the connective tissues giving rise to the bar. My own efforts to identify a similar nerve tissue requirement in plethodontid remodeling have been unsuccessful. I found that the morphogenesis of the adult epibranchial in *Eurycea bislineata* proceeded normally after all nerves to the associated musculature were proximally severed (Rose, personal observations).

Medvedeva's (1959, 1960, 1986, and references therein) work on development of the septomaxilla, lacrimal, and prefrontal bones in urodeles points to an inductive relationship between the nasolacrimal duct and these bones. These bones normally arise in late larval and metamorphic periods, after formation of the nasolacrimal duct. In hynobiids extirpation of the placode which gives rise to the nasolacrimal duct results in the incomplete development of the septomaxilla and the complete absence of the lacrimal (Medvedeva 1959, 1960). The same operation on salamandrids, which normally lack a septomaxilla and lacrimal, results in a deficient prefrontal; in ambystomatids, which lack a lacrimal, this operation causes the septomaxilla and a portion of the prefrontal not to form. Medvedeva (1986) speculates that the prefrontal in these latter families is a composite bone comprised of lacrimal and prefrontal ossification centers, the former of which is still associated with the nasolacrimal duct. In each urodele the incomplete formation or absence of a portion of the nasolacrimal duct was correlated with a deficiency in or absence of the tubular bone that later forms around that portion of the duct. In plethodontids the septomaxilla and prefrontal both form at metamorphosis (fig. 8.5c), well after the nasolacrimal duct has appeared (Wilder 1925; Alberch et al. 1986); hence a similar association may be involved. However, in some plethodontids such as *Eurycea bislineata* the nasolacrimal duct does not appear to contact the septomaxilla, as it enters the nasal capsule posterior to the anlage of this bone, the inference being that septomaxilla formation is no longer dependent on this interaction. Lastly, to confirm that Medvedeva's results signify a true inductive interaction requires further proof that the progenitor cells contributing to the bone blastemata were not also removed during the placode extirpation.

Helff, Clemen, and Medvedeva's observations suggest that epigenetic interactions may be integral to a variety of metamorphic tissue responses. However, outside Clemen's and Medvedeva's work, there is almost nothing known regarding the reliance of skeletal remodeling per se upon extrinsic, nonhormonal factors. There has been very little effort to test whether TH-induced shape changes in cranial cartilage and bone are being specified by interactions other than the initial embryonic events responsible for their larval shapes. Research on embryonic induction (see Hall 1989, and references therein) has indicated that neural crest–derived elements of the craniofacial skeleton receive their basic shape specifications prior to migration. Postmigratory cells are induced by epithelium to differentiate into either cartilage or bone, and a variable component of the final larval shape is attributed to later physical interactions, including contact with adjacent structures (e.g., Leibel 1976) and stress from movement (e.g., Hall 1986).

The evidence available for anurans points to strong intrinsic specification of many aspects of the skeletal remodeling at metamorphosis. As mentioned above, anuran jaw cartilages can be induced in vitro to undergo normal, site-specific morphogenesis at a normal rate (Summers and Hanken 1988). Some anuran bones which appear to initiate ossification and morphogenesis just prior to metamorphosis are already preformed as blastemata by this stage; their development at metamorphosis is more correctly considered a TH-induced phase of accelerated cell proliferation and differentiation (Hanken and Hall 1988a). The developmental interactions precipitating the morphogenetic responses of these cartilages and bones at metamorphosis presumably occur well before this stage.

On the other hand, various classical studies have hypothesized mechanical interactions at metamorphosis to account for several disparate aspects of cranial remodeling, the most notable being the backward rotation of the palatoquadrate in anurans (fig. 8.6) and the eye migration in flatfishes. Histological studies on the former system give evidence for crumpling in the posterior end of the quadrate bar, which have led some workers (e.g., Gaupp 1893) to suggest that lengthening in the lower jaw mechanically forces the jaw joint backward. An alternative but equally plausible source for this mechanical force is the lengthening of the pterygoid process. Eye migration in flatfishes is thought to be driven by the interplay of a subocular ligament and skull growth. Lengthening of the skull in early metamorphosis is hypothesized to cause tension in the ligament, which lifts the eye dorsally and across to the contralateral side (Mayhoff 1914; Kyle 1921). These intriguing suggestions beg for an experimental investigation of relationships between skeletal morphogenesis and physical forces that may be generated intracranially at metamorphosis.

To summarize, a mosaic model of tissues acquiring specific sensitivities and responding independently to increasing TH is clearly too simplistic to account for the disparate aspects of morphogenesis and differentiation in complex metamorphic systems. Response capacity and possibly response specificity may be partially determined by the tissue's long-term interaction with endogenous hormone during the larval and premetamorphic periods.

Moreover, mechanisms of acquiring response capacity, e.g., receptor recruitment, may themselves be products of epigenetic interactions (see, e.g., Heuberger et al. 1982). Response specificity may also be directly conferred by epigenetic interactions, as evidenced by their role in integumentary differentiation, dentitional replacement, formation of the dermal bones associated with the nasolacrimal duct, and possibly growth of the vomerine bar. Whether skeletal remodeling generally incorporates significant interplay between extrinsic factors, i.e., epigenesis, and intrinsic specifications, i.e., embryonic inductions and tissue-specific programs of TH regulation, must be determined by future investigation.

Cellular Pathways for Metamorphic Remodeling

Metamorphic ontogenies have been generally interpreted as manifesting either linear or parallel cellular pathways for transforming larval organ systems into adult ones (Cohen and Massey 1983; Cohen 1985; Fox 1983). The linear pathway involves an embryonic organ rudiment comprised of one or more clonal cell populations that have the capacity to generate the shape and differentiation state of the larval organ, and to subsequently reorganize at metamorphosis into the adult counterpart. This reorganization in skeletal tissue may conceivably draw upon all of the cellular responses mentioned above: localized cell proliferation, cell migration, cell apposition and cell death, localized cell growth and cell shrinkage, cell rearrangement or respecification, accelerated cell differentiation, including matrix secretion, mineralization, and resorption, and cell redifferentiation. In contrast, the parallel pathway involves apportioning the embryo into clonal cell populations destined either to form a larval organ or to be set aside as presumptive adult tissue. At metamorphosis the presumptive adult tissue is activated to proliferate and undergo morphogenesis and differentiation into an adult organ, while a corresponding larval organ may experience partial or complete elimination via cell death and matrix resorption.

As we are discussing vertebrate metamorphosis, wherein parts of the larval skeleton generally serve to some extent as templates for corresponding adult structures, the distinction between linear and parallel pathways becomes primarily a quantitative one, and definitions of these terms are hence appropriate only for describing the two extremes of a continuum. Nonetheless, this terminology is useful as a conceptual tool for discussing the variation in pathway by which skeletal organs are transformed at a cellular level. The linear pathway is characterized by the persistence of the majority of cells comprising a larval organ as the major constituents of the corresponding adult organ; hence, the organ exhibits essentially a biphasic development. The parallel pathway is distinguished by a general lack of cellular continuity between larval and adult organs; the adult organ is primarily derived de novo, from one or more clonal cell populations which did not comprise the major constituents of any one larval organ but may have resided as undifferentiated components of the larval morphology.

The distinction between elements engaged in parallel versus linear development is drawn independently of the embryonic tissue origin. The embryonic mesenchyme that provides the source of all musculoskeletal tissue in the larval and adult crania is derived from neural crest and paraxial mesoderm (see Noden 1982 for review). Although it is now well established for avian systems that the majority of the viscerocranium, much of the chondrocranium, and numerous dermal bones and connective tissues are derived from neural crest alone (Noden 1982), the exact interface between these two types of mesenchyme in the adult cranium seems to vary among taxa (Noden 1987). In the absence of cell lineage analyses for any metamorphic system, little can be said regarding the contributions of each type to skeletal tissues undergoing parallel versus linear development. Hence, our discussion of this topic is restricted to a comparative overview of remodeling pathways in skeletal elements, nerves, and muscles, as inferred from thymidine marking, ultrastructural analyses, and histological descriptions.

Skeleton. Anuran chondrocranial remodeling incorporates a combination of linear and parallel pathways. Remodeling in the lower jaw cartilage of *Xenopus* involves primarily linear remodeling via localized cell death, cell proliferation, and matrix secretion in the preformed larval element (Thomson 1986, 1987, 1989). Although other anuran systems have not received explicit experimental analysis, histological studies (e.g., de Jongh 1968) often show a clear demarcation of newly forming cartilage from cartilage which is retained at metamorphosis. For example, ranids retain much of the larval palatoquadrate at metamorphosis (fig. 8.6), although with major resorption and the addition of numerous adult components. The basal and adult otic processes appear to arise from de novo condensations, but the pterygoid process (fig. 8.6b–d) is derived from interstitial growth in the larval element (de Jongh 1968). Hence, the palatoquadrate itself exhibits both pathways, the interstitial growth of the pterygoid process being an extreme case of linear remodeling, whereby a large adult process is derived from a relatively small larval one. In the ranid hyobranchium, the anterior process of the adult ceratohyal develops as a de novo condensation alongside the degenerating larval process (de Jongh 1968). Other candidates for parallel development are the tympanic annulus and pars externa plectri, which in *Bufo* appear to derive their constituent cells from the eroding surface of the adjacent palatoquadrate cartilage (Barry 1956), and the cartilages of the larynx which form de novo posterior to the hyobranchium (Märtens 1898).

Among urodeles, the outgrowth of the vomerine bar in salamandrids and plethodontids represents perhaps the most conspicuous case of bone morphogenesis at metamorphosis. The bar develops from very localized and rapid osteogenic activity on the posterior border of the vomer (fig. 8.5e); it appears to form via the apposition of cells from adjacent connective tissues (Clemen 1979b). If, in fact, this element is derived entirely from cells outside the larval vomer, then this morphogenesis would be attributable to parallel development.

A remarkable case of parallel development is the hyobranchial apparatus of the caecilian *Epicrionops* (Wake 1989). The four ceratobranchials and ceratohyals of the larval hyobranchium have extensively ossified shafts which are completely resorbed at metamorphosis and replaced by newly forming cartilaginous elements.

To date, however, Alberch and Gale's (1986) study of hyobranchial transformation in *Eurycea bislineata* provides the only experimental confirmation of parallel development in skeletal morphogenesis. As first reported by Smith (1920), the larval epibranchial cartilages are replaced entirely by a new adult element (fig. 8.5g–i). The three larval epibranchial cartilages are eliminated via cell autophagocytosis and matrix resorption (Alberch et al. 1985), and a longer and slimmer adult epibranchial cartilage is generated de novo along with its helically wound subarcualis rectus muscle. The first sign of the adult epibranchial is an accentuated proliferation of cells in the antero-ventral perichondrium of the first larval epibranchial. The early growth of the adult condensation occurs by proliferation and the apposition of mesenchymal cells. As the larval cartilage disintegrates, the adult condensation develops its own perichondrium and starts to elongate by internal proliferation. Thymidine marking suggests that cells of the adult epibranchial cartilage are largely, if not exclusively, derived from the antero-ventral perichondrium of the larval element (Alberch and Gale 1986).

Skeletal remodeling in lampreys is complicated by the involvement of mucocartilage. Adult cranial cartilages have been described as arising in three different locations: in fibrous larval tissue, in degenerating larval muscles, and either alongside or inside degenerating mucocartilage elements (Johnels 1948; reviewed by Hardisty 1981). Johnels's (1948) histological study suggests that the chondrocytes of elements arising in fibrous and muscle-rich regions, e.g., the annular and anterior tectal cartilages (fig. 8.1), come from connective tissue within larval tissues. Cartilages arising at the periphery of degenerating mucocartilage elements, e.g., the extrahyal, styliform process, and subocular arch, appear to derive their constituent cells from connective tissues associated with the velum, neurocranium, and mucocartilage elements. Conversely, the adult processes of the branchial basket appear to result from localized proliferation within the larval arches. These largely inferential reports would suggest that both pathways are used in this chondrocranial system and that choice of pathway is specific to the developmental location of the remodeling, with the parallel pathway being dependent on the presence of adjacent mucocartilage, cartilage, or connective tissues.

The adult piston cartilage of lampreys is unique for having its mesenchymal blastema arise well inside the core of a mucocartilage element, the longitudinal ventro-median bar (fig. 8.1). The ultrastructural studies of Armstrong et al. (1985, 1987) indicate that in the first stages of metamorphosis, and prior to the appearance of the piston blastema, mucocartilage cells lose the tubulovesicular character of their cell membranes and start to develop auto- and/or heterophagic vacuoles. The ensuing breakdown of the extracellular matrix is accompanied by an increase in cell density inside the core of the bar and an increase in proliferative activity outside the core region. Armstrong et al. (1987) implicate centrally migrating connective tissue cells as responsible for the latter events. Meanwhile, the dedifferentiating mucocartilage cells in the core apparently lose their autophagic vacuoles and show no evidence of cell disintegration prior to the appearance of the piston blastema. Hence, it is not clear which population of cells—the dedifferentiated mucocartilage cells or the migrant connective tissue cells—makes the primary contribution of mesenchyme to the piston blastema. The subsequent growth of the blastema is marked by a high rate of cell proliferation, although many cells are also observed in various states of degeneration (Armstrong et al. 1987). Thus, from its inception, the blastema of the piston cartilage appears to contain two intermixed populations of cells, one fated to cell death and the other to chondroblast proliferation. It is plausible that the former population is comprised of the original mucocartilage cells which go on to complete their earlier process of autophagocytosis. In the absence of techniques for marking mucocartilage cells, their exact contribution to the morphogenesis of the adult piston cartilage will remain debatable.

Nerves. In conjunction with these skeletal changes, numerous neural centers undergo major revision at metamorphosis (see Kollros 1981 for review). Larval nuclei and their associated nerves can undergo complete degeneration via TH-induced cell death, as exemplified by the lateral line system in anurans (Shelton 1970; Wahnschaffe et al. 1987). There is less evidence, however, for cell proliferation in the replacement and modification of larval nuclei. Rovainen (1982) attributes metamorphic growth in most lamprey CNS centers to the enlargement of pre-existing larval cells rather than to cell division, and Kollros (1981) draws a similar conclusion for anurans.

There is also little indication that new neural centers are derived de novo from presumptive adult tissue at metamorphosis (Kollros 1981; Rovainen 1982). Marking experiments on the trigeminal nerve in *Rana pipiens* (Alley and Barnes 1983; Barnes and Alley 1983; Alley 1989, 1990) have confirmed that no additional trigeminal motoneurons are generated during larval maturation or metamorphosis, and that the majority of primary motoneurons are retained from the larval to the adult nervous system. This work demonstrates that trigeminal motoneurons are being respecified at metamorphosis, meaning that the motoneuron axons transfer their peripheral affiliation from degenerating larval myofibers to the myofibers of newly forming adult jaw muscles. Alley (1989, 1990) reports a temporal overlap between larval and adult myofibers, as well as a high degree of fidelity being maintained in the terminal distribution of motor axons; axonal sprouts generally contact developing myotubes that are adjacent to the degenerating larval myofibers. Similar conclusions are reached for the trigeminal metamorphosis in lampreys. Homma (1978) reports that the three principal motor nerves of the trigeminal do not change with respect to the region of musculature innervated or the relative positions of their cell nuclei inside the trigeminal nucleus. The nerves are not functional during any metamorphic stages; this may reflect a delay in establishing new synapses, which is expected in view of the prolonged and radical nature of remodeling in lamprey oral musculature (Homma 1978). The similarity between anuran and lamprey trigeminal nerves prompts the speculation that neuron respecification may be the characteristic mechanism for remodeling CNS nuclei that control disparate sets of larval and adult muscles.

Muscles. Cranial systems can exhibit large-scale muscle replacement at metamorphosis, as exemplified by the lampreys (Hardisty and Rovainen 1982) and anurans (de Jongh 1968; Takisawa et al. 1976). However, there have been remarkably few experimental attempts to identify the source of myoblasts contributing to the adult musculature. Histological study of anuran jaw adductor muscles (Alley and Cameron 1983; Alley 1989) suggests that adult myofibers arise from satellite cells within the larval muscles; these are distributed along the surface of larval myofibers and are scattered throughout the muscle belly. There appears to be a complete turnover of larval myofibers in the jaw musculature, which implies that larval satellite cells are the sole source for adult myofibers in this cranial region.

EVOLUTIONARY IMPLICATIONS OF CELLULAR PATHWAYS IN CRANIAL REMODELING

In broaching the issue of evolutionary opportunities and constraints afforded by these pathways, it seems appropriate to consider first their evolutionary origins. The replacement and respecification pathways implemented by muscles and neural centers probably did not evolve as specific strategies for metamorphic remodeling per se. The derivation of new myofibers from satellite cells constitutes the most plausible pathway for renewed muscle development and regeneration in nonmetamorphic systems (Mauro 1961; Carlson 1973), and the tendency of CNS centers to accommodate changes in the periphery by rearranging their synaptic connections is a widespread phenomenon outside metamorphosis (Purves 1988). Likewise, there is no evidence for regarding the cellular pathways used in skeletal remodeling at metamorphosis as qualitatively distinct from those involved in nonmetamorphic systems (see Hall 1978, 1983b; Thorogood 1983; and Marks and Popoff 1988 for reviews on bone and cartilage development in nonmetamorphic systems). The cellular processes of cell death, proliferation, apposition, growth, and shrinkage, as well as matrix secretion, mineralization, and resorption, seem to be distinguished in parallel, linear, and nonmetamorphic development only by the scale at which they occur, and their manner of hormonal mediation. There do not appear to be any qualitative factors that would predispose skeletal tissue to adopt one pathway over the other.

Once in place, however, linear and parallel pathways may confer their own developmental limits upon the degree to which any one organ system can be altered, and these limits may, in turn, govern how pervasively each pathway can be utilized in complex cranial remodeling. One important source of constraint is likely to be metabolic cost, i.e., the energy consumed by cell proliferation, differentiation, cell death, and matrix resorption. The parallel pathway invokes these cell behaviors on a larger scale than the linear pathway, and thus should entail higher metabolic costs, especially when involving the resorption of cartilage and bone matrix. The developmental and phylogenetic rarity of complete organ replacement in the skeletal system would support this contention. Conversely, the pervasiveness of organ replacement in muscle systems may reflect inherently low metabolic costs for mobilizing satellite cells and resorbing myofibers.

The tenet that differentiation is a progressive restriction of cell fate would imply that linear pathways have, as a rule, very limited potential for generating new differentiation states in the adult organ (Alberch 1987, 1989). While some cell types may reach a terminal state of larval differentiation which precipitates their replacement at metamorphosis (see Fox 1983 for erythrocytes), other cell types may conceivably embark upon a process of dedifferentiation at metamorphosis. For most tissues, partial dedifferentiation probably presents a more viable process than complete dedifferentiation; however, the former process is inevitably more restrictive in the range of cell fates available for the subsequent development of that tissue. In anuran metamorphosis, larval chondrocytes are released from their matrix and their subsequent fate remains unknown (de Jongh 1968). In lampreys, transformation of the mucocartilage bar into the adult piston cartilage presents a possible candidate for redifferentiation in skeletal tissue. However, it is equally possible that most piston chondroblasts are derived from undifferentiated connective tissue, as is suspected for most of the other cranial cartilages arising in adult lampreys. The replacement of bone by cartilage in the hyobranchium of the caecilian *Epicrionops* (Wake 1989) presents a second candidate for skeletal redifferentiation, yet one can only speculate on the cellular pathway involved.

In addition to developmental limitations, the choice of cellular pathway in metamorphic systems may bear profound consequences for evolutionary diversification owing to the plurality of contingent effects that characterize developmental sequences. In principle, the linear pathway is inherently constraining for skeletal evolution, since the shape of an adult element is, with a few notable exceptions, determined to a large extent by its larval shape, and at the same time, larval shape may be constrained by being a precursor to adult shape. For example, the adult epibranchial cartilage in ambystomatids and salamandrids forms via localized cell proliferation and cell death in the larval element; hence, its shape and function do not change substantially at metamorphosis. The evolution of parallel developmental pathways escapes this self-imposed conservatism by allowing larval and adult structures to develop de novo at different times in ontogeny and thus to evolve divergent shapes and functions. The adult epibranchial of *Eurycea bislineata* serves as a good illustration of this principle (see Alberch 1987, 1989 for a full discussion of its functional and evolutionary significance). However, cases such as the anuran palatoquadrate, which combines linear with parallel remodeling to effect an equally major shape change, lead one to question the universality of this principle.

The linear pathway is also theoretically constrained by a greater developmental burden (see Riedl 1978). Developmental programs for organ differentiation and morphogenesis are characterized by an orderly sequence of developmental events, each of which is causally related to its antecedent and succeeding events (Alberch 1985). In a linear pathway, metamorphic events in an organ are thus contingent upon earlier embryonic and larval events. Moreover, a perturbation manifesting a positive developmental effect upon a metamorphic event would be evolutionarily nullified if it has a prerequisite negative effect upon an earlier event, and vice versa. Burden thus should act to resist developmental innovation in linear metamorphic programs, and consequently to restrain the evolutionary diversification of corresponding larval and adult organs. While conceptually valuable, this theory remains difficult to test without a greater knowledge of the genetic and epigenetic bases for skeletal development in metamorphic systems. However, perturbation experiments that are designed to eliminate specific inductive interactions during embryogeny and that are continued until after metamorphosis is complete (e.g., Luther 1925) may illuminate some aspects of developmental burden as it pertains to skeletal remodeling.

Metamorphic programs that employ parallel cellular pathways experience inherently fewer contingent effects among embryonic, larval, and metamorphic events. One consequence of this is that larval and adult organs may experience greater potential for heterochronic divergence. For example, the evolution of parallel pathways not only frees an adult structure from shape constraints posed by its larval precursor, but may also allow for the complete elimination of the larval precursor in direct-developing forms. Embryos of the plethodontid *Bolitoglossa* bear no sign of recapitulating the larval epibranchial development; the single epibranchial directly assumes its adult shape and muscle configuration at an early stage (Alberch 1989). Similarly, the anuran *Eleutherodactylus* is notable for eliminating most larval structures and having most cranial cartilages directly assume an adult configuration (Lynn 1942; Hanken and Summers 1988a). Alberch (1989) uses the example of plethodontid epibranchials to argue that the complete elimination of larval structures is possible only when larval and adult morphologies have been decoupled by parallel pathways. However, other systems need to be examined to clarify whether parallel development is actually a prerequisite for, rather than merely a facilitating factor in, the complete elimination of larval morphology. For example, it is not clear yet whether instances of loss or reduction in larval morphology are always preceded by the evolution of a parallel developmental pathway for the corresponding adult part(s).

Cellular pathways may additionally influence the potential for evolving cyclical phases of metamorphic remodeling. Cyclical remodeling, which is perhaps best demonstrated by salmonids, requires that the adult morphology retain cell populations with the capacity for episodic proliferation, differentiation, and subsequent regression. Such capacity is presumably demonstrated by connective tissues in the lower jaw of *Salmo*, which repeatedly generate a large hook in spawning males (fig. 8.2). An alternative route for jaw modification evolved by *Oncorhynchus* involves the excessive ossification and fusion of tooth bases, differentiation events which are structurally more permanent and developmentally less retractable than proliferative events in connective tissue alone. Hence, the occurrence of repeated spawning among extant salmon correlates with the choice to remodel the lower jaw with nonosteogenic tissue.

This choice may have in fact developmentally predisposed *Salmo* to evolve its cyclical secondary metamorphosis.

DIRECTIONS FOR FUTURE RESEARCH

Metamorphic systems collectively illustrate an enormous potential for ontogenetic diversification in cranial skeletal morphology, yet these systems have often received inadequate morphological description, and, with the exception of anurans, almost no mechanistic investigation. Compared to embryonic development, there is little known about the developmental interactions underlying metamorphic remodeling in the skull. We have emphasized the potential roles of peripheral regulation, i.e., epigenetic interactions, hormone processing, and receptor induction, all of which may serve as important determinants of response specificity; the latter two may further serve as ontogenetic mechanisms for preparing tissues for hormonal activation. The choice of cellular pathway is also presented as a focal mechanism for exploring the constraints emplaced by development upon cranial diversification in both ontogeny and phylogeny.

Our assessment of the experimental literature yields the general conclusion that the developmental interactions and cellular behaviors employed at metamorphosis are qualitatively similar to those utilized in postembryonic nonmetamorphic development. This conclusion encourages the use of metamorphic systems as a general model for examining the roles of various kinds of developmental mechanisms, such as hormonal synergisms or antagonisms and tissue interactions, in skeletal tissue remodeling. At the same time, a more extensive comparative basis of mechanistic data is needed before we can hope to discern whether any developmental mechanisms are in fact fundamental to metamorphic systems alone and are prerequisite for expressing a midontogenetic period of complex cranial remodeling. We think three directions for future research are particularly essential.

(1) *Descriptive studies of diverse metamorphic systems.* Detailed descriptive studies of skull metamorphosis are a prerequisite to any investigation of the underlying developmental mechanisms. Adequate studies, even at a gross morphological level, currently exist only for anurans and lampreys, although particular regions of the skull have received attention in other groups (e.g., the palate and hyobranchium of urodeles). Particularly distressing is the lack of a thorough descriptive study of metamorphosis in elopomorphs and flatfishes. Descriptive studies should be taken to a histological level, as various studies have demonstrated that much insight into cellular behaviors can be inferred from the cell and matrix morphology at both LM and EM levels (e.g., Alberch et al. 1985; Alberch and Gale 1986; Armstrong et al. 1985, 1987; Thomson 1989).

(2) *Intrinsic versus epigenetic control of cranial remodeling.* The techniques of classical experimental embryology, e.g., extirpation, heterotopic and xenoplastic transplantation, are widely applicable to metamorphic systems, as demonstrated by the work of Helff, Clemen, and Medvedeva. These techniques allow one to test for metamorphic tissue inductions in a fashion analogous to testing for embryogenic inductions. Mechanical interactions at metamorphosis are also amenable to experimental investigation. For example, the hypothesis that eye migration in flatfish is driven by tension in the subocular ligament could easily be tested by bisecting the ligament. On the other hand, as illustrated by Summers and Hanken (1988), Niki et al. (1982) and Tata et al. (1991), there is a great potential offered by organ culture techniques for testing the dependence of specific tissue responses upon epigenetic interactions, for confirming the direct effects of various hormones as well as elucidating their synergistic versus antagonistic interactions, and for quantifying the development of tissue sensitivity to TH as a function of tissue type and cell fate.

The related problem of how skeletal tissues acquire their response capacity may be tackled once a technique becomes available for measuring the hormone binding capacity of skeletal tissues in situ. An in situ technique is essential, since morphogenesis in skeletal tissue generally reflects a combination of several cellular behaviors being expressed differentially in different regions of the element. In vitro techniques employing saturation binding kinetics are not applicable, since the cells must first be isolated and regional differences among cells would hence be lost. Antibodies for TH receptors (Luo et al. 1988; Puymirat et al. 1989; Macchia et al. 1990; Sasaki et al. 1991) and cDNA probes for their transcripts (Kawahara et al. 1991) have recently been employed for demonstrating the relative abundance and regional distribution of TH receptors in sectioned tissue. More research of this type is needed to determine whether skeletal tissues actively regulate their TH binding capacity during the larval period, and whether the nature of this regulation is in fact specific to cell type and/or cell fate at metamorphosis.

(3) *Linear versus parallel pathways of skeletal transformation.* Two developmental problems need to be addressed in order to clarify the extent and implication of these pathways in metamorphic remodeling. These are (a) the neural crest versus paraxial mesoderm origin for larval and presumptive adult skeletal tissues, and (b) the transfer versus turnover of skeletal cells in the transition from larval to adult morphology. Tracing cell lineages, however, requires an effective means of marking cells, the difficulties of which are compounded by the long duration of most larval periods and the extensive growth during this time. Cell marking by fixable fluorescent vital dyes, e.g., lysinated fluorescein dextran (LFD) (Gimlich and Braun 1985), may be useful when working with systems with excep-

tionally short (1 to 2 week) larval periods, as well as with direct developers. The other principle marking technique, radiography, is less reliable, since cell turnover cannot be ruled out, i.e., tritiated thymidine released by degrading cells may be taken up by nearby proliferating cells. The best solution is a two-species system of intrinsic nuclear markers analogous to the chick-quail system that has proven so valuable for studying amniote cell lineages. One such system has recently become available for *Xenopus* spp. (Thiébaud 1983), and has proved quite successful in mapping the contributions of neural crest to larval visceral cartilages (Sadaghiani and Thiébaud 1987). Interestingly, the ceratohyal and ceratobranchials of *Xenopus* are composed of cells from both neural crest and paraxial mesoderm; the question of whether this dual origin has any bearing upon the manner of metamorphic remodeling awaits future investigation.

In the absence of a viable cell-labeling technique for most metamorphic systems, marking cells in the process of division (e.g., Alberch and Gale 1986) or cells expressing a specific antigen (e.g., Williamson et al. 1991a, b) provides the next best alternative. In this way, populations of cells undergoing proliferation and conceivably apposition or migration may be identified, and the relative contributions of these processes to de novo morphogenesis may be elucidated. Extirpation (e.g., Luther 1925) and transplantation experiments may also provide insight, as long as the effects of regulation can be accounted for.

In conclusion, many techniques developed for experimental embryology can be directly applied to metamorphic systems, albeit under the constraints imposed by a long growth period preceding the events of interest. Moreover, the complexity of skeletal remodeling in metamorphic systems, and especially in poorly studied systems such as the flatfishes and lampreys, holds much promise for future research into mechanistic issues of skull development.

ACKNOWLEDGMENTS

We thank Pere Alberch for providing the conceptual inspiration, and the editors, particularly Jim Hanken, for their continued patience and support. Marvalee Wake kindly allowed one of us to examine specimens of caecilians. We also thank Kathy Brown-Wing for providing the figures.

REFERENCES

Agar, W. E. 1906. The development of the skull and visceral arches in *Lepidosiren* and *Protopterus*. Transactions of the Royal Society of Edinburgh 45: 49–64.

Ahlstrom, E. H., K. Amaoka, D. A. Hensley, H. G. Moser, and B. Y. Sumida. 1984. Pleuronectiformes: Development. In *Ontogeny and Systematics of Fishes,* H. G. Moser, W. J. Richards, D. M. Cohen, M. P. Fahay, A. W. Kendall, Jr., and S. L. Richardson, eds. Lawrence, Kans.: American Society of Ichthyologists and Herpetologists, pp. 640–670.

Ahlstrom, E. H., W. J. Richards, and S. H. Weitzman. 1984. Families Gonostomatidae, Sternoptychidae, and associated stomiiform groups: Development and relationships. In *Ontogeny and Systematics of Fishes,* H. G. Moser, W. J. Richards, D. M. Cohen, M. P. Fahay, A. W. Kendall, Jr., and S. L. Richardson. Lawrence, Kans.: American Society of Ichthyologists and Herpetologists, pp. 184–198.

Alberch, P. 1980. Ontogenesis and morphological diversification. American Zoologist 20: 653–667.

———. 1982. The generative and regulatory roles of development in evolution. In *Environmental Adaptation and Evolution,* D. Mossakowski and G. Roth, eds. Stuttgart: Gustav Fischer, pp. 19–36.

———. 1985. Problems with the interpretation of developmental sequences. Systematic Zoology 34: 46–58.

———. 1987. Evolution of a developmental process: Irreversibility and redundancy in amphibian metamorphosis. In *Development as an Evolutionary Process,* R. A. Raff and E. C. Raff, eds. New York: Alan R. Liss, pp. 23–46.

———. 1989. Development and the evolution of amphibian metamorphosis. In *Trends in Vertebrate Morphology,* H. Splechtna and H. Helge, eds. New York: Gustav Fischer Verlag, pp. 163–173.

Alberch, P., and J. Alberch. 1981. Heterochronic mechanisms of morphological diversification and evolutionary change in the neotropical salamander, *Bolitoglossa occidentalis* (Amphibia: Plethodontidae). Journal of Morphology 167: 249–264.

Alberch, P., and E. A. Gale. 1986. Pathways of cytodifferentiation during the metamorphosis of the epibranchial cartilage in the salamander, *Eurycea bislineata.* Developmental Biology 117: 233–244.

Alberch, P., E. A. Gale, and P. R. Larsen. 1986. Plasma T_4 and T_3 levels in naturally metamorphosing *Eurycea bislineata* (Amphibia; Plethodontidae). General and Comparative Endocrinology 61: 153–163.

Alberch, P., G. A. Lewbart, and E. A. Gale. 1985. The fate of larval chondrocytes during the metamorphosis of the epibranchial in the salamander, *Eurycea bislineata.* Journal of Embryology and Experimental Morphology 88: 71–83.

Allen, B. M. 1916. The results of extirpation of the anterior lobe of the hypophysis and the thyroid of *Rana pipiens* larvae. Science 44: 755–757.

———. 1938. The endocrine control of amphibian metamorphosis. Biological Review 13: 1–19.

Alley, K. E. 1989. Myofiber turnover is used to retrofit jaw muscles during metamorphosis. American Journal of Anatomy 184: 1–12.

———. 1990. Retrofitting larval neuromuscular circuits in the metamorphosing frog. Journal of Neurobiology 21: 1092–1107.

Alley, K. E., and M. D. Barnes. 1983. Birth dates of trigeminal motoneurons and metamorphic reorganization of the jaw myoneural system in frogs. Journal of Comparative Neurology 218: 395–405.

Alley, K. E., and J. A. Cameron. 1983. Turnover of anuran jaw muscles during metamorphosis. Anatomical Record 205: 7A.

Alluchon-Gérard, M.-J. 1982. Influence de la thyroidectomie et du traitement par le propylthiouracile sur l'ultrastructure du cartilage de l'embryon et de la très jeune roussette (Scyllium canicula, Chondrichthyens). Archives d'anatomie microscopique et de morphologie expérimentale 71: 51–70.

Aoyama, F. 1930. Die Entwicklungsgeschichte des Kopfskelettes des Cryptobranchus japonicus. Zeitschrift für Anatomie und Entwickslungsgeschichte 93: 106–181.

Armstrong, L. A., G. M. Wright, and J. H. Youson. 1985. The development of cartilage during lamprey metamorphosis. Anatomical Record 211: 12A.

———. 1987. Transformation of mucocartilage to a definitive cartilage during metamorphosis in the sea lamprey, Petromyzon marinus. Journal of Morphology 194: 1–21.

Aumonier, F. J. 1941. Development of the dermal bones in the skull of Lepidosteus osseus. Quarterly Journal of Microscopical Science 83: 1–33.

Ballard, W. W., and R. G. Needham. 1964. Normal embryonic stages of Polyodon spathula (Walbaum). Journal of Morphology 114: 465–478.

Barber, S., and E. J. W. Barrington. 1972. Dynamics of uptake and binding of ^{35}S-sulphate by the cartilage of Rainbow trout (Salmo gairdneri) and the influence of thyroxine. Journal of Zoology, London 168: 107–117.

Barnes, M. D., and K. E. Alley. 1983. Maturation and recycling of trigeminal motoneurons in anuran larvae. Journal of Comparative Neurology 218: 406–414.

Barry, T. H. 1956. The ontogenesis of the sound-conducting apparatus of Bufo augusticeps Smith. Morphologisches Jahrbuch 97: 477–544.

Beebe, W. 1934. Deep-sea fishes of the Bermuda Oceanographic Expeditions. Family Idiacanthidae. Zoologica, New York 16 (4): 149–241.

Belyanina, T. N. 1977. Materials on development of chauliod fishes (Chauliodontidae, Pisces). Trudy Instituta Okeanologii Akademia Nauk SSSR 109: 113–132. In Russian with English summary.

Bertelsen, E. 1951. The ceratioid fishes: Ontogeny, taxonomy, distribution, and biology. Dana-Report 39: 1–276.

———. 1984. Ceratioidei: Development and relationships. In Ontogeny and Systematics of Fishes, H. G. Moser, W. J. Richards, D. M. Cohen, M. P. Fahay, A. W. Kendall, Jr., and S. L. Richardson, eds. Lawrence, Kans.: American Society of Ichthyologists and Herpetologists, pp. 325–334.

Bertelsen, E., T. W. Pietsch, and R. J. Lavenberg. 1981. Ceratioid anglerfishes of the family Gigantactinidae: Morphology, systematics, and distribution. Natural History Museum of Los Angeles County, Contributions in Science no. 332: i–vi, 1–74.

Bertin, L. 1957. Larves et métamorphoses. In Traité de zoologie, P.-P. Grassé, ed. Paris: Masson et Compagnie, pp. 1813–1833.

Bertmar, G. 1966. The development of skeleton, blood-vessels, and nerves in the dipnoan snout, with a discussion on the homology of the dipnoan posterior nostrils. Acta zoologica 47: 81–150.

Böhlke, E. B. 1989. *Fishes of the Western North Atlantic.* Sears Foundation for Marine Research, Memoir no. 1, pt. 9, vol. 1. New Haven: Sears Foundation for Marine Research.

Bonebrake, J. E., and R. A. Brandon. 1971. Ontogeny of cranial ossification in the small-mouthed salamander, *Ambystoma texanum* (Mathes). Journal of Morphology 133: 189–204.

Breckenridge, W. R., S. Nathanael, and L. Pereira. 1987. Some aspects of the biology and development of *Ichthyophis glutinosus* (Amphibia: Gymnophiona). Journal of Zoology, London 211: 437–449.

Budgett, J. S. 1901. On the breeding habits of some West-African fishes, with an account of the external features in development of *Protopterus annectens,* and a description of the larva of *Polypterus lapradei.* Transactions of the Zoological Society of London 16: 115–136.

Burch, W. M., and H. E. Lebowitz. 1982a. Triiodothyronine stimulates maturation of porcine growth-plate cartilage in vitro. Journal of Clinical Investigation 70: 496–504.

———. 1982b. Triiodothyronine stimulation of in vitro growth and maturation of embryonic chick cartilage. Endocrinology 111: 462–468.

Burch, W. M., and J. Van Wyk. 1987. Triiodothyronine stimulates cartilage growth and maturation by different mechanisms. American Journal of Physiology: Endocrinology and Metabolism 15: E176–E182.

Canalis, E. 1983. The hormonal and local regulation of bone formation. Endocrine Reviews 4: 62–77.

Carlson, B. M. 1973. The regeneration of skeletal muscle: A review. American Journal of Anatomy 137: 119–150.

Castle, P. H. J. 1984. Notacanthiformes and Anguilliformes: Development. In *Ontogeny and Systematics of Fishes,* H. G. Moser, W. J. Richards, D. M. Cohen, M. P. Fahay, A. W. Kendall, Jr., and S. L. Richardson, eds. Lawrence, Kans.: American Society of Ichthyologists and Herpetologists, pp. 62–93.

Chen, T. L., and D. Feldman. 1978. Distinction between alpha-fetoprotein and intracellular estrogen receptors: Evidence against the presence of estradiol receptors in rat bone. Endocrinology 102: 236–244.

Chou, H. I., and J. J. Kollros. 1974. Stage-modified responses to thyroid hormone in anurans. General and Comparative Endocrinology 22: 255–260.

Clemen, G. 1978. Beziehungen zwischen Gaumenknochen und ihren Zahnleisten bei *Salamandra salamandra* (L.) während der Metamorphose. Roux's Archives of Developmental Biology 185: 19–36.

———. 1979a. Die Bedeutung des Ramus palatinus für die Vomerspangenbildung bei *Salamandra salamandra* (L.). Roux's Archives of Development Biology 187: 219–230.

———. 1979b. Untersuchungen zur Bildung der Vomerspange bei *Salamandra salamandra* (L.). Roux's Archives of Developmental Biology 185: 305–321.

———. 1987. On the determination of the oral epithelium in *Salamandra salamandra* (L.) after hetero- and homotopic transplantation—an ultrastructural analysis. Zeitschrift für mikroskopische-anatomische Forschung 101: 137–178.

———. 1988a. Competence and reactions of early- and late-larval dental laminae in original and not-original dental systems of *Ambystoma mexicanum* Shaw. Archives of Biology 99: 307–324.

———. 1988b. Experimental analysis of the capacity of dental laminae in *Ambystoma mexicanum* Shaw. Archives of Biology 99: 111–132.

Cohen, J. 1985. Metamorphosis: Introduction, usages, and evolution. In *Metamorphosis*, M. Balls and M. Bownes, eds. Oxford: Clarendon Press, pp. 1–19.

Cohen, J., and B. D. Massey. 1983. Larvae and the origins of major phyla. Biological Journal of the Linnean Society 19: 321–328.

Cole, W. C., and J. H. Youson. 1981. The effect of pinealectomy, continuous light, and continuous darkness on metamorphosis of anadromous sea lampreys, *Petromyzon marinus* L. Journal of Experimental Zoology 218: 397–404.

Corsin, J. 1966. The development of the osteocranium of *Pleurodeles waltlii* Michahelles. Journal of Morphology 119: 209–216.

Davidson, F. A. 1935. The development of the secondary sexual characters in the pink salmon (*Oncorhynchus gorbuscha*). Journal of Morphology 57: 169–183.

de Beer, G. R. 1937. *The Development of the Vertebrate Skull*. Oxford: Oxford University Press.

de Jongh, H. J. 1968. Functional morphology of the jaw apparatus of larval and metamorphosing *Rana temporaria* L. Netherlands Journal of Zoology 18: 1–103.

de Villiers, C. G. S. 1929. The development of a species of *Arthroleptella* from Jonkershoek, Stellenbosch. South African Journal of Science 26: 481–510.

Dent, J. N. 1942. The embryonic development of *Plethodon cinereus* as correlated with the differentiation and functioning of the thyroid gland. Journal of Morphology 71: 577–601.

———. 1988. Hormonal interaction in amphibian metamorphosis. American Zoologist 28: 297–308.

Devillers, C. 1965. The role of morphogenesis in the origin of higher levels of organization. Systematic Zoology 14: 259–271.

Dickhoff, W. W., C. L. Brown, C. V. Sullivan, and H. A. Bern. 1990. Fish and amphibian models for developmental endocrinology. Journal of Experimental Zoology 4(suppl.): 90–97.

Duellman, W. E., and L. Trueb. 1986. *Biology of Amphibians*. New York: McGraw-Hill.

Eagleson, G. W., and B. A. McKeown. 1978. Changes in thyroid activity of *Ambystoma gracile* (Baird) during different larval, transforming, and postmetamorphic phases. Canadian Journal of Zoology 56: 1377–1381.

Eales, J. G. 1979. Thyroid functions in cyclostomes and fishes. In *Hormones and Evolution*, E. J. W. Barrington, ed. New York: Academic Press, pp. 341–436.

Eddy, J. M. P. 1969. Metamorphosis and the pineal complex in the brook lamprey, *Lampetra planeri*. Journal of Endocrinology 44: 451–452.

Edgeworth, F. H. 1923. On the larval hyobranchial skeleton and musculature of

Cryptobranchus, Menopoma, and *Ellipsoglossa.* Journal of Anatomy 57: 97–105.

Erdmann, K. 1933. Zur Entwicklung des knöchernen Skelets von *Triton* und *Rana* unter besonderer Berücksichtigung der Zeitfolge der Ossifikationen. Zeitschrift für Anatomie und Entwicklungsgeschichte 101: 566–651.

Etkin, W. 1935. The mechanisms of anuran metamorphosis. 1. Thyroxine concentration and the metamorphic pattern. Journal of Experimental Zoology 71: 317–340.

———. 1950. The acquisition of thyroxine-sensitivity by tadpole tissues. Anatomical Record 108: 541.

———. 1955. Metamorphosis. In *Analysis of Development,* B. H. Willier, P. A. Weiss, and V. Hamburger, eds. Philadelphia: Saunders, pp. 631–663.

———. 1963. The metamorphosis activating system of the frog. Science 139: 810–814.

———. 1964. Metamorphosis. In *Physiology of the Amphibia,* J. A. Moore, ed. New York: Academic Press, pp. 427–468.

———. 1968. Hormonal control of amphibian metamorphosis. In *Metamorphosis: A Problem in Developmental Biology,* W. Etkin and L. I. Gilbert, eds. New York: Appleton-Century-Crofts, pp. 313–348.

Evans, B. I., and R. D. Fernald. 1990. Metamorphosis and fish vision. Journal of Neurobiology 21: 1037–1052.

Evans, R. M. 1988. The steroid and thyroid hormone receptor superfamily. Science 240: 889–895.

Eyal-Giladi, H., and N. Zinberg. 1964. The development of the chondrocranium of *Pleurodeles waltlii.* Journal of Morphology 114: 527–548.

Fox, H. 1965. Early development of the head and pharynx of *Neoceratodus* with a consideration of its phylogeny. Journal of Zoology 146: 470–554.

———. 1983. *Amphibian Morphogenesis.* Clifton, N.J.: Humana Press.

Fukuhara, O., and T. Fushimi. 1986. Development and early life history of the ayu reared in the laboratory. Bulletin of the Japanese Society of Scientific Fisheries 52(1): 75–80.

Galton, V. A. 1983. Thyroid hormone action in amphibian metamorphosis. In *Molecular Basis of Thyroid Hormone Action,* J. H. Oppenheimer and H. H. Samuels, eds. New York: Academic Press, pp. 445–483.

———. 1984. Putative nuclear triiodothyronine receptors in tadpole erythrocytes: Regulation of receptor number by thyroid hormone. Endocrinology 114: 735–742.

———. 1986. Thyroxine and 3,5,3′-triiodothyronine bind to the same putative receptor in hepatic nuclei of *Rana catesbeiana* tadpoles. Endocrinology 118: 1114–1118.

———. 1988. The role of thyroid hormone in amphibian development. American Zoologist 28: 309–318.

———. 1990. Mechanisms underlying the acceleration of thyroid hormone-induced tadpole metamorphosis by corticosterone. Endocrinology 127: 2997–3002.

Galton, V. A., and A. Hiebert. 1987. Hepatic iodothyronine 5-deiodinase activity in *Rana catesbeiana* tadpoles at different stages of the life cycle. Endocrinology 121: 42–47.

———. 1988. The ontogeny of iodothyronine 5′-monodeiodinase activity in *Rana catesbeiana* tadpoles. Endocrinology 122: 640–645.

Galton, V. A., and K. Munck. 1981. Metabolism of thyroxine in *Rana catesbeiana* tadpoles during metamorphic climax. Endocrinology 109: 1127–1131.

Gaupp, E. 1893. Beiträge zur Morphologie des Schädels. I. Primordial-Cranium und Kieferbogen von *Rana fusca*. Morphologische Arbeiten 2(2): 275–481.

Geigy, R. 1941. Die Metamorphose als Folge gewebsspezifischer Determination. Revue suisse de zoologie 48: 483–494.

Gimlich, R., and J. Braun. 1985. Improved fluorescent compounds for tracing cell lineage. Developmental Biology 109: 509–514.

Gorbman, A., W. W. Dickhoff, J. L. Mighell, E. F. Prentice, and F. W. Waknitz. 1982. Morphological indices of developmental progress in the parr-smolt Coho salmon, *Oncorhynchus kisutch*. Aquaculture 28: 1–19.

Gordon, A. S., E. D. Goldsmith, and H. A. Charipper. 1943. Effect of thiourea on the development of the amphibian. Nature 152: 504–505.

Gray, K. M., and P. A. Janssens. 1990. Gonadal hormones inhibit the induction of metamorphosis by thyroid hormones in *Xenopus laevis* tadpoles in vivo, but not in vitro. General and Comparative Endocrinology 77: 202–211.

Gudernatsch, J. F. 1912. Feeding experiments on tadpoles. I. The influence of specific organs given as food on growth and differentiation: A contribution to the knowledge of organs with internal secretion. Archiv für Entwicklungsmechanik der Organismen 35: 457–483.

———. 1914. Feeding experiments on tadpoles. II. A further contribution to the knowledge of organs with internal secretion. American Journal of Anatomy 15: 431–480.

Hall, B. K. 1978. *Developmental and Cellular Skeletal Biology*. New York: Academic Press.

Hall, B. K. 1983a. Epigenetic control in development and evolution. In *Development and Evolution*, B. C. Goodwin, N. Holder, and C. C. Wylie, eds. Cambridge: Cambridge University Press, pp. 353–379.

———. 1983b. Tissue interactions and chondrogenesis. In *Cartilage*, vol. 2, *Development, Differentiation, and Growth*, B. K. Hall, ed. New York: Academic Press, pp. 187–222.

———. 1986. The role of movement and tissue interactions in the development and growth of bone and secondary cartilage in the clavicle of the embryonic chick. Journal of Embryology and Experimental Morphology 93: 133–152.

———. 1989. Morphogenesis of the skeleton: Epithelial or mesenchymal control? In *Trends in Vertebrate Morphology*, H. Splechtna and H. Helge, eds. New York: Gustav Fischer Verlag, pp. 198–201.

Halme, J., J. Uitto, K. I. Kivirikko, and L. Saxén. 1972. Effect of triiodothyronine on the metabolism of collagen in cultured embryonic bones. Endocrinology 90: 1476–1482.

Hanken, J., and B. K. Hall. 1988a. Skull development during anuran metamorphosis. I. Early development of the first three bones to form: The exoccipital, the parasphenoid, and the frontoparietal. Journal of Morphology 195: 247–256.

———. 1988b. Skull development during anuran metamorphosis. II. Role of thyroid hormone in osteogenesis. Anatomy and Embryology 178: 219–227.

Hanken, J., and C. H. Summers. 1988a. Developmental basis of evolutionary success: Cranial ontogeny in a direct-developing anuran. American Zoologist 28: 12A.

———. 1988b. Skull development during anuran metamorphosis. III. Role of thyroid hormone in chondrogenesis. Journal of Experimental Zoology 246: 156–170.

Hardisty, M. W. 1981. The skeleton. In *The Biology of Lampreys*, vol. 3, M. W. Hardisty and I. C. Potter, eds. London: Academic Press, pp. 333–376.

Hardisty, M. W., and B. I. Baker. 1982. Endocrinology of lampreys. In *The Biology of Lampreys*, vol. 4b, M. W. Hardisty and I. C. Potter, eds. London: Academic Press, pp. 1–135.

Hardisty, M. W., and I. C. Potter. 1971a. The behavior, ecology, and growth of larval lampreys. In *The Biology of Lampreys*, vol. 1, M. W. Hardisty and I. C. Potter, eds. London: Academic Press, pp. 85–125.

———. 1971b. The general biology of adult lampreys. In *The Biology of Lampreys*, vol. 1, M. W. Hardisty and I. C. Potter, eds. London: Academic Press, pp. 127–206.

Hardisty, M. W., and C. M. Rovainen. 1982. Morphological and functional aspects of the muscular system. In *The Biology of Lampreys*, vol. 4a, M. W. Hardisty and I. C. Potter, eds. London: Academic Press, pp. 137–231.

Hartwig, H. 1940. Metamorphose-Reaktionen auf lokalisierten Hormonreiz. Biologisches Zentralblatt 60: 473–478.

Helff, O. M. 1927. Influence of annular tympanic cartilage on development of tympanic membrane (*Rana pipiens*). Proceedings of the Society for Experimental Biology and Medicine 25: 158–159.

———. 1928. Studies on amphibian metamorphosis. III. The influence of the annular tympanic cartilage on the formation of the tympanic membrane. Physiological Zoology 1: 463–495.

———. 1931. Studies on amphibian metamorphosis. VII. The influence of the columella on the formation of the lamina propria of the tympanic membrane. Journal of Experimental Zoology 59: 179–196.

———. 1933. Studies on amphibian metamorphosis. X. Biological Bulletin 65: 304–316.

———. 1934. Studies on amphibian metamorphosis. XII. Potential influences of the quadrate and supra-scapula on tympanic membrane formation in the anuran. Journal of Experimental Zoology 68: 305–318.

———. 1937. Studies on amphibian metamorphosis. XV. Direct tympanic membrane formation from dermal plicae integument transplanted to the ear region. Journal of Experimental Biology 14: 1–15.

———. 1940. Studies on amphibian metamorphosis. XVII. Influence of non-living annular tympanic cartilage on tympanic membrane formation in the anuran. Journal of Experimental Biology 17: 45–60.

Hensley, D. A., and E. H. Ahlstrom. 1984. Pleuronectiformes: Relationships. In *Ontogeny and Systematics of Fishes*, H. G. Moser, W. J. Richards, D. M. Cohen, M. P. Fahay, A. W. Kendall, Jr., and S. L. Richardson, eds. Lawrence, Kans.: American Society of Ichthyologists and Herpetologists, pp. 670–687.

Hetherington, T. E. 1987. Timing of development of the middle ear of Anura (Amphibia). Zoomorphology 106: 289–300.

Heuberger, B., I. Fitzka, G. Wasner, and K. Kratochwil. 1982. Induction of androgen receptor formation by epithelium-mesenchyme interaction in embryonic mouse mammary gland. Proceedings of the National Academy of Sciences, U.S.A. 79: 2957–2961.

Homma, S. 1978. Organization of the trigeminal motor nucleus before and after metamorphosis in lampreys. Brain Research 140: 33–42.

Hoskins, S. G. 1990. Metamorphosis of the amphibian eye. Journal of Neurobiology 21: 970–989.

Howes, G. J., and C. P. J. Sanford. 1987. Oral ontogeny of the ayu, *Plecoglossus altivelis* and comparisons with the jaws of other salmoniform fishes. Zoological Journal of the Linnean Society of London 89: 133–169.

Hughes, A. M., and E. B. Astwood. 1944. Inhibition of metamorphosis in tadpoles by thiouracil. Endocrinology 34: 138–139.

Inui, Y., and S. Miwa. 1985. Thyroid hormone induces metamorphosis of flounder larvae. General and Comparative Endocrinology 60: 450–454.

Jarvik, E. 1942. On the structure of Crossopterygians and Lower Gnathostomes in general. Zoologiska Bidrag Från Uppsala 21: 235–675.

Johnels, A. G. 1948. On the development and morphology of the skeleton of the head of *Petromyzon*. Acta zoologica 29: 139–279.

Jollie, M. 1980. Development of head and pectoral fin girdle skeleton and scales in *Acipenser*. Copeia (2): 226–249.

Joss, J. M. P. 1985. Pituitary control of metamorphosis in the southern hemisphere lamprey, *Geotria australis*. General and Comparative Endocrinology 60: 58–62.

Just, J. J., J. Kraus-Just, and D. A. Check. 1981. Survey of chordate metamorphosis. In *Metamorphosis: A Problem in Developmental Biology*, L. I. Gilbert and E. Frieden, eds. New York: Plenum Press, pp. 265–326.

Kaltenbach, J. C. 1953a. Local action of thyroxin on amphibian metamorphosis. I. Local action in *Rana pipiens* larvae effected by thyroxin-cholesterol implants. Journal of Experimental Zoology 122: 21–39.

———. 1953b. Local action of thyroxin on amphibian metamorphosis. II. Development of the eyelids, nictitating membrane, cornea, and extrinsic ocular muscles in *Rana pipiens* larvae effected by thyroxin-cholesterol implants. Journal of Experimental Zoology 122: 41–51.

———. 1953c. Local action of thyroxin on amphibian metamorphosis. III. Formation and perforation of the skin window in *Rana pipiens* larvae effected by thyroxin-cholesterol implants. Journal of Experimental Zoology 122: 449–467.

———. 1958. Direct steroid enhancement of induced metamorphosis in peripheral tissues. Anatomical Record 131: 569–570.

————. 1968. Nature of hormone action in amphibian metamorphosis. In *Metamorphosis: A Problem in Developmental Biology,* W. Etkin and L. I. Gilbert, eds. New York: Appleton-Century-Crofts, pp. 399–441.

————. 1982. Circulating thyroid hormone levels in amphibia. In *Gunma Symposia on Endocrinology,* vol. 19, *Phylogenetic Aspects of Thyroid Hormone Action,* G. U. Institute of Endocrinology, ed. Tokyo: Center for Academic Publications, Japan, pp. 63–74.

Kaltenbach, J. C., and A. W. Hobbs. 1972. Local action of thyroxine on amphibian metamorphosis. V. Cell division in the eye of anuran larvae effected by thyroxine-cholesterol implants. Journal of Experimental Zoology 179: 157–166.

Kan, K. W., and R. L. Cruess. 1987. Gestational changes of thyroid hormone activity in the developing fetal bovine epiphysis. Calcified Tissue International 41: 332–336.

Kawaguchi, K., and H. G. Moser. 1984. Stomiatoidea: Development. In *Ontogeny and Systematics of Fishes,* H. G. Moser, W. J. Richards, D. M. Cohen, M. P. Fahay, A. W. Kendall, Jr., and S. L. Richardson, eds., Lawrence, Kans.: American Society of Ichthyologists and Herpetologists, pp. 169–181.

Kawahara, A., B. S. Baker, and J. R. Tata. 1991. Developmental and regional expression of thyroid hormone receptor genes during *Xenopus* metamorphosis. Development 112: 933–943.

Kawamura, K., K. Yamamoto, and S. Kikuyama. 1986. Effects of thyroid hormone, stalk section, and transplantation of the pituitary gland on plasma prolactin levels at metamorphic climax in *Rana catesbeiana.* General and Comparative Endocrinology 64: 129–135.

Keller, R. 1946. Morphogenetische Untersuchungen am Skelett von *Siredon mexicanus* Shaw mit besonderer Berücksichtigung des Ossifikationsmodus beim neotenen Axolotl. Revue suisse de zoologie 53: 329–426.

Kemp, A. 1987. The biology of the Australian lungfish, *Neoceratodus forsteri* (Krefft, 1870). In *The Biology and Evolution of Lungfishes,* W. E. Bemis, W. W. Burggren, and N. E. Kemp, eds. New York: Alan R. Liss, pp. 181–198.

Kemp, N. E., and J. A. Hoyt. 1965. Influence of thyroxine on ossification of the femur in *Rana pipiens.* Journal of Cell Biology 27: 51A.

————. 1969. Ossification of the femur in thyroxine treated tadpoles of *Rana pipiens.* Developmental Biology 20: 387–410.

Kerr, J. G. 1899. The external features in the development of *Lepidosiren paradoxa,* Frit. Philosophical Transactions of the Royal Society of London 192: 299–330.

Kerr, J. G. 1909. *Normal Plates of the Development of* Lepidosiren paradoxa *and* Protopterus annectens. Jena: Gustav Fischer.

Kikuyama, S., K. Niki, M. Mayumi, R. Shibayama, M. Nishikawa, and N. Shintake. 1983. Studies on corticoid action on the tadpole tail in vitro. General and Comparative Endocrinology 52: 395–399.

Kitajima, C., T. Sato, and M. Kawanishi. 1967. On the effect of thyroxine to promote the metamorphosis of a Conger Eel: Preliminary report. Bulletin of the Japanese Society of Scientific Fisheries 33: 919–922.

Klumpp, W., and B. Eggert. 1934. Die Schilddrüse und die branchiogenen Organe von *Ichthyophis glutinosus* L. Zeitschrift für wissenschaftliche Zoologie 146: 329–381.

Knutson, T. L., and K. V. Prahlad. 1971. 3,5,3′-triiodo-L-thyronine uptake and development of metamorphic competence by *Xenopus laevis* embryonic tissues. Journal of Experimental Zoology 178: 45–58.

Kollros, J. J. 1961. Mechanisms of amphibian metamorphosis: Hormones. American Zoologist 1: 107–114.

———. 1981. Transitions in the nervous system during amphibian metamorphosis. In *Metamorphosis: A Problem in Developmental Biology*, L. I. Gilbert and E. Frieden, eds. New York: Plenum Press, pp. 445–460.

Kyle, H. M. 1921. The asymmetry, metamorphosis, and origin of flat-fishes. Philosophical Transactions of the Royal Society of London 211B: 75–129.

Langille, R. M., and B. K. Hall. 1988. Role of the neural crest in development of the trabeculae and branchial arches in embryonic sea lamprey, *Petromyzon marinus* (L.). Development 102: 301–310.

Larras-Regard, E., A. Taurog, and M. Dorris. 1981. Plasma T$_4$ and T$_3$ levels in *Ambystoma tigrinum* at various stages of metamorphosis. General and Comparative Endocrinology 43: 443–450.

Larsen, J. H., Jr. 1963. The cranial osteology of neotenic and transformed salamanders and its bearing on interfamilial relationships. Ph.D. diss., University of Washington.

Larsen, L. O. 1974. Effects of testosterone and oestradiol on gonadectomized and intact male and female river lampreys (*Lampetra fluviatilis* [L.] Gray). General and Comparative Endocrinology 24: 305–313.

———. 1980. The physiology of adult lampreys, with special reference to natural starvation, reproduction, and death after spawning. Canadian Journal of Fisheries and Aquatic Sciences 37: 1762–1779.

Leibel, W. S. 1976. The influence of the otic capsule in ambystomatid skull formation. Journal of Experimental Zoology 196: 85–104.

Leiby, M. M. 1979a. Leptocephalus larvae of the eel family Ophichthidae. I. *Ophichthus gomesi* Castlenau. Bulletin of Marine Science 29 (3): 329–343.

———. 1979b. Morphological development of the eel *Myrophis punctatus* (Ophichthidae) from hatching to metamorphosis, with emphasis on the developing head skeleton. Bulletin of Marine Science 29 (4): 509–521.

Leloup, J., and M. Buscaglia. 1977. La triiodothyronine, hormone de la métamorphose des amphibiens. Comptes rendus des séances de l'Académie des sciences, ser. D 284: 2261–2263.

Liegro, I. D., G. Savettieri, and A. Cestelli. 1987. Cellular mechanism of action of thyroid hormones. Differentiation 35: 165–175.

Lintlop, S. P., and J. H. Youson. 1983. Concentration of triiodothyronine in the sera of the sea lamprey, *Petromyzon marinus*, and the brook lamprey, *Lampetra lamottenii*, at various phases of the life cycle. General and Comparative Endocrinology 49: 187–194.

Luo, M., R. Faure, J. Ruel, and J. H. Dussault. 1988. A monoclonal antibody to the rat nuclear T$_3$ receptor: Production and characterization. Endocrinology 123: 180–186.

Luther, A. 1925. Entwicklungsmechanische Untersuchungen am Labyrinth einiger Anuren. Societas scientarum fennica Commentationes biologicae 2(1): 1–48.

Lynn, W. G. 1942. The embryology of *Eleutherodactylus nubicola,* an anuran which has no tadpole stage. Carnegie Institute of Washington, Contributions to Embryology no. 190: 27–62.

———. 1947. Effects of thiourea and phenylthiourea upon the development of *Plethodon cinereus.* Biological Bulletin 92: 199.

———. 1948. The effects of thiourea and phenylthiourea upon the development of *Eleutherodactylus ricordii.* Biological Bulletin 94: 1–15.

Lynn, W. G., and A. M. Peadon. 1955. The role of the thyroid gland in direct development in the anuran, *Eleutherodactylus martinicensis.* Growth 19: 263–286.

Macchia, E., A. Nakai, A. Janiga, A. Sakurai, M. E. Fisfalen, P. Gardner, K. Soltani, and L. J. DeGroot. 1990. Characterization of site-specific polyclonal antibodies to *c-erbA* peptides recognizing human thyroid hormone receptors α_1, α_2, and β and native 3,5,3'-triiodothyronine receptor, and study of tissue distribution of the antigen. Endocrinology 126: 3232–3239.

Maderson, P. F. A. 1975. Embryonic tissue interactions as the basis for morphological changes in evolution. American Zoologist 15: 315–327.

Marconi, M., and A. M. Simonetta. 1988. The morphology of the skull in neotenic and normal *Triturus vulgaris meridonalis* (Boulenger) (Amphibia Caudata Salamandridae). Monitore zoologico italiano, n.s., 22: 365–396.

Marks, S. C., and S. N. Popoff. 1988. Bone cell biology: The regulation of development, structure, and function in the skeleton. American Journal of Anatomy 183: 1–44.

Märtens, M. 1898. Die Entwickelung des Knorpelgerüstes im Kehlkopf unserer eimheimischen anuren Amphibien. Verhandlungen der anatomischen Gesellschaft 12: 238–240.

Matsuda, R. 1987. *Animal Evolution in Changing Environments with Special Reference to Abnormal Metamorphosis.* New York: John Wiley and Sons.

Mauro, A. 1961. Satellite cells of skeletal muscle fibers. Journal of Biophysical and Biochemical Cytology 9: 493–495.

Mayhoff, H. 1914. Zur Ontogenese des Kopfes der Plattfische. Zoologischer Anzeiger 43(9): 389–404.

Medvedeva, I. M. 1959. The naso-lacrimal duct and its connection with the lacrimal and septomaxillary bones in *Ranodon sibiricus.* Doklady: Biological Sciences Section (English translation of Doklady Akademii Nauk SSSR) 128: 789–792.

———. 1960. Connection between the developing nasolacrimal duct and the covering lacrimale and septomaxillare bones in *Hynobius kaiserlingii.* Doklady: Biological Sciences Section (English translation of Doklady Akademii Nauk SSSR) 131: 221–223.

———. 1986. On the origin of nasolacrimal duct in Tetrapoda. In *Studies in Herpetology,* Third General Meeting of the Societas Europaea Herpetologica, Z. Rocek, ed. Prague: Charles University, pp. 37–40.

Miwa, S., and Y. Inui. 1987. Effects of various doses of thyroxine and triiodothyronine on the metamorphosis of flounder (*Paralichthys olivaceus*). General and Comparative Endocrinology 67: 356–363.

Miwa, S., M. Tagawa, Y. Inui, and T. Hirano. 1988. Thyroxine surge in metamorphosing flounder larvae. General and Comparative Endocrinology 70: 158–163.

Miyauchi, H., F. T. LaRochelle, Jr., M. Suzuki, M. Freeman, and E. Frieden. 1977. Studies on thyroid hormones and their binding in bullfrog tadpole plasma during metamorphosis. General and Comparative Endocrinology 33: 254–266.

Mondou, P. M., and J. C. Kaltenbach. 1979. Thyroxine concentrations in blood serum and pericardial fluid of metamorphosing tadpoles and of adult frogs. General and Comparative Endocrinology 39: 343–349.

Mosekilde, L., E. F. Eriksen, and P. Charles. 1990. Effects of thyroid hormones on bone and mineral metabolism. Endocrinology and Metabolism Clinics of North America, Metabolic Bone Disease, pt. 2, 19 (1): 35–63.

Moser, H. G., and E. H. Ahlstrom. 1970. Development of lanternfishes (family Myctophidae) in the California Current. Part 1. Species with narrow-eyed larvae. Bulletin of the Los Angeles County Museum of Natural History, Science no. 7: 1–145.

Moser, H. G., E. H. Ahlstrom, and J. R. Paxton. 1984. Myctophidae: Development. In *Ontogeny and Systematics of Fishes,* H. G Moser, W. J. Richards, D. M. Cohen, M. P. Fahay, A. W. Kendall, Jr., and S. L. Richardson, eds. Lawrence, Kans.: American Society of Ichthyologists and Herpetologists, pp. 218–239.

Moser, H. G., W. J. Richards, D. M. Cohen, M. P. Fahay, A. W. Kendall, Jr., and S. L. Richardson, eds. 1984. *Ontogeny and Systematics of Fishes.* Lawrence, Kans.: American Society of Ichthyologists and Herpetologists.

Mundy, G. R., J. L. Shapiro, J. G. Bandelin, E. M. Canalis, and L. G. Raisz. 1976. Direct stimulation of bone resorption by thyroid hormones. Journal of Clinical Investigation 58: 529–534.

Nielsen, J. G., and E. Bertelsen. 1985. The gulper-eel family Saccopharyngidae (Pisces, Anguilliformes). Steenstrupia 11 (6): 157–206.

Nielsen, J. G., and D. G. Smith. 1978. The eel family Nemichthyidae (Pisces, Anguilliformes). Dana-Report 88: 1–71.

Niki, K., H. Namiki, S. Kikuyama, and K. Yoshizato. 1982. Epidermal tissue requirement for tadpole tail regression induced by thyroid hormone. Developmental Biology 94: 116–120.

Niki, K., K. Yoshizato, H. Namiki, and S. Kikuyama. 1984. In vitro regression of tadpole tail by thyroid hormone. Development, Growth, and Differentiation 26: 329–338.

Noble, G. K. 1929. Further observations on the life-history of the newt, *Triturus viridescens.* American Museum Novitates 348: 1–22.

Noble, G. K., and S. H. Davis. 1928. The effect on the dentition and cloaca of testicular transplants in the adult female salamander, *Desmognathus;* the effect of castration on the male. Anatomical Record 38: 24.

Noden, D. M. 1982. Patterns and organization of craniofacial skeletogenic and myogenic mesenchyme: A perspective. In *Factors and Mechanisms Influencing Bone Growth,* Progress in Clinical and Biological Research, vol. 101, A. D. Dixon and B. G. Sarnat, eds. New York: Alan R. Liss, pp. 167–203.

―――. 1987. Interactions between cephalic neural crest and mesodermal populations. In *Developmental and Evolutionary Aspects of the Neural Crest,* P. F. A. Maderson, ed. New York: John Wiley and Sons, pp. 89–119.

Norman, J. R. 1926. The development of the chondrocranium of the eel (*Anguilla vulgaris*), with observations on the comparative morphology and development of the chondrocranium in bony fishes. Philosophical Transactions of the Royal Society of London 214B: 369–464.

―――. 1934. *A Systematic Monograph of the Flatfishes (Heterosomata),* vol. 1, *Psettodidae, Bothidae, Pleuronectidae.* London: British Museum (Natural History).

Norman, M. F., J. A. Carr, and D. O. Norris. 1987. Adenohypophysial-thyroid activity of the tiger salamander, *Ambystoma tigrinum,* as a function of metamorphosis and captivity. Journal of Experimental Zoology 242: 55–66.

Norris, D. O. 1983. Evolution of endocrine regulation of metamorphosis in lower vertebrates. American Zoologist 23: 709–718.

Nutik, G., and R. L. Cruess. 1974. Estrogen receptors in bone: An evaluation of the uptake of estrogen into bone cells. Proceedings of the Society for Experimental Biology and Medicine 146: 265–268.

Parr, A. E. 1930. On the osteology and classification of the pediculate fishes of the genera *Aceratias, Rhynchoceratias, Haplophryne, Laevoceratias, Allector,* and *Lipactis.* Occasional Papers of the Bingham Oceanographic Collections 3: 1–23.

Pickford, G. E., and J. W. Atz. 1957. *The Physiology of the Pituitary Gland of Fishes.* New York: New York Zoological Society.

Puckett, W. O. 1937. X-radiation and thyroid-induced metamorphosis in anuran larvae. Journal of Experimental Zoology 76: 303–323.

Purves, D. 1988. *Body and Brain: A Trophic Theory of Neural Connections.* Cambridge, Mass.: Harvard University Press.

Puymirat, J., M. Luo, and J. H. Dussault. 1989. Immunocytochemical localization of thyroid hormone nuclear receptors in cultured hypothalamic dopaminergic neurons. Neuroscience 30: 443–449.

Ramaswami, L. S. 1947. Apodous Amphibia of the eastern Ghats, South India. Current Science 16: 8–10.

Reddi, A. H. 1982. Local and systemic mechanisms regulating bone formation and remodelling: An overview. In *Current Advances in Skeletogenesis: Development, Biomineralization, Mediators, and Metabolic Bone Disease,* M. Silbermann and H. C. Slavkin, eds. Amsterdam: Excerpta Medica, pp. 77–86.

Regan, C. T., and E. Trewavas. 1932. Deep-sea angler-fishes (Ceratioidea). Dana-Report 2: 1–113.

Regard, E., A. Taurog, and T. Nakashima. 1978. Plasma thyroxine and triiodothyronine levels in spontaneously metamorphosing *Rana catesbeiana* tadpoles and in adult anuran amphibia. Endocrinology 102: 674–684.

Reilly, S. M. 1986. Ontogeny of cranial ossification in the eastern newt, *Notoph-*

thalmus viridescens (Caudata: Salamandridae, and its relationship to metamorphosis and neoteny. Journal of Morphology 188: 315–326.

————. 1987. Ontogeny of the hyobranchial apparatus in the salamanders *Ambystoma talpoideum* (Ambystomatidae) and *Notophthalmus viridescens* (Salamandridae): The ecological morphology of two neotenic strategies. Journal of Morphology 191: 205–214.

Riedl, R. 1978. *Order in Living Organisms: A Systems Analysis of Evolution*. New York: Wiley.

Rocek, Z. 1981. Cranial anatomy of frogs of the family Pelobatidae Stannius, 1856, with outlines of their phylogeny and systematics. Acta Universitatis Carolinae biologica 1980: 1–164.

Rosenkilde, P. 1979. The thyroid hormones in amphibia. In *Hormones and Evolution*, E. J. W. Barrington, ed. New York: Academic Press, pp. 437–491.

Roth, G., and D. B. Wake. 1985. Trends in the functional morphology and sensorimotor control of feeding behavior in salamanders: An example of the role of internal dynamics in evolution. Acta biotheoretica 34: 175–192.

Rovainen, C. M. 1982. Neurophysiology. In *The Biology of Lampreys*, vol. 4a, M. W. Hardisty and I. C. Potter, eds. London: Academic Press, pp. 1–136.

Ryder, J. A. 1890. The sturgeons and sturgeon industries of the eastern coast of the United States, with an account of experiments bearing upon sturgeon culture. Bulletin of the U.S. Fisheries Commission 8: 231–328.

Sadaghiani, B., and C. H. Thiébaud. 1987. Neural crest development in the *Xenopus laevis* embryo, studied by interspecific transplantation and scanning electron microscopy. Developmental Biology 124: 91–110.

Sasaki, S., H. Nakamura, T. Tagami, Y. Osamura, and H. Imura. 1991. Demonstration of nuclear 3,5,3'-triiodothyronine receptor proteins in gonadotrophs and corticotrophs in rat anterior pituitary by double immunohistochemical staining. Endocrinology 129: 511–516.

Sassoon, D., and D. B. Kelley. 1986. The sexually dimorphic larynx of *Xenopus laevis:* Development and androgen regulation. American Journal of Anatomy 177: 457–472.

Sassoon, D., N. Segil, and D. Kelley. 1986. Androgen-induced myogenesis and chondrogenesis in the larynx of *Xenopus laevis*. Developmental Biology 113: 135–140.

Saunders, R. L., and C. B. Schom. 1985. Importance of the variation in the life history parameters of Atlantic salmon (*Salmo salar*). Canadian Journal of Fisheries and Aquatic Sciences 42: 615–618.

Schubert, M. 1926. Untersuchungen über die Weschselbeziehungen zwischen wachsenden und reduktiven Geweben. Erste Mitteilung. Zeitschrift für mikroskopisch-anatomische Forschung 6: 162–189.

Schultheiss, H. 1980. T_3 and T_4 concentrations during metamorphosis of *Xenopus laevis* and *Rana esculenta* and in the neotenic Mexican axolotl. General and Comparative Endocrinology 40: 372.

Schwartz, Z., W. A. Soskolne, T. Neubauer, M. Goldstein, S. Adi, and A. Ornoy. 1991. Direct and sex-specific enhancement of bone formation and calcification of sex steroids in fetal mice long bone in vitro (biochemical and morphometric study). Endocrinology 129: 1167–1174.

Schwind, J. L. 1933. Tissue specificity at the time of metamorphosis in frog larvae. Journal of Experimental Zoology 66: 1–14.

Sedra, S. N., and M. I. Michael. 1957. The development of the skull, visceral arches, larynx, and visceral muscles of the South African clawed toad, *Xenopus laevis* (Daudin) during the process of metamorphosis (from stage 55 to stage 66). Verhandelingen der Koninklijke Nederlandse Akademie van Wetenschappen, Afdeling Natuurkunde, Tweede Reeks 51 (4): 1–80.

Shelton, P. M. J. 1970. The lateral line system at metamorphosis in *Xenopus laevis* (Daudin). Journal of Embryology and Experimental Morphology 24: 511–524.

Silbermann, M. 1983. Hormones and cartilage. In *Cartilage,* vol. 2, *Development Differentiation, and Growth,* B. K. Hall, ed. New York: Academic Press, pp. 327–368.

Smith, L. 1920. The hyobranchial apparatus of *Spelerpes bislineata.* Journal of Morphology 33: 527–583.

Sokol, O. M. 1962. The tadpole of *Hymenochirus boettgeri.* Copeia (2): 272–284.

———. 1969. Feeding in the pipid frog *Hymenochirus boettgeri* (Tornier). Herpetologica 25: 9–24.

Summers, C. H., and J. Hanken. 1988. Site-dependent response by anuran cranial cartilages to thyroid hormone in vitro. American Zoologist 28: 12A.

Suzuki, S. 1986. Induction of metamorphosis and thyroid function in the larval lamprey. In *Frontiers in Thyroidology,* G. Medeiros-Neto and E. Gaitan, eds. New York: Plenum Press, pp. 667–670.

———. 1987a. Induction of metamorphosis and thyroid function in the larval lamprey. In *Proceedings of the First Congress of the Asia and Oceania Society for Comparative Endocrinology* (AOSCE), E. Ohnishi, Y. Nagahama, and H. Ishizaki, eds. Nagoya: Nagoya University Corp., pp. 220–221.

———. 1987b. Plasma thyroid hormone levels in metamorphosing larvae and adults of a salamander, *Hynobius nigrescens.* Zoological Science 4: 849–854.

Suzuki, S., and M. Suzuki. 1981. Changes in thyroidal and plasma iodine compounds during and after metamorphosis of the bullfrog, *Rana catesbeiana.* General and Comparative Endocrinology 45: 74–81.

Swanepoel, J. H. 1970. The ontogenesis of the chondrocranium and of the nasal sac of the microhylid frog *Breviceps adspersus pentheri* Werner. Annals of the University of Stellenbosch 45A (1): 1–119.

Szarski, H. 1957. The origin of the larva and metamorphosis in Amphibia. American Naturalist 91: 283–301.

Takisawa, A., Y. Shimura, and K. Kaneko. 1976. Metamorphic changes in anuran muscles following thyroxine treatment. Okajimas folia anatomica japonica 53: 253–278.

Tata, J. R. 1968. Early metamorphic competence of *Xenopus* larvae. Developmental Biology 18: 415–440.

———. 1970. Simultaneous acquisition of metamorphic response and hormone binding in *Xenopus* larvae. Nature 227: 686–689.

Tata, J. R., A. Kawahara, and B. S. Baker. 1991. Prolactin inhibits both thyroid hormone-induced morphogenesis and cell death in cultured amphibian larval tissues. Developmental Biology 146: 72–80.

Tchernavin, V. 1937. Preliminary account of the breeding changes in the skulls of *Salmo* and *Oncorhynchus*. Proceedings of the Linnean Society of London 14: 11–19.

———. 1938a. The absorption of bones in the skull of salmon during their migration to rivers. Fisheries Board for Scotland: Salmon Fisheries 6: 2–4.

———. 1938b. Changes in the salmon skull. Transactions of the Zoological Society of London 24: 103–184.

Thiébaud, C. H. 1983. A reliable new cell marker in *Xenopus*. Developmental Biology 98: 245–249.

Thomson, D. A. R. 1986. Meckel's cartilage in *Xenopus laevis* during metamorphosis: A light and electron microscope study. Journal of Anatomy 149: 77–87.

———. 1987. A quantitative analysis of cellular and matrix changes in Meckel's cartilage in *Xenopus laevis*. Journal of Anatomy 151: 249–254.

———. 1989. A preliminary investigation into the effect of thyroid hormones on the metamorphic changes in Meckel's cartilage in *Xenopus laevis*. Journal of Anatomy 162: 149–155.

Thorogood, P. 1983. Morphogenesis of cartilage. In *Cartilage*, vol. 2, *Development, Differentiation, and Growth*, B. K. Hall, ed. New York: Academic Press, pp. 223–254.

Trueb, L. 1985. A summary of osteocranial development in anurans with notes on the sequence of cranial ossification in *Rhinophrynus dorsalis* (Anura: Pipoidea: Rhinophrynidae). South African Journal of Science 81 (4): 181–185.

Trueb, L., and P. Alberch. 1985. Miniaturization and the anuran skull: A case study of heterochrony. Fortschritte der Zoologie 30: 113–121.

van Eeden, J. A. 1951. The development of the chondrocranium of *Ascaphus truei* Stejneger with special reference to the relations of the palatoquadrate to the neurocranium. Acta zoologica 32: 41–136.

Vilter, V. 1946. Action de la thyroxine sur la métamorphose larvaire de l'anguille. Comptes rendus des séances de la Société biologie et de ses filiales 140: 783–785.

Visser, M. H. C. 1963. The cranial morphology of *Ichthyophis glutinosus* (Linné) and *Ichthyophis monochrous* (Bleeker). Annals of the University of Stellenbosch 38: 67–102.

Vladykov, V. D., and E. Kott. 1979. Satellite species among the holoarctic lampreys (Petromyzonidae). Canadian Journal of Zoology 57: 860–867.

Wahnschaffe, U., B. Bartsch, and B. Fritzsch. 1987. Metamorphic changes within the lateral-line system of Anura. Anatomy and Embryology 175: 431–442.

Wake, D. B. 1966. Comparative osteology and evolution of the lungless salamanders, family Plethodontidae. Memoirs of the Southern California Academy of Sciences 4: 1–111.

Wake, D. B., and A. Larson. 1987. Multidimensional analysis of an evolving lineage. Science 238: 42–48.

Wake, M. H. 1989. Metamorphosis of the hyobranchial apparatus in *Epicrionops* (Amphibia: Gymnophiona: Rhinatrematidae): Replacement of bone by cartilage. Annales des sciences naturelles, zoologie 13, ser. 10: 171–182.

Wake, M. H., and J. Hanken. 1982. Development of the skull of *Dermophis mexicanus* (Amphibia: Gymnophiona), with comments on skull kinesis and amphibian relationships. Journal of Morphology 173: 203–223.

Wake T. A., D. B. Wake, and M. H. Wake. 1983. The ossification sequence of *Aneides lugubris*, with comments on heterochrony. Journal of Herpetology 17: 10–22.

Weil, M. R. 1986. Changes in plasma thyroxine levels during and after spontaneous metamorphosis in a natural population of the green frog, *Rana clamitans*. General and Comparative Endocrinology 62: 8–12.

Weinberger, C., C. C. Thompson, E. S. Ong, R. Lebo, D. J. Gruol, and R. M. Evans. 1986. The *c-erb-A* gene encodes a thyroid hormone receptor. Nature 324: 641–646.

Weiss, P., and F. Rosetti. 1951. Growth responses of opposite sign among different neuron types exposed to thyroid hormones. Proceedings of the National Academy of Sciences 37: 540–556.

Werner, E. E., and J. F. Gilliam. 1984. The ontogenetic niche and species interactions in size-structured populations. Annual Review of Ecology and Systematics 15: 393–425.

White, B. A., G. S. Lebovic, and C. S. Nicoll. 1981. Prolactin inhibits the induction of its own renal receptors in *Rana catesbeiana* tadpoles. General and Comparative Endocrinology 43: 30–38.

White, B. A., and C. S. Nicoll. 1981. Hormonal control of amphibian metamorphosis. In *Metamorphosis: A Problem in Developmental Biology*, L. I. Gilbert and E. Frieden, eds. New York: Plenum Press, pp. 363–396.

Wilder, I. W. 1925. *The Morphology of Amphibian Metamorphosis*. Northampton, Mass.: Smith College Fiftieth Anniversary Publication.

Williams, S. R. 1901. Changes accompanying the migration of the eye and observations on the tractus opticus and tectum opticum in *Pseudopleuronectes americanus*. Bulletin of the Museum of Comparative Zoology 40: 1–57.

Williamson, D. A., E. P. Parrish, and G. M. Edelman. 1991a. Distribution and expression of two interactive extracellular matrix proteins, cytotactin and cytotactin-binding proteoglycan, during development of *Xenopus laevis*. I. Embryonic development. Journal of Morphology 209: 189–202.

———. 1991b. Distribution and expression of two interactive extracellular matrix proteins, cytotactin and cytotactin-binding proteoglycan, during development of *Xenopus laevis*. II. Metamorphosis. Journal of Morphology 209: 203–213.

Wintrebert, P. 1922. La voute palatine des Salamandridae. Bulletin biologique de la France et de la Belgique 56: 275–426.

Wright, G. M. 1989. Ultrastructure of the adenohypophysis in the anadromous sea lamprey, *Petromyzon marinus*, during metamorphosis. Journal of Morphology 202: 205–223.

Wright, G. M., and J. H. Youson. 1977. Serum thyroxine concentrations in larval and metamorphosing anadromous sea lamprey, *Petromyzon marinus* L. Journal of Experimental Zoology 202: 27–32.

———. 1982. Ultrastructure of mucocartilage in the larval anadromous sea lamprey, *Petromyzon marinus* L. American Journal of Anatomy 165: 39–51.

Yaoita, Y., and D. D. Brown. 1990. A correlation of thyroid hormone receptor gene expression with amphibian metamorphosis. Genes and Development 4: 1917–1924.

Yaoita, Y., Y.-B. Shi, and D. D. Brown. 1990. *Xenopus laevis* α and β thyroid hormone receptors. Developmental Biology 87: 7090–7094.

Youson, J. H. 1980. Morphology and physiology of lamprey metamorphosis. Canadian Journal of Fisheries and Aquatic Sciences 37: 1687–1710.

———. 1988. First metamorphosis. In *Fish Physiology,* W. S. Hoar and D. J. Randall, eds. San Diego: Academic Press, pp. 135–196.

9

Preconception of Adult Structural Pattern in the Analysis of the Developing Skull

ROBERT PRESLEY

INTRODUCTION

THE STRUCTURAL PATTERN of adults dominates the classical analytical methods used in morphology and phylogenetics. Traditional descriptive accounts of ontogeny adopt concepts and terminology appropriate to adults as early as possible in development. This method treats the embryo as if its functional components were constrained only by an imperative to arrive at an adult anatomy. In reality, many detailed features of embryonic anatomy have a vital but transient role. The judgment as to when the change from ontogenetic to adult terminology should take place must, of course, be subjective at least until we have a very full knowledge of the biological role of each feature in question. But care must be taken not to prejudice our insights into how embryos adapt by misapplying adult terms that prejudge the homology involved by conveying an aura of precision based on an adult anatomy not appropriate to the embryonic stage.

Experimental science now gives a great deal of insight into the processes and kinetics of development at the cell and genetic level. Such insight was only just beginning when de Beer (1937) wrote his great synthesis on skull development. Much of our new insight needs to be integrated more fully into the classical analyses of developmental morphology. Changing developmental patterns are very complicated when compared with adult anatomy. Probably more cells degenerate in development, having performed a vital function restricted to early morphogenesis, than directly form into the components of adult anatomy. Each individual must be viable at each instant in developmental life, requiring a full functional biology within the organ systems at that instant. This functional biology is not always that of the adult. My theme in this chapter is that a tendency to describe developing structures using quasi-adult terms has on occasion led workers to overlook important differences. It is likely that the classical literature contains many more such errors, and my purpose is to alert all who use it to look very carefully at the reasoning explicitly or implicitly used by past authors.

The components at any anatomical locus at instants in development do not necessarily have the significance of their adult equivalents, and it is important that they should not be homologized fortuitously with entities of adult anatomy. In amniotes, such precursor units are more likely to be miniatures of adult anatomy (but with major metabolic specializations because of scaling effects) than in forms with free-living larvae, whose anatomy must be adapted to immediate function. It is therefore ironic that the development of amniotes, especially that of *Homo,* has had the strongest influence on our terminological approach to embryology. In classical analysis blastemata have often been explained by their prospective fate, with less than proper emphasis on transient vital function. The effect has been to describe embryonic anatomy as if it were largely a fate map of a somewhat generalized adult vertebrate, a homunculus such as would have been familiar to the preformationist school of embryology (Needham 1934). It is my view that a principal weakness of developmental craniology is the persistent influence of such a homunculus, trapping the homology of developmental components within an archetypic framework founded on adult structure and function. My best guess as to the anatomy of the homunculus which still haunts us is a miniature skeleton of neonatal *Homo,* slightly contaminated with lizard bones! The homology of soft tissues is often mutilated to give flesh to this specter!

The simplest (and abundantly criticized) distortion produced by seeing illusory images of the adult has been naive recapitulation theory. We now reject recapitulation but live on with more subtle distortions, by relying on terminological definitions which retain some reference to position within the homunculus rather than to position within the embryo. For the sake of clear explanation, the special terminology used to describe embryos has often been effectively rendered equivalent to easily recognized adult terms. Such practices have given rise to a number of errors or misunderstandings which have had a permanent influence on morphological literature. The elimination of this kind of error is a useful line along which experimental and morphological science could blend.

EXEMPLARY CASES

I shall present examples of each of what I see as four major kinds of error that have arisen from relying on the false accuracy of anatomical terms relating an embryo too directly to a miniature of adult pattern. The four kinds of error are: (1) confusing of synonymy with homology in topographic analysis; (2) neglecting soft-tissue precursor detail in the analysis of skeletal components; (3) assuming serial homology in linear arrays of structures having a similar appearance at an instant in development; (4) neglecting the developmental process of neomorphic extensions.

I do not present these errors with any intended disrespect to the workers involved: it is only my opinion that they are wrong. The point is that each case represents the scholarly application of the methodology and assumptions prevailing in its time: the "preconception" in my title. In every cited case, much further work arose from the hypotheses advanced. My intention is not to provide a universal method for correction, but to show that such classes of problem exist. The examples are chosen from cranial topics which were discussed by Goodrich (1930) or by de Beer (1937) in syntheses which are still justly regarded as encyclopedic and are used as a definitive source in many more modern papers. Each example seems to me to demonstrate the influence of my supposed homunculus in analysis at that time and to leave some problems still unresolved. I suggest possible lines along which better insights could be developed.

CONFUSION OF SYNONYMY WITH HOMOLOGY IN TOPOGRAPHIC ANALYSIS

The Reference Frame for Homology in Young Embryos

It is vital for accurate comparative anatomy to ensure that false homologies are not consolidated in the literature because the same term was employed by different authors with different meanings. This becomes much more difficult to avoid when developmental stages are compared. In precartilage and cartilaginous embryos the homology of soft-tissue structures such as vessels, nerves, and muscle anlagen has always been by reference to prospective fate and to position with respect to the adult skeleton when this has emerged. Unless the detailed reasoning of each embryologist is thoroughly checked, it becomes very easy unwittingly to carry to one organism an implied suite of features associated with another usage in another organism. In my view, it would have been much safer if we had adopted conventions based on several developmental reference frames for our anatomical definitions, instead of two, namely the chondrocranium at its "optimal stage" (de Beer 1937) and the adult osteocranium. I suggest also using the cranial nerves and their sensory ganglia as a descriptive reference for stages with mesenchymatous anlagen, and possibly also the primary head vein for stages where procartilage centers are visible.

I illustrate this in a detailed treatment of the example of the so-called lateral head vein. That of adult squamates and its homonym in amniote embryos are homologous only in a restricted part of their courses, a part included in the primary head vein. Use of "lateral head vein" for subtly different and nonhomologous parts has led to some anatomical confusion. There are very many craniological papers which refer to "the lateral head vein (vena capitis lateralis)," but seldom is it defined. This matter needs attention, and could well exemplify similar problems for many other soft-tissue structures. More generally, it has given rise to the morphological concept of "intramural" (de Beer 1937), which while pragmatically effective in dealing with the homological problem under study, by its nature reduces the resolving power of pattern analysis. The term is almost the literal equivalent of "sitting on the fence."

Developmental Dynamics and the Nomenclature of Major Head Veins

The structure of the vascular system is very labile both during development and in adults. We take this for granted in wound-healing, surgery, and many physiological experimental systems, but descriptive morphologists often discuss blood vessels as if they were rigidly conserved structures, constant in development and reliable as landmarks across widespread taxonomic groups. Although the practice is almost universal, it is rare to find precise definitions of the terms used in description of the vascular system. Instead, the tradition has been to cite some previous author, often without reference to the homological doubts the latter may himself have expressed.

The common cardinal veins (Ducts of Cuvier) are the first to collect blood from the systemic circulation (as distinct from the embryonic membranes) and return it to the heart. They are probably homologous by function, position, and phylogeny throughout the embryos of vertebrates. The principal tributaries, the anterior and posterior cardinal veins, are also obvious in early development. During later development the cardinal veins are often replaced divergently, in whole or in part. The "lateral head vein" of adult squamate reptiles is an example of this replacement process, as will be shown later.

The basis of the nomenclature of adult and embryonic veins in this region can be appreciated from the general review of Hofmann (1901), that of O'Donoghue (1920) on *Sphenodon*, used as a reference for much subsequent work on squamates, and the developmental synthesis of Goodrich (1930, esp. fig. 245A, B). Early developmental anatomy seems to be similar in a wide range of vertebrates. I shall describe the structures involved in some detail, because I believe that there is still much confusion about which parts of the anatomy are consistent and which are very labile.

In this region, probably in all vertebrates, a longitudinal plexus of veins forms in the meninx primitiva, close to the neural tube and medial to the nerve roots (fig. 9.1a). It is of capillary or sinusoidal structure, and expands caudally. It joins, and provides most of the blood in, the anterior cardinal vein. If veins mature in this initial position they lie in the lepto-

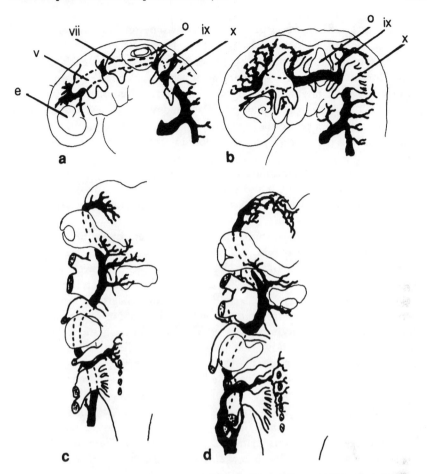

Fig. 9.1. Dynamic pattern of developing cephalic veins. Schematic diagrams of brain, cranial nerves, and head veins in early human development. a. Ca. 2.5 mm CRL shows the course of the primordial head channel. b. Ca. 6 mm CRL shows the primary head vein. c. Ca. 7 mm shows a ventral view of the primary head vein. d. Ca. 10 mm shows this, but with "drift" to outside the vagus ganglion. Abbreviations: e, optic vesicle; o, otocyst; V, VII, IX, X, the ganglia of those cranial nerves.

meninges of an adult: internal to the dura and to the cranial and vertebral skeleton and close to or upon the brain surface. Recognizing that the plexus was therefore not strictly homologous with any major vein in adult vertebrates, Streeter (1918) proposed, initially for human embryology, to replace the century-old term for it, "vena capitis medialis," by "primordial hindbrain channel." Skeletal anlagen soon condense within the mesenchyme and the primordial veins are eclipsed by larger vessels. These develop substantially thicker walls and were thus termed the primary head veins (Streeter 1918). Descriptively this is much better English, but it is not strictly acceptable in international scientific nomenclature.

Lying more lateral than the primordial channel, in the early embryological literature Streeter's "primary head vein" was called the lateral head vein (vena capitis lateralis; e.g., Hofmann 1901). This older use was anatomically confusing, since some parts lay medial and others lateral to the emerging cranial nerve roots (fig. 9.1b). Because of the continuing confusion in modern literature, I provide below an account of the primary head vein applicable to the anatomy of vertebrate embryos at a procartilaginous stage. I find it a useful landmark in comparing the anatomy of procartilage embryos. More generally, it shows the problems created by the dynamics of development which can apply to homologizing veins anywhere else in the head or body.

It is important to appreciate that in development major vessels do not simply appear and disappear, as, on first reading, classical descriptions suggest. Rather, in a tiny embryo, channels of the largest, lowest-resistance vessels (which would be classified as capillaries in adult histology) are accorded the name "artery" or "vein." As the embryo grows, organs may increase tenfold to a hundredfold in a matter of days. New pathways form among substantially larger vessels which, by offering a more favorable route for efficient blood flow, take over from the earlier channels. In some cases it is the early channels themselves which enlarge, and whose walls mature, but in other cases the bypassed flow in the early channels becomes relatively and then absolutely diminished as new vessels take over. The major veins of the head show these effects well (Padget 1957). The crucial problem, often totally ignored, is how to use a nomenclature accurately to describe every stage of this dynamic process, with a minimum of terms. The primary head vein is but one example of this difficulty affecting precise homological analysis.

The Primary Head Vein of Streeter and Venous "Drift" in Development

Anterior tributaries from the orbit, nose, and anterior part of the forebrain typically combine to form a trunk on each side of the pituitary and anastomose in front of and beneath it. They are medial to the maxillary and mandibular nerves, with the ophthalmic nerve following them dorsally.

At the level of the pro-otic incisure (usually also the level of the maxillo-mandibular ganglion) they move laterally to pass outside the otic capsule and lateral to the trunk of the facial nerve. This transitional part of the vein, the post-trigeminal part (Padget 1957) is often a single vein passing between mandibular and facial nerves, but during early phases of its development it can be a plexus around the maxillary, mandibular, and facial nerves, and variations in adult form can thus be explained.

The lateral part, that which probably attracted the use of "vena capitis lateralis" for this vein, lies under the crista parotica. It is dorso-lateral to the facial nerve and usually (not always) passes dorsal to the stapes or its homologue. In my view, the reason for the attention given to this part of the vein is that it regresses during the development of marsupial and placental mammals (Hofman 1901). Since most other amniotes retain it in the adult, from the early days of comparative anatomy this "vena capitis lateralis" appeared to have great morphological significance.

The most caudal part of the vein (continuing as the anterior cardinal vein in the neck) during human development (Padget 1957) nicely illustrates the dynamics of development and the associated problems of nomenclature and homology. Initially the vein runs lateral to the glossopharyngeal nerve, passes in front of, then medial to, the vagus, the hypoglossal, and the spinal nerves. This is the classical relationship of the anterior cardinal vein (fig. 9.1c): medial to the nerves (therefore classically "medial head vein"). But from about 5 mm crown-rump length (CRL) small vessels anastomose and enlarge lateral to the vagus nerve, until by 10 mm CRL (fig. 9.1d) they become greater than the medial vein, and by 14 mm CRL the medial vein has become insignificant (and presumably stagnates and reduces to capillary size or degenerates). The effect is to produce a lateral head vein emerging (in *Homo*) from the skull lateral to the vagus, being the major tributary of the adult internal jugular vein.

This process can vary, and often does further caudally, as is shown in *Homo* by the accessory nerve. Without obvious heritability, about two-thirds of adults are found with the vein medial to it, one third with the vein lateral, and a small percentage with the nerve transfixing the vein (Parsons and Keith 1897). Thus the detailed anatomy is epigenetically determined, perhaps by the effects on vessel size of the volume delivered by tributaries and local tissue pressures at some determining instant. Such factors may readily vary with alterations in size and shape and posture during growth.

It follows that even within *Homo* the terms "lateral head vein" and "medial head vein" need to be read and used with very great care in different accounts. At a commonsense level no one has doubted the homology of the structures involved, but the outcome has been the use of apparently contrasting terms for the same vein (see Padget 1957 for a full discussion). Unfortunately, discrepant use of the terminology is widespread. By seeming to propose an accurate distinction between a lateral and a medial vein this usage has set a trap in the literature into which has fallen, as one example, the snake laterosphenoid. There can be no doubt (Goodrich 1930; de Beer 1937) that Streeter's image of the human veins was firmly imprinted on the subsequent English-language synthesizers of comparative developmental analysis. But the term "lateral head vein" was widely used, and seems to have carried with it an image of its relations to the bony elements of a lizardlike homunculus which could not possibly emerge from the actual developmental anatomy.

The Veins and the Laterosphenoid Bone of Snakes

The following passage concerning the laterosphenoid, from de Beer (1926, 315) but with emphasis added, illustrates the way the vessels were used in general comparisons at that time. "It is not a processus ascendens, for it does not arise from and has no relations with the palatoquadrate. . . . It is not a pila prootica, because it lies behind the profundus; it is not a pila lateralis as in *Amia, for it is situated median to the vena capitis lateralis.* Consequently its homologue is not to be found in the pterosphenoid of Teleostomes, the epipterygoid of reptiles, the true laterosphenoid of crocodiles, nor the alisphenoid of mammals. . . . I regard it as part of the original cranial wall."

The reasoning homologizes the vena capitis lateralis in snakes with that in a fish (*Amia*), and extends it to other tetrapods. If skeletal elements are differently placed with respect to this vein in two forms, then they are not homologues.

The problem of the snake laterosphenoid is made difficult partly because in snakes the bony cranial wall is exceptionally thick and partly because the cartilage framework (including pila antotica, and processus ascendens) found in the orbitotemporal region of other squamates is not shown clearly at any stage of development. Workers have therefore looked for small elements to homologize with relics of this framework.

The problem of such skeletal components, of which the laterosphenoid is an example, is now usually discussed in terms of the developmental anatomy of the region, accepting de Beer's view (1926, 1937) that the trigeminal ganglion, lying medial to the laterosphenoid, is intramural, i.e., in a recess in a thickened but truly neurocranial skull wall, and not in the cavum epiptericum as in other vertebrates. In lizards, a classical morphotype for amniote head structure, the trigeminal ganglia do lie in the cavum epiptericum, outside the plane of the fibrous and cartilaginous neurocranium but inside the plane occupied by the epipterygoid and its associated fascia. The laterosphenoid problem is more generally important because the concept of intramural was introduced by de Beer in direct response to his rejection of the laterosphenoid as a homologue of the lateral wall of the cavum. As shown above, de Beer's rejection of the pila lateralis comparison for snakes was based on the position of the lateral head vein. His authority is cited or implicitly accepted by many subsequent workers (Brock 1929, 1941; Pringle 1954; Kamal and Hammouda 1965; Rieppel 1976) in setting out the position from which their discussions of the problem start. The analysis depends vitally on the correct homology of

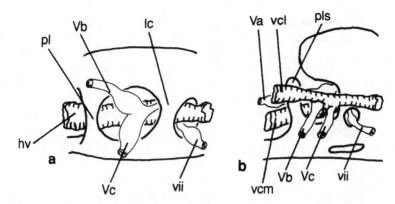

Fig. 9.2. Pila lateralis, laterosphenoid, and the primary head vein. *Amia* (a) and *Natrix* (b) after de Beer (1926) but much simplified. Contrary to his statement, the pila lateralis (pl) and the laterosphenoid (pls) are not differently placed with respect to his "hv" and "vcm." His "vcl" is not represented in his figure of *Amia* as judged by the relations of ophthalmic (Va), maxillary or ophthalmicus superficialis (Vb), mandibular (Vc), and facial (VII) nerves. His "vcm" and "hv" seem similar and have the properties of the primary head vein as set out here. The lateral commissure (lc) in *Amia* is not relevant to the present discussion.

the snake lateral head vein, in effect requiring it to be exactly homologous with the vein in *Amia*.

Oddly, his own figures (de Beer 1926, figs. 38, 85) cast doubt on this. He shows a head vein (labeled hv) with clear relations to the basicranium, otic capsule, trigeminal and facial ganglia, and lateral commissure. In a 10 mm long (*sic*, presumably head length) *Tropidonotus* (= *Natrix*) embryo he illustrates a vena capitis lateralis (vcl) lateral to the trigeminal ganglion and laterosphenoid (pls: his "pleurosphenoid"). But he does not show this in *Amia* (fig. 9.2a), and he also labels, in *Natrix*, a vena capitis medialis (vcm) passing medial to the trigeminal ganglion between maxillary and mandibular nerves and then medial to the laterosphenoid. This vessel (fig. 9.2b) has a very similar course to what he calls the head vein (hv) in *Amia*. Clearly the true homologues must be his vcm of *Natrix* and his hv of *Amia*: they have similar relations to trigeminal, pituitary, and otic capsule. My interpretation is that de Beer tripped in the snare of the dual usage of "vena capitis lateralis," and inadvertently homologized what is a special feature of snakes with the primary head vein of vertebrates because the latter had been and still frequently is called the lateral head vein. So named, it carried with it a suite of general anatomical relationships to the bones of the homunculus which quite overrode the detail which indicated that the vein, and not necessarily the bone, was discrepant.

In my specimens of *Natrix* the primary head vein is replaced (before chondrogenesis) in its post-trigeminal section by an anastomosis running from the orbital sinus to the lateral segment of the primary head vein (sensu Streeter). The anastomosis lies in a plane among the deeper layers of the mandibular adductors and must therefore be superficial to any cavum epiptericum. Descriptively and logically, this can be called the lateral head vein in snakes, although it clearly is not comparable with the lateral head vein in *Homo*. It must not be confused with the normal forward continuation of the primary head vein in other vertebrates running medially into the post-trigeminal section. In his argument about the laterosphenoid, this is exactly what de Beer (1926) seems to have done. Because of the nonhomology of the veins, his argument as to the morphology of the laterosphenoid must be invalid: positionally it could well be a pila lateralis, using his own logic. The argument of Brock (1929) that it is a relic of the epipterygoid may not be ruled out simply on these grounds, as was done by de Beer (1937) and accepted by Brock (1941).

Broader Implications of This Example

The message implicit in the above example seems simple: we should look carefully at the developmental anatomies of all the forms included in our comparisons, and must never assume that all prior authors adopted identical usage. We should look at the nerves to homologize the veins, and at both the nerves and the veins to homologize the skeletal blastemata.

Nevertheless, there may be deeper residual difficulties. It seems likely from my own and other (e.g., Rieppel 1976, 1988, 1990) observations that the laterosphenoid problem in snakes is an example of the still very severe difficulty of defining a general framework of reference structures capable of establishing homology for neomorphic features in the developing vertebrate head. Rieppel's work on muscles suggests that the problems associated with bony elements, as exemplified here, may be trivial when compared with those of soft tissues. This case study shows clearly that the concept of loci within the skeletal framework, i.e., positions actually or potentially occupied by skeletal elements, although implicit in the traditions of comparative analysis, cannot be used to test homologies independently of soft-tissue relationships which are themselves even more dynamic and capable of reversal during development.

No easy solution can be suggested. Careful illustration of each stage, not simply textual listing of terms, must become mandatory. We are obliged to keep terminology simple and comprehensible and it is here that the homunculus is most likely to haunt us. It seems appropriate to use descriptive criteria for choosing the name of a structure and in most cases this means positionally descriptive. This was the standard reasoning of topographical anatomy. Therefore a name such as "lateral head vein" must refer to a vein at a locus in the head defined by a suite of topographical features. But for embryologists and pheneticists particularly the problems of dynamics and variance arise. The reference framework within which the locus is defined must itself be regarded as capable of movements which will be manifest as alternates. Traditional morphology favors the skeletal elements as a reliable rigid framework, and the soft tissues as labile. My purpose in this chapter is to question this as a universal assumption.

NEGLECT OF SOFT-TISSUE PRECURSOR DETAIL IN THE ANALYSIS OF SKELETAL COMPONENTS

Complexity of Developmental Events Affecting Pattern Analysis

Phylogenetic reasoning using development ought to give the early pattern of soft tissue at least equal weight to that given to the comparison of skeletal features which emerge later. But the classical practice has been, much more, to make direct deductions from features of the bony units of adults, frequently moving directly between such very different forms as lizards and placental mammals. Paradoxically (or the homunculus again?) certain other obvious factors for comparison were traditionally neglected. For example, in the coming case study one should remember the relatively large size of the orbit and small size of the trigeminal ganglion in the lizard embryo when comparing with the mammal—this sort of allometric difference is almost universally neglected in the literature synthesized by de Beer (1937) or Goodrich (1930).

In mammals, as in all other vertebrates, the skeletal anlagen chondrify, ossify, and mature only after the nerve pattern is established. To recommend the use of the pattern of such embryonic soft tissues is easy. Less clear is how to present the analysis formally. A balance must be held in our understanding between pattern and process. It is a fundamental assumption of phylogenetic methodology that the number of occasions when a foramen or sheet of bone in the cranium appears in evolution is minimal—the principle af parsimony. A great many of the character states used for living forms, and most of those in fossils, are handled by analytic procedures which assume that such features can be precisely diagnosed and homologized. Such a feature is either present or absent, giving a true-or-false, Boolian character statement applicable as an absolute truth in comparison of taxa. A more sophisticated corollary is the convention, which creates special difficulty for palaeontologists, of supposing that parallelism has been demonstrated if different developmental paths are shown leading to the same end.

From a practical point of view, this is the best we can do. But in this section I show two examples, drawn from mammalian osteology, each recognized as problematic by de Beer (1937), which remain problematic and are illustrative of a potential host of other craniological characters whose solidity may be only an illusion. Additionally, the help provided by developmental studies need not be simple. From this, I draw the conclusion that many osteological character states often used with binary logic may be more like probability distributions than clear dichotomies. If this is true, the theoretical structure of parsimonious cladistic analysis as applied to osteological features, using the mathematics of binary decisions, may be unsound because the data are insufficient to indicate the most probable set of relationships.

The Mammalian Alisphenoid and Foramen Rotundum

The case of the alisphenoid shows an osteological "unit" treated as a homologous entity in the braincase and used to diagnose a particular group of mammals, setting them apart from other mammals. Within it, the second case, the foramen rotundum, is an apparently clear-cut osteological feature classically recorded as present or absent in the description and phylogenetic analysis of mammals. In both cases, development shows that the true analysis, and the inferences drawn, are much more complex and uncertain. I suggest that in both cases the homunculus, here more like a little man and less like a lizard, has haunted the analysis. *Homo* possesses both an alisphenoid (strictly the greater wing or ala temporalis of the sphenoid in human anatomy) with a foramen rotundum in it. So, ran the canon, his ancestors can be easily recognized by these features, and they may be "higher" forms than those without. Their anlagen can be easily seen within human embryos, and—in a slightly different place with respect to soft tissues—in lizards. So let us not overburden ourselves by worrying about that slightly different place. But I caution that we must be prepared to account for every detail of anatomy, however tedious, or we may be lost.

The Epipterygoid-Alisphenoid Homology. When I was taught comparative anatomy, the proof that the mammalian alisphenoid (apparently an element unique to the braincase of so-called higher mammals but not present in monotremes) was homologous with the epipterygoid of other tetrapods (Broom 1914; Watson 1916; Goodrich 1930; Starck 1967) ranked second only to the establishment of the Reichert theory of the auditory ossicles (Gaupp 1913) as the paradigm of classical comparative anatomy. Features of mammalian structure which had seemed unique—the alisphenoid (a bone sheet lying directly between cranial cavity and temporal fossa with no extracranial cavum epiptericum; a wholly intracranial trigeminal ganglion) and the suspensorium (three auditory ossicles; a jaw joint between two membrane bones)—had been given a full explanation using stages both from development and from the fossil record to display a continuous

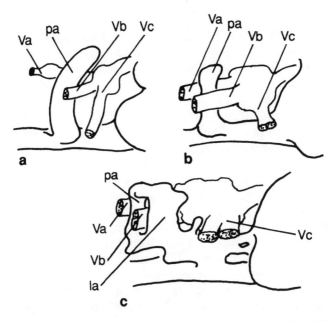

Fig. 9.3. Positional detail in the region of the foramen rotundum. Schematic drawings from reconstructions of chondrocrania of (a) *Sphenodon*, stage R, (b) *Didelphis marsupialis* 14 mm CRL, (c) *Potamogale velox* 29 mm CRL. The nerve relations of processus ascendens (pa) and lamina ascendens (la) should be compared. Va, Ophthalmic nerve; Vb, maxillary nerve; Vc, mandibular nerve, with anterior and posterior rami.

transform in each case. This is the ideal requirement for applying anatomy to test evolutionary theory.

It is important to recognize that the above homologies cannot be unambiguously established using detailed adult topographical anatomy alone. For the alisphenoid this was the cause both of early disputes (Fuchs 1915; Kesteven 1918; Gregory and Noble 1924) and certain problems which persist (Barry 1965; Crompton and Jenkins 1979; Novacek 1980; Zeller 1989). An obvious soft-tissue discrepancy was the course of maxillary and mandibular nerves (fig. 9.3). These pass laterally from the cavum epiptericum behind the processus ascendens of the typical amniote epipterygoid. But adult mammals show a bar of bone which is termed the "lamina ascendens" between maxillary and mandibular nerves (Goodrich 1930; de Beer 1937). In marsupials and placentals this is in the alisphenoid, but may partly or wholly be petrosal in monotremes (Kuhn 1971; Griffiths 1978; Presley 1981; Kuhn and Zeller 1987) and in multituberculates (Clemens and Kielan-Jaworowska 1979; Miao 1988). There is now general agreement (Starck 1967) that the true neurocranium is represented in the connective tissue of the dura mater, vestigeal cartilages, or ossified pila antotica medial to the trigeminal ganglion. But continuing disagreement exists (Maier 1987) over the phylogenetic implications of the lamina ascendens.

Mammalian Development: Special Features of the ala temporalis. When Gaupp (1902) set out his component analysis of the developmental morphology of this region in vertebrate skulls, no mammal embryo was then known which did not have an (initially) cartilaginous lamina ascendens developing between the two nerves. He took this to be true for all mammals. In lizards the processus ascendens of the reptilian epipterygoid lay anterior to both maxillary and mandibular nerves. Gaupp thus reasoned that the lamina ascendens, and therefore the mammalian ala temporalis of which it was a component, could not be homologues of the epipterygoid, and were therefore probably specialized developments of the basal process. The cartilage processes of the mammalian ala temporalis were upgrowths of the floor of the cavum epiptericum, whose primitive side wall had been reduced to a fibrous tissue sheet termed the "membrana sphenoobturatoria."

Subsequently Fuchs (1915) found a different pattern in young *Didelphis* where a well-developed process of cartilage ran between ophthalmic and maxillary nerves, but no cartilage lay between maxillary and mandibular nerves. The similarity to a processus ascendens of the epipterygoid seemed obvious to Fuchs. He argued that this was the mammalian ala temporalis in its primitive form, homologous with the epipterygoid. For Fuchs, the evolution of the cartilaginous lamina ascendens in higher mammals could be understood as a modified expression of the bony lamina ascendens found in the opossum.

It is important to understand that there is a bony lamina ascendens in the alisphenoid of adult *Didelphis*. Fuchs's point was therefore not obvious to most osteologists, who seemed to prefer to project the concept of the adult lamina back into the embryo: the effect of the homunculus again. Unfortunately Gaupp and Fuchs had bitter and polemic disagreements which affected their successors. It should have been clear at that time that a simple statement of homology or nonhomology with the epipterygoid could not be wholly correct. Two distinct anatomical problems apply here to mammals and warn of the need for the qualification of any homology statement: first, the shape of both cartilage and bone is much more variable than that of the typical reptilian epipterygoid; and second, there is a wide separation of the exit points of the maxillary and mandibular nerves which is not seen in typical squamates.

Histogenesis and Skeletal Anatomy. Well before chondrification in mammals the maxillary and mandibular nerves diverge almost at right angles (fig. 9.3b, c), the maxillary running forward below and parallel with the ophthalmic, while the mandibular runs infero-laterally from the trigeminal ganglion to reach the anlagen of jaw adductors and lower jaw. This divergence is less marked in other vertebrates (except in amphisbaenids; Bellairs and Kamal 1981). Later, in *Didelphis,* incremental bone, *zuwachsknochen,* ossifies between those nerves, within the membrana spheno-obturatoria, to form the lamina ascendens, vide Presley (1981). The cartilaginous processus ascendens of Fuchs (1915) appears prior to this. Two separable histogenetic components are assimilated into the alisphenoid: only one, or neither, can possibly be simply homologous with the epipterygoid.

My preference (Presley 1981) has been to regard the processus ascendens as the homologue of the epipterygoid and to suppose that this element is extremely reduced in monotremes (Kuhn and Zeller 1987; Zeller 1989). The field of *zuwachsknochen* may be treated (simplistically) as a distinct element, incorporated into the alisphenoid in marsupial and placental mammals, but into the petrosal in monotremes and fossil nontherian mammals (Kermack and Kielan-Jaworowska 1971; Griffiths 1978; Presley 1981). Additional anatomical features, such as the lamina ascendens of Gaupp (1902), Goodrich (1930), and de Beer (1937), may best be treated as apomorphic features in phylogenetic analysis. But the nonmammalogist should appreciate that the monotremes show more sign of a lamina ascendens (i.e., the apomorphy) than the processus ascendens (i.e., the plesiomorphy), so that the phylogeny cannot be simple. This awkward but obvious truth, I suspect, lay behind much of the classical discussion; there was probably a universal reluctance to regard the monotremes as advanced. In this case, the unwritten preference was that the monotreme homunculus should be more like the lizard than the man!

In an extensive and detailed study of the problem, Maier (1987) has shown that no simple statement can be made about whether a cartilaginous processus ascendens (and by implication for phylogenetics a bony one) exists in any group of mammals. Even within small groups such as the dasyurids or didelphids there is complete variation between presence of "processus ascendens" and presence only of a "lamina ascendens." Maier strongly advocates that the formal distinction between the two terms should be abandoned, since the distinction reinforces the idea of a phylogenetic dichotomy which has no simple validity. He presents developmental differences especially in terms of function and process, and seeks to deflect attention from simple but false homologies. While having great force, his recommendation leaves two problems: how to educate subsequent readers to cope with past literature; and how to write sentences in prose which convey the detailed difference in anatomy, especially with respect to adjacent soft tissues. My preference is to retain the use of both "processus ascendens" and "lamina ascendens" in order to convey the nervous anatomy, but at the same time to recognize that not all homonyms are phylogenetic homologues. The last statement is nicely shown by a feature of the alisphenoid, the foramen rotundum.

The Foramen Rotundum. The foramen rotundum exemplifies the diagnostic use of an apparently clear-cut bony feature within the alisphenoid. It is easy to recognize in fossil as well as in Recent mammals, if present. If the medial (rostral) margin is absent, the character state can be objectively scored as "foramen rotundum confluent with spheno-orbital fissure." These are the only two character states, according to the classical view.

Multituberculates, monotremes, some marsupials, and some of the earliest placentals show confluence (Kermack and Kielan-Jaworowska 1971; Kielan-Jaworowska 1984). Thus it seems easiest to hypothesize, using accepted phylogenetic reasoning, that this is the primitive mammalian condition and that possession of the foramen rotundum is an advanced feature. However, careful within-group comparisons cause difficulty (Novacek 1980). For example, in the case of primates the character is unstable. Some lemurs show the foramen, while others show confluence. Tarsiers and all simians show the foramen. The tree shrews present a similar problem: *Ptilocercus* has confluence, while the other living forms have a discrete foramen rotundum. It would seem reasonable to seek a developmental insight into how such a traditional landmark could oscillate. In practice, this insight proved misleading, and the example provides a warning to all scholars comparing skeletal development.

Pioneering the approach, Spatz (1966), treating the problem of the relationship of tree shrews to primates, suggested that development upheld a phylogenetic distinction between the primate and tupaiid forms. In his youngest specimen of *Tupaia* the foramen showed its caudal margin in cartilage; the rostral margin was in fibrous tissue only. In comparable embryos of higher primates the foramen was always fully enclosed by cartilage. An older *Tupaia* showed that the bony rostral margin was formed by ossification directly in membrane. It was argued that this developmental difference indicated that the tupaiid bony foramen must have evolved convergently. This was reinforcing evidence for the trend, not at that time fully established, away from affiliating tree shrews with primates: a separation now well supported by many other characters. Embryology thus seemed to add greater resolving power in confirming a suspected dissimilarity between two apparently similar but nonhomologous character states seen in adult bone.

But recently Zeller (1985, 1987) has shown that in a full developmental series of *Tupaia* there is a stage at which the foramen rotundum is completely surrounded by cartilage. The rostral margin then reduces to fibrous tissue in which ossification later completes the bony foramen rotundum in membrane, complementing the endochondral ossification in its caudal margin. One very important aspect of Zeller's work is that it highlights the greatest methodological problem in comparative embryology: the scarcity of complete, close-coupled developmental series to uphold deductions and categorizations. In this example he has shown Spatz's simple and apparently elegant developmental discriminant to be unusable: *Tupaia* in fact commences with a primatelike character state (complete cartilaginous foramen), but this state then oscillates. Zeller's observation shows a general problem which could well become even more difficult to handle if equally thorough developmental studies undertaken in other mammals show repeated within-species reversal for other character states.

General Implications. It is possible that, using more information, we could nevertheless recognize a difference in pattern. For example, is the fact that the margin in *Tupaia* is entirely *zuwachsknochen* (incremental bone) a phylogenetically significant difference from the primate pattern, or can regression to membrane be found also among the primates? After the work of Zeller, no answer of this sort could be sufficiently certain until the development of all primates has been studied with the same degree of thoroughness. This is a very improbable achievement for living primates, and of course it is impossible for fossils. The logical impact is bleak: this example shows that an apparently clear-cut feature of osteology can arise through different developmental processes, many of which can never be known, and which could oscillate within the individual's life history. Therefore apparently identical osteological conditions could include indistinguishable parallelisms and reversals. Such a conclusion in principle applies to most osteological features used in taxonomy. Can any solution other than a vast body of tedious observation be prescribed? Let us use the above example as a test case.

The Mammalian Morphotype. The complexity and uncertainty which emerge from the above considerations are capable of resolution by the following statements:

1. In all mammals there is a functional foramen rotundum. This is the primitive mammalian state, but it implies only the existence of some sort of connective tissue between ophthalmic and maxillary nerves, which need not be bone. It is the locus of the typical reptilian processus ascendens.

2. In cases where it is absent in bone it is present in dense fibrous connective tissue or cartilage. In those cases it is sufficient functionally

(apart from the histology) to represent homology with, and to understand the fate of, the morphotypic epipterygoid.

3. "Cases" in (2) may mean either species (after development is complete), or transient developmental stages thereof, or sporadic occurrences at any stage.

4. The range found for (3), or its potential observability, is a measure of the strength or the weakness of this character state in phylogenetic reasoning.

I believe that the above statements distill the essence of a solution for the analytic problem, but notice that the effect is to invalidate any assumption that allows parsimony to be applied in cladistic analysis—the character can oscillate, has done so, and must be expected to.

Statement (3) can account for any erratic form, for example the thin rostro-medial bony margin of a "foramen rotundum" present in a skull of *Tachyglossus* in my possession. On the argument above this foramen is the equivalent of the foramen rotundum in *Homo*. The vast majority of human skulls possess the foramen, formed in endochondral bone in the ala temporalis and then incorporated into the alisphenoid. By contrast only a small proportion of *Tachyglossus* have it, probably formed by late extension of *zuwachsknochen* into the spheno-obturator membrane. Under the classical rules it is not acceptable to speak of homology. But in reality the ala temporalis of mammals, as shown by Zeller's studies, is a labile chondrified zone continuous with the spheno-obturator membrane. It fully surrounds the maxillary nerve in the case of the classical foramen rotundum, but even within species it need not always do so. It does not do so in the many cases of confluence, of which the normal *Tachyglossus* form is one example. But a phylogeny asserting simply that *Tachyglossus,* and by implication its near precursors, must always lack a foramen rotundum is rendered a guess, not a fact.

Thus an apparently clear diagnostic bony feature reduces to slight, sometimes variable, adjustments of boundaries between different tissue types in a connective-tissue continuum. Seen in this way, morphological discriminants become more dynamic and less reliable than has been assumed by many phylogeneticists. This renders uncertain the principal method of phylogenetic analysis: the deduction of character-state polarities using out-groups and parsimony. By examining the detail of the process of development and its dynamics, an element of uncertainty has been introduced into each character-state attribution. When a character state of this sort is used to compare two forms it must represent a probability value, not a certainty, of being a true synapomorphy. It is the solidity and seeming permanence of bone which has given rise to its apparent reliability, but this is more a reflection of the needs of the human mind than of the processes of development and evolution.

Phylogenetic hypotheses have much to offer if set within the context of development: first let us deduce at which stage in phylogeny ancestral mammalian embryos got their small eyes, divergent maxillary and mandibular nerves, and large trigeminal ganglia—or whether it is possible that there were several similar steps within different phylogenies. This reasoning will be easier to achieve if it becomes the practice to treat osteological details rather more as indicators of a suite of developmental features than as clear-cut diagnostic items to be checked off a list of equivalences. But this requires us to support phylogenetic hypotheses by means of developmental scenarios, and reject unweighted cladistic methods. The reader may judge how likely this is to be accepted in the near future.

ASSUMING SERIAL HOMOLOGY IN LINEAR ARRAYS OF STRUCTURES

General Significance of Linear Arrays in Development

At present there is great interest in linear arrays in development. This is aroused both by the use of molecular probes demonstrating segmentation in development, for example linear patterns of the *Hox* gene family (Hunt et al. 1991), and by the great resolving power available to modern microscopists, for example the somitomeres (Jacobson and Meier 1984). But history shows that we should not assume that each member of a series of apparently similar structures at one stage in development is necessarily equivalent to its neighbors in the series. At the start of comparative anatomy, skull segments were formally treated in mammals, often as quasi-serial units. Almost a century later a tendency persisted to treat the landmark terms of these "segments" with an almost mesmerized rigidity of thought, as if they were indeed a linear series reflecting a process of iterative homology (Ghiselin 1976). Consequently, apparent loss or gain of such a unit within the skull was treated as a major change, and a major phylogenetic event: especial suspicion was accorded to hypothesized loss or gain of nonterminal units within the series. In principle, the reasoning is acceptable. In practice, one should always look carefully at such a series to ensure that each unit does in fact involve the same developmental pattern as the others: if not, the series is not iterative, and intrusive events must clearly be suspected.

I suggest that this reasoning applies to any linear array of whatever tissue at whatever stage of development the array is manifest. However, testing is not easy, and appearances can be deceptive. Two examples taken from mammalian craniology (remember that the mammalian skull is the prime source of our broadly applied terminology: another place in which the homunculus lurks!) show that even in a midline series of skull bones, difficulties can arise through looking at too restricted a range in development.

The Basicranial Series

Classical craniology recognized four skull segments: mesethmoid, presphenoid, basisphenoid, and basioccipital. These terms were established by extension from the human skull (Flower 1885). The row of cylindroid bones so-named suggested serial homology, especially given the history of the segmental theory of vertebrates. Further projection of the terminology back to "lower forms" was considered possible. With the acceptance of evolutionary theory, there were attempts to use the series as phylogenetic evidence. Broom (1930), using the observation that "lower" mammals did not possess the presphenoid, subdivided mammals into palaeotheres with three elements and neotheres with four. The logic here was that a new member had been inserted into a series, and this occurred at a significant point in phylogeny. This was a standard way of treating such an anatomical series wherever it occurred.

Roux (1947) formally refuted the scheme, showing that Broom's groups were internally inconsistent, and supporting previous doubts (Goodrich 1930) about the phylogenetic implications of the dichotomy. But most important, he also applied embryology and affirmed what ought to have been emphasized previously (e.g., Parker 1885): although seeming to be in a linear series, the presphenoid center is not single or midline. Unlike the others, it is formed by the spread inward of bilateral ossifications (arising in the roots of the orbitosphenoid). The presphenoid, the defining synapomorphy of the neotheres proposed by Broom, was not a true element in a hypothetical basicranial linear series, and therefore did not represent a diagnostic change in the array.

From a more functional viewpoint the presphenoid has a wide but sporadic incidence within mammals, making it a probable case of parallel evolution. Therefore presphenoids are not all homologous. (Its bilateral origin removes it from the midline basicranial series, but to disprove its phylogenetic significance in- and out-group comparisons are needed.) It may be explicable in terms of biomechanics and the growth kinetics of the neurocranium and its support of nasal capsule, but much more study of developmental series is needed.

The Homology of the Vomer

The use of the concept of a linear series with the nonterminal elements strongly conserved has caused other difficulties. In accounting for the

mammalian vomer, de Beer and Fell (1936) homologized it with the dumb-
bell bone of *Ornithorhynchus*. Using the prevailing concepts of the conservation of the central elements of a sequence, they were then bound to
homologize the vomer of monotremes and mammals with the cultriform
process of the parasphenoid of reptiles, and the paired vomers of reptiles
and fishes were termed "pre-vomers."

Parrington and Westoll (1940), citing Green's (1930) clear demonstration (now confirmed in other specimens; Presley and Steel 1978) that the
dumbbell develops by detachment from the palatine process of the premaxilla, homologized the single mammalian vomer with the paired reptilian vomers (which according to de Beer's serial rules became pre-vomers).
A corollary was the reduction and loss of the parasphenoid as a midline
element in mammals. Traces of the parasphenoid can be seen in mammalian embryos (Toeplitz 1920; Reinbach 1951), apparently clinching the
matter. De Beer (1937) somewhat polemically dismissed these observations (incompatible with his homologies) of a parasphenoid vestige on the
illogical ground that they were not reported in some other specimens,
making the existence of the vestige "doubtful." This fallacy is almost un-
forgiveable: the existence of a structure described in a specimen cannot be
denied until that specimen has been examined.

General Implications

Simple acceptance that the Parrington-Westoll view has been proved is an
insufficient response to the last parable. Since the cultriform process of the
parasphenoid is a mechanical component of the neurocranium in other
tetrapods, should not the implications of its loss in development be considered in analyzing the pattern of the evolving mammalian skull? At present
this is not the case. More generally, where any set of similar developmental
units seems to form a series at one stage, scrupulous examination of the
prior developmental stages should always be undertaken to ensure that the
sequence truly indicates iterative homology. It is important to check all
traditional accounts to be sure that the line of proof does not rest automatically upon the nested assumptions: that such series are strongly conserved, the members may never become subdivided, and deletions in the
middle of the series are impossible. Such assumptions are almost instinc-
tive and yet are clearly too rigid for our current perceptions of developmental process: they are associated with the homunculus concept, but
strangely with one that has no mechanism for change during its phylogeny.

The resolution of the example of the presphenoid is deceptively simple
and trivial in its effects on classification and literature. Our current appreciation is that there is no residual problem, but the standard morphological
assumptions implicated have not been fully explored. For osteology in general a well-known problem, so far unsolved, is what precise logical rela-

tionship exists between a single bone and what often are its several centers of ossification. In other words, we have an exact image of the number of bones in our homunculus, and tend to dismiss, or not look for, detailed differences in the developmental pattern of each. To take the basicranial series again, in my embryo collection covering a broad range of mammals, the basioccipital starts to ossify from bilateral centers in a number of species without obvious phylogenetic linkage. We may guess at a biomechanical or biochemical epigenetic cause, but until we have more insight we cannot be sure. And the occurrences seem to invalidate the logical method of Roux's (1947) argument, at least in its appealingly simple form, since now the basioccipital and the presphenoid vie equally to be taken out of the basicranial series of ostensibly similar bones. Clearly the concept of any equivalence of simple units in a series of bones must always be carefully questioned. If this is so, how much more so for linear series of soft tissue such as somitomeres, or biochemical events such as *Hox*-gene expression?

NEGLECTING THE DEVELOPMENTAL PROCESS OF NEOMORPHIC EXTENSIONS

The Growth Process and the Analysis of New Structures

Embryonic growth in early stages is rapid, and the absolute size of developing structures is small. In the case of noncalcified connective tissues (which usually grow or remodel interstitially in adults) apposition from mesenchyme is widespread in early cranial growth (Enlow 1968). This is indicated for early cartilage by its ill-defined perichondrium, where mesenchymatous cells are not only added to the pre-existing centers, but can also condense as small satellite centers of chondrified matrix which later fuse with the primary center (fig. 9.4a, b).

Standard morphological treatments, in explaining the adult pattern, usually do not mention this accretion of satellite elements. Their terminology is that of the homunculus: it assumes that the information exists in the embryo to produce a predetermined number of basic centers and that development simply subserves their ultimate manifestation. On this basis they are permitted on limited occasions to "advance" phylogenetically by developing outgrowths or processes. The formal handling of such features traditionally implies centrifugal development: each process develops by extension from the center. Under standard rules it may not be homologized with a similar-looking structure fused to another center, or one existing independently. Thus each homologous center is an atom, indivisible, identified by phylogenetic methods—it is a component of the homunculus and neomorphic features are extra ornaments upon the homunculus.

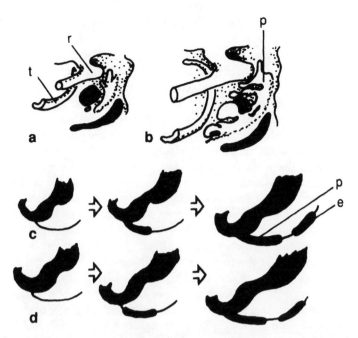

Fig. 9.4. Appositional growth of cartilaginous elements in the tympanic bulla.
a. *Homo*, 107 mm CRL. b. *Homo* 165 mm CRL. Note how the small tympanic
process (p) of the petrosal grows to buttress Reichert's cartilage (r) and the
ectotympanic (t) with an irregular front suggestive of the apposition of satellite
cartilages. c. The classical treatment of such processes as outgrowths from the petrosal,
quite different from a free-standing entotympanic. d. The same anatomy represented
as addition of satellites, showing how the difference between process and
entotympanic is not in kind, but in timing.

The problem is that the subsequent use of these atoms in phylogenetic
reasoning risks circularity. Each process is defined by its anatomy within
its taxon and is also a defining character state of that taxon. I suggest that
for any such neomorphic feature some consideration of the developmental
processes by which it could have arisen is obligatory before using the feature as a phylogenetic discriminant. I illustrate this using the example of
the entotympanic of primates and tupaiids (tree shrews).

The Homology of the Entotympanic

The middle ear apparatus of mammals is a unique feature. The bony elements enclosing it are therefore regarded as neomorphic additions to older
skull bones. By this logic, the separate entotympanic found in many groups
of mammals (van Kampen 1905; van der Klaauw 1931) is a neomorphic
cranial component. It is assumed that the evolution of a new skull bone is
a rare event. Hence possession of the entotympanic is used as strong

evidence of phylogenetic affinity (Spatz 1966) or, where this seems improbable, is explained as a symplesiomorphic condition for placental mammals, independently lost in various derived groups (Novacek 1977).

After considering the complexities extensively displayed and discussed in MacPhee (1981), it seems quite reasonable to accept that the lemurs and tree shrews must be distinct groups. Despite the superficially striking similarity in the placement of a slender tympanic ring within the middle ear cavity, the apparently clinching argument is that because the tree shrews have an entotympanic, while in its place lemurs have a tympanic process of the petrosal, the walls of the tympanic bulla contain nonhomologues. Close phylogenetic relationship is unlikely; any similarity is thus deceptive.

A corollary of this form of analysis is that petrosal plates (van der Klaauw 1931) or tympanic processes (MacPhee 1981) are formations quite distinct in homology from entotympanics. The cartilage capsule of the petrosal has the fibrous membrane of the tympanic cavity attached to its perichondrium, but the two can be distinguished (MacPhee 1977). Petrosal tympanic processes are described as cartilaginous extensions from the petrosal into the fibrous membrane, or ossifications upon its outer surface. MacPhee considers the chondrification within the plane of the fibrous membrane a diagnostic criterion of an entotympanic. He (1977, 1979, 1981) has made careful studies of the development of the tympanic processes in lemurine primates and concludes that they are extensions, chondrified within or ossified upon the outer surface of the fibrous membrane of the tympanic cavity. In this view, entotympanics are distinctly different. They arise as chondrifications satellite to the petrosal, within the membrane.

At the base of this reasoning is an assumption that an entotympanic may not become a tympanic plate of the petrosal or vice versa. However, even within the present literature empirical assumptions are needed to make a character statement. In the case of tupaiids (Spatz 1966; MacPhee 1981; Zeller 1987) it is clear that although in many specimens distinct entotympanics (as defined above) exist prior to birth, they fuse, initially with the petrosal, during the perinatal period. From the viewpoint of developmental process this is not surprising, and it is wise to remember that synostosis between skull bones is quite frequent where growth is reaching completion in mammals.

The problem is the exact logic used in phylogenetics by which the entotympanics in tupaiids, behaving in this way, may be distinguished from the petrosal tympanic processes of primates. Without experiments on cell kinetics, no certainty is possible, but from the shape and cellular appearance of the tympanic processes (fig. 9.4 a, b) it appears extremely unlikely that chondrocytes and matrix are forced out into the membrane by interstitial growth pressure within the body of the petrosal. It is only sensible to suppose that development and expansion of the processes involve some apposition of chondrocytes and matrix from cells initially in fibrous tissue close to the petrosal. There is nothing heretical in this: appositional growth of cartilage has long been recognized, and in many specimens the irregular edge of the expanding processes in this region is extremely suggestive of apposition.

The morphological problem presented is that the distinction between the behavior of the primate tympanic process and the tupaiid entotympanic becomes one of timing only: it is not possible by any other criterion (relations, histology, or—without circularity—phylogeny) to separate the two (fig. 9.4c, d). Once this is admitted, ready interconversion between the two by heterochronic or allometric effects becomes feasible. Recognizing this, the power of the entotympanic as a phylogenetic discriminant is greatly diminished. Its analytic power has been reduced to that of one of several possible manifestations of a single therian autapomorphy: possession of an auditory bulla (or more exactly, a fibrous membrane of the tympanic cavity in development). Without great caution, presence or absence of entotympanics should not be used as a single character state to discriminate between bullae.

OVERALL CONCLUSIONS: THE EFFECT OF DEVELOPMENT ON PHYLOGENETIC STATEMENTS

At the start of this chapter, to form a frame for its examples, I listed four types of fallacy possibly leading to false homologies. It is easy to find many other instances of the kinds of fallacy illustrated here throughout comparative anatomy. The initial impression on thinking of such case studies is negative: criticisms seem destructive without offering any guarantee of improvement in clarity or insight. The use of developmental considerations appears to have obscured rather than enhanced some apparently simple evolutionary insights.

However, they are all reflections of one methodological weakness, which I suggest has been our failure to develop a descriptive method which adequately copes with the dynamics of development. For this reason I have frequently referred to the homunculus. Every anatomical term we use is fixed in shape and relationships. Without such a convention, description is probably impossible. But all my examples illustrate how easy it is in thought to transpose this arbitrarily imposed rigidity to inappropriate situations. This mistake is one which has been prevalent in the use of developmental analysis in our current insights (and disputes) concerning evolution. We have failed to include additional terms reflecting developmental dynamics in descriptive morphology. To a large extent this has been an inevitable consequence of our lacking the necessary techniques to clarify exactly what processes are taking place in development. This is now beginning to change. It may be that molecular probes will provide a much more accurate clock within the embryo, by which we may be able to make much more appropriate comparisons and depart from the "optimum chondrocranium" and the "homunculus," or nerves and vessels.

Our perception of phylogeny has always been of changing form. This change in form must reflect effects on developmental processes of which adult form is only the final manifestation. The classical concept of homology expresses this. In my view the main cause of the difficulties attributed to biological homology has been neglect of detail, and in particular, neglect of the whole range of developmental forms not directly visualizable as adult equivalents: egg structure, epibolic movements, embryonic membranes, and zones of programmed degeneration are largely ignored in cladistics except when used to resolve a conflict previously established using adult anatomy.

The structures touched on in this chapter (e.g., epipterygoid, alisphenoid, laterosphenoid, foramen rotundum, presphenoid, entotympanic) represent typical operators in phylogenetic analysis and in arguments on homology. Whereas most classical analysis has assumed that they are precisely defined by reference to bone and are robust in phylogeny, as shown here they can be transitory and reversible. While some analyses treat their anatomy with respect to cartilage, very few take account of mesenchymal anatomy, or of the number of centers of histodifferentiation assimilated into each "homologous" entity. Surely it must be an absolute requirement to consider information from these precursor stages, which are an essence of Van Valen's (1982) concept of the "continuity of information" underlying homology. I feel that attempts to create subsets of homology such as phylogenetic, iterative, ontogenetic, or polymorphic (Roth 1991) represent pragmatic methodological approaches to an overall problem which is much greater than that perceived by any one isolated discipline. It should be remembered that specific gene loci do not seem to effect codable changes in characters such as those treated here (Berry and Searle 1963; Johnson 1986); the main burden of this chapter is to show that the coding of such morphological characters for use in phylogenetic analysis may be much more difficult than is usually assumed. The background to both these cautions is that evolution and selection forces act on a continuum of whole life cycles, not discrete events of enzyme production or bone-modeling.

Drawing attention to the process of development and its dynamics must often introduce an element of uncertainty into each character-state attribution. When such a character state is then used to compare two forms, the act must represent a probability value, not a certainty, of being a true categorization. Of course, good phylogenies will be based on many such character states. But the probability of a sound phylogeny being so derived will be a function of the product of the probability values of these character states (and also a probability factor estimating whether all truly discrepant character states have been correctly identified and rejected, i.e., the adequacy of available methodology in detecting primary observer error). The current practice of preferring a phylogeny with the best support from character states, counting each as a binary unit, may be unsound: because of the process-dependent uncertainties it may be that a phylogeny with fewer, sounder, units of support is more probable.

The conclusion of this study seems gloomy for cladistics as presently practiced, because it implies that many of our established character states have unknown values as a result of our neglect of developmental studies. While this reasoning makes structure and homology potentially understandable and better testable in extant species and for future workers, it makes equivalent valuing of the fossil record impossible. But common sense suggests that development, the fossil record, and phylogenetics are capable of reconciliation. To achieve this, each must consider the detailed problems of the others.

References

Barry, T. H. 1965. On the epipterygoid-alisphenoid transition in therapsida. Annals of the South African Museum 48: 399–426.

De Beer, G. R. 1926. Studies on the vertebrate head. II. The orbitotemporal region of the skull. Quarterly Journal of Microscopical Science 70: 263–370.

———. 1937. *The Development of the Vertebrate Skull,* London: Oxford University Press.

De Beer, G. R., and W. A. Fell. 1936. The development of the skull of *Ornithorhynchus.* Transactions of the Zoological Society, London 23: 1–43.

Bellairs, A. d'A., and A. M. Kamal. 1981. The chondrocranium and the development of the skull in Recent reptiles. In *Biology of the Reptilia,* vol. II, C. Gans and T. S. Parsons, eds. London: Academic Press, pp. 1–263.

Berry, R. J., and A. G. Searle. 1963. Epigenetic polymorphism of the rodent skeleton. Proceedings of the Zoological Society of London 140: 577–615.

Brock, G. T. 1929. On the development of the skull of *Leptodeira hotamboia.* Quarterly Journal of Microscopial Science 73: 289–334.

———. 1941. The skull of *Acontias meleagris,* with a study of the affinities between lizards and snakes. Journal of the Linnean Society, Zoology 41: 71–88.

Broom, R. 1914. Croonian Lecture: On the origin of mammals. Philosophical Transactions of the Royal Society of London 206: 1–48.

———. 1930. On the structure of the mammal-like reptiles of the sub-order Gorgonopsia. Philosophical Transactions of the Royal Society of London B 218: 345–370.

Cartmill, M., and R. D. E. MacPhee. 1980. Tupaiid affinities: The evidence of the carotid arteries and cranial skeleton. In *Comparative Biology and Evolutionary Relationships of Tree Shrews,* W. P. Luckett, ed. New York: Plenum Press, pp. 95–132.

Clemens, W., and Z. Kielan-Jaworowska. 1979. Multituberculata. In *Mesozoic Mammals,* J. A. Lillegraven, Z. Kielan-Jaworowska, and W. A. Clemens, eds. Berkeley: University of California Press, pp. 99–149.

Crompton, A. W., and F. A. Jenkins. 1979. Origin of mammals. In *Mesozoic Mammals,* J. A. Lillegraven, Z. Kielan-Jaworowska, and W. A. Clemens, eds. Berkeley: University of California Press, pp. 58–73.

Enlow, D. H. 1968. *The Human Face.* New York: Harper and Row.

Flower, H. 1885. *Osteology of the Mammalia.* 3d Ed. London: Macmillan.

Fuchs, H. 1915. Über den Bau und die Entwicklung des Schädels der *Chelone imbricata.* In *Reise in Ostafrika in den Jahren 1903–1905, wissenschaftliche Ergebnisses,* vol. 5, A. Voeltzkow, ed. Stuttgart: Schweitzerbart'sche Verlagsbuchhandlung pp. 1–325.

Gaupp, E. 1902. Uber das ala temporalis des Saugerschadels und die Regio orbitalis einiger anderer Wirbeltierschadel. Anatomisches Heft, 1 Abt. 19: 155–230.

———. 1913. Die Reichertsche Theorie (Hammer-, Amboss und Kieferfrage). Archiv für Anatomie und Physiologie 1912 (suppl.): 1–416.

Ghiselin, M. T. 1976. The nomenclature of correspondence: A new look at "homology" and "analogy." In *Evolution, Brain, and Behaviour: Persistent Problems,* R. B. Masterton, W. Hodos, and H. Jerison, eds. Hillsdale, N.J.: Lawrence Erlbaum, pp. 129–142.

Goodrich, E. S. 1930. *Studies on the Structure and Development of Vertebrates.* Macmillan: London.

Green, H. L. H. H. 1930. A description of the egg tooth of *Ornithorhynchus,* together with some notes on the development of the palatine process of the premaxilla. Journal of Anatomy 64: 512–522.

Gregory, W. K., and G. K. Noble. 1924. The origin of the mammalian alisphenoid bone. Journal of Morphology and Physiology 39: 435–463.

Griffiths, M. 1978. *The Biology of Monotremes.* London: Academic Press.

Hofmann, M. 901. Zur vergleichenden Anatomie der Gehirn und Ruckenmarksvenen der Vertebraten. Zeitschrift für Morphologie und Anthropologie 3: 239–299.

Hunt, P., D. Wilkinson, and R. Krumlauf. 1991. Patterning the vertebrate head: Murine Hox genes mark distinct subpopulations of premigratory and migrating neural crest. Development 112: 43–51.

Jacobson, A. G., and S. Meier. 1984. Morphogenesis of the head of a newt: Mesodermal segments, neuromeres, and distribution of the neural crest. Developmental Biology 106: 181–193.

Johnson, D. R. 1986. *The Genetics of the Skeleton.* Oxford: Oxford University Press.

Kamal, A. M., and H. G. Hammouda. 1965. On the laterosphenoid bone in Ophidia. Anatomischer Anzeiger 116: 116–123.

Kampen, P. N. van. 1905. Die tympanalgegend des saugertierschädels. Morphologisches Jahrbuch 34: 321–722.

Kermack, K. A., and Z. Kielan-Jaworowska. 1971. Therian and non-therian mammals. In Early Mammals. Zoological Journal of the Linnean Society 50 (suppl. 1), D. M. Kermack and K. A. Kermack, eds. London: Linnean Society, pp. 103–115.

Kesteven, H. L. 1918. The homology of the mammalian alisphenoid and of the echidna pterygoid. Journal of Anatomy 52: 223–238.

Kielan-Jaworowska, Z. 1984. Evolution of the therian mammals in the late Cretaceous of Asia. Part VII. Synopsis. Palaeontologia polonica 46: 173–183.

Klaauw, C. J., van der. 1931. The auditory bulla in some fossil mammals. Bulletin of the Museum of Natural History 62: 1–352.

Kuhn, H.-J. 1971. Die Entwicklung und Morphologie des Schädels von Tachyglossus aculeatus. Abhandlungen, Senckenbergische Naturforschende Gesellschaft 528: 1–224.

Kuhn, H.-J., and U. Zeller. 1987. The cavum epiptericum in monotremes and therian mammals. In Morphogenesis of the Mammalian Skull: Mammalia Depicta, H.-J. Kuhn and U. Zeller, eds. Berlin: Verlag Paul Parey, pp. 51–70.

MacPhee, R. D. E. 1977. Ontogeny of the ectotympanic-petrosal plate relationship in strepsirhine prosimians. Folia primatologica 27: 245–283.

———. 1979. Entotympanics, ontogeny, and primates. Folia primatologica 31: 23–47.

———. 1981. Auditory regions of primates and eutherian insectivores. Contributions to Primatology 18: 1–282.

Maier, W. 1987. The ontogenetic development of the orbitotemporal region in the skull of Monodelphis domestica (Didelphidae, Marsupialia) and the problem of the mammalian alisphenoid. In Morphogenesis of the Mammalian Skull: Mammalia Depicta, H.-J. Kuhn, and U. Zeller, eds. Berlin: Verlag Paul Parey, pp. 71–90.

Miao, D. 1988. Skull morphology of Lambdopsalis bulla (Mammalia, Multituberculata) and its implications to mammalian evolution. Contribution to Geology, University of Wyoming, Special Paper 4: 1–104.

Needham, J. 1934. A History of Embryology. Cambridge: Cambridge University Press.

Novacek, M. 1977. Aspects of the problem of variation, origin, and evolution of the eutherian auditory bulla. Mammal Review 7: 131–149.

———. 1980. Cranioskeletal features in tupaiids and selected Eutheria as phylogenetic evidence. In Comparative Biology and Evolutionary Relationships of Tree Shrews, W. P. Luckett, ed. New York: Plenum Press, pp. 35–93.

O'Donoghue, C. H. 1920. The blood vascular system in the tuatara, Sphenodon punctatus. Philosophical Transactions of the Royal Society of London B 210: 175–252.

Padget, D. H. 1957. The development of the cranial venous system in man, from the viewpoint of comparative anatomy. Contributions to Embryology 36: 81–151.

Parker, W. K. 1885. The structure and development of the skull in mammalia (part

2, Edentata; part 3, Insectivora). Philosophical Transactions of the Royal Society of London B 176: 1–275.

Parrington, F. R., and T. S. Westoll. 1940. Evolution of the mammalian palate. Proceedings of the Royal Society of London B 230: 305–355.

Parsons, F. G., and A. Keith. 1897. The position of the spinal accessory nerve. Journal of Anatomy 32: 177.

Presley, R. 1981. Alisphenoid equivalents in placentals, marsupials, monotremes, and fossils. Nature, London 294: 668–670.

Presley, R., and F. L. D. Steel. 1976. On the homology of the alisphenoid. Journal of Anatomy 121: 441–459.

———. 1978. The pterygoid and extopterygoid in mammals. Anatomy and Embryology 154: 95–110.

Pringle, J. A. 1954. The cranial development of certain South African snakes and the relationships of these groups. Proceedings of the Zoological Society of London 123: 813–865.

Reinbach, W. 1951. Uber einen Rest des Parasphenoids bei einem rezenten Saugetier. Zeitschrift für Morphologie und Anthropologie 43: 195–205.

Rieppel, O. 1976. The homology of the laterosphenoid bone in snakes. Herpetologica 32: 426–429.

———. 1988. The development of the trigeminal jaw adductor musculature in the grass snake Natrix natrix. Journal of Zoology, London 216: 743–770.

———. 1990. The structure and development of the jaw adductor musculature in the turtle Chelydra serpentina. Zoological Journal of the Linnean Society 98: 27–62.

Roth, V. L. 1991. Homology and hierarchies: Problems solved and unresolved. Journal of Evolutionary Biology 4: 167–194.

Roux, G. H. 1974. The cranial development of certain Ethiopian insectivores and its bearing on the mutual affinities of the group. Acta zoologica, Stockholm 28: 165–397.

Spatz, W. B. 1966. Zur ontogenese der bulla tympanica von Tupaia glis Diard 1820 (Prosimiae, Tupaiiformes). Folia primatologica 4: 26–50.

Starck, D. 1967. Le crâne des mammifères. In Traité de Zoologie, vol. 16 (1), P. P. Grassé, ed. Paris: Masson, pp. 405–549.

Streeter, G. L. 1918. The developmental alterations in the vascular system of the brain of the human embryo. Contributions to Embryology 8: 5–38.

Toeplitz, C. 1920. Bau und Entwicklung des Knorpelschädels von Didelphys marsupialis. Zoologica Heft, Stuttgart 70: 1–83.

Van Valen, L. 1982. Homology and causes. Journal of Morphology 173: 305–312.

Watson, D. M. S. 1916. The monotreme skull: A contribution to mammalian morphogenesis. Philosophical Transactions of the Royal Society of London B 207: 311–374.

Zeller, U. 1985. Die Ontogenese und Morphologie der Fenestra rotunda und des Aquaeductus cochleae von Tupaia und anderen Saugern. Morphologische Jahrbuch 131: 179–204.

———. 1987. Morphogenesis of the mammalian skull with special reference to

Tupaia. In *Morphogenesis of the Mammalian Skull: Mammalia Depicta*, H.-J. Kuhn and U. Zeller, eds. Berlin: Verlag Paul Parey, pp. 17–50.

———. 1989. Die Entwicklung und Morphologie des Schädels von *Ornithorhynchus anatinus* (Mammalia: Prototheria: Monotremata). Abhandlungen senckenbergische naturforschende Gesellschaft 545: 1–188.

10

Bibliography of Skull Development, 1937–89

BRIAN K. HALL AND JAMES HANKEN

INTRODUCTION

IN THIS CHAPTER we present a list, with accompanying indices, of studies containing information about skull development in vertebrates published between the years 1937 and 1989. These 53 years span the interval between the publication of Sir Gavin de Beer's (1937) *The Development of the Vertebrate Skull,* which is generally regarded as the primary guide (at least in the English language) to earlier literature, and the appearance of and widespread access to computerized bibliographic data bases, such as Zoological Record (1978–) and Biosis Previews (1969–). The famous embryologist Conrad Waddington, in discussing the fantastic rate of accumulation of scientific information in the modern world, conjectured in 1977 that in some branches of science, "it becomes easier to rediscover a fact . . . than to find out whether somebody else has already discovered and described it" (1977, 33). Based on our experience in preparing this bibliography, which has involved literally hundreds of hours spent deep in the bowels of libraries both in North America and Europe, we are there, at least as far as the development of the vertebrate skull is concerned.

We initially intended to restrict our coverage to studies that concerned embryonic development exclusively. This, however, would have omitted significant developmental phenomena that occur after birth or hatching, such as the profound morphological rearrangements that accompany amphibian metamorphosis, as well as a large number of more subtle developmental events, e.g., bone fusions, that occur relatively late in the ontogeny of many taxa. At the same time, it became increasingly evident that for the vast majority of vertebrate species, few if any features of skull development have been formally documented, and most of these are based on static descriptions of the skull in one or only a few juvenile stages. Given that our principal aim in preparing this bibliography was to organize the existing literature in such a way as to facilitate future studies of both comparative and mechanistic aspects of cranial development, we decided to include these studies as well. Exceptions to this policy were made in the case of a few species that are extensively used in biomedical research into mechanisms of postembryonic skull growth, and for which there is a vast recent literature. These are the common fowl (*Gallus domesticus*), the laboratory rat (*Rattus rattus*) and mouse (*Mus domesticus*), and humans (*Homo sapiens*). By and large, these studies were not included, as they would have increased the size of the present bibliography to the point where it no longer would have been manageable, and doing so would simply have exceeded the abilities, resources, and patience of the compilers. Similarly, we omitted studies of a clinical nature as well as those pertaining to teratology and developmental mutants, except where they contribute basic knowledge about normal cranial development.

The reference list is indexed in two ways. The subject index organizes references according to major structural, functional, and developmental categories. Within each major structural category (e.g., neurocranium) references are indexed for each of the eight extant vertebrate classes as commonly recognized (cyclostomes—Class Myxini and Class Cephalaspidomorphi—are for convenience listed as "agnathans," and separate listings are provided for humans, marsupials, monotremes, and other mammals) as well as for major developmental categories such as growth. Cross-referencing between categories, entered as "See also," should facilitate both the usage and the utility of the index. Common synonyms are listed with the appropriate entry; for example, "Chondrocranium. *See* Neurocranium."

The systematic index organizes references according to genera considered therein, listed in alphabetical order by class. References that provide general descriptions of skull development in major groups are identified as such at the beginning of each section. Finally, an attempt was made to index taxa by their current generic designation, as provided by recent standardized checklists when available (e.g., fishes—Nelson 1984; amphibians—Frost 1985; birds—Gruson and Forster 1976; Howard and Moore 1991; mammals—Corbet and Hill 1990; Honacki et al. 1982; Nowak and Paradiso 1983). In cases where the appropriate current generic name could not be determined with certainty, the genus provided in the original reference is listed.

As authors of this bibliography, we would like to think that our list is complete and exhaustive. We know, however, that this is not true. The potentially relevant literature is simply too vast, the scope of our topic is too broad, and there have been too many close judgments concerning which references to include for us to think otherwise. Nevertheless, we hope that students of the vertebrate skull find this list useful, and an aid in their studies of its development.

REFERENCES

Corbet, G. B., and J. E. Hill. 1990. *World List of Mammalian Species*. 3d ed. New York: Oxford University Press.

de Beer, G. R. 1937. *The Development of the Vertebrate Skull*. Oxford: Oxford University Press. Paperback reprint. Chicago: University of Chicago Press, 1985.

Frost, D., ed. 1985. *Amphibian Species of the World*. Lawrence, Kans.: Association of Systematic Collections.

Gruson, E. S., and R. A. Forster. 1976. *Checklist of the World's Birds: A Complete List of the Species, with Names, Authorities, and Areas of Distribution*. New York: Quadrangle/New York Times Book Co.

Honacki, J. H., K. E. Kinman, and J. W. Koeppl, eds. 1982. *Mammal Species of the World: A Taxonomic and Geographic Reference*. Lawrence, Kans.: Allen Press, and Association of Systematic Collections.

Howard, R., and A. Moore. 1991. *A Complete Checklist of the Birds of the World*. 2d ed. London: Academic Press.

Nelson, J. S. 1984. *Fishes of the World*. 2d ed. New York: John Wiley and Sons.

Nowak, R. M., and J. L. Paradiso. 1983. *Walker's Mammals of the World*. 4th ed., vols. 1 and 2. Baltimore: Johns Hopkins University Press.

Waddington, C. H. 1977. *Tools for Thought: How to Understand and Apply the Latest Scientific Techniques of Problem Solving*. New York: Basic Books.

SUBJECT INDEX

SYSTEMATIC INDEX: GENERAL

Phylum Chordata

Class Mammalia

REFERENCES

1. Abe, N., and O. Kurosawa. 1984. The moult and age determination of *Parus palustris* and *P. montanus* ringed in Hokkaido. Journal of the Yamashina Institute of Ornithology 16: 136–141.
2. Abeloos, M. 1946. Croissance relative du squelette de la face chez les Ruminants. Comptes rendus des séances de la Société de biologie, et de ses filiales, Paris 140: 957–958.
3. Able, K. W., D. F. Markle, and M. P. Fahay. 1984. Cyclopteridae: Development. In *Ontogeny and Systematics of Fishes*, American Society of Ichthyologists and Herpetologists Special Publication no. 1, H. G. Moser, ed. Lawrence, Kans.: Allen Press, pp. 428–437.
4. Aboussouan, A. 1968. Oeufs et larvae de téléostéens de l'ouest africain. VII. Larvae de *Syacium guineensis* (Blkr.) Bothidaeå. Bulletin, Institut fondamental d'Afrique noire, ser. A, Sciences naturelles 30: 1188–1197.
5. Aboussouan, A., and J. M. Leis. 1984. Balistoidei: Development. In *Ontogeny and Systematics of Fishes*, American Society of Ichthyologists and Herpetologists Special Publication no. 1, H. G. Moser, ed. Lawrence, Kans.: Allen Press, pp. 450–459.
6. Academica Sinica, Institute of Zoology, Department of Animal Ecology Group I. 1978. Age investigations of Brandt's voles populations. Acta zoologica sinica 24: 344–358.
7. Adamczewska-Andrzejewska, K. 1973. Growth, variations, and age criteria in *Apodemus agrarius* (Pallas, 1771). Acta theriologica 18: 353–394.
8. Adamson, L., R. G. Harrison, and I. Bayley. 1960. The development of the

whistling frog *Eleutherodactylus martinicensis* of Barbados. Proceedings of the Zoological Society of London 133: 453–469.

9. Adelmann, H. B. 1937. Experimental studies on the development of the eye. IV. The effect of the partial and complete excision of the prechordal substrate on the development of the eyes of *Amblystoma punctatum*. Journal of Experimental Zoology 75: 199–227.

10. Ahlstrom, E. H., and O. P. Ball. 1954. Description of eggs and larvae of jack mackeral (*Trachurus symmetricus*) and distribution and abundance of larvae in 1950 and 1951. U.S. National Marine Fisheries Service, Fishery Bulletin 56: 209–245.

11. Ahlstrom, E. H., K. Amaoka, D. A. Hensley, H. G. Moser, and B. Y. Sumida. 1984. Pleuronectiformes: Development. In *Ontogeny and Systematics of Fishes*, American Society of Ichthyologists and Herpetologists Special Publication no. 1, H. G. Moser, ed. Lawrence, Kans.: Allen Press, pp. 641–670.

12. Airoldi, J. P., and R. S. Hoffmann. 1984. Age variation in voles (*Microtus californicus, Microtus ochrogaster*) and its significance for systematic studies. ICES Publications-CM 111: 1–45.

13. Alberch, P. 1980. Ontogenesis and morphological diversification. American Zoologist 20: 653–667.

14. Alberch, P. 1983. Morphological variation in the neotropical salamander genus *Bolitoglossa*. Evolution 37: 906–919.

15. Alberch, P. 1985. Problems with the interpretation of developmental sequences. Systematic Zoology 34: 46–58.

16. Alberch, P. 1987. Evolution of a developmental process: Irreversibility and redundancy in amphibian metamorphosis. In *Development as an Evolutionary Process*, R. A. Raff and E. C. Raff, eds. New York: Alan R. Liss, pp. 23–46.

17. Alberch, P. 1989. Development and the evolution of amphibian metamorphosis. Fortschritte der Zoologie 35: 163–173.

18. Alberch, P., and J. Alberch. 1981. Heterochronic mechanisms of morphological diversification and evolutionary change in the neotropical salamander, *Bolitoglossa occidentalis* (Amphibia: Plethodontidae). Journal of Morphology 167: 249–264.

19. Alberch, P., and E. A. Gale. 1986. Pathways of cytodifferentiation during the metamorphosis of the epibranchial cartilage in the salamander *Eurycea bislineata*. Developmental Biology 117: 233–244.

20. Alberch, P., E. A. Gale, and P. R. Larsen. 1986. Plasma T_4 and T_3 levels in naturally metamorphosing *Eurycea bislineata* (Amphibia: Plethodontidae). General and Comparative Endocrinology 61: 153–163.

21. Alberch, P., S. J. Gould, G. F. Oster, and D. B. Wake. 1979. Size and shape in ontogeny and phylogeny. Paleobiology 5: 296–317.

22. Alberch, P., and E. Kollar. 1988. Strategies of head development: Workshop report. Development 103 (suppl.): 25–30.

23. Alberch, P., G. A. Lewbart, and E. A. Gale. 1985. The fate of larval chondrocytes during the metamorphosis of the epibranchial in the salamander *Eurycea bislineata*. Journal of Embryology and Experimental Morphology 88: 71–83.

24. Aliverti, V., L. Bonanomi, E. Giavini, V. G. Leone, and L. Mariani. 1979. The

extent of fetal ossification as an index of delayed development in teratogenic studies on the rat. Teratology 20: 237–242.

25. Allis, E. P. 1938. Concerning the development of the prechordal portion of the vertebrate head. Journal of Anatomy, London 72: 584–607.

26. Altaba, A. R., and D. A. Melton. 1989. Involvement of the *Xenopus* homeobox gene Xhox3 in pattern formation along the anterior-posterior axis. Cell 57: 317–326.

27. Altig, R. 1969. Notes on the ontogeny of the osseous cranium of *Ascaphus truei*. Herpetologica 25: 59–62.

28. Amaoka, K. 1970. Studies on the larval and juveniles of the sinistral flounders. I. *Taeniopsetta ocellata* (Gunther). Japanese Journal of Ichthyology 17: 95–104.

29. Amaoka, K. 1971. Studies on the larval and juveniles of the sinistral flounders. II. *Chascanopsetta lugubris*. Japanese Journal of Ichthyology 18: 25–32.

30. Amaoka, K. 1972. Studies on the larval and juveniles of the sinistral flounders. III. *Laeops kitaharae*. Japanese Journal of Ichthyology 19: 154–165.

31. Amaoka, K. 1973. Studies on the larval and juveniles of the sinistral flounders. IV. *Arnoglossus japonicus*. Japanese Journal of Ichthyology 20: 145–156.

32. Ambrosi, G., M. E. Camosso, and L. Roncali. 1973. Morphological data regarding conjunctival papillae and scleral ossicles in chick embryos. Bollettino della Società italiana di biologia sperimentale 49: 135–140.

33. Amer, F. I., M. H. Ismail, and R. M. Elbalshy. 1987. The development of the skull in *Gambusia affinis affinis* (Baired & Girard). 1. The development of the chondral neurocranium. Journal of the University of Kuwait, Science 14: 137–160.

34. Anagnostopoulou, S., D. D. Karamaliki, and M. N. Spyropoulos. 1988. Observations on the growth and orientation of the anterior cranial base in the human fetus. European Journal of Orthodontics 10: 143–148.

35. Anan'eva, N. B. 1977. Taxonomic differences in the structure of cranium and dental system in agamid lizards (Sauria, Agamidae) of the fauna of the USSR. Zoologicheskii zhurnal 56: 1062–1070.

36. Andersen, T., and O. Wiig. 1984. Growth of the skull of Norwegian lynx (*Lynx lynx*). Acta theriologica 29: 89–110.

37. Anderson, C. L., and S. Meier. 1981. The influence of the metameric pattern in the mesoderm on migration of cranial neural crest cells in the chick embryo. Developmental Biology 85: 385–402.

38. Anderson, M. E. 1984. Zoarcidae: Development and relationships. In *Ontogeny and Systematics of Fishes,* American Society of Ichthyologists and Herpetologists Special Publication no. 1, H. G. Moser, ed. Lawrence, Kans.: Allen Press, pp. 578–582.

39. Ando, A., S. Shiraishi, N. Higashibara, and T. A. Uchida. 1988. Relative growth of the skull in the laboratory-reared Smith's red-backed vole, *Eothenomys smithii* and so-called "Kage" red-backed vole, *Eothenomys kageus*. Journal of the Faculty of Agriculture, Kyushu University 33: 297–304.

40. Andres, G. 1945. Über die Entwicklung des Anurenlabyrinths in Urodelen (Xenoplasticher Austausch zwischen *Bombinator* und *Triton alpestris*). Revue suisse de zoologie 52: 400–406.

41. Andres, G. 1946. Über Induktion und Entwicklung von Kopforganen aus Unkenektoderm in Molch (Epidermis, Plakoden und Derivate der Neuralleiste). Revue suisse de zoologie 53: 502–510.

42. Andres, G. 1949. Untersuchungen an chimaren von *Triton* und *Bombinator*. Genetica 24: 387–534.

43. Angst, R. 1985. Beitrag zur Kenntnis des Elefantenschädels (Mammalia: Proboscoidea): Stosszahnlose afrikanische Elefanten in den Landessammlungen für Naturkunde. Carolinea 42: 129–137.

44. Anonymous. 1986. Handbuch der Saugetiere Europas: Familie Cervidae Gray, 1821–Hirsche. In *Handbuch der Saugetiere Europas, Band 2/2: Paarhufer-Artiodactyla (Suidae, Cervidae, Bocidae)*, J. Niethammer and F. Krapp, eds. Wiesbaden: Aula-Verlag, pp. 67–89.

45. Anson, B. J., E. W. Cauldwell, and A. F. Reiman. 1944. The human stapes: A nonconformist among bones. Quarterly Bulletin of the Northwestern University Medical School 18: 33–40.

46. Anson, B. J., J. S. Hanson, and S. F. Richany. 1960. Early embryology of the auditory ossicles and associated structures in relation to certain anomalies observed clinically. Annals of Otology, Rhinology, and Laryngology 69: 427–448.

47. Ansorge, H. 1986. Analyse einer Population der Bandmaus, *Apodemus agrarius,* aus der ostlichen Oberlausitz. Abhandlungen und Berichte, Naturkundemuseums Goerlitz 59: 1–20.

48. Anthony, J., and D. Robineae. 1976. On some juvenile characters of *Latimeria chalumnae* (Pisces, Crossopterygii, Coelacanthidae). Comptes rendus hedbomadaires des séances de l'Académie des sciences, Paris, ser. D, Science Naturelle 283: 1739–1742.

49. Aprieto, V. L. 1974. Early development of the five carangid fishes of the Gulf of Mexico and the south Atlantic coast of the United States. U.S. National Marine Fisheries Service, Fishery Bulletin 72: 415–443.

50. Arata, G. F., Jr. 1954. A contribution to the life history of the swordfish *Xiphias gladius* Linnaeus, from the South Atlantic coast of the United States and the Gulf of Mexico. Bulletin of Marine Science of the Gulf and Caribbean 4: 183–243.

51. Armstrong, L. A., G. M. Wright, and J. H. Youson. 1987. Transformation of a mucocartilage to a definitive cartilage during metamorphosis in the sea lamprey *Petromyzon marinus*. Journal of Morphology 194: 1–22.

52. Arsdel, I. W. C., and H. H. Hillemann. 1951. The ossification of the middle and internal ear of the golden hamster (*Cricetus auratus*). Anatomical Record 109: 673–689.

53. Arvy, L. 1979. Les rhythms de croissance et des lamellations de la mandibule et des dents (dentine, cément, ivoire) chez les odontocètes. Annales, Société des sciences naturelles de la Charente-Maritime 6: 483–494.

54. Asling, C. W., G. van Wagenen, and W. F. Marovitz. 1963. Roentgenographic demonstration of skeletal development in the foetal monkey (*Macaca mulatta*). Journal of Anatomy, London 97: 477–478.

55. Aspis, M. E. 1949. Methods of replacement of cartilage with bone in Teleostei.

Comptes rendus hedbomadaires des séances de l'Académie des sciences, Moscow, n.s., 68: 153–156.

56. Atchley, W. R. 1987. Developmental quantitative genetics and the evolution of ontogenies. Evolution 41: 316–330.

57. Atchley, W. R., S. W. Herring, B. Riska, and A. A. Plummer. 1984. Effects of the muscular dysgenesis gene on developmental stability in the mouse mandible. Journal of Craniofacial Genetics and Developmental Biology 4: 179–189.

58. Atchley, W. R., A. A. Plummer, and B. Riska. 1985. Genetics of mandible form in the mouse. Genetics 111: 555–577.

59. Atchley, W. R., B. Riska, L. A. P. Kohn, A. A. Plummer, and J. J. Rutledge. 1984. A quantitative genetic analysis of brain and body size associations, their origin, and ontogeny: Data from mice. Evolution 38: 1165–1179.

60. Atchley, W. R., and J. J. Rutledge. 1980. Genetic components of size and shape. I. Dynamics of components of phenotypic variability and covariability during ontogeny in the laboratory rat. Evolution 34: 1161–1173.

61. Atchley, W. R., J. J. Rutledge, and D. E. Crowley. 1981. Genetic components of size and shape. II. Multivariate covariance patterns in the rat and mouse skull. Evolution 35: 1037–1055.

62. Augier, M. 1937. Pré-conditions chondrales de l'ostéogenèse et types tecto-occipitaux chez *Sus scrofa dom.* Archives of Anatomy, Histology, and Embryology, Strasbourg 23: 249–280.

63. Aumonier, F. J. 1941. Development of the dermal bones in the skull of *Lepidosteus osseus.* Quarterly Journal of Microscopical Science 82: 1–33.

64. Avery, J. K. 1987. Developmental prenatal craniofacial skeleton. In *Oral Development and Histology,* J. K. Avery, ed. Baltimore: Williams and Wilkins, pp. 42–53.

65. Aziz, I. A. 1965a. Absorption of some parts of the chondrocranium among teleostean fishes during later stages of development. Bulletin of the Faculty of Science, Cairo University, no. 39: 135–142.

66. Aziz, I. A. 1965b. The chondrification of the parachordals in *Tilapia nilotica.* Bulletin of the Faculty of Science, Cairo University, no. 39: 143–148.

67. Aziz, I. A. (1965c). The development of the hyoid arch in some Nile bony fishes larvae. Bulletin of the Faculty of Science, Cairo University, no. 39: 149–157.

68. Aziz, I. 1960. The chondrocranium of *Hydrocyon forskalii* Laria (9 mm). II. Branchial arches. Proceedings of the Egyptian Academy of Science 15: 65–69.

69. Azzarello, M. Y. 1989. The pterygoid series in *Hippocampus zosterae* and *Syngnathus scoveli* (Pisces: Syngnathidae). Copeia: 621–628.

70. Bacon, W., and R. Mathis. 1983. Craniofacial characteristics of cyclopia in man and swine: Implications on role of medial structures in normal growth and development. Angle Orthodontist 53: 290–310.

71. Badenhorst, A. 1989a. Development of the chondrocranium of the shallow-water Cape hake *Merluccius capsensis* (Cast.). Part 1: Neurocranium. South African Journal of Zoology 24: 33–48.

72. Badenhorst, A. 1989b. Development of the chondrocranium of the shallow-

water Cape hake *Merluccius capsensis* (Cast.). Part 2: Viscerocranium. South African Journal of Zoology 24: 49–57.

73. Baer, M. J. 1954. Patterns of growth of the skull as revealed by vital staining. Human Biology 26: 80–126.

74. Bahl, K. N. 1937. The skull of *Varanus monitor* (Linn.). Records of the Indian Museum 39: 133–174.

75. Bailey, D. W. 1956. A comparison of genetic and environmental principal components of morphogenesis in mice. Growth 20: 63–74.

76. Bailey, D. W. 1985. Genes that affect the shape of the murine mandible: Congenic strain analysis. Journal of Heredity 76: 107–114.

77. Bailey, D. W. 1986a. Genetic programming of development: A model. Differentiation 33: 89–100.

78. Bailey, D. W. 1986b. Genes that affect morphogenesis of the murine mandible. Journal of Heredity 77: 17–25.

79. Bailey, D. W. 1986c. Mandibular-morphogenesis gene linked to the H-2 complex in mice. Journal of Craniofacial Genetics and Developmental Biology 2 (suppl.): 33–39.

80. Bailey, J. W., and G. A. Heidt. 1984. Postnatal osteology of the northern grasshopper mouse, *Onychomys leucogaster*. Proceedings of the Arkansas Academy of Science 38: 13–16.

81. Bailey, L. T. J., R. Minkoff, and W. E. Koch. 1988. Relative growth rates of maxillary mesenchyme in the chick embryo. Journal of Craniofacial Genetics and Developmental Biology 8 (suppl.): 167–177.

82. Baker, L. W. 1941. The influence of the formative dental organs on the growth of the bones of the face. American Journal of Orthodontics 27: 489–506.

83. Balabai, P. P. 1937. Zur Frage über die Homologie der visceralen Bogen der Cyclostomen und Gnathostomen. Travaux sur la morphologie des animaux, Kieff 4: 27–45.

84. Balabai, P. P. 1946. Metamorphosis of the visceral apparatus of the lamprey. Comptes rendus hedbomadaires des séances de l'Académie des sciences, Moscow, n.s., 53: 765–768.

85. Balabai, P. P. 1948. On the problem of transformation of the "mucous cartilage" into the definitive cartilaginous tissue in the ontogenesis of the minnow. Zoologicheskii zhurnal, Moscow 27: 219–230.

86. Balabai, P. P. 1956. *Morphology and Phylogenetic Development of the Agnatha* (Morfologiya i filogenetichesokye razvitiye gruppy bezchelyustnykh). Kiev.

87. Balart, E. F. 1985. Osteological development of the hyobranchial apparatus in *Engraulis japonicus*. Bulletin of the Japanese Society of Scientific Fisheries 51: 515–519.

88. Baldwin, G. F., and P. J. Bentley. 1980. Calcium metabolism in bullfrog tadpoles. Journal of Experimental Biology 88: 357–365.

89. Balinsky, B. I. 1948. Korrelation in der Entwicklung der Mund- und Kiemenregionen und des Darmkanals bei Amphibien. Wilhelm Roux' Archiv für Entwicklungsmechanik der Organismen 143: 365–395.

90. Ballard, K. A., R. L. Pickett, and J. G. Sivak. 1987. Comparison of the musculoskeletal structure of the orbits of the migrating and non-migrating eyes in

the winter flounder (*Pseudopleuronectes americanus*). Experimental Biology 47: 23–26.

91. Balling, R., G. Mutter, P. Gross, and M. Kessel. 1989. Craniofacial abnormalities induced by ectopic expression of the homeobox gene Hox 1.1 in transgenic mice. Cell 58: 337–347.

92. Balon, E. K. 1980a. Early ontogeny of the lake charr, *Salvelinus (Cristivomer) namaycush*. In *Charrs: Salmonid Fishes of the Genus* Salvelinus, E. K. Balon, ed. The Hague: W. Junk, pp. 485–562.

93. Balon, E. K. 1980b. Early ontogeny of the North American landlocked arctic charr-sunapee, *Salvelinus (Salvelinus) alpinus oquassa*. in *Charrs: Salmonid Fishes of the Genus* Salvelinus, E. K. Balon, ed. The Hague: W. Junk, pp. 563–606.

94. Balon, E. K. 1980c. Early ontogeny of the European landlocked charr—altricial form, *Salvelinus (Salvenlinus) alpinus alpinus*. In *Charrs: Salmonid Fishes of the Genus* Salvelinus, E. K. Balon, ed. The Hague: W. Junk, pp. 607–630.

95. Balon, E. K. 1980d. Early ontogeny of the brook charr, *Salvelinus (Baione) fontinalis*. In *Charrs: Salmonid Fishes of the Genus* Salvelinus, E. K. Balon, ed. The Hague: W. Junk, pp. 631–666.

96. Balon, E. K. 1980e. Comparative ontogeny of charrs. In *Charrs: Salmonid Fishes of the Genus* Salvelinus, E. K. Balon, ed. The Hague: W. Junk, pp. 703–720.

97. Balon, E. K. 1980f. The juvenilization process in phylogeny and the altricial to precocious forms in the ontogeny of fishes. Environmental Biology of Fishes, The Hague 4: 193–198.

98. Baltzer, F. 1950. Chimären und merogone bei Amphibien. Revue suisse de Zoologie 57 (suppl. 1): 93–114.

99. Baltzer, F. 1952. Experimentelle Beitrag zur Frage der Homologie. Experientia 8: 285–297.

100. Bamford, T. W. 1948. Cranial development of *Galeichthys felis*. Proceedings of the Zoological Society of London 118: 364–391.

101. Banks, W. J. 1974. The ossification process of the developing antler in the white-tailed deer (*Odocoileus virginianus*). Calcified Tissue Research 14: 257–274.

102. Banks, W. J., and J. W. Newbrey. 1983a. Antler development as a unique modification of mammalian endochondral ossification. In *Antler Development in Cervidae*, R. D. Brown, ed. Kingsville, Tex.: Caesar Kleberg Wildlife Research Institute, pp. 279–306.

103. Banks, W. J., and J. W. Newbrey. 1983b. Light microscopic studies of the ossification process in developing antlers. In *Antler Development in Cervidae*, R. D. Brown, ed. Kingsville, Tex.: Caesar Kleberg Wildlife Research Institute, pp. 231–260.

104. Barbu, P. 1961. Contributions à l'étude monographique de *Miniopterus schreibersii* Kühl. Analele, Universitatii C. I. Parhon 10: 196–203.

105. Barel, C. D. N. 1984. Form-relations in the context of constructional morphology: The eye and suspensorium of lacustrine Cichlidae (Pisces, Teleostei). Netherlands Journal of Zoology 34: 439–502.

106. Barghusen, H. R., and J. A. Hopson. 1979. The endoskeleton: The comparative anatomy of the skull and the visceral skeleton. In *Hyman's Comparative Vertebrate Anatomy,* M. H. Wake, ed, 3d ed. Chicago: University of Chicago Press, pp. 265–326.

107. Barr, M., Jr. 1982. Facial duplication: Case, review, and embryogenesis. Teratology 25: 153–159.

108. Barry, T. H. 1953. Contributions to the cranial morphology of *Agama hispida.* Annals of the University of Stellenbosch 29A: 55–80.

109. Barry, T. H. 1956a. The ontogenesis of the sound-conducting apparatus of *Bufo angusticeps* Smith. Gegenbaurs Morphologisches Jahrbuch, Leipzig 97: 477–544.

110. Barry, T. H. 1956b. Origin and development of the septomaxillary in *Bufo angusticeps* Smith. South African Journal of Science 53: 28–32.

111. Bartelmez, G. W., and M. P. Blount. 1954. The formation of neural crest from the primary optic vesicle in man. Contributions to Embryology of the Carnegie Institute 35: 55–91.

112. Bartolucci, L. 1975. Biparietal diameter of the skull and fetal weight in the second trimester: An allometric relationship. American Journal of Obstetrics and Gynecology 122: 439–445.

113. Bartosiewicz, L. 1980a. Relationship between the cranial measurements of cattle. Ossa 7: 3–18.

114. Bartosiewicz, L. 1980b. Changes in skull proportions of cattle during ontogeny. Ossa 7: 19–32.

115. Bartosiewicz, L. 1987. Sexual dimorphism in the cranial development of Scandinavian moose (*Alces alces* [L] *alces*). Canadian Journal of Zoology 65: 747–750.

116. Barus, V., C. Babicka, and J. Zejda. 1982. On the morphology of a feral population of sika deer (*Cervus nippon*) in Czechoslovakia. Folia zoologica 31: 195–208.

117. Basit, A., and M. A. Beg. 1978. Nongeographic variations in *Fynambulus pennanti.* Biologia, Lahore 24: 297–304.

118. Basoglu, M., and S. Zaloglu. 1964. Morphological and osteological studies in *Pelobates syriacus* from Izmir region, Western Anatolia. Senckenbergiana biologica 45: 233–242.

119. Bassin, P. 1985. Jeune pie-grièche grise, *Lanius excubitor,* avec le bec croisé. Nos oiseaux 38: 148.

120. Bast, T. H., and B. J. Anson. 1949. *The Temporal Bone and the Ear.* Springfield: Charles C. Thomas.

121. Bast, T. H., B. J. Anson, and S. F. Richany. 1956. The development of the second branchial arch (Reichert's cartilage), facial canal, and associated structures in man. Quarterly Bulletin of the Northwestern University Medical School 30: 235–250.

122. Batcheler, C. L., and M. J. McClennan. 1977. Craniometric study of allometry, adaptation, and hybridism of red deer (*Cervus elaphus scoticus,* L.) and Wapiti (*C. e. nelsoni,* Bailey) in Fiordland, New Zealand. New Zealand Ecological Society Proceedings 24: 57–75.

123. Bauchot, M. L. 1959. Étude des larves leptocéphales du groupe *Leptocephalus lanceolatus* Stromann et identification à la famille des Serrivomeridae. Dana Reports, Carlsberg Foundation, no. 48: 1–148.

124. Baume, L. J. 1962a. Embryogenesis of the human temporomandibular joint. Science 138: 904–905.

125. Baume, L. J. 1962b. The prenatal and postnatal development of the human temporomandibular joint. Transactions of the European Orthodontic Society: 1–11.

126. Baume, L. J. 1962c. Ontogenesis of the human temporomandibular joint. 1. Development of the condyles. Journal of Dental Research 41: 1327–1339.

127. Baume, L. J. 1968. Patterns of cephalofacial growth and development. A comparative study of the basicranial growth centers in rat and man. International Dental Journal 18: 489–513.

128. Baume, L. J., J. C. Franquin, and W. W. Körner. 1972. The prenatal effects of maternal vitamin A deficiency on the cranial and dental development of the progeny. American Journal of Orthodontics 62: 447–460.

129. Baume, L. J., and J. Holz. 1970. Ontogenesis of the human temporomandibular joint. 2. Development of the temporal components. Journal of Dental Research 49: 864–875.

130. Beacham, T. D., and C. B. Murray. 1986. Sexual dimorphism in length of upper jaw and adipose fin of immature and maturing Pacific salmon (*Oncorhynchus*). Aquaculture 58: 269–276.

131. Beale, G. 1985. A radiological study of the kiwi, *Apteryx australis mantelli*. Journal of the Royal Society of New Zealand 15: 187–200.

132. Beatty, M. D., and H. H. Hillemann. 1950. Osteogenesis in the golden hamster. Journal of Mammalogy 31: 121–134.

133. Beaver, T. D., G. A. Feldhamer, and J. A. Chapman. 1982. Dental and cranial anomalies in the river otter (Carnivora: Mustelidae). Brimleyana 7: 101–109.

134. Beden, M. 1983. Données nouvelles sur le dimorphisme et la croissance du crâne les éléphantides actuels et fossiles. Bulletin de la Société zoologique de France 108: 654–663.

135. Bednjakov, T. A. 1947a. The formative influence of chorda on development of parachordalia in Amphibia. Comptes rendus hebdomadaires des séances de l'Académie des sciences, Moscow 56: 977–979.

136. Bednjakov, T. A. 1947b. Character of formative influence of chorda on the skeletogenic mesenchyme of Amphibia. Comptes rendus hebdomadaires des séances de l'Académie des sciences, Moscow. 57: 875–878.

137. Bee, J., and D. Newgreen. 1988. Cellular and molecular aspects of cephalic neural crest development: Workshop report. Development 103 (suppl.): 95–100.

138. Bee, J., and P. Thorogood. 1980. The role of tissue interactions in the skeletogenic differentiation of avian neural crest cells. Developmental Biology 78: 47–62.

139. Behramm, G., and M. Klima. 1985. Cartilaginous structures in the forehead of the sperm whale *Physeter macrocephalus*. Zeitschrift für Saeugetierkunde 50: 357–356.

140. Behrents, R. G., and L. E. Johnston. 1984. The influence of the trigeminal nerve on facial growth and development. American Journal of Orthodontics 85: 199–206.

141. Bell, G. L., and M. A. Sheldon. 1986. Description of a very young mosasaur from Greene County, Alabama. Journal of the Alabama Academy of Science 57: 76–82.

142. Bellairs, A. d'A. 1949a. The anterior brain-case and interorbital septum of Sauropsida, with a consideration of the origin of snakes. Zoological Journal of the Linnean Society 41: 482–512.

143. Bellairs, A. d'A. 1949b. Observations on the snout of Varanus, and a comparison with that of other lizards and snakes. Journal of Anatomy, London 83: 116–146.

144. Bellairs, A. d'A. 1949c. Orbital cartilages in snakes. Nature 163: 106.

145. Bellairs, A. d'A. 1950. Observations on the cranial anatomy of Anniella, and a comparison with that of other burrowing lizards. Proceedings of the Zoological Society of London 119: 887–904.

146. Bellairs, A. d'A. 1955. Skull development in chick embryos after ablation of one eye. Nature 176: 658–659.

147. Bellairs, A. d'A. 1958. The early development of the interorbital septum and the fate of the anterior orbital cartilages in birds. Journal of Embryology and Experimental Morphology 6: 68–85.

148. Bellairs, A. d'A. 1965. Cleft palate, microphthalmia, and other malformations in embryos of lizards and snakes. Proceedings of the Zoological Society of London 144: 239–251.

149. Bellairs, A. d'A. 1972. Comments on the evolution and affinities of snakes. In Studies in Vertebrate Evolution, K. A. Joysey and T. S. Kemp, eds. Edinburgh: Oliver and Boyd, pp. 157–172.

150. Bellairs, A. d'A. 1977. The nose and Jacobson's organ in reptiles: A review. Cotswold Herpetology Symposium Report 3: 27–36.

151. Bellairs, A. d'A. 1983. Partial cyclopia and monorhinia in turtles. In Advances in Herpetology and Evolutionary Biology, A. G. J. Rhodin and K. Miyata, eds. Cambridge, Mass.: Museum of Comparative Zoology, pp. 150–158.

152. Bellairs, A. d'A. 1984. Closing address: With comments on the organ of Jacobson and the evolution of Squamata, and on the intermandibular connections in Squamata. In The Structure, Development, and Evolution of Reptiles, M. W. J. Ferguson, ed. London: Academic Press, pp. 665–683.

153. Bellairs, A. d'A., and J. D. Boyd. 1947. The lachrymal apparatus in lizards and snakes. I. The brille, the orbital glands, lachrymal canaliculi, and origin of the lachrymal duct. Proceedings of the Zoological Society of London 117B: 81–108.

154. Bellairs, A. d'A., and J. D. Boyd. 1950. The lachrymal apparatus in lizards and snakes. II. The anterior part of the lachrymal duct and its relationship with the palate and with the nasal and vomeronasal organs. Proceedings of the Zoological Society of London 120: 269–310.

155. Bellairs, A. d'A., and J. D. Boyd. 1957. Anomalous cleft palate in snake embryos. Proceedings of the Zoological Society of London 129: 525–539.

156. Bellairs, A. d'A., and H. J. Gamble. 1960. Cleft palate, microphthalmia and other anomalies in an embryo lizard (*Lacerta vivipara* Jacquin). British Journal of Herpetology 2: 171–176.

157. Bellairs, A. d'A., and C. Gans. 1983. A reinterpretation of the amphisbaenian orbitosphenoid. Nature 302: 243–244.

158. Bellairs, A. d'A., and C. R. Jenkin. 1960. The skeleton of birds. In *Biology and Comparative Physiology of Birds*, A. J. Marshall, ed, vol. 1. New York: Academic Press, pp. 241–300.

159. Bellairs, A. d'A., and A. M. Kamal. 1981. The chondrocranium and the development of the skull in recent reptiles. In *Biology of the Reptilia*, vol. 11, *Morphology F*, C. Gans and T. S. Parsons, eds. New York: Academic Press, pp. 1–264.

160. Bellairs, R., D. A. Ede, and J. W. Lash, eds. 1986. *Somites in Developing Embryos*. NATO Advanced Studies Institutes Series, vol. 118. New York: Plenum Press.

161. Bellmer, E. H. 1963. The time of embryonic fusion of the malleus and incus of the guinea pig. American Midland Naturalist 69: 426–434.

162. Bemis, W. E. 1984a. Morphology and growth of lepidosirenid lungfish tooth plates (Pisces: Dipnoi). Journal of Morphology 179: 73–93.

163. Bemis, W. E. 1984b. Paedomorphosis and the evolution of the Dipnoi. Paleobiology 10: 293–307.

164. Benjamin, M. 1986. The oral sucker of *Gyrinocheilus aymonieri* (Teleostei: Cypriniformes). Journal of Zoology, London, pt. B, 1: 211–254.

165. Benjamin, M. 1988. Mucochondroid (mucous connective) tissues in the heads of teleosts. Anatomy and Embryology 178: 461–474.

166. Benjamin, M. 1989a. The development of hyaline cell cartilage in the head of the black molly, *Poecilia sphenops:* Evidence for secondary cartilage in a teleost. Journal of Anatomy 164: 145–154.

167. Benjamin, M. 1989b. Hyaline-cell cartilage (chondroid) on the heads of teleosts. Anatomy and Embryology 179: 285–303.

168. Benoit, J. A. A. 1955. De l'excision de l'otocyste chez l'embryon de Poulet, et ses conséquences sur la morphogenèse de la capsule otique. Comptes rendus, Société de biologie 149: 998–1000.

169. Benoit, J. A. A. 1957a. Irradiation localisée de l'otocyste chez les embryons de poulet et de truite. Bulletin de la Société zoologique de France 82: 238–243.

170. Benoit, J. A. A. 1957b. Sur un example de cascade d'inductions dans l'organogenèse des vertébrés: La genèse de l'oreille interne. L'année biologique, 3d ser., 61: 385–412.

171. Benoit, J. A. A. 1959. Action inductrice de l'extrait d'otocystes dans la différenciation en cartilage du mésenchyme otique de l'embryon de poulet. Comptes rendus hebdomadaires des séances de l'Académie des sciences, Paris 248: 1705–1707.

172. Benoit, J. A. A. 1960a. Étude expérimentale des facteurs de l'induction du cartilage otique chez les embryons de poulet et de truite. Annales des Sciences Naturelles, Zoologie, ser. 2, 12: 323–385.

173. Benoit, J. A. A. 1960b. Induction de cartilage *in vitro* par l'extrait d'otocystes

d'embryons de poulet. Journal of Embryology and Experimental Morphology 8: 33–38.

174. Benoit, J. A. A. 1960c. L'otocyste exerce-t-il une action inductrice sur le mésenchyme somatique chez l'embryon de poulet? Journal of Embryology and Experimental Morphology 8: 39–46.

175. Benoit, J. A. A. 1963. Chronologie de l'induction du cartilage otique chez l'embryon de poulet. Archives d'anatomie microscopique et de morphologie expérimentale 52: 573–590.

176. Benoit, J. A. A. 1964. Étude expérimentale de l'origine de la columelle auriculaire de l'embryon de poulet. Archives d'anatomie microscopique et de morphologie expérimentale 53: 357–366.

177. Benoit, J. A. A. 1982. Origine du mésenchyme squelettogène et induction du cartilage et de l'os. In Traite de zoologie: anatomie, systématique, biologie, P-P. Grassé and J. A. A. Benoit, eds., vol. 76(7), Mammifères, embryologie. Paris: Masson, pp. 392–440.

178. Benoit, J. A. A., and J. Schowing. 1970. Morphogenesis of the Neurocranium. In Tissue Interactions during Organogenesis, E. Wolff, ed. New York: Gordon and Breach, pp. 105–130.

179. Bentley, P. J. 1984. Calcium metabolism in the Amphibia. Comparative Biochemistry and Physiology 79A: 1–5.

180. Benton, M. J., and R. Kirkpatrick. 1989. Heterochrony in a fossil reptile: Juveniles of the Rhynchosaur Scaphonyx fischeri from the late Triassic of Brazil. Palaeontology 32: 335–354.

181. Benzer, P. 1944. Morphology of calcification in Squalus acanthias. Copeia: 217–224.

182. Beresford, W. A. 1981. Chondroid Bone, Secondary Cartilage, and Metaplasia. Munich: Urban and Schwarzenberg.

183. Bergsma, D., ed. 1975. Morphogenesis and Malformation of Face and Brain. New York: Alan R. Liss.

184. Berkovitz, B. B. B., and P. Sloan. 1979. Attachment tissues of the teeth in Caiman sclerops (Crocodilia). Journal of Zoology, London 187: 179–194.

185. Berman, D. S. 1976. Cranial morphology of the lower Permian lungfish Gnathorhiza (Osteichthyes, Dipnoi). Journal of Paleontology 50: 1020–1033.

187. Bernasconi, A. F. 1951. Über den Ossifikationsmodus bei Xenopus laevis Daud. Denkschriften der schweizerische naturforschende Gesellschaft 79: 189–252.

187. Bernot, C. 1955. Beiträge zur Entwicklung des Primordial craniums bei Bitterling (Rhodeus amarus Bl.). Bioloski vestnik, Ljubljana 4: 23–36.

188. Berrill, N. J. 1987a. Early chordate evolution. Part 1. Amphioxus, the riddle of the sands. International Journal of Invertebrate Reproduction and Development 11: 1–14.

189. Berrill, N. J. 1987b. Early chordate evolution. Part 2. Amphioxus and Ascidians: To settle or not to settle. International Journal of Invertebrate Reproduction and Development 11: 15–28.

190. Berry, F. H. 1964. Aspects of the development of the upper jaw bones in teleosts. Copeia: 375–384.

191. Bersch, W., and W. Reinbach. 1970. Das Primordialcranium eines mensch-

lichen Embryo von 52 mm Sch.-St.-Länge. Zur Morphologie des Cranium älterer menschlicher Feten II. Zeitschrift für Anatomie Entwicklungsgeschichte 132: 240–251.

192. Bertelsen, E., and J. G. Nielsen. 1987. The deep sea eel family Monognathidae (Pisces, Anguilliformes). Steenstrupia 13: 141–197.

193. Bertin, L. 1958. Tissus squelettiques. In *Traité de zoologie,* vol. 13(1), *Agnathes et Poissons, anatomie, éthologie, systématique,* P.-P. Grassé, ed. Paris: Masson et Cie, pp. 532–550.

194. Bertmar, G. 1959. On the ontogeny of the chondral skull in Characidae, with a discussion of the chondrocranial base and the visceral chondrocranium in fishes. Acta zoologica, Stockholm 40: 203–364.

195. Bertmar, G. 1962a. Homology of the ear ossicles. Nature 193: 393–394.

196. Bertmar, G. 1962b. On the ontogeny and evolution of the arterial vascular system in the head of the African characidean fish *Hepsetus odoe.* Acta zoologica, Stockholm 43: 255–295.

197. Bertmar, G. 1963a. Finns det kotor i huvudet? (Are there vertebrae in the vertebrate head?). Zoologisk Revy: 47–54.

198. Bertmar, G. 1963b. The trigemino-facialis chamber, the cavum epiptericum and the cavum orbitonasale, three serially homologous extracranial spaces in fishes. Acta zoologica, Stockholm 44: 329–344.

199. Bertmar, G. 1965a. The olfactory organ and upper lips in Dipnoi, an embryological study. Acta zoologica, Stockholm 44: 1–40.

200. Bertmar, G. 1965b. On the development of the jugular and cerebral veins in fishes. Proceedings of the Zoological Society of London 144: 87–130.

201. Bertmar, G. 1966a. On the ontogeny and homology of the choanal tubes and choanae in urodela. Acta zoologica, Stockholm 47: 43–59.

202. Bertmar, G. 1966b. The development of skeleton, blood-vessels, and nerves in the dipnoan snout, with a discussion on the homology of the dipnoan posterior nostrils. Acta zoologica, Stockholm 47: 81–150.

203. Bertmar, G. 1968a. Phylogeny and evolution in lungfishes. Acta zoologica, Stockholm 49: 189–201.

204. Bertmar, G. 1968b. Lungfish phylogeny. In *Current Problems of Lower Vertebrate Phylogeny,* Nobel Symposium, vol. 4, T. Ørvig, ed. Stockholm: Almqvist and Wiksell, pp. 259–283.

205. Bertmar, G. 1969. The vertebrate nose: Remarks on its structural and functional adaptation and evolution. Evolution 23: 131–152.

206. Bevelander, G., and P. L. Johnson. 1950. A histochemical study of the development of membrane bone. Anatomical Record 108: 1–21.

207. Beveridge, M. C. M., M. R. P. Briggs, M. E. Northcutt, and L. G. Ross. 1988. The occurrence, structure, and development of microbranchiospines among the tilapias (Cichlidae, Tilapiini). Canadian Journal of Zoology 66: 2564–2572.

208. Bhargava, H. N. 1957. Studies on the development and morphology of the chondrocranium of *Mastacembelus armatus* (Cuv. et Val.). Journal of the University of Saugar (2B) 6: 86–89.

209. Bhargava, H. N. 1958. The development of the chondrocranium of *Mastacembelus armatus* (Cuv. et Val.). Journal of Morphology 102: 401–426.

210. Bhargava, H. N. 1959. The morphology of the chondrocranium of *Mastacembelus armatus* (Cuv. et Val.). Journal of Morphology 104: 237–267.
211. Bhaskar, S. N. 1953. Growth patterns of the rat mandible from 13 days insemination to 30 days after birth. American Journal of Anatomy 92: 1–33.
212. Bianco, P., G. Silvestrini, J. D. Termine, and E. Bonucci. 1988. Immunohistochemical localization of osteonectin in developing human and calf bone using monoclonal antibodies. Calcified Tissue International 43: 155–161.
213. Biegert, J. 1957. Der Formwandel des Primatenschadels und seine Beziehungen zur ontogenetischen (Entwicklung und den phylogenetischen specialisationen der Kopforgane). Gegenbaurs Morphologische Jahrbuch 98: 77–199.
214. Birkmann, K. 1940. Morphologisch-anatomische Untersuchungen zur Entwicklung des hautigen Labyrinths der Amphibiens. Zeitschrift für Anatomie und Entwicklungsgeschichte 110: 443–465.
215. Biseswar, R. 1980. A comparative study of the morphology of the chondrocranium of *Dendroaspis angusticeps* and *D. p. polylepis*. South African Journal of Zoology 15: 205–216.
216. Biur, K., and J. P. Thapliyal. 1972. Cranial pneumatization in the Indian weaver bird, *Ploceus philippinus*. Condor 74: 198–200.
217. Bjerring, H. C. 1967. Does a homology exist between the basicranial muscle and the polar cartilage? Colloque international du Centre national de la recherche scientifique 163: 223–267.
218. Bjerring, H. C. 1968. The second somite with special reference to the evolution of its myotomic derivatives. In *Current Problems of Lower Vertebrate Phylogeny*, Nobel Symposium, vol. 4, T. Ørvig, ed. Stockholm: Almqvist and Wiksell, pp. 341–357.
219. Bjerring, H. C. 1971. The nerve supply to the second metamere basicranial muscle in osteolepiform vertebrates, with some remarks on the basic composition of the endocranium. Acta zoologica, Stockholm 52: 189–225.
220. Bjerring, H. C. 1972. The rhinal bone and its evolutionary significance. Zoologica scripta 1: 193–201.
221. Bjerring, H. C. 1977. A contribution to structural analysis of the head of craniate animals: The orbit and its contents in 20–22 mm embryos of the North American actinopterygian *Amia calva* L., with particular reference to the evolutionary significance of an aberrant, nonocular, orbital muscle innervated by the oculomotor nerve and notes on the metameric character of the head in craniates. Zoologica scripta 6: 127–183.
222. Bjerring, H. C. 1978. The "intracranial joint" versus the "ventral otic fissure." Acta zoologica, Stockholm 59: 203–214.
223. Bjerring, H. C. 1984a. Major anatomical steps towards craniotedness: A heterodox view based largely on embryological data. Journal of Vertebrate Paleontology 4: 17–29.
224. Bjerring, H. C. 1984b. The term "fossa bridgei" and five endocranial fossae in teleostome fishes. Zoologica scripta 13: 231–238.
225. Bjerring, H. C. 1985. The question of a presupracleithrum in brachiopterygian fishes. Acta zoologica, Stockholm 66: 171–174.
226. Blackwood, H. J. J. 1965. Vascularization of the condylar cartilage of the human mandible. Journal of Anatomy, London 99: 551–564.

227. Blair, A. F. 1961. Metamorphosis of *Pseudotriton palleucus* with iodine. Copeia: 499.

228. Blanc, M. 1945. L'ossification des arcs branchiaux chez les Poissons Téléostéens. Bulletin de la Société zoologique de France 69: 226–230.

229. Blanc, M. 1953. Contribution à l'étude de l'ostéogenèse chez les poissons téléostéens. Mémoires du Muséum nationale d'histoire naturelle, Paris 7A: 1–146.

230. Blaney, S. P. A. 1986. An allometric study of the frontal sinus in *Gorilla, Pan,* and *Pongo*. Folia primatologica 47: 81–96.

231. Blaxter, J. H. S., E. J. Denton, and J. A. B. Gray. 1981. The auditory bullae-swimbladder system in late stage herring larvae. Journal of the Marine Biological Association of the United Kingdom 61: 315–326.

232. Blechschmidt, E. 1961. *Die Vorgeburtlichen Entwicklungsstadien des Menschen*. Basel: Karger.

233. Blechschmidt, E. 1965. Das Antlitz des menschlichen Embryo. Die Waage 4: 139–151.

234. Blechschmidt, E. 1976a. Principles of biodynamic differentiation. In *Development of the Basicranium*, J. F. Bosma, ed. Bethesda: U.S. Department of Health, Education, and Welfare, pp. 54–76.

235. Blechschmidt, E. 1976b. The biokinetics of the basicranium. In *Development of the Basicranium*, J. F. Bosma, ed. Bethesda: U.S. Department of Health, Education, and Welfare, pp. 44–53.

236. Blin, P.-C., J. D. Souteyrand-Boulenger, and J. Benoit. 1982. Squelette, articulations, muscles. In *Traité de Zoologie: Anatomie, systématique, biologie*, vol. 16(7), *Mammifères, embryologie*, P.-P. Grassé and J. Benoit, eds. Paris: Masson et Cie, pp. 327–440.

237. Blinov, V. A. 1937. On the time of beginning of chondrogenesis and its rate in various organs of avian embryos. Bulletin de biologie et de médecine expérimentale de l'URSS, Moscow 3: 392–394.

238. Blood, B. R., J. O. Matson, and D. R. Patten. 1985. Multivariate analysis of allometry in a single population of coyotes (Canidae: *Canis latrans* Say). Australian Mammal 8: 221–231.

239. Bluzma, P. P. 19074. Morphology of the skull in the Roe deer (*Capreolus capreolus*). Zoologischeskii zhurnal 53: 263–271.

240. Bock, W. J. 1960. The palatine process in the premaxilla in the Passeres: A study of the variation, function, evolution, and taxonomic value of a single character throughout an avian order. Bulletin of the Museum of Comparative Zoology, Harvard 122: 361–488.

241. Bock, W. J. 1963. The cranial evidence for ratite affinities. Proceedings of the Eighth International Ornithological Congress: 39–54.

242. Bock, W. J. 1974. The avian skeletomuscular system. In *Avian Biology*, vol. 4, D. S. Farner, J. R. King, and K. C. Parkes, eds. New York: Academic Press, pp. 119–259.

243. Bock, W. J., and J. Morony. 1978. The preglossale of *Passer* (Aves: Passeriformes): A skeletal neomorph. Journal of Morphology 155: 99–110.

244. Bol'shakov, V. N., and Z. D. Epifantseva. 1972. The bent-nose mutation in the vole *Promethromys schaposchnikovi*. Soviet Genetics 4: 1404.

245. Bonebrake, J. E., and R. A. Brandon. 1971. Ontogeny of cranial ossification in the small-mouthed salamander, *Ambystoma texanum* (Matthes). Journal of Morphology 133: 189–204.

246. Bordet, G. 1981. Analyse ultrastructurale de la croissance supra-linguale des processus palatins chez *Oryctolagus cuniculus* (Fauve de Bourgogne). Journal de biologie buccale 9: 253–270.

247. Borgen, U. J. 1983. Homologization of skull roofing bones between tetrapods and osteolepiform fishes. Palaeontology 26: 735–754.

248. Borkhvardt, V. G. 1983. The development of the cranio-vertebral joint in salamanders. Vestnik Leningradskogo Universiteta, Biologiya: 26–33.

249. Borsuk-Bialynicka, M. 1973. Studies on the Pleistocene rhinoceros *Coelodonta antiquitatis* (Blumenbach). Palaeontologia polonica 29: 1–97.

250. Bosch, H. A. J. in den, and C. J. M. Musters. 1987. Scalation and skull morphology of a cyclopian *Natrix maura*. Journal of Herpetology 21: 107–114.

251. Bosma, J. F., ed. 1976a. *Symposium on Development of the Basicranium.* DHEW Publication (NIH) 76-989. Bethesda: U.S. Department of Health, Education, and Welfare.

252. Bosma, J. F. 1976b. Introduction. In *Symposium on Development of the Basicranium,* DHEW Publication (NIH) 76-989. Bethesda: U.S. Department of Health, Education and Welfare, pp. 3–28.

253. Bourne, G. H., ed. 1969. *The Chimpanzee,* vol. 1, *Anatomy, Behavior, and Diseases of Chimpanzees.* Basel: S. Karger.

254. Boy, J. A. 1974. Die larven der rhachitomen Amphibien (Amphibia: Temnospondylii; Karbon-Trias). Palaeontologische Zeitschrift 48: 236–268.

255. Boy, J. A. 1988. Über einige Vertrerer der Erypoidea (Amphibia: Temnospondylii) aus dem Europaischen Rotliegend (?hoechstes Oberkarbon-Perm). 1. *Sclerocephalus.* Palaeontologische Zeitschrift 62: 107–132.

256. Boy, J. A. 1989. Über einige Vertrerer der Erypoidea (Amphibia: Temnospondylii) aus dem Europaischen Rotliegend (?hoechstes Oberkarbon-Perm). 2. *Acanthostomatops.* Palaeontologische Zeitschrift 63: 133–151.

257. Boyd, J. S. 1976a. Studies on the appearance of the centers of ossification of the axial skeleton in the feline fetus. Anatomy, Histology, and Embryology 5: 193–205.

258. Boyd, J. S. 1976b. Radiographic studies on the developing feline skull. I. The foetal skull. British Veterinary Journal 132: 354–362.

259. Boyd, M. J. 1982. Morphology and relationships of the Upper Carboniferous aistopod amphibian, *Ophiderpeton nanum*. Palaeontology, London 25: 209–214.

260. Bragg, A. N. 1956. Dimorphism and cannibalism in tadpoles of *Scaphiopus bombifrons* (Amphibia, Salientia). Southwest Naturalist 1: 105–108.

261. Bragg, A. N., and W. N. Bragg. 1959. Variations in the mouth parts in tadpoles of *Scaphiopus* (*Spea*) *bombifrons* Cope (Amphibia: Salientia). Southwest Naturalist 3: 55–69.

262. Brandon, R. A., J. Jacobs, A. Wynn, and D. M. Sever. 1986. A naturally metamorphosed Tennessee cave salamander (*Gyrinophilus palleucus*). Journal of the Tennessee Academy of Science 61: 1–2.

263. Branson, B. A., and G. A. Moore. 1962. The lateralis components of the

acoustico-lateralis system in the sunfish family Centrarchidae. Copeia: 1–108.

264. Breder, C. M., Jr. 1944. Ocular anatomy and light sensitivity studies on the blind fish from Cueva de los Sabinos, Mexico. Zoologica 29: 131–144.

265. Breder, C. M., Jr. 1945. Compensating reactions to the loss of the lower jaw in a cave fish. Zoologica, New York 30: 95–100.

266. Breitwieser, B. 1969. Studies on the intraspecific variability of the skull of *Bathyergys suillus suillus* (Schreber, 1782, Mammalia, Rodentia, Bathyergidae). Zeitschrift für Saeugetierkunde 34: 321–347.

267. Brewster, B. 1987. Eye migration and cranial development during flatfish metamorphosis: A reappraisal (Teleostei: Pleuronectiformes). Journal of Fish Biology 31: 805–833.

268. Briel, W. 1979. Alterbestimmung mach Zahn- und Kiefermerkmalen an Siegerländer Rehböcken und Rothirschen und Sauerländer Sikahirschen. Zeitschrift Jagdwiss 24: 167–177.

269. Brinkley, L. L., and M. M. Vickermann. 1978. The mechanical role of the cranial base in palatal shelf movement: An experimental reexamination. Journal of Embryology and Experimental Morphology 48: 93–100.

270. Brock, G. T. 1937. The morphology of the ostrich chondrocranium. Proceedings of the Zoological Society of London. 107B: 225–243.

271. Brock, G. T. 1941a. The skull of *Acontias meleagris*, with a study of the affinities between lizards and snakes. Zoological Journal of the Linnean Society 41: 71–88.

272. Brock, G. T. 1941b. The skull of the chameleon, *Lophosaura ventralis* (Gray): Some developmental stages. Proceedings of the Zoological Society of London 110: 219–241.

273. Brodie, A. G. 1941. On the growth patterns of the human head: From the third month to the eighth year of life. American Journal of Anatomy 68: 209–262.

274. Bromage, T. G. 1980. A brief review of cartilage and controlling factors in chondrocranial morphogenesis. Acta morphologica Neerlando Scandinavica 18: 317–322.

275. Bromage, T. G. 1982. The scanning electron microscope in craniofacial remodeling research: Application of the topographic principle. Progress in Clinical and Biological Research 101: 143–153.

276. Bromage, T. G. 1989. Ontogeny of the early hominid face. Journal of Human Evolution 18: 751–773.

277. Broman, I. 1939. Über die Entwicklung der Geruchsorgane bei den Lungenfischen. Morphologische Jahrbuch 83: 85–106.

278. Bronner-Fraser, M. 1988. Distribution and function of tenascin during cranial neural crest development in the chick. In *Journal of Neuroscience Research*, J. D. Vellis, G. Ciment, and J. Lauder, eds. New York: Alan R. Liss, pp. 135–147.

279. Broom, R. 1946. Notes on a late Gorilla fetus. Annals of the Transvaal Museum 20: 347–350.

280. Brown, R. D., ed. 1983. *Antler Development in Cervidae*. Kingsville: Caeser Kleberg Wildlife Research Institute, Texas A & I University.

281. Bruce, J. A. 1941. Time and order of appearance of ossification centres and

their development in the skull of the rabbit. American Journal of Anatomy 68: 41–67.

282. Brylski, P. 1989. The ontogeny of morphological diversity in geomyoid rodents. Fortschritte der Zoologie 35: 220–223.

283. Bub, H. 1984. Kennzeichen und Mauser europäischer Singvögel, 3. Teil Seidenschwanz, Wasseramsel, Zaunkönig, Braunellen, Spötter, Laubsänger, Goldhähnchen (Bombycillidae, Cinclidae, Troglodytidae, Prunellidae, Sylviidae I). Die neue Brehm-Bücherei, no. 550: 1–200.

284. Bubenik, A. B. 1959. Ein weiterer Beitrag zu den Besonderheiten der Geweihtrophik beim Ren. Zeitschrift für Jagdwissenschaft 5: 51–55.

285. Bubenik, A. B. 1979. Zum Beitrag von E. ueckermann über die Spiesserstufe hinausgehende Geweihentwicklung beim Damhirsch (Dama dama [I.]) vom 1. Kopf. Zeitschrift für Jagdwissenschaft 25: 32–33.

286. Bubenik, G. A., and A. B. Bubenik. 1987. Recent advances in studies of antler development and neuroendocrine regulation of the antler cycle. In Biology and Management of the Cervidae, C. M. Wemmer, ed. Washington, D.C.: Smithsonian Institution Press, pp. 99–109.

287. Bubenik, G. A., A. B. Bubenik, G. M. Brown, and D. A. Wilson. 1975. The role of sex hormones in the growth of antler bone tissues. 1. Endocrine and metabolic effects of antiandrogen therapy. Journal of Experimental Zoology 194: 349–358.

288. Bubenik, G. A., A. B. Bubenik, E. D. Stevens, and A. G. Binnington. 1982. The effect of neurogenic stimulation on the development and growth of bony tissues. Journal of Experimental Zoology 219: 205–216.

289. Bubenik, G. A., A. J. Sempere, and J. Hamr. 1987. Developing antler, a model for endocrine regulation of bone growth: Consideration of a gradient of T_3, T_4, and alkaline phosphatase in the antler, jugular, and the saphenous veins. Calcified Tissue International 41: 38–43.

290. Buchalczyk, T., and A. L. Ruprecht. 1977. Skull variability of Mustela putorius Linnaeus, 1758. Acta theriologica 22: 87–120.

291. Buffetaut, E. 1977. Eugène Eudes-Deslongchamps et le parallélisme entre formes et stades embryonnaires chez les Crocodiliens (1868). Histoire et nature 11: 81–94.

292. Bühler, P. 1970. Schädelmorphologie und Kiefermechanik der Caprimulgidae (Aves). Zeitschrift für Morphologie der Tiere 66: 337–399.

293. Bühler, P. 1985. On the morphology of the skull of Archaeopteryx. In The Beginnings of Birds, Proceedings of the International Archaeopteryx Conference, Eichstatt, 1984, M. K. Hecht, J. H. Ostrom, G. Viohl, and P. Wellnhofer, eds. Eichstatt: Freunde des Jura-Museums Eichstatt, pp. 135–140.

294. Burdi, A. R. 1968. Morphogenesis of mandibular dental arch shape in human embryos. Journal of Dental Research 47: 50–58.

295. Burdi, A. R. 1976. Early development of the human basicranium: Its morphogenetic controls, growth patterns, and relations. In Development of the Basicranium, J. F. Bosma, ed. Bethesda: U.S. Department of Health, Education, and Welfare, pp. 81–90.

296. Burdi, A. R., and M. N. Spyropoulos. 1978. Prenatal growth patterns of the

human mandible and masseter muscle complex. American Journal of Orthodontics 74: 380–387.

297. Burgess, A. M. C. 1982. The developmental effect of calcitonin on the interocular distance in early *Xenopus* embryos. Journal of Anatomy 135: 745–751.

298. Burgess, A. M. C. 1985. The effect of calcitonin on the prechordal mesoderm, neural plate, and neural crest of *Xenopus laevis*. Journal of Anatomy 140: 49–55.

299. Burgin, T. 1987. Asymmetry and functional design: The pharyngeal apparatus in Solenoid flatfishes (Pisces: Pleuronectiformes). Netherlands Journal of Zoology 37: 322–364.

300. Buscalioni, A. D., E. Buffetaur, and J. L. Sanz. 1984. An immature specimen of the crocodilian *Bernissartia* from the Lower Cretaceous of Gaive (province of Teruel, Spain). Palaeontology, London 27: 809–814.

301. Butler, H. 1983. The embryology of the lesser galago (*Galago senegalensis*). Contributions of Primatology 19: 1–156.

302. Butler, J. L. 1960. Development of the weberian apparatus of a catostomid fish. Proceedings of the Iowa Academy of Science 67: 532–543.

303. Byrd, K. E., and D. R. Swindler. 1980. Palatal growth in *Macaca nemestrina*. Primates 21: 253–261.

304. Cadenat, H. 1952. Problème du rangement de l'arcade temporaire. Cahiers odontostomatologiques 2: 19.

305. Camperio Ciani, A. 1989. Cranial morphology and development: New light on the evolution of language. Human Evolution 4: 9–32.

306. Canavase, B. 1987. Variabilità e corrispondenza numerica degli ossicini sclerali negli occhi di tacchino, pollo e quaglia. Summa 4: 27–31.

307. Canavase, B., P. Durio, S. Bellardi, and P. Porporato. 1986. Caratteristiche morfologiche degli ossicini sclerali e dell'os opticus in alcune specie di uccelli domestici e selvatici. Annali della Facoltà di Medicina Veterinaria di Torino 31: 1–23.

308. Cantrell, C., G. Baskin, and J. Blanchard. 1987. Craniosynostosis in two African green monkeys. Laboratory Animal Science 37: 631–634.

309. Capel-Williams, G., and D. Pratten. 1978. The diet of adult and juvenile *Agama bibroni* (Reptilia, Lacertae) and a study of the jaw mechanisms in the two age groups. Journal of Zoology, London 185: 309–318.

310. Caronna, E. W. 1984. Dati preliminari sull'evoluzione dell'ossifazione embrionale in *Cleithrionomys glareolus* Schr. Atti della Società italiana di scienze naturali, e del Museo civile di storia naturale, Milan 125: 121–131.

311. Carroll, R. L. 1986. Developmental processes and the origin of lepospondyls. In *Studies in Herpetology*, Z. Roček, ed. Prague: Charles University, pp. 45–48.

312. Carvalho, F. M. 1980. Alimentação do mapará (*Hypophthalmus edentalus* Spix, 1829) do Lago do Castanho, Amazonas (Siliriformes, Hypophthalmidae). Acta amazonica 10: 379–387.

313. Cassarà, A. 1958. Gli effetti d'asportazione totale di endoderma in *Discoglossus pictus* allo stadio di tappovitellino, con particolare riguardo alla

formazione della cartilagini dello scheletto ce falico. Atti dell'Accademia, Palermo 17: 247–267.

314. Cassin, C. 1975. Crête neurale et capacité morphogénétique du stomodeum chez *Pleurodeles waltlii* (Amphibien Urodèle). Revue stomato-odontologique du nord de la France 118: 149–162.

315. Cassin, C., and A. Capuron. 1972. Obtention d'ouvertures buccales et de bouches complètes par implantation, dans le blastocoèle, de tissus embryonnaires de *Pleurodeles waltlii* Michah. (Amphibien Urodèle). Comptes rendus Académie des sciences, Paris, ser. D, 275: 2953–2956.

316. Cassin, C., and A. Capuron. 1977. Évolution de la capacité morphogénétique de la région stomodéale chez l'embryon de *Pleurodeles waltlii* Michah. (Amphibien Urodèle): Étude par transplantation intrablastocéienne et par culture *in vitro*. Wilhelm Roux Archives of Developmental Biology 181: 107–112.

317. Cassin, C., and A. Capuron. 1979. Buccal organogenesis in *Pleurodeles waltlii* Michah. (Urodele, Amphibian): Study by intrablastocoelic transplantation and *in vitro* culture. Journal de biologie buccale 7: 61–76.

318. Catt, D. C. 1979. Age determination in Bennett's wallaby, *Macropus rufogriseus fruticus* (Marsupialia), in South Canterbury, New Zealand. Australian Wildlife Research 6: 13–18.

319. Cave, A. J. E. 1964. Cranial epiphyses in mammals. Nature 204: 838–839.

320. Cave, A. J. E., and J. E. King. 1964. The ossiculum mastoideum of the otariid skull. Annals and Magazine of Natural History 7: 235–240.

321. Chacko, T. 1965a. The hyolaryngeal apparatus of two anurans. Acta zoologica, Stockholm 46: 83–108.

322. Chacko, T. 1965b. The development and metamorphosis of the hyobranchial skeleton in *Rana tigrina*, the Indian bull frog. Acta zoologica, Stockholm 46: 311–328.

323. Chacko, T. 1976. Development of chondrocranium in *Rana tigrina* (Daubin). Journal of the Zoological Society of India 28: 103–138.

324. Chan, W. Y., and P. P. L. Tam. 1988. A morphological and experimental study of the mesencephalic neural crest cells in the mouse embryo using wheat germ agglutinin-gold conjugate as the cell marker. Development 102: 427–442.

325. Chang, J. 1985. Study on the division of age group and the age composition of population of striped hamster in Beijing area. Acta theriologica sinica 5: 141–150.

326. Chang, T. K. 1949a. Skeletal growth in Ancon sheep. Growth 13: 221–267.

327. Chang, T. K. 1949b. Morphological study on the skeleton of Ancon sheep. Growth 13: 269–297.

328. Chang, T. K., and W. Landauer. 1950. Observations on the skeleton of African dwarf goats. Journal of Morphology 86: 367–379.

329. Chanin, P. 1983. Observations on two populations of feral mink in Devon, U.K. Mammalia 47: 463–476.

330. Chapman, N. 1984. *Fallow Deer*. Oswestry, U.K.: Mammal Society.

331. Chardon, M., and P. Vandewalle. 1971. Comparaison de la région céphalique chez cinq espèces du genre *Tilapia*, dont trois incubateurs buccaux. Annales de la Société royale zoologique de Belgique, Brussels 101: 3–24.

332. Chekanovskaia, O. V. 1937. Development of the skull in the water snake (*Tropidonotus natrix*). Russkii arkhiv anatomii, gistologii i émbriologii 15: 3–33.

333. Chen, P. S., and F. Baltzer. 1954. Chimarische Haftfaden nach xenoplastichen Ektodermaustausch zwischen *Triton* und *Bombinator*. Wilhelm Roux Archives of Developmental Biology 147: 214–258.

334. Cherepanov, G. U. 1988. Theory of thecal and epithecal ossifications in the context of morphogenetic data. Zoologicheskii zhurnal 67: 729–738.

335. Chernousova, N. F. 1984. Analysis of morphological characters and growth features of three forms of voles of the group *Microtus juldaschi-carruthersi*. In *Population Ecology and Morphology of Mammals*, L. N. Dobrinskij, ed. Sverdlovsk: Academy of Sciences, USSR, Urals Scientific Center, pp. 124–141.

336. Cheverud, J. M. 1982a. Phenotypic, genetic, and environmental morphological integration in the cranium. Evolution 36: 499–516.

337. Cheverud, J. M. 1982b. Relationships among ontogenetic, static, and evolutionary allometry. American Journal of Physical Anthropology 59: 139–149.

338. Cheverud, J. M., L. J. Leamy, W. R. Atchley, and J. J. Rutledge. 1983. Quantitative genetics and the evolution of ontogeny. 1. Ontogenetic changes in quantitative genetic variance components in randombred mice. Genetical Research, Cambridge 42: 65–75.

339. Cheverud, J. M., and J. T. Richtsmeier. 1986. Finite-element scaling applied to sexual dimorphism in Rhesus macaque (*Macaca mulatta*) facial growth. Systematic Zoology 35: 381–399.

340. Chiakulas, J. J. 1957. The specificity and differential fusion of cartilage derived from mesoderm and mesectoderm. Journal of Experimental Zoology 136: 287–299.

341. Chibon, P. 1964. Analyse par la méthode de marquage nucléaire a la thymidine tritiée des dérivés de la crête neurale céphalique chez l'Urodèle *Pleurodeles waltlii* Michah. Comptes rendus hebbomadaires des séances de l'Académie des sciences, Paris 259: 3624–3627.

342. Chibon, P. 1966. Analyse expérimentale de la régionalisation et des capacités morphogénétiques de la crête neurale chez l'amphibien urodèle *Pleurodeles waltlii* Michah. Mémoires de la Société zoologique de France 36: 1–107.

343. Chibon, P. 1967. Marquage nucléaire par la thymidine tritiée des dérivés de la crête neurale chez l'amphibien urodèle *Pleurodeles waltlii* Michah. Journal of Embryology and Experimental Morphology 18: 343–358.

344. Chopra, S. R. K. 1957. The cranial suture closure in monkeys. Proceedings of the Zoological Society of London 128: 67–112.

345. Christ, B., M. Jacob, H. J. Jacob, and F. Wachtler. 1989. On the origin and development of the cranial connective tissue, bones, and muscles in avian chimeras. In *Trends in Vertebrate Morphology*, Fortschritte der Zoologie, 35, H. Splechtna and H. Hilgers, eds. Stuttgart: Gustav-Fischer Verlag, pp. 416–420.

346. Christophorov, O. L. 1983. Some morphological abnormalities in natural populations of Atlantic salmon and sea trout. Sbornki Nauchnykh trudov

(Gosudarstvennyi) Nauchno-Isslednatelskii Institut Ozernogo i Rechnogo rybnogo Khoziaistva. 195: 140–143.

347. Chung, H-M., A. W. Neff, and G. M. Malacinski. 1989. Autonomous death of amphibian (*Xenopus laevis*) cranial myotomes. Journal of Experimental Zoology 251: 290–299.

348. Claeys, H., and W. Verraes. 1984. Note on the development of a temporary interbranchial IV in *Salmo gairdneri* Richardson, 1836 (Teleostei: Salmonidae). Netherlands Journal of Zoology 34: 418–425.

349. Clemen, G. 1978. Relations between osseous palate and its dental laminae in *Salamandra salamandra* (L.) during metamorphosis. Wilhelm Roux Archives of Developmental Biology 185: 19–36.

350. Clemen, G. 1979a. Experimental alterations to the osseous palate in the larval axolotl and their results during metamorphosis. Zoologischer Anzeiger 203: 23–34.

351. Clemen, G. 1979b. Untersuchungen zur Bildung der Vomerspange bei *Salamandra salamandra* (L.) Wilhelm Roux Archives of Developmental Biology 185: 305–321.

352. Clemen, G. 1979c. Die Bedeutung des Ramus palatinus für die Vomerspangenbildung bie *Salamandra salamandra*. Wilhelm Roux Archives of Developmental Biology 187: 219–230.

353. Clemen, G. 1988a. Competence and reactions of early- and late-larval dental laminae in original and not-original dental systems of *Ambystoma mexicanum* Shaw. Archives de biologie, Brussels 99: 307–324.

354. Clemen, G. 1988b. Experimental analysis of the capacity of dental laminae in *Ambystoma mexicanum* (L.) Shaw. Archives de biologie, Brussels 99: 111–132.

355. Clemen, G., and H. Greven. 1979. Morphological studies on the mouth cavity of urodeles. V. The teeth of the upper jaw and the palate in *Triturus vulgaris* (L.) (Salamandridae: Amphibia). Zoologische Jahrbücher, Anatomie 102: 170–186.

356. Clemen, G., and H. Greven. 1980. Morphologische untersuchungen au der mundhohle von urodelen. VII. Die munddachbeyahnung von *Amphiuma* (Amphiumidae: Amphibia). Bonner Zoologische Beiträge 31: 357–362.

357. Clemen, G., and H. Greven. 1988. Morphological studies on the mouth cavity of Urodela. IX. Teeth of the palate and splenials in *Siren* and *Pseudobranchus* (Sirenidae: Amphibae). Zeitschrift für zoologische Systematik und Evolutionsforschung 26: 135–143.

358. Cleveland, L., D. R. Buckler, F. L. Mayer, and D. R. Branson. 1982. Toxicity of three preparations of pentachlorophenol to fathead minnows: A comparative study. Environmental Toxicology and Chemistry 6: 205–212.

359. Cochard, L. R. 1985. Ontogenetic allometry of the skull and dentition of the Rhesus monkey (*Macaca mulatta*). In *Size and Scaling in Primate Biology*, W. L. Jungers, ed. New York: Plenum Press, pp. 231–255.

360. Coffin-Collins, P. A., and B. K. Hall. 1989. Chondrogenesis of mandibular mesenchyme from the embryonic chick is inhibited by mandibular epithelium and by epidermal growth factor. International Journal of Developmental Biology 33: 297–311.

361. Collette, B. B. 1982. Recognition of two species of double-lined mackerels (*Grammatorcynus:* Scombridae). Proceedings of the Biological Society of Washington 96: 715–718.

362. Collette, B. B., G. E. McGowen, N. V. Parin, and S. Mito. 1984. Beloniformes: Development and relationships. In *Ontogeny and Systematics of Fishes,* American Society of Ichthyologists and Herpetologists Special Publication no. 1, H. G. Moser, ed. Lawrence, Kans.: Allen Press, pp. 335–354.

363. Collette, B. B., T. Potthoff, W. J. Richards, S. Ueyanagi, J. L. Russo, and Y. Nishikawa. 1984. Scombroidei: Development and relationships. In *Ontogeny and Systematics of Fishes,* American Society of Ichthyologists and Herpetologists Special Publication no. 1, H. G. Moser, ed. Lawrence, Kans.: Allen Press, pp. 591–620.

364. Coman, B. J. 1989. The age structure of a sample of red foxes (*Vulpes vulpes* L.) taken by hunters in Victoria. Australian Wildlife Research 15: 223–229.

365. Cong, L., L. Hou, and X. Wu. 1984. Age variation in the skull of *Alligator sinensis* (Chinensis) Fauvel in topographic anatomy. Acta herpetologica sinica 3: 1–13.

366. Conroy, G. C. 1980. Ontogeny, auditory structures, and primate evolution. American Journal of Physical Anthropology 52: 443–451.

367. Coochi, U. 1944. Die Ossifikations des skelettes beim Star und Mauersegler und deren Beziehung zur Frage des Unterschiedes zwischen Nestflüchter und Nesthocker. Neujahrsblatt herausgegeben von der Naturoforschenden Gesellschaft in Zürich 89: 122–133.

368. Cooke, J. 1988. The early embryo and the formation of body pattern. American Scientist 76 (1): 35–41.

369. Cooke, J. 1989. Induction and organization of the body plan in *Xenopus* development. In *Cellular Basis of Morphogenesis,* D. Evered and J. Marsh, eds. New York: John Wiley and Sons, pp. 187–194.

370. Cooper, J. E. 1981. Development and replacement order of pharyngeal teeth in the golden shiner, *Notemigonus crysoleucas.* Ohio Journal of Science 8: 14–18.

371. Cooper, J. E., L. Arnold, and G. M. Henderson. 1982. A developmental abnormality in the Round Island skink *Leiolopisma telfarii.* Dodo 19: 78–81.

372. Copray, J. C. V. M., J. M. N. Dibbets, and T. Kantomaa. 1988. The role of condylar cartilage in the development of the temporomandibular joint. Angle Orthodontist 58: 369–380.

373. Cordier, R., and A. Dalcq. 1954. Organs stato-acoustique. In *Traité de Zoologie,* vol. 12, *Vertébrés, embryologie, grands problèmes d'anatomie comparée, caracteristiques biochemiques,* P. P. Grassé, ed. Paris: Masson et Cie, pp. 451–521.

374. Corruccini, R. S., and R. L. Ciochon. 1979. Primate facial allometry and interpretations of australopithecine variation. Nature 281: 62–64.

375. Corruccini, R. S., and A. M. Henderson. 1978. Multivariate dental allometry in primates. American Journal of Physical Anthropology 48: 203–208.

376. Corsin, J. 1961. Étude de quelques corrélations morphogénétiques dans le développement du chondrocrâne de *Salmo.* Bulletin de la Société zoologique de France. 86: 772–785.

377. Corsin, J. 1966a. The development of the osteocranium of *Pleurodeles waltlii* Michahelles. Journal of Morphology 119: 209–216.

378. Corsin, J. 1966b. Quelques problèmes de morphogenèse du crâne chez les urodèles. In *Problèmes actuels de paléontologie (évolution des vertébrés)*, Colloque international du Centre national de la recherche scientifique 163: 295–300.

379. Corsin, J. 1968a. Influence des placodes et des ébauches optiques sur la morphogenèse du squelette crânien chez *Pleurodeles waltlii* Michah. Annales d'embryologie et de morphogenèse 1: 41–48.

380. Corsin, J. 1968b. Rôle de la compétition osseuse dans la forme des os du toit crânien des urodèles. Journal of Embryology and Experimental Morphology 19: 103–108.

381. Corsin, J. 1972. Rôle des ébauches sensorielles au cours de la morphogenèse du chondrocrâne chez *Pleurodeles waltlii* Michah. Archives d'anatomie microscopique et de morphologie expérimentale 61: 47–60.

382. Coulombre, A. A., and J. L. Coulombre. 1973. The skeleton of the eye. II. Overlap of the scleral ossicles of the domestic fowl. Developmental Biology 33: 257–267.

383. Coulombre, A. J., J. L. Coulombre, and H. Mehta. 1962. The skeleton of the eye. 1. Conjunctival papillae and scleral ossicles. Developmental Biology 5: 382–401.

384. Coulombre, A. J., and E. S. Crelin. 1958. The role of the developing eye in the morphogenesis of the avian skull. American Journal of Physical Anthropology 16: 25–37.

385. Couly, G. F., and N. M. Le Douarin. 1985. Mapping of the early neural primordium in quail-chick chimeras. 1. Developmental relationships between placodes, facial ectoderm, and prosencephalon. Developmental Biology 110: 422–439.

386. Couly, G. F., and N. M. Le Douarin. 1987. Mapping of the early neural primordium in quail-chick chimeras. II. The prosencephalic neural plate and neural folds: Implications for the genesis of cephalic human congenital abnormalities. Developmental Biology 120: 198–214.

387. Cousin, P. O., R. Fenart, and R. Deblock. 1981. Ontogenetic variations of basicranial and facial angles: Comparative studies on *Homo* and *Pan*. Bulletin et mémoires de la Société d'anthropologie de Paris 13: 189–212.

388. Cousin, R. 1972. Biparietal spherization during human ontogenesis: First statistical approach. Comptes rendus, Association des Anatomistes 154: 995–1004.

389. Cozzi, B., I. de Francesco, L. Cagnolaro, and L. Leonardi. 1985. Radiological observations on the skeletal development in fetal and newborn specimens of *Delphinus delphis* L. and *Stenella coeruleoalba* P (Meyen) (Mammalia Cetacea). Atti della Società italiana di scienza naturali 126: 120–136.

390. Crabtree, C. B. 1985. Sexual dimorphism of the upper jaw in *Gallichthys mirabilis*. Bulletin of the Southern California Academy of Science 94: 96–103.

391. Crelin, E. S. 1981. Development of the musculoskeletal system. Clinical Symposium 33 (1): 1–36.

392. Crelin, E. S. 1987. *The Human Vocal Tract: Anatomy, Function, Development, and Evolution.* New York: Vantage Press.

393. Crompton, A. W. 1953. The development of the chondrocranium of *Spheniscus demersus* with special reference to the columella auris. Acta zoologica, Stockholm 34: 72–146.

394. Croucher, S. J., and C. Tickle. 1989. Characterization of epithelial domains in the nasal passages of chick embryos: Spatial and temporal mapping of a range of extracellular matrix and cell surface molecules during development of the nasal placode. Development 106: 493–509.

395. Cunat, J. J., S. N. Bhasker, and J. P. Weinmann. 1956. Development of the squamoso-mandibular articulation in the rat. Journal of Dental Research 35: 533–546.

396. Curran, B. K., and D. C. Weaver. 1982. The use of the coefficient of agreement and likelihood ratio test to examine the development of the skeletons. American Journal of Physical Anthropology 58: 343–346.

397. Cusimano, T., A. Fagone, and G. Reverberi. 1962. On the origin of the larval mouth in the anurans. Acta embryologiae et morphologiae experimentalis 5: 82–103.

398. Cusimano-Carollo, T. 1962. Sulla capacità organo-formative delle pieghe neurali degli Anuri: Richerche su *Discoglossus pictus* Otth. Accademia Nazionale dei Lincei. Atti. Classe di Scienze Fisiche, Matematiche, e Naturali. Rendiconti 33: 354–358.

399. Cusimano-Carollo, T. 1963. Investigation of the ability of the neural folds to induce a mouth in *Discoglossus pictus* embryos. Acta embryologiea et morphologiae experimentalis 6: 158–168.

400. Cusimano-Carollo, T. 1967. La piega neurale trasversa e la formazione della bocca nelle larve di *Discoglossus pictus*. Accademia Nazionale dei Lincei. Atti. Classe di Scienze Fisiche, Matematiche, e Naturali. Rendiconti 43: 252–258.

401. Cusimano-Carollo, T. 1969. Phenomena of induction by the transverse neural fold during the formation of the mouth in *Discoglossus pictus*. Acta embryologiae et morphologiae experimentalis 1: 97–110.

402. Cusimano-Carollo, T. 1972. On the mechanism of the formation of the larval mouth in *Discoglossus*. Acta embryologiae et morphologiae experimentalis 4: 289–332.

403. Cussac, V. E., and M. C. Maggese. 1988. Ontogeny of the maxillary barbels and palatine-maxillary mechanism in the catfish *Rhamdia sapo* (Pisces, Pimelodidae). Revista brasileira de biologia 48: 195–201.

404. Czaplewski, N. J. 1987. Deciduous teeth of *Thyroptera tricolor*. Bat Research News 28: 23–25.

405. Daget, J. 1964. La crâne des Téléostéens. Mémoires du Muséum national d'histoire naturelle, ser. A, Zoologie 31: 163–340.

406. Daget, J., and J. Arnault. 1965. Étude de la croissance chez *Polypterus senegalus* Cuvier. Acta zoologica, Stockholm 46: 297–309.

407. Daget, J., and F. d'Aubenton. 1957. Développement et morphologie du crâne d'*Heterotis niloticus* Ehr. Bulletin de l'Institut française d'Afrique Noire, Ser. A, Sciences naturelles 3: 881–936.

408. Daget, J., M.-L. Bauchot, R. Bauchot, and J. Arnault. 1964. Développement

du chondrocrâne et des arcs aortiques chez *Polypterus senegalus* Cuvier. Acta zoologica, Stockholm 46: 201–244.

409. Dahinten, S. L., H. M. Pucciarelli, and F. R. Moreno. 1988. Effect of gonadal activity on the cranial dimorphism of the rat. Acta anatomica 132: 324–331.

410. Dalcq, A., and J. Pasteels. 1954. Le développment des vertébrés. In *Traité de Zoologie*, vol. 12, *Vertébrés: Généralités, embryologie, topographique anatomie comparée*, P. P. Grassé, ed. Paris: Masson et Cie, pp. 35–201.

411. Dalrymple, G. H. 1977. Intraspecific variation in the cranial feeding mechanism of turtles of the genus *Trionyx* (Reptilia, Testudines, Trionychidae). Journal of Herpetology 11: 255–286.

412. Damas, H. 1942. Le développement de la tête de la lamproie (*Lampetra fluviatilis* L.). Annales de la Société royale zoologique de Belgique, Brussels 73: 201–211.

413. Damas, H. 1944. Recherches sur le développement de *Lampetra fluviatilis* L.: Contribution à l'étude de la céphalogenèse des Vertébrés. Archives de biologie 55: 1–284.

414. Damas, H. 1958. Crâne des Agnathes. In *Traité de Zoologie*, vol. 13(1), *Agnathes et poissons: Anatomie, éthologie, systématique*, P.-P. Grassé, ed. Paris: Masson, pp. 22–39.

415. Dambricourt Malasse, A. 1988. Hominisation et foetalisation (Bolk, 1926). Comptes rendus, Académie des sciences, ser. 2, Mécanique, physique, chimie, sciences de l'univers, Sciences de la Terre 307: 199–204.

416. D'Amico-Martel, A., T. R. van de Water, J. A. M. Wotton, and R. R. Minor. 1987. Changes in the types of collagen synthesized during chondrogenesis of the mouse otic capsule. Developmental Biology 120: 542–555.

417. D'Angelo, S., and H. A. Charipper. 1939. The morphology of the thyroid gland in the metamorphosing *Rana pipiens*. Journal of Morphology 64: 355–372.

418. Danielson, M., and I. Kihlstrom. 1986. Calcification of the rabbit fetal skeleton. Growth 50: 378–384.

419. Datta, N. C., A. K. Saha, and A. Baiyda. 1975. Comparative study of osteocranium and Weberian apparatus of *Clarias batrachus* (Linn.) and *Heteropneustes fossilis* (Bl.) (Pisces). Zoologisches Anzeiger 195: 374–386.

420. Davidson, D. 1988. Segmentation in frogs. Development 104 (suppl.): 221–230.

421. Davies, M. 1989. Ontogeny of bone and the role of heterochrony in the myobatrachine genera *Uperoleia*, *Crinia*, and *Pseudophryne* (Anura: Leptodactylidae: Myobatrachinae). Journal of Morphology 200: 269–300.

422. Davies, M., and M. J. Littlejohn. 1986. Frogs of the genus *Uperoleia* Gray (Anura: Leptodactylidae) in south-eastern Australia. Transactions of the Royal Society of South Australia 109: 111–143.

423. Davies, M., K. R. McDonald, and C. Corben. 1986. The genus *Uperoleia* Gray (Anura: Leptodactylidae) in Queensland, Australia. Proceedings of the Royal Society of Victoria 98: 147–188.

424. Davis, D. D. 1964. The giant panda: Morphological studies of evolutionary mechanisms. Fieldiana: Zoology, Memoirs 3: 1–339.

425. Davis, D. E. 1947. Size of bursa of Fabricius compared with ossification of skull and maturity of gonads. Journal of Wildlife Management 11: 244–3251.
426. Dawson, J. A. 1963. The oral cavity, the "jaws" and the horny teeth of Myxine glutinosa. In The Biology of Myxine, A. Brodal and R. Fange, eds. Oslo: Universitets Forlaget, pp. 231–255.
427. Dean, J. N., J. L. Glenn, and R. C. Straight. 1980. Bilateral cleft labial and palate in the progeny of a Crotalus viridis viridis. Rafinesque. Herpetological Review 11: 91–92.
428. Dean, M. C., and B. A. Wood. 1981. Developing pongid dentition and its use for ageing crania in comparative cross-sectional growth studies. Folia primatologica 36: 111–127.
429. Dean, M. C., and B. A. Wood. 1984. Phylogeny, neoteny, and growth of the cranial base in hominoids. Folia primatologica 43: 157–180.
430. de Beer, G. R. 1937. The Development of the Vertebrate Skull. London: Oxford University Press. Reissued. Chicago: University of Chicago Press, 1985.
431. de Beer, G. R. 1938. Embryology and Evolution. In Evolution: Essays on Aspects of Evolutionary Biology, G. R. de Beer, ed. Oxford: Clarendon Press, pp. 55–77.
432. de Beer, G. R. 1939. The identity of morphological units. In À la mémoire de A. N. Sewertzoff, vol. 1. Moscow, pp. 81–96.
433. de Beer, G. R. 1947. The differentiation of neural crest cells into visceral cartilages and odontoblasts in Amblystoma, and a re-examination of the germ-layer theory. Proceedings of the Royal Society of London 134B: 377–398.
434. de Beer, G. R. 1948. Embryology and the evolution of man. Royal Society of South Africa, Robert Broom Commemorative Volume: 181–190.
435. de Beer, G. R. 1949a. Caruncles and egg-teeth: Some aspects of the concept of homology. Proceedings of the Linnean Society of London 161: 218–224.
436. de Beer, G. R. 1949b. Les trabecules du crâne. Comptes rendus, 13e Congrès international de zoologie, Paris, 1948: 287–289.
437. de Beer, G. R. 1955. The continuity between the cavities of the premandibular somites and of Rathke's pocket in Torpedo. Quarterly Journal of Microscopical Science 96: 279–283.
438. de Beer, G. R. 1958. Embryos and Ancestors. 3d ed. London: Oxford University Press.
439. de Beer, G. R., and W. A. Fell. 1937. The development of the Monotremata—part III. The development of the skull of Ornithorhynchus. Transactions of the Zoological Society of London 23: 1–42.
440. de Blase, A. F. 1980. The bats of Iran: Systematics, distribution, ecology. Fieldiana: Zoology 4: 1–424.
441. de Block, R., and R. Fenart. 1977. Basal cranial angles in chimpanzees. Bulletin of the Association of Anatomy 61: 183–188.
442. de Buffrénil, V. 1982a. Morphogenesis of bone ornamentation in extant and extinct crocodiles. Zoomorphology 99: 155–166.

443. de Buffrénil, V. 1982b. Données preliminaires sur la presence de lignes d'arrêt de croissance periostiques dans le mandible du marsouin commun, *Phocaena phocaena* (L.) et leur utilisation comme indicateur de l'age. Canadian Journal of Zoology 60: 2557–2567.

444. de Buffrénil, V., and E. Buffetaut. 1981. Skeletal growth lines in an Eocene crocodilian skull from Wyoming as an indicator of ontogenetic age and paleoclimatic conditions. Journal of Vertebrate Paleontology 1: 57–66.

445. de Buffrénil, V., and A. Collet. 1983. Donneés methodologiques sur l'emploi de la technique squelettochronologique chez le dauphin commun (*Delphinus delphis* L.). Annales de sciences naturelles, Zoologie et biologie animale 5: 269–284.

446. de Buffrénil, V., A. Collet, and M. Pascal. 1985. Ontogenetic development of skeletal weight in a small delphinid, *Delphinus delphis* (Cetacea, Odontoceti). Zoomorphology 105: 335–344.

447. de Buffrénil, V., and M. Pascal. 1984. Croissance et morphogenèse postnatales de la mandibule du vison (*Mustela vison* Schreiber): Données sur la dynamique et l'interprétation fonctionelle des dépôts osseux mandibulaires. Canadian Journal of Zoology 62: 2026–2037.

448. Degn, H. J. 1974. Wormian bones in a sample of Danish squirrels, *Sciurus vulgaris fuscoater* Linne, 1758. Saeugetierkundliche Mitteilungen 22: 236–238.

449. de Haven, R. W., F. T. Crase, and M. R. Miller. 1974. Aging tricolored blackbirds by cranial ossification. Bird Banding 45: 156–159.

450. de Jager, E. F. J. 1939. The gymnophione quadrate and its processes with special reference to the processus ascendens in a juvenile *Ichthyophis glutinosus*. Anatomisches Anzeiger 88: 223–232.

451. de Jager, E. F. J. 1947. Some points in the development of the stages of the *Ichthyophis glutinosus*. Anatomisches Anzeiger 96: 203–210.

452. de Jongh, H. J. 1968. Functional morphology of the jaw apparatus of larvae and metamorphosing *Rana temporaria* L. Netherlands Journal of Zoology 18: 1–103.

453. de Kock, J. M. 1955. The cranial morphology of *Sturnus vulgaris vulgaris* Linnaeus. Annals of the University of Stellenbosch 31A: 153–177.

454. de Kock, J. M. 1987. The development of the chondrocranium of *Melopsittacus undulatus*. Advances in Anatomy, Embryology, and Cell Biology 104: 1–80.

455. Delaire, J. 1972. The base of the skull and maxillary morphology (data obtained and research perspectives). Fortschritte der Kieferorthopaedie 33: 375–386.

456. Delaire, J., and D. Precious. 1987. Interaction of the development of the nasal septum, the nasal pyramid, and the face. International Journal of Pediatric Otorhinolaryngology 12: 311–326.

457. Delattre, A., and R. Fenart. 1955. Le développement du crâne du gorilla et du chimpanze comparé au développement du crâne humain. Bulletin et mémoires de la Société d'anthropologie de Paris 60: 159–173.

458. Demes, B., N. Creel, and H. Preuschoft. 1986. Functional significance of allometric trends in the hominoid masticatory apparatus. In *Primate Evolu-*

tion, J. G. Else and P. C. Lee, eds. Cambridge: Cambridge University Press, pp. 229–237.

459. Dencker, L., R. d'Argy, B. R. G. Danielsson, H. Ghantous, and G. O. Sperber. 1987. Saturable accumulation of retinoic acid in neural and neural crest derived cells in early embryonic development. Developmental Pharmacology and Therapeutics 10: 212–223.

460. Dent, J. N. 1942. The embryonic development of *Plethodon cinereus* as correlated with the differentiation and functioning of the thyroid gland. Journal of Morphology 71: 577–601.

461. Dent, J. N., and J. S. Kirby-Smith. 1963. Metamorphic physiology and morphology of the cave salamander *Gyrinophilus palleucus.* Copeia: 119–130.

462. Deraniyagala, P. E. P. 1958. Reproduction in the monitor lizard *Varanus bengalensis* (Daudin). Spolia zeylanica 28: 161–166.

463. de Ricqles, A., and J. R. Bolt. 1983. Jaw growth and tooth replacement in *Captorhinus aguti* (Reptilia, Captorhinomorpha): A morphological and histological analysis. Journal of Vertebrate Paleontology 3: 7–24.

464. De Sa, R. O. 1988. Chondrocranium and ossification sequence of *Hyla lanciformis.* Journal of Morphology 195: 345–356.

465. De Sylva, D. P., and W. N. Eschmeyer. 1977. Systematics and biology of the deep-sea fish family Gibberichthyidae, a senior synonym of the family Kasidoroidae. Proceedings of the California Academy of Sciences, ser. 4, 41: 215–231.

466. Dethlefsen, V. 1988. Skelettdeformationen des Kabeljau (*Gadus morthua*) in der sudlichen Nordsee. Informationen für die Fischwirtschaft 35: 70–74.

467. Devillers, C. 1944a. Morphogenèse de quelques os craniens chez la truite arc-en-ciel, *Salmo irideus* (Gibb). Annales des sciences naturelles, Zoologie et biologie animale 6: 25–31.

468. Devillers, C. 1944b. Le rôle des pit-organs dans la morphogenèse de l'ostéocrâne des téléostéens: Le problème du squamosal. Bulletin du Muséum d'histoire naturelle, Paris 16: 295–297.

469. Devillers, C. 1944c. Le système sensoriel céphalique du Gardon (*Leuciscus rutilus* L.). Bulletin de la Société de France 69: 94–97.

470. Devillers, C. 1947. Recherches sur la crâne dermique des téléostéens. Annales de paleontologie, Paris 33: 1–94.

471. Devillers, C. 1949a. Le rôle système sensoriel céphalique dans l'edification du crâne dermiques des poissons. Comptes rendus, 13e Congrès international de zoologie, Paris, 1948: 290–293.

472. Devillers, C. 1949b. Rapport des os dermiques avec le système latéral. Comptes rendus, 13e Congrès international de zoologie, Paris, 1948: 293–297.

473. Devillers, C. 1950. Quelques aspects de l'évolution du crâne chez les poissons. L'année biologique, 3d ser., 54: 145–180.

474. Devillers, C. 1958. Le crâne des poissons. In *Traité de Zoologie,* vol. 13(1), *Agnathes et poissons: anatomie, éthologie, systématique, biologie,* P.-P. Grassé, ed. Paris: Masson et Cie, pp. 551–687.

475. Devillers, C. 1965. The role of morphogenesis in the origin of higher levels of organization. Systematic Zoology 14: 259–271.

476. Devillers, C., and J. Corsin. 1968. Les os dermiques crânien des poissons et des amphibiens: Pointe de vue embryologique sur les "territoires osseux" et les "fusions." In *Current Problems of Lower Vertebrate Phylogeny*, T. Ørvig, ed. Stockholm: Almqvist and Wiksell, pp. 413–428.

477. Devillers, C., J. Mahe, D. Ambroise, R. Bauchot, and E. Chatelain. 1984. Allometric studies on the skull of living and fossil Equidae (Mammalia: Perissodactyla). Journal of Vertebrate Paleontology 4: 471–480.

478. Dierbach, A. R. 1985a. Zur Morphogenese des Craniums von *Cavia porcellus* L. Teil 1: Einfuhrung, Systematik und beschreibender Teil. Gegenbaurs Morphologische Jahrbuch 131: 441–476.

479. Dierbach, A. R. 1985b. Zur Morphogenese des Craniums von *Cavia porcellus* L. Teil 2: Vergleichender Teil und Schrifyyum. Gegenbaurs Morphologische Jahrbuch 131: 617–642.

480. Diersing, V. E. 1980. Systematics and evolution of the pygmy shrews subgenus *Microsorex* of North America. Journal of Mammalogy 61: 76–101.

481. Diewert, V. M. 1976. Graphic reconstructions of craniofacial structures during secondary palate development in rats. Teratology 14: 291–313.

482. Diewert, V. M. 1982a. A comparative study of craniofacial growth during secondary palate development in four strains of mice. Journal of Craniofacial Genetics and Developmental Biology 2: 247–263.

483. Diewert, V. M. 1982b. Contribution of differential growth of cartilages to changes in craniofacial morphology. In *Factors and Mechanisms Influencing Bone Growth*, A. D. Dixon and B. G. Sarnat, eds. New York: Alan R. Liss, pp. 229–242.

484. Diewert, V. M. 1983. A morphometric analysis of craniofacial growth and changes in spatial relations during secondary palate development in human embryos and fetuses. American Journal of Anatomy 167: 495–522.

485. Diewert, V. M. 1985. Growth movements during prenatal development of human facial morphology. In *Normal and Abnormal Bone Growth: Basic and Clinical Research*, vol. 187, *Progress in Clinical and Biological Research*, A. D. Dixon and B. G. Sarnat, eds. New York: Alan R. Liss, pp. 57–66.

486. Disney, H. J. de S. 1980. Skull pneumatization in African birds with reference to ageing and breeding and some comparisons with Australian species. In *Proceedings of the Fourth Pan-African Ornithological Congress*, D. N. Johnson, ed. South Africa: Southern African Ornithological Society, pp. 43–50.

487. Dodson, P. 1975a. Relative growth in two sympatric species of *Sceloporus*. American Midland Naturalist 94: 421–450.

488. Dodson, P. 1975b. Functional and ecological significance of relative growth in *Alligator*. Journal of Zoology, London 175: 315–355.

489. Dodson, P. 1975c. Taxonomic implications of relative growth in lambeosaurine hadrosaurs. Systematic Zoology 24: 37–54.

490. Dodson, P. 1976. Quantitative aspects of relative growth and sexual dimorphism in *Protoceratops andrewsi*. Journal of Paleontology 50: 929–940.

491. Dodson, P. 1978. On the use of ratios in growth studies. Systematic Zoology 27: 62–67.

492. Dodson, P., and P. J. Currie. 1988. The smallest ceratopsid skull: Judith River

formation of Alberta [Canada]. Canadian Journal of Earth Sciences 25: 926–930.

493. Dolan, K. J. 1971. Cranial suture closure in two species of South American monkeys. American Journal of Physical Anthropology 35: 109–118.

494. Domashevskaya, E. I. 1989. Pecularities of the periosteal structure in anuran amphibians. Vestnik zoologii: 42–46.

495. Dorenbos, J. 1973. Morphogenesis of the spheno-occipital and the presphenoidal synchondrosis in the cranial base of the fetal Wistar rat. Acta morphologica Neerlando-Scandinavica 11: 63–74.

496. Dornesco, G. T., M. Dornesco, H. Marco, and C. Soresco. 1969. Contribution to the study of cartilaginous neurocranial development in Cyprinus carpio L. Anatomisches Anzeiger 125: 296–302.

497. Dornesco, G. T., and C. Soresco. 1971a. Développement de quelques os du neurocrâne chez Cyprinus carpio. L. Anatomisches Anzeiger 128: 16–38.

498. Dornesco, G. T., and C. Soresco. 1971b. Sur le développement et la valeur morphologique de la région ethmoïdale de la carpe. Anatomisches Anzeiger 129: 33–52.

499. Dornesco, G. T., and C. Soresco. 1973. L'origine et le développement des os de la région otique du neurocrâne de la carpe. Anatomisches Anzeiger 133: 305–330.

500. Dornesco, G. T., and C. Soresco. 1974. L'origine et le développement des os de la région occipitale du neurocrâne de la carpe. Anatomisches Anzeiger 136: 318–333.

501. dos Reis, S. F., J. F. da Cruz, and C. J. von Zulen. 1988. Multivariate analysis of skull evolution in caviine rodents: Convergence of ontogenetic trajectories. Revista brasileira de genetica 11: 633–642.

502. Dragoo, J. W., J. R. Chaote, and T. P. O'Farrell. 1987. Intrapopulational variation in two samples of arid-land foxes. Texas Journal of Sciences 39: 223–232.

503. Drews, U., U. Kocher-Becker, and U. Drews. 1972. Die Induktion von Kiemenknorpel aus Kopfneuralleistenmaterial durch präsumptiven Kiemendarm in der Gewebekultur und das Bewegungsverhalten der Zellen während ihrer Entwicklung zu Knorpel. Wilhelm Roux Archives of Developmental Biology 171: 17–37.

504. Dschawachischwili, G. A. 1940. Uber gewisse Fragen der Entwicklung der Schädel von Säugetieren. Bulletin du Muséum de Géorgie, Tiflis 10A: 1–70.

505. Du Brul, E. L. 1950. Posture, locomotion, and the skull in Lagomorpha. American Journal of Anatomy 87: 277–313.

506. Du Brul, E. L. 1964. Evolution of the temporomandibular joint. In The Temporomandibular Joint, B. G. Sarnat ed., 2d ed. Springfield: C. C. Thomas, pp. 3–27.

507. Du Brul, E. L. 1965. The skull of the lion marmoset Leotides rosalia Linnaeus. A study in biomechanical adaptation. American Journal of Physical Anthropology 23: 261–276.

508. Du Brul, E. L., and D. M. Laskin. 1961. Preadaptive potentialities in the mammalian skull: An experiment in growth and form. American Journal of Anatomy 109: 117–132.

509. Dudzinski, M. L., A. E. Newsome, J. C. Merchant, and B. L. Bolton. 1977. Comparing the two usual methods for aging Macropodidae on tooth-classes in the agile wallaby. Australian Wildlife Research 4: 219–222.

510. Duellman, W. E., and L. Trueb. 1966. Neotropical frogs of the genus *Smilisca*. University of Kansas Publications, Museum of Natural History 17: 281–375.

511. Duellman, W. E., and L. Trueb. 1986. *Biology of Amphibians*. New York: McGraw-Hill Co.

512. Dullemeijer, P. 1971. Comparative ontogeny and cranio-facial growth. In *Cranio-Facial Growth in Man*, R. E. Moyers and W. Krogman, eds. Oxford: Pergamon Press, pp. 45–75.

513. Dullemeijer, P. 1972. Methodology in craniofacial biology. Acta morphologica neerlando-scandinavica 10: 9–23.

514. Dullemeijer, P. 1974. *Concepts and Approaches in Animal Morphology*. Assen, The Netherlands: Van Gorcum.

515. Dullemeijer, P. 1985. The significance of van Limborgh's approach to craniofacial biology. Acta morphologica neerlando-scandinavica 23: 317–324.

516. Dundee, H. A. 1957. Partial metamorphosis induced in *Typhlomolge rathbuni*. Copeia: 52–53.

517. Dundee, H. A. 1961. Response of the neotenic salamander, *Haideotriton wallacei*, to a metamorphic agent. Science 135: 1060–1061.

518. Dunn, J. R. 1983a. Development and distribution of the young of northern smoothtongue *Leuroglossus schmidti* (Bathylagidae) in the northeast Pacific, with comments on the systematics of the genus *Leuroglossus* Gilbert. U.S. National Marine Fisheries Service, Fishery Bulletin 81: 23–40.

519. Dunn, J. R. 1983b. The utility of developmental osteology in taxonomic and systematic studies of teleost larvae: A review. NOAA Technical Report, NMFS Circular no. 450.

520. Dunn, J. R. 1984. Developmental osteology. In *Ontogeny and Systematics of Fishes*, American Society of Ichthyologists and Herpetologists Special Publication no. 1, H. G. Moser, ed. Lawrence, Kans.: Allen Press, pp. 48–50.

521. Du Plessis, S. S. 1945. Cranial anatomy and ontogeny of the South African cordylid *Chamaesaura anguina*. South African Journal of Science 41: 245–268.

522. Durkin, J. F., J. Heeley, and J. T. Irvine. 1973. The cartilage of the mandibular condyle. Oral Science Reviews 2: 29–99.

523. Duterloo, H. S., and D. H. Enlow. 1970. A comparative study of cranial growth in *Homo* and *Macaca*. American Journal of Anatomy 127: 357–368.

524. Duterloo, H. S., and H. W. B. Jansen. 1969. Chondrogenesis and osteogenesis in the mandibular condylar blastema. Transactions of the European Orthodontic Society: 1–10.

525. Du Toit, A. E. 1942. The nasal region of the chondrocranium of *Elephantulus*. South African Journal of Medical Science 7 (Biology supplement): 33–49.

526. Eales, N. B. 1950. The skull of foetal narwhal, *Monodon monoceras* L. Philosophical Transactions of the Royal Society of London B 235: 1–33.

527. Earle, R. D., and K. R. Kramm. 1980. Techniques for age determination in the Canadian porcupine (*Erethizon dorsatum dorsatum*). Journal of Wildlife Management 44: 413–419.

528. Eaton, T. H. 1939. Development of the frontoparietal bones in frogs. Copeia: 95–97.

529. Eavey, R. D., T. M. Schmid, and T. F. Linsenmayer. 1988. Intrinsic and extrinsic controls of the hypertrophic programme of chondrocytes in the avian columella. Developmental Biology 126: 57–62.

530. Ede, D. A., and W. A. Kelly. 1964. Developmental abnormalities in the head region of the talpid mutant of the fowl. Journal of Embryology and Experimental Morphology 12: 161–182.

531. Egorov, Y. E. 1979. The correlated pleiades and stabilization of ontogenesis in minks (*Mustela vison*). Zhurnal Obschchei biologii 40: 579–586.

532. Eikamp, H. 1979. Schwarzmilan (*Milvus migrans*) schlagt Saatkrähen (*Corvus frugilegus*) mit Schnabelmissbildungen. Ornithologische Mitteilungen, Gottingen 31: 120.

533. Eisentraut, M. 1976. The palatal ridge pattern of mammals and its significance for phylogenetic and taxonomic studies. Bonner Zoologische Monographien, no. 8: 5–214.

534. Elliott, C. L., and J. T. Flinders. 1984. Cranial measurements of the Columbian ground squirrel, *Spermophilus columbianus columbianus*, with special reference to subspecies taxonomy and juvenile skull development. Great Basin Naturalist 44: 505–508.

535. Ellis, C. J. 1977. Syringeal history. 7. Unhatched and one-day old meadowlark (*Sturnella* sp.). Iowa State Journal of Research 52: 19–30.

536. El-Najjar, M. Y., and G. L. Dawson. 1977. The effect of artificial cranial deformation on the incidence of Wormian bones in the lambdoidal suture. American Journal of Physical Anthropology 46: 155–160.

537. Eloff, F. C. 1948. The early development of the skull of *Otomys tropicalis*. Annals of the Transvaal Museum 21: 103–152.

538. Eloff, F. C. 1950a. The homology of the mammalian pterygoid in the light of some new evidence. Proceedings of the Linnean Society of London 162: 56–63.

539. Eloff, F. C. 1950b. On the relations of the vomer to the ethmoidal skeleton in certain rodents. Annals of the Transvaal Museum 21: 217–222.

540. Eloff, F. C. 1950c. On the nasal region of the chondrocranium of the Cape Hare, *Lepus capensis*. Annals of the Transvaal Museum 21: 222–233.

541. Eloff, F. C. 1951a. On the organ of Jacobson and the nasal-floor cartilages in the chondrocranium of *Galago senegalensis*. Proceedings of the Zoological Society of London 121: 651–655.

542. Eloff, F. C. 1951b. Observations on the Chondrocranium of *Rhabdomys pumilio*. Annals of the Transvaal Museum 21: 369–380.

543. Eloff, F. C. 1952. On the relations of the human vomer to the anterior paraseptal cartilages. Journal of Anatomy, London 86: 16–19.

544. Eloff, F. C. 1953. On the occurrence of pineal cartilages in the chondrocranium of a mammal. Zoological Journal of the Linnean Society 42: 269–272.

545. El Raham, A. A., and A. I. El Moghraby. 1984. Use of the frontal bone in age determination of *Labeo horie* (Pisces, Cyprinidae) in Jebel Aulia Reservoir, Sudan. Hydrobiologia 110: 281–286.

546. El-Toubi, M. R. 1939. The osteology of the lizard *Scincus scincus* (Linn.). Bulletin of the Faculty of Science of the Egyptian University, Cairo, no. 14: 1–38.

547. El-Toubi, M. R. 1945. Notes on the cranial osteology of *Uromastix aegyptia* (Forskal). Bulletin of the Faculty of Science of Fouad I University, Cairo, no. 25: 1–10.

548. El-Toubi, M. R. 1947. The development of the spiracular cartilages of the spiny dogfish, *Acanthias vulgaris* (*Squalus acanthias*). Biological Bulletin 93: 287–295.

549. El-Toubi, M. R. 1949. The development of the chondrocranium of the Spiny dogfish, *Acanthias vulgaris* (*Squalus acanthias*). Part I. Neurocranium, mandibular, and hyoid arches. Journal of Morphology 84: 227–279.

550. El-Toubi, M. R. 1952. The development of the chondrocranium of the spiny dogfish, *Acanthias vulgaris* (*Squalus acanthias*). Part II. Branchial arches and extravisceral cartilages. Journal of Morphology 90: 33–64.

551. El-Toubi, M. R., and A. M. Kamal. 1959a. The development of the skull of *Chalcides ocellatus*. I. The development of the chondrocranium. Journal of Morphology 104: 269–306.

552. El-Toubi, M. R., and A. M. Kamal. 1959b. The development of the skull of *Chalcides ocellatus*. II. The fully formed chondrocranium and the osteocranium of a late embryo. Journal of Morphology 105: 55–104.

553. El-Toubi, M. R., and A. M. Kamal. 1961a. The development of the skull of *Ptyodactylus hasselquistii*. I. The development of the chondrocranium. Journal of Morphology 108: 63–94.

554. El-Toubi, M. R., and A. M. Kamal. 1961b. The development of the skull of *Ptyodactylus hasselquistii*. II. The fully formed chondrocranium. Journal of Morphology 108: 165–192.

555. El-Toubi, M. R., and A. M. Kamal. 1961c. The development of the skull of *Ptyodactylus hasselquistii*. III. The osteocranium of a late embryo. Journal of Morphology 108: 193–202.

556. El-Toubi, M. R., and A. M. Kamal. 1965. The origin of the tectum of the occipito-auditory region in Squamata. Proceedings of the Egyptian Academy of Science 18: 73–75.

557. El-Toubi, M. R., and A. M. Kamal. 1970. The origin of lizards in the light of the developmental study of the skull. Zeitschrift für Zoologische Systematik und Evolutionsforschung 8: 47–52.

558. El-Toubi, M. R., A. M. Kamal, and H. G. Hammouda. 1965a. The phylogenetic relationship between the ophidian families Boidae, Colubridae, and Viperidae in the light of the developmental study of the skull. Zoologischer Anzeiger 175: 289–294.

559. El-Toubi, M. R., A. M. Kamal, and H. G. Hammouda. 1965b. The origin of the Ophidia in the light of the developmental study of the skull. Zeitschrift für Zoologische Systematik und Evolutionsforschung 3: 94–102.

560. El-Toubi, M. R., A. M. Kamal, and H. G. Hammouda. 1968. The common characters of the ophidian chondrocranium. Bulletin of the Faculty of Science of the Egyptian University, Cairo 41: 109–118.

561. El-Toubi, M. R., A. M. Kamal, and F. M. Mokhtar. 1970. The chondrocra-

nium of late embryos of the Egyptian cobra, *Naja haje*. Anatomisches Anzeiger 127: 288–289.

562. El-Toubi, M. R., A. M. Kamal, and M. M. Zaher. 1973a. The development of the chondrocranium of the snake *Malpolon monspessulana*. I. The early and intermediate stages. Acta anatomica 85: 275–299.

563. El-Toubi, M. R., A. M. Kamal, and M. M. Zaher. 1973b. The development of the chondrocranium of the snake *Malpolon monspessulana*. II. The fully formed stage. Acta anatomica 85: 593–619.

564. Engelbrecht, D. van Z. 1958. The development of the chondrocranium of *Pyromelana orix orix*. Acta zoologica, Stockholm 39: 115–199.

565. Engels, H. 1979a. Das postnatale Schädelwachstum bei der Hausmaus *Mus musculus* Linne 1758, und bei zwei verschieden grossen Unterarten der Feldmaus *Microtus arvalis* Pallas 1779. Teil 1. Einleitung Materiel und Methoden. Gegenbaurs Morphologische Jahrbuch 125: 218–237.

566. Engels, H. 1979b. Das postnatale Schädelwachstum bei der Hausmaus *Mus musculus* Linne 1758, und bei zwei verschieden grossen Unterarten der Feldmaus *Microtus arvalis* Pallas 1779. Teil 2. Ergebnisse (1). Gegenbaurs Morphologische Jahrbuch 125: 324–348.

567. Engels, H. 1979c. Das postnatale Schädelwachstum bei der Hausmaus *Mus musculus* Linne 1758, und bei zwei verschieden grossen Unterarten der Feldmaus *Microtus arvalis* Pallas 1779. Teil 3. Ergebnisse (2), Diskussion, Zusammenfassung und Literatur. Gegenbaurs Morphologische Jahrbuch 125: 550–571.

568. Engstrom, M. D., D. J. Schmidly, and P. K. Fox. 1982. Nongeographic variation and discrimination of species within the *Peromyscus leucopus* species group (Mammalia: Cricetinae) in eastern Texas. Texas Journal of Science 34: 149–192.

569. Enlow, D. H. 1969. The bone of reptiles. In *Biology of the Reptilia*, vol. 1, C. Gans, A. d'A. Bellairs, and T. S. Parsons, eds. New York: Academic Press, pp. 45–80.

570. Enlow, D. H. 1975. *Handbook of Facial Growth*. Philadelphia: W. B. Saunders.

571. Enlow, D. H. 1976. The prenatal and postnatal growth of the human basicranium. In *Development of the Basicranium*, J. F. Bosma, ed. Bethesday: U.S. Department of Health, Education, and Welfare, pp. 192–205.

572. Enlow, D. H. 1978. Normal maxillofacial growth. In *Symposium on Reconstruction of Jaw Deformities*, L. A. Whitaker, ed. St. Louis: C. V. Mosby, pp. 13–23.

573. Enlow, D. H. 1986. Normal craniofacial growth. In *Craniosynostosis: Diagnosis, Evaluation, and Management*, M. M. Cohen, Jr., ed. New York: Raven Press, pp. 131–156.

574. Enlow, D. H., and M. Azuma. 1975. Functional growth boundaries in the human and mammalian face. In *Morphogenesis and Malformations of the Face and Brain*, J. Langman, ed. White Plains: National Foundations.

575. Enlow, D. H., and J. A. McNamara. 1973. The neurocranial basis for facial form and pattern. Angle Orthodontist 43: 256–270.

576. Epperlein, H. H., and R. Lehmann. 1975. Ectomesenchymal-endodermal in-

teraction system (EEIS) of *Triturus alpestris* in tissue culture. II. Observations on differentiation of visceral cartilage. Differentiation 4: 159–174.

577. Erdmann, K. 1940. Zur Entwicklungsgeschichte der Knochen im Schädel des Huhnes bis zum Zeitpunktdes Ausschlüpfen aus dem Ei. Zeitschrift für Morphologie und Okologie der Tiere, Berlin 36: 315–400.

578. Erickson, L. C., and A. L. Ogilvie. 1958. Aspects of growth in the cranium, mandible, and teeth of the rabbit as revealed through the use of alizarin and metallic implants. Angle Orthodontist 28: 47–56.

579. Erritzoe, J. 1985. Geschlechts-und Altersbestimmung bei Vogeln. Preparator 31: 81–93.

580. Evans, H. E. 1955. The osteology of a worm snake, *Typhlops jamaicensis* (Shaw). Anatomical Record 122: 381–396.

581. Evans, H. E. 1982. Anatomy of the budgerigar. In *Diseases of Cage and Aviary Birds*, M. L. Petrak, ed. 2d ed. Philadelphia: Lea and Febiger, pp. 111–187.

582. Evans, H. E. 1986. Reptiles: Introduction and anatomy. In *Zoo and Wild Animal Medicine*, M. E. Fowler, ed. 2d ed. Philadelphia: W. B. Saunders, pp. 108–132.

583. Evseenko, S. A. 1978. Some data on metamorphosis of larvae of the genus *Bothus* (Pisces, Bothidae) from the Caribbean Sea. Zoologischeskii zhurnal 57: 1040–1047.

584. Evseenko, S. A. 1979. Larvae of the founder (*Cyclopsetta fimbriata* and *Cyclopsetta chittendeni*) (Bothidae, Pisces) from the northwestern Atlantic. Biologiya morya no. 2: 67–75.

585. Ewert, M. A. 1979. The embryo and its egg: Development and natural history. In *Turtles: perspectives and research,* M. Harless and H. Morlock, eds. New York: John Wiley and Sons, pp. 333–413.

586. Ewert, M. A. 1985. Embryology of turtles. In *Biology of the Reptilia,* C. Gans, F. Billett, and P. F. A. Maderson, eds., vol. 14, development A. New York: John Wiley and Sons, pp. 75–267.

587. Eyal-Giladi, H. 1964. The development of the chondrocranium of *Agama stellio*. Acta zoologica, Stockholm 45: 139–165.

588. Eyal-Giladi, H., and N. Zinberg. 1964. The development of the chondrocranium of *Pleurodeles waltlii*. Journal of Morphology 114: 527–548.

589. Fagen, R. M., and K. S. Wiley. 1978. Field paedomorphosis, with special reference to *Leopardus*. Carnivore 1: 78–81.

590. Fagone, A. 1959. Ricerche sperimentali sulla formazione della bocca in *Discoglossus pictus*. Acta embryologiae et morphologiae experimentalis 2: 133–150.

591. Fagone, A. 1960. Ulteriori ricerche sperimentali sulla formazione della bocca in *Discoglossus pictus*. Atti, Accademia nazionale dei Lincei, Rendiconti 28: 249–253.

592. Faha, M. P., and P. Berrien. 1979. Preliminary description of larval tilefish (*Lophatilus chamaeoleonticeps*). Rapports et procès-verbaux des réunions, Conseil international pour l'exploration de la mer 178: 600–602.

593. Fairall, N. 1980. Growth and age determination in the hyrax, *Procavia capensis*. South African Journal of Zoology 15: 16–21.

594. Faleev, V. I. 1982. To the study of geographic variation of morphometric indications of water vole (*Arvicola terrestris* L.) with the method of general components. Izvestiya Sibirskogo Otdeleniya Akademii NAUK SSR Seriya Biologicheskikh NAUK: 92–97.

595. Farkas, L. G., J. S. James, and B. M. Vanderby. 1977. Quantitative assessment of the morphology of the pig's head used as a model in surgical experimentation: 2. Results of measurements. Canadian Journal of Comparative Medicine 41: 455–459.

596. Fearnhead, R. W., C. C. D. Shute, and A. d'A. Bellairs. 1955. The temporomandibular joint in shrews. Proceedings of the Zoological Society of London 125: 795–806.

597. Fenart, R. 1973. Biparietal spherization in chimpanzees: Ontogenesis and sexual differences; comparison with human skull in vestibular orientation. Bulletin et mémoires de la Société d'anthropologie de Paris 9: 213–233.

598. Fenart, R., and R. de Block. 1978. Ontogenetic development of the surface of the angular sagittal cranio-facial sectors in man and chimpanzee. Bulletin de l'Association des anatomistes 62: 85–88.

599. Ferembach, D. 1962. Contribution à l'étude de la croissance du crâne du chimpanzé. Biotypologie 23: 95–118.

600. Ferembach, D. 1963. Contribution à l'étude de la croissance du crâne du chimpanzé. Anthropos 7: 39–45.

601. Ferguson, M. W. J. 1981a. The structure and development of the palate in *Alligator mississippiensis*. Archives of Oral Biology 26: 427–443.

602. Ferguson, M. W. J. 1981b. The value of the American alligator (*Alligator mississippiensis*) as a model for research in craniofacial development. Journal of Craniofacial Genetics and Developmental Biology 1: 123–144.

603. Ferguson, M. W. J. 1984. Craniofacial development in *Alligator mississippiensis*. In *The Structure, Development, and Evolution of Reptiles*, M. W. J. Ferguson, ed. London: Academic Press, pp. 223–274.

604. Ferguson, M. W. J. 1985. Reproductive biology and embryology of the crocodilians. In *Biology of the Reptilia*, vol. 14, *Development A*, C. Gans, F. Billett, and P. F. A. Maderson, eds. New York: John Wiley and Sons, pp. 329–492.

605. Ferguson, M. W. J. 1988. Palate development. Development 103 (suppl.): 41–60.

606. Ferguson, M. W. J., and L. S. Honig. 1984. Epithelial-mesenchymal interactions during vertebrate palatogenesis. Current Topics in Developmental Biology 19: 138–165.

607. Ferguson, M. W. J., and L. S. Honig. 1985. Experimental fusion of the naturally cleft embryonic chick palate. Journal of Craniofacial Genetics and Developmental Biology 1 (suppl.): 323–337.

608. Ferguson, M. W. J., L. S. Honig, P. Bringas, Jr., and H. C. Slavkin. 1982. *In vivo* and *in vitro* development of first branchial arch derivatives in *Alligator mississippiensis*. In *Factors and Mechanisms Influencing Bone Growth*, A. D. Dixon and B. G. Sarnat, eds. New York: Alan R. Liss, pp. 275–286.

609. Ferguson, M. W. J., L. S. Honig, P. Bringas, Jr., and H. C. Slavkin. 1983. Alligator mandibular development during long term organ culture. In Vitro 19: 385–393.

610. Ferguson, M. W. J., L. S. Honig, and H. C. Slavkin. 1983. *In vitro* development of alligator first branchial arch derivatives. Journal of Anatomy 136: 618–619.

611. Ferguson, M. W. J., L. S. Honig, and H. C. Slavkin. 1984. Differentiation of cultured palatal shelves from alligator, chick, and mouse embryos. Anatomical Record 209: 231–249.

612. Ferigolo, J. 1981. The mesethmoid bone and the Edentata. Anais, Academia brasiliera de ciencias 53: 817–824.

613. Ferron, R. R., R. S. Miller, and W. P. McNulty. 1976. Estimation of fetal age and weight from radiographic skull diameters in the Rhesus monkey (*Macaca mulatta*). Journal of Medical Primatology 5: 41–48.

614. Fields, H. W., Jr., L. Metzner, J. D. Garol, and V. G. Kokich. 1978. The craniofacial skeleton in anencephalic human fetuses. I. Cranial floor. Teratology 17: 57–66.

615. Finch, R. A. 1969. The influence of the nerve on lower jaw regeneration in the adult newt, *Triturus viridescens*. Journal of Morphology 129: 401–414.

616. Findlay, G. H. 1944. The development of the auditory ossicles in the elephant shrew, the tenrec, and the golden mole. Proceedings of the Zoological Society of London 114B: 91–99.

617. Fineman, G. 1939. Zur Entwicklungsgeschichte des Kopfskel bei *Chamaeleon bitaeniatus* Elliott. Gegenbaurs Morphologisches Jahrbuch, Leipzig. 83: 544–568.

618. Fineman, G. 1941. Zur Entwicklungsgeschichte des Kopfskelets bei *Chamaeleon bitaeniatus* Elliott. Gegenbaurs Morphologisches Jahrbuch, Leipzig 85: 91–114.

619. Fischer, K., and H. Schnare. 1986. Einflusse experimenteller Veranderungen im Jahresgang der Photoperiode auf morphogenetische und physiologische Prozesse beim Damhirsch (*Dama dama* L.). 1. Der Geweihzyklus mit stoffwechselphysiologischen Grundlagen. Zeitschrift für Jagdwissenschaft 32: 1–13.

620. Fisk, A. 1954. The early development of the ear and acoustico-facialis complex of ganglia in the lamprey *Lampetra planeri* Bloch. Proceedings of the Zoological Society of London 124: 125–151.

621. Fitch, J. M., A. Mentzer, R. Mayne, and T. F. Linsenmayer. 1989. Independent deposition of collagen types II and IX at epithelial-mesenchymal interfaces. Development 105: 85–95.

622. Flint, O. P., and D. A. Ede. 1978. Facial development in the mouse: A comparison between normal and mutant (*amputated*) mouse embryos. Journal of Embryology and Experimental Morphology 48: 249–267.

623. Ford, E. H. 1956. The growth of the foetal skull. Journal of Anatomy, London 90: 63–72.

624. Ford, E. H. 1958. Growth of the human cranial base. American Journal of Orthodontics 44: 498–506.

625. Ford, E. H., and G. Horn. 1959. Some problems in the evaluation of differential growth in the rat skull. Growth 23: 191–204.

626. Fordyce, R. E., R. H., Mattlin, and J. M. Dixon. 1985. Second record of

spectacled porpoise from subantarctic southwest Pacific. Scientific Report of the Shales Research Institute, Tokyo 35: 159–164.

627. Fourie, S. 1955. A contribution to the cranial morphology of *Nyctisyrigmus pectoralis pectoralis* with special reference to the palate and cranial kinesis. Annals of the University of Stellenbosch 31A: 178–215.

628. Fox, G. Q., G. P. Richardson, and C. Kirk. 1985. Torpedo electromotor system development: Neuronal cell death and electric organ development in the fourth branchial arch. Journal of Comparative Neurology 236: 274–281.

629. Fox, H. 1954. Development of the skull and associated structures in the Amphibia, with special reference to the urodeles. Transactions of the Zoological Society of London. 28: 241–304.

630. Fox, H. 1957. The occipital crest and anterior spinal nerves in the larval urodele, *Hynobius nebulosus*. Proceedings of the Zoological Society of London 128: 365–368.

631. Fox, H. 1959. A study of the development of the head and pharynx of the larval urodele *Hynobius* and its bearing on the evolution of the vertebrate head. Philosophical Transactions of the Royal Society of London 242B: 151–204.

632. Fox, H. 1961a. The occipital crest and anterior spinal nerves in the larval urodele *Salamandra maculosa*. British Journal of Herpetology 2: 211–213.

633. Fox, H. 1961b. The segmentation of components in the hind region of the head of *Neoceratodus* and their relation to the pronephric tubules. Acta anatomica 47: 156–163.

634. Fox, H. 1963a. The hyoid of *Neoceratodus* and a consideration of its homology in urodele Amphibia. Proceedings of the Zoological Society of London 141: 803–819.

635. Fox, H. 1963b. Prootic anatomy of the *Neoceratodus* larva. Acta anatomica 52: 126–129.

636. Fox, H. 1965. Early development of the head and pharynx of *Neoceratodus* with a consideration of its phylogeny. Journal of Zoology, London 146: 470–554.

637. Fox, W., C. Gordon, and M. H. Fox. 1961. Morphological effects of low temperature during the embryonic development of the garter snake *Thamnophis elegans*. Zoologica, New York 46: 57–71.

638. Francillon, H. 1974. Développement de la partie postérieure de la mandibule de *Salmo trutta fario* L. (Pisces, Teleostei, Salmonidae). Zoologica scripta 3: 41–51.

639. Francillon, H. 1977. Développement de la partie anterieure de la mandibule de *Salmo trutta fario* (Pisces, Teleostei, Salmonidae). Zoologica scripta 6: 245–251.

640. Francillon, H., F. Meunier, D. Ngo Tuan Phong, and A. de Ricqlès. 1975. Données préliminaires sur les structures histologiques du squelette de *Latimeria chalumnae*. II. Tissues osseux et cartilages. In *Problèmes actuels de paléontologie (évolution des vertébrés)*, J.-P. Lehman, ed. Colloque international du Centre national de la recherche scientifique 218: 169–174.

641. Frangioni, G. 1970. The chondrocranium of *Proteles cristatus* and of *Genetta genetta* (Mammalia, Carnivora). Monitore zoologico italiano 3 (suppl.): 173–192.

642. Frank, G. H. 1954. The development of the chondrocranium of the Ostrich. Annals of the University of Stellenbosch 30: 179–248.

643. Frank, G. H., and A. L. Smit. 1974. The early ontogeny of the columella auris of *Crocodilus niloticus* and its bearing on problems concerning the upper end of the reptilian hyoid arch. Zoologica africana 9: 59–88.

644. Frank, G. H., and A. L. Smit. 1976. The morphogenesis of the avan columella auris with special reference to *Struthio camelus*. Zoologica africana 11: 159–182.

645. Franklin, M. A. 1945. The embryonic appearance of centres of ossification in the bones of snakes. Copeia: 68–72.

646. Franzmann, A. W. 1978. Moose. In *Big Game of North America: Ecology and Management*, J. L. Schmidt and D. L. Gilbert, eds. Harrisburg: Stackpole Books, pp. 67–81.

647. Frazetta, T. H. 1970. From hopeful monster to bolyerine snakes. American Naturalist 104: 55–72.

648. Freedman, L. 1962. Growth of muzzle length relative to calvaria length in *Papio*. Growth 26: 117–128.

649. Freer, V., and B. Belanger. 1981. A technique for distinguishing the age classes of adult bank swallows (*Riparia riparia*). Journal of Field Ornithology 52: 341–343.

650. Freye, H. A. 1952–53. Das Gehörorgan der Vögel. Wissenschaftliche Zeitschrift der Martin-Luther-Universität, Halle-Wittenberg 2: 267–297.

651. Friant, M. 1959. Sur l'ossification enchondrale du cartilage de Meckel chez les Rongeurs. Bulletin du Groupement international pour la recherche scientifique en stomatologie 4: 1–11.

652. Friant, M. 1960. L'évolution du cartilage de Meckel humain, jusqu'à la fin du sixième mois de la vie foetale. Acta anatomica 41: 228–239.

653. Friant, M. 1964a. Sur l'ossification du cartilage de Meckel d'une chauve-souris, le grand Murin (Chiroptera, *Myotis myotis* [Borkh]). Acta anatomica 57: 66–71.

654. Friant, M. 1964b. Sur l'évolution du cartilage de Meckel d'une chauve-souris frugivore, *Epomops franqueti strepitans* Andersen (Macrochiroptera, Pteropodidae). Journal of the Nihon University School of Dentistry 6: 139–142.

655. Friant, M. 1965. Le développement des dents temporaires des Chiroptères. Revue mensuelle suisse d'odonto-stomatologie 75: 208–212.

656. Friant, M. 1966a. Vue d'ensemble sur l'évolution du "cartilage de Meckel" de quelques groupes de Mammifères: Insectivores, Chiroptères, Rongeurs. Acta zoologica, Stockholm 47: 67–80.

657. Friant, M. 1966b. Development of Meckel's cartilage in the tiger. Folia morphologica, Prague 14: 130–134.

658. Friant, M. 1968. L'évolution du cartilage de Meckel du porc (*Sus scrofa* dom. Gray). Annali della Facoltà di medicina veterinaria Università di Pisa 21: 1–17.

659. Friant, M. 1969. L'évolution du cartilage de Meckel du cheval (*Equus cabal-*

lus L.). Annali della Facoltà di medicina veterinaria Università di Pisa 22: 253–275.

660. Friant, M. 1970. Le début de l'évolution du cartilage de Meckel du boeuf (*Bos taurus* L.). Annali della Facoltà di medicina veterinaria Università di Pisa 23: 321–330.

661. Friant, M. 1974a. Le cartilage de Meckel d'un singe, le Douroucouli (*Aotus*). Archives, Institut Grand-Ducal de Luxembourg 36: 369–371.

662. Friant, M. 1974b. Meckel's cartilage of *Tupaia javanica* Horsf.: A stage of its evolution. Folia morphologica, Prague 22: 389–396.

663. Friant, M. 1974c. Sur le cartilage de Meckel des Vespertillionidae chauves-souris insectivores. Archives, Institut Grand-Ducal de Luxembourg 36: 359–367.

664. Frick, H. 1952a. Zur Morphogenese der Fenestra rotunda. Verhandlungen der Anatomischen Gesellschaft, Jena 50: 194–203.

665. Frick, H. 1952b. Über die Aufteilung des Foramen perilymphaticum in der Ontogenese der Säuger. Zeitschrift für Anatomie Entwicklungsgeschichte 116: 523–551.

666. Frick, H. 1953. Über die Entwicklung der Schneckenfensternische (Fossula fenestrae rotundae) beim Menschen. Archiv für Ohren-, Nasen-, und Kehlkopfheilkunde, Leipzig. 162: 520–534.

667. Frick, H. 1954. *Die Entwicklung und Morphologie des Chondrocraniums von* Myotis *Kaup*. Stuttgart: George Thieme Verlag.

668. Frick, H. 1986. On the development of chondrocranium in the albino mouse. In *Craniogenesis and Craniofacial Growth,* Nova acta Leopoldina 58, no. 262, G.-H. Schumacher, ed. Halle: Deutsche Akademie der Naturforscher Leopoldina, pp. 305–317.

669. Frick, H., and U. Heckmann. 1955. Ein Beitrag zur Morphogenese des Kaninchenschädels. Acta anatomica 24: 268–314.

670. Friede, H. 1981. Normal development and growth of the human neurocranium and cranial base. Scandinavian Journal of Plastic and Reconstructive Surgery 15: 163–170.

671. Friedenstein, A. Y. 1949. On histogenesis of some bones of Mammals. Comptes rendus hebdomadaires des séances de l'Académie des sciences, Moscow, n.s., 68: 931–933.

672. Friedenstein, A. Y. 1950. Histogenesis of the basic bones of the visceral skeleton of mammals and birds. Doklady akademiya Nauk, SSSR 71: 159–161.

673. Frindt, A., W. Empel, M. Sobczyk, M. Bednary, and H. Sadowska. 1981. Investigation on the course of ossification and the skeletal growth of some selected weasel (Mustelidae) species. Zeszyty Problemone Postepow Nauk Roiniczych, no. 259: 107–110.

674. Frith, C. B., and D. W. Frith. 1978. Bill growth and development in the northern pied hornbill *Anthracoceros malabaricus*. Avicultural Magazine 84: 20–31.

675. Fritz, H. 1975. Prenatal ossification in rabbits as indicative of fetal maturity. Teratology 11: 313–320.

676. Fritz, H., and R. Hess. 1970. Ossification of the rat and mouse skeleton in the perinatal period. Teratology 3: 331–338.

677. Fritzche, R. A., and G. D. Johnson. 1980. Early osteological development of white perch and striped bass with emphasis on identification of their larvae. Transactions of the American Fisheries Society 109: 387–406.

678. Frommer, J. 1964. Prenatal development of the mandibular joint in mice. Anatomical Record 150: 449–462.

679. Frommer, J., and C. W. Monroe. 1966. Development and distribution of elastic fibers in the mandibular joint of the mouse. A comparison of fetal, suckling, juvenile, and adult stages. Anatomical Record 156: 333–346.

680. Fuiman, L. A. 1983. Growth gradients in fish larvae. Journal of Fish Biology 23: 117–123.

681. Fujioka, T. 1955. Time and order of appearance of ossification centres in the chicken skeleton. Acta anatomica nipponica 30: 140–150.

682. Fukuhara, O., and M. Tanaka. 1987. Staining techniques for bone and scale formation of larval fishes. Aquabiology, Tokyo 9: 97–99.

683. Fuller, T. K., D. W. Kuechn, and R. K. Markl. 1985. Physical characteristics of striped skunks in northern Minnesota. Journal of Mammalogy 66: 371–374.

684. Funmilayo, O. 1976. Age determination, age distribution, and sex ratio in mole populations. Acta theriologica 21: 207–215.

685. Furtwängler, J. A., S. H. Hall, and L. K. Koshinen-Moffett. 1985. Sutural morphogenesis in the mouse calvaria: The role of apoptosis. Acta anatomica 124: 74–80.

686. Futch, C. R. 1977. Larvae of *Trichopsetta ventralis* (Pisces: Bothidae) with comments on intergeneric relationships with the Bothidae. Bulletin of Marine Science 27: 740–757.

687. Futch, C. R., and F. H. Hoff, Jr. 1971. Larval development of *Syacium papillosum* (Bothidae) with notes on adult morphology. Florida Department of Natural Resources Leaflet Series 4, pt. 1, no. 2.

688. Fyfe, D. M., M. W. J. Ferguson, and R. Chiquet-Ehristmann. 1988. Immunochemical localization of tenascin during the development of scleral papillae and scleral ossicles in the embryonic chick. Journal of Anatomy 159: 117–127.

689. Fyfe, D. M., and B. K. Hall. 1981. A scanning electron microscopic study of the developing epithelial scleral papillae in the eye of the embryonic chick. Journal of Morphology 167: 201–209.

690. Fyfe, D. M., and B. K. Hall. 1983. The origin of the ectomesenchymal condensations which precede the development of the bony scleral ossicles in the eyes of embryonic chicks. Journal of Embryology and Experimental Morphology 73: 69–86.

691. Gaffney, E. S. 1979. Comparative cranial morphology of Recent and fossil turtles. Bulletin of the American Museum of Natural History 164: 69–376.

692. Galkina, L. I., and I. V. Nadeev. 1980. Some questions of the morphology, distribution, and history of *Myospalax* (Rodentia, Myospalacinae) of western Siberia. Trudy Biologischeskogo Instituta Akademiya Nauk SSSR Sibirskoe Otdelenie 44: 162–176.

693. Galton, P. M., and R. T. Bakker. 1985. The cranial anatomy of the prosauropod dinosaur *Efraasia diagnostica*, a juvenile individual of *Sellosaurus gra-*

cilis from the Upper Triassic of Nordwuerttemberg, West Germany. Stuttgart Beiträge zur Naturkunde, ser. B, Geologie und Palaeontologie 117: 1–15.

694. Ganguly, D. N., and K. K. Singh-Roy. 1965a. A study on the cranio-vertebral joint in the vertebrates. I. In the mammals, as illustrated by its structure in the guinea pig and development in the guinea pig and *Talpa*. Anatomisches Anzeiger 117: 421–429.

695. Ganguly, D. N., and K. K. Singh-Roy. 1965b. A study on the cranio-vertebral joint in the vertebrates. II. In the birds, as illustrated by its structure in the *Struthio* and *Gallus* as well as development in *Gallus* and *Psittacula*. Anatomisches Anzeiger 117: 430–446.

696. Ganguly, D. N., K. K. Singh-Roy, and B. Mitra. 1966. A study on the cranio-vertebral joint in the vertebrates. III. In the reptiles, as illustrated by its structure in the *Hemidactylus flaviviridis* and development in both *Hemidactylus* and *Chelydra* sp. Anatomisches Anzeiger 118: 122–131.

697. Gans, C. 1980. Allometric changes in the skull and brain of *Caiman crocodilus*. Journal of Herpetology 14: 297–301.

698. Gans, C. 1987. The neural crest: A spectacular invention. In *Developmental and Evolutionary Aspects of the Neural Crest*, P. F. A. Maderson, ed. New York: John Wiley and Sons, pp. 361–370.

699. Gans, C. 1989. Stages in the origin of vertebrates: Analysis by means of scenarios. Biological Reviews of the Cambridge Philosophical Society 64: 221–268.

700. Gans, C., and R. G. Northcutt. 1983. Neural crest and the origin of vertebrates: A new head. Science 220: 268–274.

701. Gans, C., and R. G. Northcutt. 1985. Neural crest: The implications for comparative anatomy. In *Functional Morphology in Vertebrates*, Fortschritte der Zoologie 30, H.-R. Duncker and G. Fleischer, eds. Stuttgart: Gustav-Fischer Verlag, pp. 507–514.

702. Garcia-Arteaga, J. P., and Y. S. Reshetnikov. 1985. Age and growth of the bar jack, *Caranx ruber*, off the coast of Cuba. Voprosy Ikhtiologii 25: 844–854.

703. Gardner, E. 1950. Physiology of moveable joints. Physiological Reviews 30: 127–176.

704. Gardner, E. 1956. Osteogenesis in the human embryo and fetus. In *The Biochemistry and Physiology of Bone*, G. H. Bourne, ed. New York: Academic Press, pp. 359–400.

705. Gardner, E. 1971. Osteogenesis in the human embryo and fetus. In *The Biochemistry and Physiology of Bone*, G. H. Bourne, ed., 2d ed., vol. 3. New York: Academic Press, pp. 77–118.

706. Garol, J. D., H. W. Fields, Jr., L. Metener, and V. G. Kokich. 1978. The craniofacial skeleton in anencephalic human fetuses. II. Calvarium. Teratology 17: 67–74.

707. Garrod, D. R. 1986. Specific inductive flypaper. BioEssays 5: 172–173.

708. Gartner, L. P., J. L. Hiatt, M. A. Khan, and D. V. Provenza. 1979. Development of the squamosomandibular articulation in the Mongolian gerbil (*Meriones unguiculatus*). II. Succinate dehydrogenase activity. Histochemistry Journal 11: 553–559.

709. Gartner, L. P., J. L. Hiatt, and D. V. Provenza. 1976. Development of the squamosomandibular articulation in the Mongolian gerbil (*Meriones unguiculatus*). Acta anatomica 96: 404–417.

710. Gasc, J.-P. 1966. Contribution à l'ostéologie et à la myologie de *Dibamus novaeguineae* Gray (Sauria, Reptilia): Discussion systématique. Annales des sciences naturelles, Zoologie et biologie animale 10: 127–150.

711. Gasc, J.-P. 1967. Squelette hyobranchial. In *Traité de zoologie: Anatomie, systématique, biologie*, vol. 16(1), *Mammifères: Téguments squelette*, P.-P. Grassé, ed. Paris: Masson et Cie, pp. 550–583.

712. Gasser, R. F. 1976. Early formation of the basicranium in man. In *Development of the Bisicranium*, J. F. Bosma, ed. Bethesda: U.S. Department of Health, Education, and Welfare, pp. 29–43.

713. Gaston, A. J. 1984. How to distinguish 1st-year murres *Uria* spp. from older birds in winter. Canadian Field Naturalist 98: 52–55.

714. Gaudin, A. J. 1973. The development of the skull in the Pacific tree frog, *Hyla regilla*. Herpetologica 29: 205–218.

715. Gaudin, A. J. 1978. The sequence of cranial ossification in the Californian toad, *Bufo boreas* (Amphibia, Anura, Bufonidae). Journal of Herpetology 12: 309–318.

716. Gaunt, W. A. 1959. The development of the deciduous cheek teeth of the rat. Acta anatomica 38: 188–212.

717. Gaunt, W. A. 1961. The growth of the teeth and jaws in the golden hamster. Acta anatomica 47: 301–327.

718. Gaunt, W. A. 1964a. The development of the teeth and jaws of the albino mouse. Acta anatomica 57: 115–151.

719. Gaunt, W. A. 1964b. A note on the pre- and post-natal location of the molar teeth of the mouse. Acta anatomica 57: 267–277.

720. Gaunt, W. A. 1964c. Changes in the form of the jaws of the albino mouse during ontogeny. Acta anatomica 58: 37–61.

721. Gaunt, W. A. 1964d. Post-optimal changes in the chondro-facial skeleton of the albino mouse. Acta anatomica 59: 212–228.

722. Gaunt, W. A. 1965. Growth of the facial region of the albino mouse as revealed by the mesh diagram. Acta anatomica 61: 574–588.

723. Gaunt, W. A. 1967. Observations upon the developing dentition of *Hipposideros caffer* (Microchiroptera). Acta anatomica 68: 9–25.

724. Gautier, A. 1976. A skull of musk ox (*Ovibos moschatus* Zimmerman, 1780) from the Lower Wuermian at Dendermonds (Oost-Vlaanderen Belgium). Natuurwetenschappelikj tijdschrift 58: 183–193.

725. Gemmell, R. T., G. Johnston, and M. M. Bryden. 1988. Osteogenesis in two marsupial species, the bandicoot *Isodon macrourus* and the possum *Trichosurus vulpecula*. Journal of Anatomy 159: 155–164.

726. Genest-Villard, H. 1966. Développement du crâne d'un boide: *Sanzinia madagascariensis*. Mémoires du Muséum national d'histoire naturelle 40A: 207–262.

727. Getmanov, S. N. 1981. Some cranial growth mechanisms in benthosuchids. Palaeontologicheskii zhurnal, no. 2: 110–116.

728. Getmanov, S. N. 1989. Triassic Amphibia of the eastern European platform. Trudy Paleontoolicheskogo Instituta Akademiya Nauk SSSR 236: 1–100.

729. Gibson, R. N. 1988. Development, morphometry, and particle retention capability of the gill rakers in the herring, *Clupea harengus* L. Journal of Fish Biology 32: 949–962.

730. Gilbert, P. W. 1952. The origin and development of the head cavities in the human embryo. Journal of Morphology 90: 149–173.

731. Gilbert, P. W. 1954. The premandibular head cavities in the opossum, *Didelphys virginiana*. Journal of Morphology 95: 47–75.

732. Giles, E. 1956. Cranial allometry in the great apes. Human Biology 28: 43–58.

733. Ginsburg, A. S. 1939. Some data on the determination of the ear in *Triton taeniatus*. Comptes rendus hebdomadaires des séances de l'Académie des sciences, Moscow, n.s., 22: 370–373.

734. Gipouloux, J. D., and J. J. Brustis. 1986. Crâne et musculature cephalique. In *Traité de zoologie: Anatomie, systématique, biologie*, vol. 14(1B), *Batraciens*, P.-P. Grassé and M. Delsol, eds. Paris: Masson, pp. 160–188.

735. Girgis, F. G., and J. J. Pritchard. 1958. Effects of skull damage on the development of sutural patterns in the rat. Journal of Anatomy, London 92: 39–51.

736. Glasstone, S. 1971. Differentiation of the mouse embryonic mandible and squamo-mandibular joint in organ culture. Archives of Oral Biology 16: 723–729.

737. Glenn, L. P. 1975. Big game investigations. Comparison of brown/grizzly bear skulls by size, age, sex, and geographic location. Project Progress Reports, Alaska Department of Fish and Game 15, Job no. 4.6R: 1–10.

738. Gluecksohn-Waelsch, S., S. D. Hagedora, and B. F. Sisken. 1956. Genetics and morphology of a recessive mutation in the house mouse affecting head and limb skeleton. Journal of Morphology 99: 465–479.

739. Godfrey, S. J. 1989. Ontogenetic changes in the skull of the Carboniferous tetrapod *Greererpeton burkemorani*. Romer, 1969. Philosophical Transactions of the Royal Society B 323: 135–153.

740. Goedbloed, J. F. 1964. The early development of the middle ear and the mouth cavity. A study of the interaction of processes in the epithelium and the mesenchyme. Archives of Biology 75: 207–244.

741. Gogan, P. J. P. 1985. Cleft palate in a tule elk calf. Journal of Wildlife Diseases 21: 463–466.

742. Goldschmid, A. 1972a. Die Entwicklung des Craniums der Mausvögel (Coliidae, Coliiformes, Aves). I. Die Frühentwicklung des Chondrocranium. Gegenbaurs Morphologisches Jahrbuch, Leipzig 118: 105–138.

743. Goldschmid, A. 1972b. Die Entwicklung des Craniums der Mausvögel (Coliidae, Coliiformes, Aves). 2. Die Entwicklung des Chondrocraniums bis zum Auftreten der dermalen Verknöcherungen. Gegenbaurs Morphologisches Jahrbuch, Leipzig 118: 274–305.

744. Goldschmid, A. 1972c. Die Entwicklung des Craniums der Mausvögel (Coliidae, Coliiformes, Aves). 3. Ausgestaltung und Umbau des Chondrocraniums

bis zum Auftreten der Ersatzverknöcherungen. Gegenbaurs Morphologisches Jahrbuch, Leipzig 118: 369–413.

745. Goldschmid, A. 1972d. Die Entwicklung des Craniums der Mausvögel (Coliidae, Coliiformes, Aves). 4. Die Entwicklungs des Osteocraniums. Gegenbaurs Morphologisches Jahrbuch, Leipzig 118: 553–569.

746. Goldstein, C. D., J. J. Jankiewicz, and M. E. Desmond. 1986. Identification of glycosaminoglycans in the chondrocranium of the chick embryo before and at the onset of chondrogenesis. Journal of Embryology and Experimental Embryology 93: 29–49.

747. Goliner, K. 1982. Untersuchungen uber die vom *n. trigeminus innervierte* Kiefermuskulatur des Schimpansen (*Pan troglodytes,* Blumenbach 1799) und des Gorilla (*Gorilla gorilla gorilla,* Savage and Wyman 1847). Gegenbaurs Morphologische Jahrbuch 128: 851–903.

748. Goni, R., and F. Abdala. 1988. Considerations of skull-teeth morphology of *Rusconiodon mignonei* (Cynodontia Traversodontidae): Diagnosis, relationships, and ontogenetic variations. Ameghiniana 25: 237–244.

749. Gonsales, P. D. 1982. Age and growth determination of the red grouper, *Epinephilus morio* (Valencienne), from the Campeche Bank of the Gulf of Mexico. Trudy Zoologicheskogo Instituta, Leningrad 114: 57–66.

750. Goose, D. H., and J. Appleton. 1982. *Human Dentofacial Growth.* Oxford: Pergamon Press.

751. Gopal Rao, K. 1977. Development of the latero-sensory system and its association with the bones in the cranium of a cyprinodont *Xiphophorus helleri* (Haeckel). Matsya 3: 15–26.

752. Gorbman, A., and A. Tamarin. 1985a. Early development of oral, olfactory, and adenohypophyseal structures of agnathans and its evolutionary implications. In *Evolutionary Biology of Primitive Fishes,* R. E. Foreman, A. Gorbman, J. M. Dodd, and R. Olsson, eds. New York: Plenum Press, pp. 165–185.

753. Gorbman, A., and A. Tamarin. 1985b. Head development in relation to hypophysial development in a myxinoid, *Eptatretus,* and a petromyzontid, *Petromyzon.* In *The Pars Distalis: Structure, Function, and Regulation,* F. Oshimura and A. Gorbman, eds. Amsterdam: Elsevier.

754. Goret-Nicaise, M. 1981a. Über das Wachstum des unterkiefers beim Menschen. Fortschritte der Kieferorthopädie 42: 405–427.

755. Goret-Nicaise, M. 1981b. Tierexperimentelle Vergleichsuntersuchung mittels zweier extraoraler mandibulärer Krafte. Fortschritte der Kieferorthopädie 42: 429–440.

756. Goret-Nicaise, M. 1986. L'ontogenèse de la mandibule humaine. In *Définition et origines de l'homme,* M. Sakka, ed. Paris: CNRS, pp. 74–84.

757. Goret-Nicaise, M., and A. Dhem. 1982. Presence of chondroid tissue in the symphyseal region of the growing human mandible. Acta anatomica 113: 189–195.

758. Goret-Nicaise, M., B. Lengele, and A. Dhem. 1984. The function of Meckel's and secondary cartilage in the histomorphogenesis of the cat mandibular symphysis. Archives d'anatomie microscopique et de morphologie experimentale 73: 291–304.

759. Goret-Nicaise, M., M. C. Manzanares, P. Bulpa, E. Nolmans, and A. Dhem.

1988. Calcified tissues involved in the ontogenesis of the human cranial vault. Anatomy and Embryology 178: 399–406.

760. Gorlin, R. J., ed. 1980. *Morphogenesis and Malformation of the Ear*. New York: Alan R. Liss.

761. Gorshkov, S. A. 1979. Comparative morphological description of the chum salmon, *Oncorhynchus keta*, of various local stocks. Voprosy Ikhtiologii 19: 209–222.

762. Goss, A. N., J. White, and G. C. Townsend. 1983. Craniofacial growth in young marmosets (*Callithrix jacchus*). Laboratory Animals 17: 303–306.

763. Goss, R. J. 1954. The role of the central cartilaginous rod in the regeneration of the catfish taste barbel. Journal of Experimental Zoology 127: 181–199.

764. Goss, R. J. 1961. Experimental investigations of morphogenesis in the growing antler. Journal of Embryology and Experimental Morphology 9: 342–354.

765. Goss, R. J. 1963. The deciduous nature of deer antlers. In *Mechanisms of Hard Tissue Destruction*, R. Sognnaes, ed., AAAS Publication no. 75. Washington, D.C.: American Association for the Advancement of Science, pp. 339–369.

766. Goss, R. J. 1964a. The role of the skin in antler regeneration. Advances in the Biology of the Skin 5: 194–207.

767. Goss, R. J. 1964b. *Adaptive Growth*. New York: Academic Press.

768. Goss, R. J. 1969. *Principles of Regeneration*. New York: Academic Press.

769. Goss, R. J. 1970. Problems in antlerogenesis. Clinical Orthopedics and Related Research 69: 227–238.

770. Goss, R. J. 1978. *The Physiology of Growth*. New York: Academic Press.

771. Goss, R. J. 1983. *Deer Antlers: Regeneration, Function, and Evolution*. New York: Academic Press.

772. Goss, R. J. 1985. Tissue differentiation in regenerating antlers. Bulletin of the Royal Society of New Zealand 22: 229–238.

773. Goss, R. J. 1987. Induction of deer antlers by transplanted periosteum. 2. Regional competence for velvet transformation in ectopic skin. Journal of Experimental Zoology 244: 101–111.

774. Goss, R. J., and L. N. Grimes. 1972. Tissue interactions in the regeneration of rabbit ear holes. American Zoologist 12: 151–157.

775. Goss, R. J., and R. S. Powel. 1985. Induction of deer antlers by transplanted periosteum. I. Graft size and shape. Journal of Experimental Zoology 235: 359–373.

776. Goss, R. J., C. W. Severinghaus, and S. Free. 1964. Tissue relationships in the development of pedicles and antlers in the Virginia deer. Journal of Mammalogy 45: 61–68.

777. Goss, R. J., and M. W. Stagg. 1958a. Regeneration of the lower jaw in adult newts. Journal of Morphology 102: 289–309.

778. Goss, R. J., and M. W. Stagg. 1958b. Regeneration in lower jaws of newts after excision of the intermandibular regions. Journal of Experimental Zoology 137: 1–12.

779. Gosztonyi, A. E. 1988. The intercalar bone in the eel-pout family Zoarcidae (Osteichthyes). Zoologisches Anzeiger 221: 134–144.

780. Gottfried, M. D. 1986. Developmental transition in feeding morphology of the Midas cichlid. Copeia: 1028–1030.

781. Gradwell, N. 1968. The jaw and hyoidean mechanism of the bullfrog tadpole during aqueous ventilation. Canadian Journal of Zoology 46: 1041–1052.

782. Gradwell, N. 1970. The function of the ventral velum during gill irrigation in *Rana catesbeiana*. Canadian Journal of Zoology 48: 1179–1186.

783. Gradwell, N. 1971. *Xenopus* tadpoles: On the water pumping mechanism. Herpetologica 27: 107–123.

784. Gradwell, N. 1972a. Comments on gill irrigation in *Rana fuscigula*. Herpetologica 28: 122–124.

785. Gradwell, N. 1972b. Gill irrigation in *Rana catesbeiana*. Part I. On the anatomical basis. Canadian Journal of Zoology 50: 481–499.

786. Gradwell, N. 1972c. Gill irrigation in *Rana catesbeiana*. Part II. On the musculoskeletal mechanism. Canadian Journal of Zoology 50: 501–521.

787. Gradwell, N. 1973. On the functional morphology of suction and gill irrigation in the tadpole of *Ascaphus,* and notes on hibernation. Herpetologica 29: 84–93.

788. Gradwell, N., and V. M. Pasztor. 1968. The jaw and hyoidean mechanism of one bullfrog during aqueous ventilation. Canadian Journal of Zoology 46: 1041–1052.

789. Graham-Smith, W. 1978. On the lateral lines and dermal bones in the parietal region of some Crossopterygian and Dipnoan fishes. Philosophical Transactions of the Royal Society of London 282B: 41–105.

790. Grainger, J. P., and J. S. Fairley. 1978. Studies on the biology of the pygmy shrew *Sorex minutus* in the west of Ireland. Journal of Zoology, London 186: 109–141.

791. Granström, G. 1986. Isoenzyme changes during rat facial development. Scandinavian Journal of Dental Research 94: 1–14.

792. Granström, G., and B. C. Magnusson. 1986. Changes in alkaline phosphatase isoenzymes of hard tissue origin during facial development in the rat. Archives of Oral Biology 31: 513–519.

793. Graumann, W. 1951. Topogenese der Bindegewebsknochen an Schädelknochen menschlicher Embryonen. Zeitschrift für Anatomie und Entwicklungsgeschichte 116: 14–26.

794. Graver, H. T. 1973. The polarity of the dental lamina in the regenerating salamander jaw. Journal of Embryology and Experimental Morphology 30: 635–646.

795. Graver, H. T. 1978. Re-regeneration of lower jaws and the dental lamina in adult urodeles. Journal of Morphology 157: 269–280.

796. Graveson, A. C., and J. B. Armstrong. 1987. Differentiation of cartilage from cranial neural crest in the axolotl (*Ambystoma mexicanum*). Differentiation 35: 16–20.

797. Green, H. L., and R. Presley. 1978. The dumb-bell bone of *Ornithorhynchus*. Journal of Anatomy, London 127: 216.

798. Greene, R. M. 1989. Signal transduction during orofacial development. Critical Reviews in Toxicology 20: 137–152.

799. Greene, R. M., and R. M. Pratt. 1976. Developmental aspects of secondary

palate formation. Journal of Embryology and Experimental Morphology 36: 225–245.

800. Greene, R. M., R. M. Shah, M. R. Lloyd, B. J. Crawford, R. Sven, J. L. Shanfield, and Z. Davodivitch. 1983. Differentiation of the avian secondary palate. Journal of Experimental Zoology 225: 43–52.

801. Greven, H., and G. Clemen. 1979. Morphological studies on the mouth cavity in urodeles. IV. The teeth of the upper jaw and the palate in *Necturus maculosus* (Rafinesque) (Proteidae: Amphibia). Archivum histologicum japonicum 42: 445–457.

802. Greven, H., and G. Clemen. 1980a. Observations on the teeth and the dental laminae of the upper jaw and palate in *Siphonops annulatus* (Mikan) (Amphibia: Gymnophiona). Anatomisches Anzeiger 147: 270–279.

803. Greven, H., and G. Clemen. 1980b. Morphological studies on the mouth cavity of urodeles. VI. The teeth of the upper jaw and the palate in *Andrias davidianus* (Blanchard) and *A. japonicus* (Temminck) (Cryptobranchidae: Amphibia). Amphibia-Reptilia 1: 49–59.

804. Greven, H., and G. Clemen. 1985a. Changes of teeth and dentigerous bones in the mouth roof of *Salamandra salamandra* (L.) (Amphibia, Urodela) during metamorphosis. Verhandlungen der Deutschen zoologischen Gesellschaft 78: 162.

805. Greven, H., and G. Clemen. 1985b. Morphological studies on the mouth cavity of Urodela. VIII. The teeth of the upper jaw and the palate in two *Hynobius* species (Hynobiidae: Amphibia). Sonderdruck aus Zeitschrift für zoologische Systematik und Evolutionsforschung 23: 136–147.

806. Griffioen, F. M. M., and J. H. Smit-Vis. 1985. The skull: Mould or cast? Acta morphologica Neerlando-Scandinavica 23: 325–335.

807. Griffiths, I. 1954a. On the nature of the fronto-parietal in Amphibia, Salientia. Proceedings of the Zoological Society of London 123: 781–792.

808. Griffiths, I. 1954b. On the "otic element" in Amphibia, Salientia. Proceedings of the Zoological Society of London 124: 35–50.

809. Griffiths, M. 1978. *The Biology of Monotremes.* New York: Academic Press.

810. Grigson, C. 1978. The craniology and relationships of four species of *Bos.* 4. The relationship between *Bos primegenius* Boj. and *B. taurus* L. and its implication for the phylogeny of the domestic breeds. Journal of Archaeological Science 5: 123–152.

811. Grigson, C. 1980. The craniology and relationships of four species of *Bos.* 5. *Bos indicus.* Journal of Archaeological Science 7: 3–32.

812. Grobman, A. B. 1943. The appearance during ontogeny of a suture between previously fused dermal bones. Anatomical Record 87: 211–213.

813. Grobman, A. B. 1959. The anterior cranial elements of the salamanders *Pseudotriton* and *Gyrinophilus.* Copeia: 60–63.

814. Groves, C. P. 1982. The skulls of Asian rhinoceroses: Wild and captive. Zoo Biology 1: 251–261.

815. Grube, D., and W. Reinbach. 1976. The cranium of a human embryo 80 millimeters long from head to hip: The morphology of the cranium of older human fetuses. III. Anatomy and Embryology 149: 183–208.

816. Gruber, G. B. 1952a. Über das Wesen den Cerviden-Geweihe. Deutsche Tier-ärzliche Wochenschruft 59: 225–228, 241–243.

817. Gruber, G. B. 1952b. Studienergebnisse am Geweih des *Cervus capreolus*. Zentralblatt für Allgemeine pathologie und pathologische Anatomie 88: 336–345.

818. Grüneberg, H. 1938. An analysis of the "pleiotropic" effects of a new lethal mutation in the rat. Proceedings of the Royal Society of London 125B: 123–144.

819. Grüneberg, H. 1953. Genetical studies on the skeleton of the mouse. VII. Congenital hydrocephalus. Journal of Genetics 51: 327–358.

820. Grüneberg, H. 1963. *The Pathology of Development: A Study of Inherited Skeletal Disorders in Animals*. Oxford: Blackwell Scientific Publications.

821. Grüneberg, H. 1975. How do genes affect the skeleton? In *New Approaches to the Evaluation of Abnormal Embryonic Development*, D. Neuberg and H. J. Merker, eds. Stuttgart: George Thieme, pp. 354–359.

822. Grüneberg, H., and G. M. Truslove. 1960. Two closely linked genes in the mouse. Genetical Research 1: 69–90.

823. Grüneberg, H., and G. A. des Wickramaratne. 1974. A re-examination of two skeletal mutants of the mouse, vestigial tail (*vt*) and congenital hydro-cephalus (*ch*). Journal of Embryology and Experimental Morphology 31: 207–222.

824. Grunz, H., and L. Tacke. 1986. The inducing capacity of the presumptive endoderm of *Xenopus laevis* studied by transfilter experiments. Wilhelm Roux Archives of Developmental Biology 195: 467–473.

825. Guardabassi, A. 1960. The utilization of the calcareous deposits of the en-dolymphatic sacs of *Bufo bufo bufo* in the mineralization of the skeleton: Investigations by means of ^{45}Ca. Zeitschrift für Zellforschung und mikroskopische Anatomie 51: 278–282.

826. Guerrier, Y. 1989. The branchial apparatus and its role in morphogenesis of the neck. Acta oto-rhino-laryngologica belgica 43: 554–558.

827. Guibé, J. 1970a. Le squelette céphalique. In *Traité de Zoologie*, vol. 14(2), *Reptiles: Caractères géneraux et anatomie*, P.-P. Grassé, ed. Paris: Masson et Cie, pp. 78–143.

828. Guibé, J. 1970b. Les organes de l'olfaction. In *Traité de Zoologie*, vol. 14(2), *Reptiles: Caractères géneraux et anatomie*, P.-P. Grassé, ed. Paris: Masson et Cie, pp. 347–359.

829. Guibé, J. 1970c. Les organes stato-acoustique. In *Traité de Zoologie*, vol. 14(2), *Reptiles: Caractères géneraux et anatomie*, P.-P. Grassé, ed. Paris: Masson et Cie, pp. 360–375.

830. Guihard-Costa, A.-M. 1984. Croissance du squamosal chez la souris: Étude des processus d'ossification par injection d'alizarine S *in vivo*. Mammalia 48: 275–280.

831. Guihard-Costa, A.-M. 1988. Discontinuity in the rhythm of growth of the human foetus' skull bones about thirty weeks old. Comptes rendus, Académie des sciences, Paris 306: 433–436.

832. Guihard-Costa, A.-M., and M. Sakka. 1982. Développement de l'os frontal

chez la souris: Étude par coloration vitale au rouge d'alizarine S. Mammalia 46: 101–106.

833. Guihard-Costa, A.-M., and M. Sakka. 1983. Développement de l'os pariétal: Étude par coloration vitale au rouge d'alizarine S. Mammalia 47: 257–264.

834. Guihard-Costa, A.-M., and M. Sakka. 1988. Post-natal ossification of the interparietal bone in the mouse. Mammalia 52: 93–100.

835. Guiler, E. R. 1984. A young strap-toothed whale in Tasmanian waters. Papers and Proceedings of the Royal Society of Tasmania 118: 65–68.

836. Gunchak, N. S. 1978. Morphometric characteristics of Sus scrofa in Ukrainian Carpathiana. Zoologicheskii zhurnal 57: 1870–1877.

837. Gurskii, I. G. 1973. Determination of Canis lupis (L.) age by the skull. Vestnik zoologii 7: 55–59.

838. Gussen, R. 1968. The labyrinthine capsule: Normal structure and pathogenesis of otosclerosis. Acta oto-laryngologica 235 (suppl).: 1–55.

839. Guth, C. 1960. L'arc hyoïdien. Bulletin du Muséum d'histoire naturelle, Paris 32: 473–483.

840. Gutherz, E. J. 1970. Characteristics of some larval bothid flatfish and development and distribution of larval spotfish flunder, Cyclopsetta fimbriata (Bothidae). U.S. National Marine Fisheries Service, Fishery Bulletin 68: 261–283.

841. Haardick, H. 1941. Wachstumsstufen in der Embryonalentwicklung des Hühnchens. Biologia generalis, Vienna 15: 30–74.

842. Hafner, J. C., and M. S. Hafner. 1983. Evolutionary relationships of heteromyid rodents. Great Basin Naturalist, Memoirs 7: 3–29.

843. Hafner, M. S., and J. C. Hafner. 1984. Brain size, adaptation, and heterochrony in geomyoid rodents. Evolution 38: 1088–1098.

844. Hagelin, L.-O. 1974. Development of the membranous labyrinth in lampreys. Acta zoologica, Stockholm (suppl.): 1–218.

845. Haines, R. W. 1937. The posterior end of Meckel's cartilage and related ossifications in bony fishes. Quarterly Journal of Microscopical Science 80: 1–38.

846. Haldiman, J. T., and H. T. Gier. 1981. Bovine notochord origin and development. Anatomia, Histologia, Embryologia 10: 1–14.

847. Hale, L. J. 1956a. Mitotic activity during the early differentiation of the scleral bones in the chick. Quarterly Journal of Microscopial Science 97: 333–353.

848. Hale, L. J. 1956b. Mesodermal cell death during the early development of the scleral bones in the chick. Quarterly Journal of Microscopial Science 97: 355–368.

849. Hall, B. K. 1967. The distribution and fate of adventitious cartilage in the skull of the eastern rosella, Platycercus eximius (Aves: Psittaciformes). Australian Journal of Zoology 15: 685–698.

850. Hall, B. K. 1968a. The fate of adventitious and embryonic articular cartilage in the skull of the common fowl, Gallus domesticus (Aves: Phasianidae). Australian Journal of Zoology 16: 795–806.

851. Hall, B. K. 1968b. Studies on the nature and evocation of the articular cartilage on the avian pterygoid. Australian Journal of Zoology 16: 815–821.

852. Hall, B. K. 1978. *Developmental and Cellular Skeletal Biology*. New York: Academic Press.

853. Hall, B. K. 1980a. Tissue interactions and the initiation of osteogenesis and chondrogenesis in the neural crest–derived mandibular skeleton of the embryonic mouse as seen in isolated murine tissues and in recombinations of murine and avian tissues. Journal of Embryology and Experimental Morphology 58: 251–264.

854. Hall, B. K. 1980b. Chondrogenesis and osteogenesis in cranial neural crest cells. In *Current Research Trends in Prenatal Craniofacial Development*, R. M. Pratt and R. L. Christiansen, eds. New York: Elsevier/North Holland, pp. 47–63.

855. Hall, B. K. 1981. Specificity in the differentiation and morphogenesis of neural crest–derived scleral ossicles and of epithelial scleral papillae in the eye of the embryonic chick. Journal of Embryology and Experimental Morphology 66: 175–190.

856. Hall, B. K. 1982a. Mandibular morphogenesis and craniofacial malformations. Journal of Craniofacial Genetics and Developmental Biology 2: 309–322.

857. Hall, B. K. 1982b. The role of tissue interactions in the growth of bone. In *Factors and Mechanisms Influencing Bone Growth*, A. D. Dixon and B. G. Sarnat, eds. New York: Alan R. Liss, pp. 205–216.

858. Hall, B. K. 1982c. How is mandibular growth controlled during development and evolution? Journal of Craniofacial Genetics and Developmental Biology 2: 45–49.

859. Hall, B. K. 1983a. Epigenetic control in development and evolution. In *Development and Evolution*, B. C. Goodwin, N. J. Holder, and C. C. Wylie, eds. Cambridge: Cambridge University Press, pp. 353–379.

860. Hall, B. K. 1983b. Tissue interactions and chondrogenesis. In *Cartilage*, vol. 2, *Development, Differentiation, and Growth*, B. K. Hall, ed. New York: Academic Press, pp. 187–222.

861. Hall, B. K. 1983c. Epithelial-mesenchymal interactions in cartilage and bone development. In *Epithelial-Mesenchymal Interactions in Development*, R. H. Sawyer and J. F. Fallon, eds. New York: Praeger Press, pp. 189–214.

862. Hall, B. K. 1984a. Developmental processes underlying the evolution of cartilage and bone. In *The Structure, Development, and Evolution of Reptiles*, M. W. J. Ferguson, ed. London: Academic Press, pp. 155–176.

863. Hall, B. K. 1984b. Genetic and epigenetic control of connective tissues in the craniofacial skeleton. Birth Defects, Original Article Series 20: 1–17.

864. Hall, B. K. 1984c. Developmental processes and heterochrony as an evolutionary mechanism. Canadian Journal of Zoology 62: 1–7.

865. Hall, B. K. 1986. Initiation of chondrogenesis from somitic, limb, and craniofacial mesenchyme: Search for a common mechanism. In *Somites in Developing Embryos*, R. Bellairs, D. A. Ede, and J. W. Lash, eds. NATO Advanced Study Institutes Series 118. New York: Plenum Publishing, pp. 247–260.

the vertebrate head. In *Developmental and Evolutionary Aspects of the Neural Crest*, P. F. A. Maderson, ed. New York: John Wiley and Sons, pp. 215–259.

867. Hall, B. K. 1987b. Sodium fluoride as an initiator of osteogenesis from embryonic mesenchyme. Bone 8: 111–116.

868. Hall, B. K. 1987c. Development of the mandibular skeleton in the embryonic chick as evaluated using the DNA-inhibiting agent 5-fluoro-2'-deoxyuridine (FUDR). Journal of Craniofacial Genetics and Developmental Biology 7: 145–159.

869. Hall, B. K. 1987d. Earliest evidence of cartilage and bone development in embryonic life. Clinical Orthopaedics and Related Research 225: 255–272.

870. Hall, B. K. 1988a. Mechanisms of craniofacial development. In *Craniofacial Morphogenesis and Dysmorphogenesis*, K. W. L. Vig and A. P. Burdi, eds. Craniofacial Growth Monograph Series 21. Ann Arbor: Center for Human Growth and Development, University of Michigan, pp. 1–21.

871. Hall, B. K. 1988b. The embryonic development of bone. American Scientist 76 (2): 174–181.

872. Hall, B. K. 1988c. Patterning of connective tissues in the head: Discussion report. Development 103 (suppl.): 171–174.

873. Hall, B. K. 1989. Morphogenesis of the Skeleton: Epithelial or mesenchymal control? Fortschritte der Zoologie 35: 198–201.

874. Hall, B. K., and J. Hanken. 1985a. Repair of fractured lower jaws in the spotted salamander: Do amphibians form secondary cartilage? Journal of Experimental Zoology 233: 359–368.

875. Hall, B. K., and J. Hanken 1985b. Foreword to reissue of *The Development of the Vertebrate Skull*, by G. R. de Beer. Chicago: University of Chicago Press, pp. vii–xxviii.

876. Hall, B. K., and S. Hörstadius. 1988. *The Neural Crest*. Oxford: Oxford University Press.

877. Hall, B. K., and H. N. Jacobson. 1975. The repair of fractured membrane bones in the newly hatched chick. Anatomical Record 181: 55–70.

878. Hall, B. K., and R. J. van Exan. 1982. Induction of bone by epithelial cell products. Journal of Embryology and Experimental Morphology 69: 37–46.

879. Hall, B. K., R. J. van Exan, and S. L. Brunt. 1983. Retention of epithelial basal lamina allows isolated mandibular mesenchyme to form bone. Journal of Craniofacial Genetics and Developmental Biology 3: 253–267.

880. Hall, E. K. 1950. Experimental modifications of muscle development in *Ambylstoma punctatum*. Journal of Experimental Zoology 113: 355–377.

881. Hall, P. M. 1985a. Brachycephalic growth and dental anomalies in the New Guinea crocodile *Crocodylus novaeguineae*. Journal of Herpetology 19: 300–303.

882. Hall, P. M. 1985b. Embryo growth curves as a method of determining the age of clutches of New Guinea crocodiles (*Crocodylus novaeguineae*). Journal of Herpetology 19: 538–541.

883. Haluska, F., and P. Alberch. 1983. The cranial development of *Elaphe obsoleta* (Ophidia, Colubridae). Journal of Morphology 178: 37–56.

884. Hamdy, A. R. 1956. The development of the hyoid arch in Rhinobatidae. Proceedings of the Egyptian Academy of Science 12: 58–71.

885. Hamdy, A. R. 1959. The structure and development of the nasal cartilages in Selachii. Proceedings of the Egyptian Academy of Science 13: 18–22.

886. Hamdy, A. R. 1961. The development of the branchial arches of *Rhinobatus halavi*. Publications, Marine Biological Station, Ghardaqa, Red Sea 11: 205–213.

887. Hamdy, A. R. 1964. The development of the mandibular arch of *Rhynchobatus djiddensis*. Proceedings of the Egyptian Academy of Science 17: 1–3.

888. Hamdy, A. R. 1974. Studies on the structure and development of the rostral cartilages in Selachii. Proceedings of the Egyptian Academy of Science 25: 17–19.

889. Hamel, P. B., J. L. Beacham, and A. E. Ross. 1983. A laboratory study of cranial pneumatization in Indigo buntings. Journal of Field Ornithology 54: 58–66.

890. Hammarberg, F. 1937. Zur Kenntnis der ontogenetischen Entwicklung des Schädels von *Lepidosteus platystomus*. Acta zoologica, Stockholm 18: 209–337.

891. Hammond, W. S., and C. L. Yntema. 1964. Depletions of pharyngeal arch cartilages following extirpation of cranial neural crest in chick embryos. Acta anatomica 56: 21–34.

892. Hammouda, H. G. 1980. On the origin and fate of the cranial ribs in birds. Bulletin of the Faculty of Science of Cairo University, no. 49: 163–174.

893. Hammouda, H. G., and F. M. Mokhtar. 1980. The development of the skull of *Upupa epops major* C. L. Brehm (the Egyptian hoopoe) Order Coraciiformes. 3. The post-hatching development of the cartilaginous nasal capsule. Bulletin to the Faculty of Science of Cairo University, no. 49: 199–218.

894. Hampton, S. H., and E. P. Volpe. 1963. Development and interpopulation variability of the mouthparts of *Scaphiopus holbrooki*. American Midland Naturalist 70: 319–328.

895. Hanken, J. 1983. Miniaturization and its effects on cranial morphology in plethodontid salamanders, genus *Thorius* (Amphibia, Plethodontidae). II. The fate of the brain and sense organs and their role in skull morphogenesis and evolution. Journal of Morphology 177: 255–268.

896. Hanken, J. 1984. Miniaturization and its effects on cranial morphology in plethodontid salamanders, genus *Thorius* (Amphibia, Plethodontidae). I. Osteological variation. Biological Journal of the Linnean Society 23: 55–75.

897. Hanken, J. 1989. Development and evolution in amphibians. American Scientist 77: 336–343.

898. Hanken, J., and B. K. Hall. 1984. Variation and timing of the cranial ossification sequence of the Oriental fire-bellied toad, *Bombina orientalis* (Amphibia, Discoglossidae). Journal of Morphology 182: 245–255.

899. Hanken, J., and B. K. Hall. 1988a. Skull development during anuran metamorphosis. I. Early development of the first three bones to form—the exoccipital, the parasphenoid, and the frontoparietal. Journal of Morphology 195: 247–256.

900. Hanken, J., and B. K. Hall. 1988b. Skull development during anuran meta-

morphosis. II. Role of thyroid hormone in osteogenesis. Anatomy and Embryology 178: 219–227.

901. Hanken, J., and C. H. Summers. 1988. Skull development during anuran metamorphosis. III. Role of thyroid hormone in chondrogenesis. Journal of Experimental Zoology 246: 156–170.

902. Hanken, J., C. H. Summers, and B. K. Hall. 1989. Morphological integration in the cranium during anuran metamorphosis. Experientia 45: 872–875.

903. Hanmer, D. B. 1978. Measurements and molt of five species of bulbul from Mozambique and Malawi. Ostrich 49: 116–131.

904. Hanmer, D. B. 1980a. Mensural and molt data on six species of bee-eater (*Merops*) in Mozambique and Malawi. Ostrich 51: 25–38.

905. Hanmer, D. B. 1980b. Mensural and molt data of eight species of kingfishers from Mozambique and Malawi. Ostrich 51: 129–150.

906. Hanmer, D. B. 1984. The brownthroated golden weaver *Ploceus xanthopterus* from Mozambique and Malawi. In *Proceedings of the Fifth Pan-African Ornithological Congress*, J. Ledger, ed. Johannesburg: Southern African Ornithological Society, pp. 121–148.

907. Hansen, C. G., and O. V. Deming. 1980. Growth and development. In *The Desert Bighorn: Its Life History, Ecology, and Management*, G. Monson and L. Sumner, eds. Tucson: University of Arizona Press, pp. 152–171.

908. Happold, D. C. D. 1979. Age structure of a population of *Praomys tullbergi* (Muridae, Rodentia) in Nigerian rain forests. Terre et la vie 33: 253–274.

909. Hardisty, M. W. 1979. *Biology of the Cyclostomes*. London: Chapman and Hall.

910. Hardisty, M. W. 1981. The skeleton. In *The Biology of Lampreys*, M. W. Hardisty and I. C. Potter, eds., vol. 3. London: Academic Press, pp. 333–376.

911. Harris, S. 1978. Age determination in the red fox (*Vulpes vulpes*)—an evaluation of technique efficiency as applied to a sample of suburban foxes. Journal of Zoology, London 184: 91–117.

912. Harrison, D. F. N., and S. Denny. 1983. Ossification within the primate larynx. Acta otolaryngologica 95: 440–446.

913. Harrison, J. G., and D. L. Harrison. 1949. Some developmental peculiarities in the skulls of birds and bats. Bulletin of the British Ornithological Club 69: 61–70.

914. Harrison, R. G. 1945. Relations of symmetry in the developing embryo. Transactions of the Connecticut Academy of Arts and Science 36: 277–330.

915. Harrison, R. G. 1978. *Clinical Embryology*. London: Academic Press.

916. Hartwig, H. 1967. Experimentelle Untersuchungen zur Entwicklungsphysiologie der Stangenbildung beim Reh (*Capreolus c. capreolus* L. 1758). Wilhelm Roux Archives of Developmental Biology 158: 358–384.

917. Hartwig, H., and J. Schrudde. 1974. Experimentelle Untersuchungen zur Bildung der primären Stirnauswüchse beim Reh (*Capreolus capreolus* L). Zeitschrift für Jagdwissenschaft, Hamburg 20: 1–13.

918. Hartwig, H., J. Schrudde, H. Kierdorf, and U. Kierdorf. 1989. The formation of a bony protuberance on the skull of a female roe deer (*Capreolus capreolus* L.) due to unspecific local stimulation of the frontal-crest periosteum. Zeitschrift für Jagdwissenschaft, Hamburg 35: 130–136.

919. Hasurkar, S. S. 1957. The nature of the septomaxillary in the frog, *Rana tigrina*. (Daud.). Journal of the Zoological Society of India 8: 235–243.
920. Hattori, J. 1988. Ontogenetic changes of the pharyngeal bones of the scarid, *Scarus sordidus Forsskai*. Journal of Tokyo University of Fisheries 75: 263–274.
921. Hauschild, R. 1937. Rassenunterschiede zwischen negriden und Europiden Primordialcranien des 3. Fetalmonats. Zeitschrift für Morphologie und Anthropologie, Stuttgart 36: 215–279.
922. Hay, K. A. 1980. Age determination of the narwhal, *Monodon monoceros* L. Report of the International Whaling Commission, Special Issue 3: 119–132.
923. Heath, L, and P. Thorogood. 1989. Keratan sulfate expression during avian craniofacial morphogenesis. Wilhelm Roux Archives of Developmental Biology 198: 103–113.
924. Hecht, M. K., and S. Tarsitano. 1983. On the cranial morphology of the Protosuchia, Notosuchia, and Eosuchia. Neues Jahrbuch für Geologie und Palaeontologie, Abhandlungen: 657–668.
925. Heggberget, T. M. 1984. Age determination in the European otter *Lutra lutra*. Zeitschrift Saugetiere 49: 229–305.
926. Heintz, A. 1963. Phylogenetic aspects of myxinoids. In *The Biology of Myxine*, A. Brodal and R. Fange, eds. Oslo: Universitetsforlaget Oslo, pp. 9–21.
927. Heintz, N. P.-M. 1970. Morphogenesis of the cranium in primates. Comptes rendus hebdomadaires des séances de l'Académie des sciences, ser. D, Science naturelle, Paris 271: 1384–1386.
928. Helff, O. M. 1940. Studies on amphibian metamorphosis. XVII. Influence of non-living annular tympanic cartilage on tympanic membrane formation. Journal of Experimental Biology 17: 45–60.
929. Hell, P., and L. Paule. 1983. Systematic position of the West Carpathian [Czechoslovakia] wild hog *Sus scrofa*. Prirodovedna Prace Ustavu Ceskoslovenske Akademie Ved v Brne 17: 1–54.
930. Hennig, R. 1988. Doppelkopfbildung beim Damhirsch. Zeitschrift für Jagdwissenschaft 34: 132–133.
931. Hensel, K. 1978. Morphology of lateral-line canal system of the genera *Abramis, Blicca,* and *Vimba* with regard to their ecology and systematic position. Acta Universitatis Carolinae biologica 1975–76: 105–149.
932. Hensel, K., and J. Holcik. 1983. On the identity of *Hucho hucho* and *Hucho taimen* (Pisces, Salmonidae). Folia zoologica 32: 67–83.
933. Hensley, D. A. 1977. Larval development of *Engyophrys senta* (Bothidae), with comments on intermuscular bones in flatfishes. Bulletin of Marine Sciences 27: 681–703.
934. Hensley, D. A., and E. H. Ahlstrom. 1984. Pleuronectiformes: Relationships. In *Ontogeny and Systematics of Fishes*, American Society of Ichthyologists and Herpetologists Special Publication no. 1, H. G. Moser, ed. Lawrence, Kans.: Allen Press, pp. 670–687.
935. Heran, I. 1981. Comments on interrelations between some characters of neu-

rocranium and development of zygomatic arch in Mustelidae. Sbornik Narodniho Musea v Praze, Rada B, Priodni Vedy 37: 193–204.

936. Heran, I. 1984. Comments on the age-conditioned changes of skull proportions in some species of Mustelidae. Lynx, Prague 22: 11–14.

937. Herring, S. W. 1972. Sutures: Tool in functional cranial analysis. Acta anatomica 83: 222–247.

938. Herring, S. W. 1974. A biometric study of suture fusion and skull growth in peccaries. Anatomy and Embryology 146: 167–180.

939. Herring, S. W. 1985. The ontogeny of mammalian mastication. American Zoologist 25: 339–349.

940. Herring, S. W., and T. C. Lakars. 1981. Craniofacial development in the absence of muscle contraction. Journal of Craniofacial Genetics and Developmental Biology 1: 341–357.

941. Hetherington, T. E. 1987. Timing of development of the middle ear of Anura (Amphibia). Zoomorphology 106: 289–300.

942. Hildman, H., and F. J. Schmidt. 1980. Ossification of the skull of the growing hamster: Autoradiographic observations. Archives of Oto-Rhino-Laryngology 228: 265–270.

943. Hilfer, S. R., R. A. Esteves, and J. F. Sanzo. 1989. Invagination of the otic placode: Normal development and experimental manipulation. Journal of Experimental Zoology 251: 253–264.

944. Hillman-Smith, A. K. K., N. Owen-Smith, J. L. Anderson, A. J. Hall-Martin, and J. P. Selaladi. 1986. Age estimation of the white rhinoceros *Ceratotherium simum*. Journal of Zoology, ser. A, 210: 355–380.

945. Hilton, W. A. 1947. The hyobranchial skeleton of Plethodontidae. Herpetologica 3: 191–194.

946. Hilton, W. A. 1950a. The development of the chondrocranium in *Ambystoma* (preliminary remarks). Journal of Entomology and Zoology, Claremont, California 42: 2–4.

947. Hilton, W. A. 1950b. Review of the chondrocrania of tailed amphibia. Herpetologica 6: 125–135.

948. Hinrichsen, K. 1985. The early development of morphology and patterns of the face in the human embryo. Advances in Anatomy, Embryology, and Cell Biology 98: 1–79.

949. Hochstetter, F. 1939. Über die Entwicklung und Differenzierung der Hüllen des menschlichen Gehirns. Gegenbaurs Morphologisches Jahrbuch 83: 359–494.

950. Hodges, P. C., Jr. 1953. Ossification in the fetal pig: A radiographic study. Anatomical Record 116: 315–325.

951. Hoedeman, J. J. 1960a. Studies on Callichthyid fishes. 3. Notes on the development of *Callichthys* (2) (Pisces-Siluriformes). Bulletin of Aquatic Biology 1: 57–68.

952. Hoedeman, J. J. 1960b. Studies on Callichthyid fishes. 4. Development of the skull of *Callichthys* and *Haplosternum* (Pisces-Siluriformes). Bulletin of Aquatic Biology 1: 73–84.

953. Hoedeman, J. J. 1960c. Studies on Callichthyid fishes. 5. Development of the

skull of *Callichthys* and *Haplosternum* (Pisces-Siluriformes). 6. The axial skeleton of *Callichthys* and *Haplosternum* (Pisces-Siluriformes). Bulletin of Aquatic Biology 2: 21–44.

954. Hofer, H. 1945. Untersuchungen über den Bau des Vogelschädels, besonders über den der Spechte und Steisshühner. Zoologische Jahrbücher, Abteilung für Anatomie und Ontogenie der Tiere 69: 1–158.

955. Hofer, H. 1952. Der Gestaltwandel des Schädels der Säugetiere und Vögel, mit besonderer Berücksichtigung der Knickungstypen und der Schädelbasis. Verhandlungen der Anatomischen Gesellschaft, Jena 50: 102–113.

956. Hofer, H. 1955. Neuere Untersuchungen zur Kopfmorphologie der Vögel. In *Acta XI Congressus Internationalis Ornithologici*, A. Portmann and E. Sutter, eds. Basel: Birkhauser Verlag, pp. 104–137.

957. Hofer, H. 1956. Die morphologische Analyse des Schädels des Menschen. In *Menschliche Abstammungslehre Fortschritte der Anthropogenie*, G. Heberer, ed. Stuttgart: Fisher, pp. 145–226.

958. Hogan, B. L. M., G. Horsburgh, J. Cohen, C. M. Hetherington, G. Fisher, and M. F. Lyon. 1986. Small eyes (*Sey*): A homozygous lethal mutation on chromosome 2 which affects the differentiation of both lens and nasal placode in the mouse. Journal of Embryology and Experimental Morphology 97: 95–110.

959. Holbrook, S. J. 1982. Ecological inferences from mandibular morphology of *Peromyscus maniculatus*. Journal of Mammalogy 63: 399–408.

960. Holland, P. W. H. 1988. Homeobox genes and the vertebrate head. Development 103 (suppl.): 17–24.

961. Holland, P. W. H. 1989. Pursuing the functions of vertebrate homeobox genes: Progress and prospects. Trends in Neuroscience 12: 206–209.

962. Holland, P. W. H., and B. L. M. Hogan. 1988a. Expression of homeobox genes during mouse development: A review. Genes and Development 2: 773–782.

963. Holland, P. W. H., and B. L. M. Hogan. 1988b. Spatially restricted patterns of expression of the homeobox-containing gene Hox 2.1 during mouse embryogenesis. Development 102: 159–174.

964. Holmgren, N. 1939. Note on the fate of the premandibular somite in sharks and rays. In *À la Mémoire de A. N. Sewertzoff*, vol. 1. Moscow, pp. 137–140.

965. Holmgren, N. 1940. Studies on the head in fishes: An embryological, morphological, and phylogenetical study. Part I. Development of the skull in sharks and rays. Acta zoologica, Stockholm 21: 51–267.

966. Holmgren, N. 1941. Studies on the head in fishes: An embryological, morphological, and phylogenetical study. Part II. Comparative anatomy of the adult selachian skull, with remarks on the dorsal fins in sharks. Acta zoologica, Stockholm 22: 1–100.

967. Holmgren, N. 1942a. Studies on the head in fishes: An embryological, morphological, and phylogenetical study. Part III. The phylogeny of elasmobranch fishes. Acta zoologica, Stockholm 23: 129–261.

968. Holmgren, N. 1942b. General morphology of the lateral sensory line system of the head in fish. Kungliga Svenska vetenskapsakademiens handlingar (3) 20: 1–46.

969. Holmgren, N. 1943. Studies on the head of fishes: An embryological, morphological, and phylogenetical study. Part IV. General morphology of the head in fishes. Acta zoologica, Stockholm 24: 1–188.

970. Holmgren, N. 1946. On two embryos of *Myxine glutinosa*. Acta zoologica, Stockholm 27: 1–90.

971. Holmgren, N. 1949. Contributions to the question of the origin of tetrapods. Acta zoologica, Stockholm 30: 459–484.

972. Holmgren, N., and T. Pehrson. 1949. Some remarks on the ontogenetical development of the sensory lines on the cheek in fishes and amphibians. Acta zoologica, Stockholm 30: 249–314.

973. Homolka, M. 1980. Biometric comparison of two populations of *Sorex araneus*. Prirodovedne Prace Ustavu Ceskoslovenska Akademie Ved v Brne 14: 1–34.

974. Honda, K., Y. Fujise, R. Tatsukawa, and N. Miyazaki. 1984. Composition of chemical components in bone of striped dolphin *Stenella coeruleoalba*: Distribution characteristics of major inorganic and organic components in various bones, and their age-related changes. Agricultural Biological Chemistry 48: 409–418.

975. Hoogerhoud, R. J. C. 1989. Prey processing and predator morphology in molluscivorous cichlid fishes. Fortschritte der Zoologie 35: 19–21.

976. Horacek, I. 1979. Comments on methods in craniomorphological studies in bats. Lynx, Prague 20: 111–112.

977. Horner, J. R., and D. B. Weishampel. 1988. A comparative embryological study of two ornithischian dinosaurs. Nature 332: 256–257.

978. Hörstadius, S. 1950. *The Neural Crest: Its Properties and Derivatives in the Light of Experimental Research*. Oxford: Oxford University Press. Reprinted. New York: Hafner Press, 1960.

979. Hörstadius, S., and S. Sellman. 1942. Experimental studies on the determination of the chondrocranium in *Ambystoma mexicanum*. Arkiv för Zoologi, Uppsala 33A: 1–8.

980. Hörstadius, S., and S. Sellman. 1946. Experimentelle untersuchungen über die Determination des Knorpeligen Kopfskelettes bei Urodelen. Nova acta Regiae societatis scientiarum Upsaliensis, ser. 4, 13: 1–170.

981. Hotta, H. 1958. Abnormal development of the cranial bones of "Jack mackeral" *Trachurus japonicus* Temminck & Schlegel with the growth. Japanese Journal of Ichthyology 7: 115–117.

982. Houde, E. D., C. R. Futch, and R. Detwyler. 1970. Development of the lined sole, *Achirus lineatus*, described from laboratory reared and Tampa Bay specimens. Florida Department of Natural Resources Marine Research Laboratory Technical Series 62: 1–43.

983. Houde, E. D., and T. Potthoff. 1976. Egg and larval development of the sea bream *Archosargus rhomboidalis* (Linnaeus): Pisces, Sparidae. Bulletin of Marine Science 26: 506–529.

984. Houde, E. D., W. J. Richards, and V. P. Saksena. 1974. Description of eggs and larvae of scaled sardine, *Harengula jaguana*. U.S. National Marine Fisheries Service, Fishery Bulletin 72: 1106–1122.

985. Howes, G. J., and C. P. J. Sanford. 1987. Oral ontogeny of the Ayu, *Pleco-*

glossus altivelis, and comparisons with the jaws of other salmoniform fishes. Zoological Journal of the Linnean Society 89: 133–169.

986. Howes, G. J., and G. G. Teugels. 1989. Observations on the ontogeny and homology of the pterygoid bones in *Corydoras paleatus* and some other catfishes. Journal of Zoology, London 219: 441–456.

987. Howes, R. I., and E. C. Eakers. 1984. Augmentation of tooth and jaw regeneration in the frog with a digital transplant. Journal of Dental Research 63: 670–674.

988. Howgate, M. E. 1985. Problems of the osteology of *Archaeopteryx:* Is the Eichstatt specimen a distinct genus? In *The Beginnings of Birds: Proceedings of the International Archaeopteryx Conference, Eichstatt 1984,* M. K. Hecht, J. H. Ostrom, G. Viohl, and P. Wellhofer, eds. Eichstatt: Freunde des Jura-Museums Eichstatt, pp. 10–112.

989. Hoyte, D. A. N. 1966. Experimental investigations of skull morphology and growth. International Review of General and Experimental Zoology 2: 345–407.

990. Hoyte, D. A. N. 1971a. The modes of growth of the neurocranium: The growth of the sphenoid bone in animals. In *Cranio-Facial Growth in Man,* R. E. Moyers and W. M. Krogman, eds. Oxford: Pergamon Press, pp. 77–105.

991. Hoyte, D. A. N. 1971b. Mechanisms of growth in the cranial vault and base. Journal of Dental Research 6 (suppl.): 1447–1461.

992. Hrabe, V. 1976a. Variation in cranial measurements of *Erinaceus europaeus occidentalis* (Insectivora, Mammalia). Zoologicke Listy 25: 303–314.

993. Hrabe, V. 1976b. Variation in cranial measurements of *Erinaceus concolor roumanicus* (Insectivora, Mammalia). Zoologicke Listy 25: 315–326.

994. Hrabe, V., and J. Zejda. 1981. Age determination and mean length of life in *Citellus citellus.* Folia zoologica 30: 117–123.

995. Hubbs, C. L. 1958. *Dikellorhynchus* and *Kanazawaichthys:* Nominal fish genera interpreted as based on prejuveniles of *Malacanthus* and *Antennarius,* respectively. Copeia: 282–285.

996. Hubendick, B. 1942. Zur Kenntnis der Entwicklung des Primordialcraniums bei *Leuciscus rutilus.* Arkiv för Zoologi, Uppsala 34A: 1–35.

997. Hublin, J.-J. 1980. La chaise suard, Engis 2 et la Quina H 18: Développement de la morphologie occipitale externe chez l'enfant prénéandertalien et néandertalien. Comptes rendus hebdomadaires des séances de l'Académie des sciences, ser. D, Paris 291: 669–672.

998. Huggins, R. A., S. E. Huggins, and I. H. Hellwig. 1943. Heterogony of ossification in the house wren. Growth 7: 427–437.

999. Huggins, R. A., S. E. Huggins, I. H. Hellwig, and G. Deutschlander. 1942. Ossification in the nestling house wren. Auk 59: 532–543.

1000. Huggins, S. E., and D. H. Thompson. 1942. Relative growth in several species of fresh-water gar. Growth 6: 163–171.

1001. Hughes, A. 1959. Studies in embryonic and larval development in Amphibia. I. The embryology of *Eleutherodactylus ricordii,* with special reference to the spinal cord. Journal of Embryology and Experimental Morphology 7: 22–38.

1002. Hulet, W. H. 1978. Structure and functional development of the eel leptocephalus *Ariosoma balearicum* (De La Roche, 1809). Philosophical Transactions of the Royal Society of London 282: 107–138.

1003. Hull, A. M. 1940. Development of the hyobranchial skeleton of the chick. University of Colorado Studies, General Series A 26: 56–57.

1004. Hulscher, J. B. 1985. Growth and abrasion of the oystercatcher bill in relation to dietary switches. Netherlands Journal of Zoology 35: 124–154.

1005. Hung, Sun Koh. 1983. A study on age variation and secondary sexual dimorphism in morphometric characters of Korean rodents. 1. An analysis on striped field mice, *Apodemus agrarius coreae* Thomas from Cheongju. Korean Journal of Zoology 26: 125–134.

1006. Hunt, R. M., Jr. 1974. The auditory bulla in Carnivora: An anatomical basis for reappraisal of carnivore evolution. Journal of Morphology 143: 21–76.

1007. Hunt, R. M., Jr. 1987. Evolution of the seluroid carnivora: Significance of auditory structure in the nimravid cat *Dinictis*. American Museum Novitates, no. 2886: 1–74.

1008. Hunt, T. J. 1958. Epimorphic regeneration during hibernation. Nature 181: 290.

1009. Huson, L. W., and R. J. C. Page. 1980. Age related variability of cranial measurements in the red fox (*Vulpes vulpes*). Journal of Zoology, London 191: 427–429.

1010. Huysseune, A. 1983. Observations on tooth development and implantation in the upper pharyngeal jaws in *Astatotilapia elegans* (Teleostei, Cichlidae). Journal of Morphology 175: 217–234.

1011. Huysseune, A. 1985. The opercular cartilage in *Astatotilapia elegans*. Fortschritte der Zoologie 30: 371–373.

1012. Huysseune, A. 1986. Late skeletal development at the articulation between upper pharyngeal jaws and neurocranial base in the fish, *Astatotilapia elegans*, with the participation of a chondroid form of bone. American Journal of Anatomy 177: 119–137.

1013. Huysseune, A. 1989. Morphogenetic aspects of the pharyngeal jaws and neurocranial apophysis in postembryonic *Astatotilapia elegans* (Trewavas, 1933) (Teleostei; Cichlidae). Mededelingen van de Koninklijke Academie voor Wetenschappen, Letteren en Schone Kunsten van Belgie 51: 11–35.

1014. Huysseune, A., M. H. Ismail, and W. Verraes. 1981. Some histological, histochemical, and ultrastructural aspects of the development of the articulation between neurocranial base and upper pharyngeal jaws in *Haplochromis elegans* (Teleostei: Cichlidae). Verhandlungen der Anatomischen Gesellschaft, Jena 75S: 499–500.

1015. Huysseune, A., W. Van den Berghe, and W. Verraes. 1986. The contribution of chondroid bone in the growth of the parasphenoid bone of a cichlid fish as studied by oblique computer-aided reconstructions. Biologisch Jaarboek, Antwerpen 54: 131–141.

1016. Huysseune, A., and W. Verraes. 1986. Chondroid bone on the upper pharyngeal jaws and neurocranial base in the adult fish, *Astatotilapia elegans*. American Journal of Anatomy 177: 527–535.

1017. Huysseune, A., and W. Verraes. 1987. Relationships between cartilage and bone growth in pharyngeal jaw development in a cichlid fish. Biologisch Jaarboek Dodonaea 55: 121–135.

1018. Huysseune, A., W. Verraes, and K. Desender. 1988. Mechanisms of branchial cartilage growth in *Astatotilapia elegans* (Teleostei: Cichlidae). Journal of Anatomy 158: 13–30.

1019. Ichikawa, M. 1937. Experiments on the amphibian mesectoderm, with special reference to the cartilage formation. Memoirs of the College of Science, Kyoto University 12B: 311–351.

1020. Inman, V. T., and J. B. de C. M. Saunders. 1937. The ossification of the human frontal bone, with special reference to its presumed pre- and postfrontal elements. Journal of Anatomy, London 71: 383–394.

1021. Iordansky, N. N. 1973. The skull of the Crocodilia. In *Biology of the Reptilia,* vol. 4, C. Gans and T. S. Parsons, eds. London: Academic Press, pp. 201–262.

1022. Irish, F. J. 1989. The role of heterochrony in the origin of a novel bauplan: Evolution of the ophidian skull. In *Ontogenèse et évolution,* B. David, J. L. Dommergues, J. Chaline, and B. Laurin, eds., Geobios, Mémoire spéciale 12. Lyon: Université Claude-Bernard, pp. 227–234.

1023. Irish, F. J., and P. Alberch. 1989. Heterochrony in the evolution of bolyeriid snakes. Fortschritte der Zoologie 35: 205.

1024. Irwin, C. R., and M. W. J. Ferguson. 1986. Fracture repair of reptilian dermal bones: Can reptiles form secondary cartilage? Journal of Anatomy, London 146: 53–64.

1025. Ismail, M. H. 1984. The postembryonic development of the olfactory organs in *Sarotherodon galilaeus* Linn. (Teleostei, Cichlidae). Annals of Zoology, Agra 21: 183–194.

1026. Ismail, M. H. 1986. Observations on the postembryonic development of the olfactory organs in *Sarotherodon galilaeus* Linnaeus (Teleostei, Cichlidae). Arab Gulf Journal of Scientific Research 4: 313–325.

1027. Ismail, M. H., W. Verraes, and A. Huysseune. 1982. Developmental aspects of the pharyngeal jaws in *Astatotilapia elegans* (Trewavas, 1933) (Teleostei: Cichlidae). Netherlands Journal of Zoology 32: 513–543.

1028. Isotopa, K. 1972. Alizarin trajectories in experimental studies of skull growth. Proceedings of the Finnish Dental Society 68 (suppl.): 1–56.

1029. Jacob, M., F. Wachtler, H. J. Jacob, and B. Christ. 1986. On the problem of metamerism in the head mesenchyme of chick embryos. In *Somites in Developing Embryos,* R. Bellairs, D. A. Ede, and J. W. Lash, eds. NATO Advanced Studies Institutes Series 118. New York: Plenum Press, pp. 79–90.

1030. Jacobson, A. G. 1987. Determination and morphogenesis of axial structures: Mesodermal metamerism, shaping of the neural plate and tube, and segregation and functions of the neural crest. In *Developmental and Evolutionary Aspects of the Neural Crest,* P. F. A. Maderson, ed. New York: John Wiley and Sons, pp. 147–180.

1031. Jacobson, A. G. 1988. Somitomeres: Mesodermal segments of vertebrate embryos. Development 104 (suppl.): 209–220.

1032. Jacobson, A. G., and S. Meier. 1984. Morphogenesis of the head of a newt:

Mesodermal segments, neuromeres, and distribution of neural crest. Developmental Biology 106: 181–193.

1033. Jacobson, A. G., and S. Meier. 1986. Somitomeres: The primordial body segments. In *Somites in Developing Embryos,* R. Bellairs, D. A. Ede, and J. W. Lash, eds. NATO Advanced Studies Institutes Series 118. New York: Plenum Press, pp. 1–16.

1034. Jacobson, W., and H. B. Fell. 1941. The developmental mechanics and potencies of the undifferentiated mesenchyme of the mandible. Quarterly Journal of Microscopical Science 82: 563–586.

1035. Jaczewski, Z. 1955. Regeneration of antlers in red deer, *Cervus elaphus* L. Bulletin of the Academy of Polish Science, ser. 2, 3: 273–278.

1036. Jaczewski, Z. 1956a. Free transplantation of antler in red deer (*Cervus elaphus* L.). Bulletin of the Academy of Polish Science, ser. 2, 4: 107–110.

1037. Jaczewski, Z. 1956b. Further observations on transplantation of antler in red deer (*Cervus elaphus* L.). Bulletin of the Academy of Polish Science, ser. 2, 4: 289–291.

1038. Jaczewski, Z. 1961. Observations on the regeneration and transplantation of antlers in deer Cervidae. Folia biologica, Krakow 9: 47–99.

1039. Jaczewski, Z. 1985. Hormonal regulation of antler casting in red deer. Fortschritte der Zoologie 30: 167–171.

1040. Jain, S. L. 1985. Variability of dermal bones and other parameters in the skull of *Amia calva.* Zoological Journal of the Linnean Society 84: 385–395.

1041. James, M. S. 1946. The role of the basibranchial cartilages in the early development of the thyroid of *Hyla regilla.* University of California Publications in Zoology 51: 215–228.

1042. James, P. S. B. R., and R. Soundararajan. 1981. An osteological study of the sperm whale, *Physeter macrocephalus* from the Indian Ocean. Indian Journal of Fisheries 28: 217–232.

1043. Jarosova, J., and Z. Roček. 1982. The incrassatio frontoparietalis in frogs, its origin and phylogenetic significance. Amphibia-Reptilia 3: 111–124.

1044. Jarvik, E. 1947. Notes on the pit-lines and dermal bones of the head in *Polypterus.* Zoologiska bidrag fram Uppsala 25: 60–78.

1045. Jarvik, E. 1954. On the visceral skeleton in *Eusthenopteron,* with a discussion of the parasphenoid and palatoquadrate in fishes. Kungliga Svenska vetenskapsakademiens handlingar, Uppsala & Stockholm 5: 1–104.

1046. Jarvik, E. 1967a. The homologies of frontal and parietal bones in fishes and tetrapods. Colloques internationaux du Centre national de la recherche scientifique 163: 181–213.

1047. Jarvik, E. 1967b. On the structure of the lower jaw in dipnoans, with a description of an early Devonian dipnoan from Canada, *Melanognathus canadensis* gen. et sp. nov. Zoological Journal of the Linnean Society 47: 155–183.

1048. Jarvik, E. 1975. On the saccus endolymphaticus and adjacent structures in Osteolepiformes, anurans, and urodeles. Colloques internationaux du Centre national de la recherche scientifique 218: 191–211.

1049. Jarvik, E. 1980. *Basic Structure and Evolution of Vertebrates,* vols. 1 and 2. London: Academic Press.

1050. Jarvik, E. 1986. The origin of the Amphibia. In *Studies in Herpetology*, Z. Roček, ed. Prague: Charles University, pp. 1–24.

1051. Jaskoll, T. F. 1980. Morphogenesis and teratogenesis of the middle ear in animals. Birth Defects, Original Article Series 16 (7): 9–28.

1052. Jaskoll, T. F., and P. F. A. Maderson. 1978. A histological study of the development of the avian middle ear and tympanum. Anatomical Record 190: 177–200.

1053. Jaskoll, T., and M. Melnick. 1982. The effects of long-term fetal constraint *in vitro* on the cranial base and other skeletal components. American Journal of Medical Genetics 12: 289–300.

1054. Jaskoll, T., M. Melnick, M. MacDougall, A. G. Brownell, and H. C. Slavkin. 1981. Spatiotemporal patterns of fibronectin distribution during embryonic development. II. Chick branchial arches. Journal of Craniofacial Genetics and Developmental Biology 1: 203–212.

1055. Jaspers, R., and F. de Vree. 1978. Trends in the development of the skull of *Okapia johnstoni*. Acta zoologica pathologica antverpiensia, no. 71: 107–129.

1056. Jefferies, R. P. S. 1986. *The Ancestry of the Vertebrates*. Cambridge: Cambridge University Press.

1057. Jenni, L., and S. Jenni-Eirmann. 1987. Der Herbstzug der Gartengrasmucke *Sylvia borin* in der Schweig. Ornithologische Beobachter 84: 173–206.

1058. Jenni, L., and R. Winkler. 1983. Altersbestimmung und Umfang der Jugendmauser in Abhangigkeit von der Jahreszeit beim Zaunkonig *Troglodytes troglodytes*. Ornithologische Beobachter 80: 203–207.

1059. Jimenez, J. 1972. Comparative postnatal growth in five species of the genus *Sigmodon*. II. Cranial character relationships. Revista de biologia tropical 20: 5–27.

1060. Johansen, V. A., and S. H. Hall. 1982. Morphogenesis of the mouse cranial suture. Acta anatomica 114: 58–67.

1061. John, M. A. 1951. Pelagic fish eggs and larvae of the Madras coast. Journal of the Zoological Society of India 3: 41–69.

1062. Johnels, A. G. 1948. On the development and morphology of the skeleton of the head of *Petromyzon*. Acta zoologica, Stockholm 29: 139–279.

1063. Johnels, A. G. 1950. On the dermal connective tissue of the head of *Petromyzon*. Acta zoologica, Stockholm 31: 177–185.

1064. Johnson, C. R. 1973. Hyperostosis in fishes of the genus *Platycephalus* (Platycephalidae). Japanese Journal of Ichthyology 20: 178.

1065. Johnson, D. R. 1976. The interfrontal bone and mutant genes in the mouse. Journal of Anatomy, London 121: 507–513.

1066. Johnson, D. R. 1983. Abnormal cartilage from the mandibular condyle of stumpy (*stm*) mutant mice. Journal of Anatomy 137: 715–728.

1067. Johnson, D. R. 1986. *The Genetics of the Skeleton: Animal Models of Skeletal Development*. Oxford: Clarendon Press.

1068. Johnson, G. D. 1984. Percoidei: Development and relationships. In *Ontogeny and Systematics of Fishes*, American Society of Ichthyologists and Herpetologists Special Publication no. 1, H. G. Moser, ed. Lawrence, Kans.: Allen Press, pp. 464–498.

1069. Johnston, M. C. 1966. A radioautographic study of the migration and fate of the cranial neural crest cells in the chick embryo. Anatomical Record 156: 143–155.

1070. Johnston, M. C., A. Bhakdinaronk, and Y. C. Reid. 1973. An expanded role of the neural crest in oral and pharyngeal development. In *Fourth Symposium on Oral Sensation and Development: Development in the Fetus and Infant,* J. F. Bosma, ed. Bethesda: National Institutes of Health, pp. 37–52.

1071. Johnston, M. C., and M. A. Listgarten. 1972. Observations on the migration, interaction, and early differentiation of orofacial tissues. In *Developmental Aspects of Oral Biology,* H. C. Slavkin and L. A. Bavetta, eds. New York: Academic Press, pp. 53–80.

1072. Johnston, M. C., G. M. Morriss, D. Kushner, and G. J. Bingle. 1977. Abnormal organogenesis of facial structures. In *Handbook of Teratology,* vol. 2, J. G. Wilson and F. C. Fraser, eds. New York: Plenum Press, pp. 421–451.

1073. Johnston, M. C., D. M. Noden, R. D. Hazelton, J. L. Coulombre, and A. J. Coulombre. 1979. Origins of avian ocular and periocular tissues. Experimental Eye Research 29: 27–45.

1074. Johnston, M. C., and R. M. Pratt. 1975. The neural crest in normal and abnormal craniofacial development. In *ECM Influences on Gene Expression,* H. C. Slavkin and R. Greulich, eds. New York: Academic Press, pp. 773–777.

1075. Joleaud, L. 1937. Sur l'évolution morphologique très récente d'un groupe d'Ongules archaïques, les Damans. Comptes rendus, Academie des sciences, Paris 204: 791–793.

1076. Jollie, M. T. 1957. The head skeleton of the chicken and remarks on the anatomy of this region in other birds. Journal of Morphology 100: 389–436.

1077. Jollie, M. T. 1958. Comments on the phylogeny and skull of the Passeriformes. Auk 75: 26–35.

1078. Jollie, M. T. 1960. The head skeleton of the lizard. Acta zoologica, Stockholm 41: 1–64.

1079. Jollie, M. T. 1962. *Chordate Morphology.* New York: Reinhold.

1080. Jollie, M. T. 1968a. Some implications for the acceptance of a delamination principle. In *Current Problems in Lower Vertebrate Phylogeny,* T. Ørvig, ed. Nobel Symposium 4. Stockholm: Almqvist and Wiksell, pp. 89–107.

1081. Jollie, M. T. 1968b. The head skeleton of a new-born *Manis javanica* with comments on the ontogeny and phylogeny of the mammal head skeleton. Acta zoologica, Stockholm 49: 227–305.

1082. Jollie, M. T. 1971a. Some developmental aspects of the head skeleton of the 35–37mm *Squalus acanthias* foetus. Journal of Morphology 133: 17–40.

1083. Jollie, M. T. 1971b. A theory concerning the early evolution of the visceral arches. Acta zoologica, Stockholm 52: 85–96.

1084. Jollie, M. T. 1975. Development of the head skeleton and pectoral girdle in *Esox.* Journal of Morphology 147: 61–88.

1085. Jollie, M. T. 1977. Segmentation of the vertebrate head. American Zoologist 17: 323–333.

1086. Jollie, M. T. 1980. Development of the head and pectoral girdle skeleton and scales in *Acipenser.* Copeia: 226–249.

1087. Jollie, M. T. 1981. Segment theory and the homologizing of cranial bones. American Naturalist 118: 785–802.

1088. Jollie, M. T. 1984a. The vertebrate head—segmented or a single morphogenetic structure? Journal of Vertebrate Paleontology 4: 320–329.

1089. Jollie, M. T. 1984b. Development of the head skeleton and pectoral girdle of salmons, with a note on the scales. Canadian Journal of Zoology 62: 1756–1778.

1090. Jollie, M. T. 1984c. Development of the head and pectoral skeleton of *Polypterus* with a note on scales (Pisces: Actinopterygii). Journal of Zoology, London 204: 469–507.

1091. Jollie, M. T. 1984d. Development of cranial and pectoral girdle bones of *Lepisosteus* with a note on scales. Copeia: 476–501.

1092. Jollie, M. T. 1984e. Development of the head and pectoral skeleton of *Amia* with a note on the scales. Gegenbaurs Morphologisches Jahrbuch, Leipzig 130: 315–351.

1093. Jollie, M. T. 1986. A primer of bone names for the understanding of the actinopterygian head and pectoral girdle skeletons. Canadian Journal of Zoology 64: 365–379.

1094. Jones, P. H. 1988. Post-fledgling wing and bill development in the razorbill *Alca torda islandica*. Ringing and Migration 9: 11–17.

1095. Jones, S., and M. Kumaran. 1967. Notes on eggs, larvae, and juveniles of fishes from Indian waters. XV. *Pegasus volitans* Linnaeus; XVI. *Dactyloptena orientalis* (Cuvier and Valenciennes); and XVII. *Dactyloptena macracanthus* (Beeker). Indian Journal of Fisheries 11: 232–246.

1096. Jones, S., and V. R. Pantulu. 1958. On some larval and juvenile fishes from the Bengal and Orissa coasts. Indian Journal of Fisheries 5: 118–143.

1097. Joslin, P. 1982. Status, growth, and other facets of the Iranian wolf. In *Wolves of the World: Perspectives of Behavior, Ecology, and Conservation,* F. H. Harrington and P. C. Paquet, eds. New Jersey: Noyes Publications, pp. 196–203.

1098. Jouventin, P., J.-L. Mougin, J.-C. Stahl, and H. Weimerskirch. 1985. Comparative biology of the burrowing petrels of the Crozet Islands. Notornis 32: 157–220.

1099. Junge, R., and D. F. Hoffmeister. 1980. Age determination in raccoons from cranial suture obliteration. Journal of Wildlife Management 44: 725–729.

1100. Jurgens, J. D. 1963. Contribution to the description and comparative anatomy of the cranium of the Cape fruit-bat, *Rousettus aegyptiacus leach* Smith. Annals of the University of Stellenbosch, ser. A, 38: 3–37.

1101. Juriloff, D. M., and M. J. Harris. 1983. Abnormal facial development in the mouse mutant first arch. Journal of Craniofacial Genetics and Developmental Biology 3: 317–337.

1102. Kaan, H. W. 1938. Further studies on the auditory vesicle and cartilaginous capsule of *Amblystoma punctatum*. Journal of Experimental Zoology 78: 159–180.

1103. Kadam, K. M. 1958. The development of the chondrocranium in the seahorse, *Hippocampus* (Lophobranchii). Zoological Journal of the Linnean Society 43: 557–573.

1104. Kadam, K. M. 1961. The development of the skull in *Nerophis* (Lophobranchii). Acta zoologica, Stockholm 42: 257–298.

1105. Kadam, K. M. 1972. The development of the skull in the Indian gerbil, *Tatera indica cuvieri* (Waterhouse). Part I. Gegenbaurs Morphologische Jahrbuch, Leipzig 118: 309–325.

1106. Kadam, K. M. 1973a. The development of the skull in the Indian gerbil, *Tatera indica cuvieri* (Waterhouse). Part II. Gegenbaurs Morphologische Jahrbuch, Leipzig 119: 47–71.

1107. Kadam, K. M. 1973b. The development of the skull in the Indian gerbil, *Tatera indica cuvieri* (Waterhouse). Part III. Gegenbaurs Morphologische Jahrbuch, Leipzig 119: 153–171.

1108. Kadam, K. M. 1976. The development of the chondrocranium in the golden hamster, *Mesocricetus auratus* (Waterhouse). Gegenbaurs Morphologische Jahrbuch, Leipzig 122: 796–814.

1109. Kadanoff, D. D., and S. S. Mutafov. 1981. Manifestation of the proatlas. Comptes rendus de l'Académie bulgare des sciences 34: 867–870.

1110. Kadosaki, M., A. Kawahara, J. Iizuka, and H. Fujioka. 1989. Comparative morphological studies of the skulls and teeth of brown and black bears of Japan. 4. Skulls (1). Annual Reports of the History Museum of Hokkaido 17: 13–43.

1111. Kahmann, H. 1981. Zur Naturgeschichte des Loffelbilches, *Eliomys melanurus* Wagner, 1840 (Mammalia, Rodentia, Gliridae). (Eine Vorlaufige Untersuchung). Spixiana, Munich 4: 1–38.

1112. Kahmann, H., and I. Vesmanis. 1979. *Erinaceus algirus* on the island of Formentera (Spain) and in north African countries. Spixiana, Munich 1: 105–136.

1113. Kälin, J., and A. Bernasconi. 1949. Über den Ossifikationsmodus bei *Xenopus laevis* Daud. Revue suisse de zoologie 56: 359–364.

1114. Kamal, A. M. 1960. The chondrocranium of *Tropiocolotes tripolitanus*. Acta zoologica, Stockholm 41: 297–312.

1115. Kamal, A. M. 1961a. The chondrocranium of *Hemidactylus turcica*. Anatomisches Anzeiger 109: 89–108.

1116. Kamal, A. M. 1961b. The common characters of the geckonid chondrocranium. Anatomisches Anzeiger 109: 109–113.

1117. Kamal, A. M. 1961c. The phylogenetic position of the Geckonidae in the light of the developmental study of the skull. Anatomisches Anzeiger 109: 114–116.

1118. Kamal, A. M. 1964a. Notes on the chondrocranium of the gecko, *Tropiocolotes steudneri*. Bulletin of the Zoological Society of Egypt 19: 73–83.

1119. Kamal, A. M. 1964b. Note on the relation between the dorsal and ventral components of the mandibular arch in early embryos of Squamata. Bulletin of the Zoological Society of Egypt 19: 84–86.

1120. Kamal, A. M. 1964c. Note on an aberrant intracapsular course of the facial nerve in early stages of the snake *Psammophis sibilans*. Bulletin of the Zoological Society of Egypt 19: 87–88.

1121. Kamal, A. M. 1965a. The chondrocranium of the gecko *Stenodactylus stenodactylus*. Proceedings of the Egyptian Academy of Science 18: 59–69.

1122. Kamal, A. M. 1965b. The fully formed chondrocranium of *Eumeces schneideri*. Proceedings of the Egyptian Academy of Science 19: 13–20.

1123. Kamal, A. M. 1965c. Observations on the chondrocranium of *Tarentola mauritanica*. Proceedings of the Egyptian Academy of Science 19: 1–9.

1124. Kamal, A. M. 1965d. The relation between the auditory capsule and the basal plate, and the commissures between them in Squamata. Zoologischer Anzeiger 175: 281–285.

1125. Kamal, A. M. 1965e. The mode of formation of the fenestrae basicranialis, X and ovalis in Squamata. Zoologischer Anzeiger 175: 285–288.

1126. Kamal, A. M. 1965f. The origin of the interorbital septum of Lacertilia. Proceedings of the Egyptian Academy of Science 18: 70–72.

1127. Kamal, A. M. 1965g. On the cranio-vertebral joint and the relation between the notochord and occipital condyle in Squamata. Proceedings of the Egyptian Academy of Science 19: 11–12.

1128. Kamal, A. M. 1966a. The single origin of the parachordal plate in Squamata. Anatomisches Anzeiger 176: 3–5.

1129. Kamal, A. M. 1966b. The sphenoid bone in Lacertilia. Anatomisches Anzeiger 118: 82–86.

1130. Kamal, A. M. 1966c. On the process of rotation of the quadrate cartilage in Ophidia. Anatomisches Anzeiger 118: 87–90.

1131. Kamal, A. M. 1966d. On the hypoglossal foramina in Squamata. Anatomisches Anzeiger 118: 91–96.

1132. Kamal, A. M. 1968. On the concha nasalis of Squamata. Bulletin of the Faculty of Science of the Egyptian University 41: 97–108.

1133. Kamal, A. M. 1969a. The differences between the lacertilian and ophidian chondrocrania. Bulletin of the Zoological Society of Egypt 22: 121–129.

1134. Kamal, A. M. 1969b. The development and morphology of the chondrocranium of *Chalcides* species. Proceedings of the Egyptian Academy of Science 22: 37–48.

1135. Kamal, A. M. 1969c. On the trabeculae cranii and trabecula communis in early embryos of Squamata. Proceedings of the Egyptian Academy of Science 22: 49–51.

1136. Kamal, A. M. 1969d. The fused posterior orbital cartilages in lizards. Proceedings of the Egyptian Academy of Science 22: 53–55.

1137. Kamal, A. M. 1969e. The phylogenetic position of the family Elapidae in the light of the developmental study of the skull. Zeitschrift für Zoologische Systematik und Evolutionsforschung 7: 254–259.

1138. Kamal, A. M. 1969f. The relation between the glossopharyngeal nerve and the chondrocranium in Squamata. Proceedings of the Zoological Society of the United Arab Republic 3: 23–29.

1139. Kamal, A. M. 1970. The distinctive characters of the elapid chondrocranium. Anatomisches Anzeiger 127: 171–175.

1140. Kamal, A. M. 1971. On the fissura metotica in Squamata. Bulletin of the Zoological Society of Egypt 23: 53–57.

1141. Kamal, A. M. 1972. The pterygoquadrate cartilage in Squamata. Zeitschrift für wissenschaftliche Zoologie 185: 69–75.

1142. Kamal, A. M. 1973a. The position of the prefacial commissure and facial foramen in Squamata. Anatomisches Anzeiger 133: 283–286.

1143. Kamal, A. M. 1973b. On the connection between the chondrocranium and vertebral column in embryos of Squamata. Anatomisches Anzeiger 133: 287–290.

1144. Kamal, A. M., and A. M. Abdeen. 1972. The development of the chondro-cranium of the lacertid lizard, *Acanthodactylus boskiana*. Journal of Morphology 137: 289–334.

1145. Kamal, A. M., and H. G. Hammouda. 1965a. The development of the skull of *Psammophis sibilans*. I. The development of the chondrocranium. Journal of Morphology 116: 197–246.

1146. Kamal, A. M., and H. G. Hammouda. 1965b. The development of the skull of *Psammophis sibilans*. II. The fully formed chondrocranium. Journal of Morphology 116: 247–296.

1147. Kamal, A. M., and H. G. Hammouda. 1965c. The development of the skull of *Psammophis sibilans*. III. The osteocranium of a late embryo. Journal of Morphology 116: 297–310.

1148. Kamal, A. M., and H. G. Hammouda. 1965d. The columella auris of the snake, *Psammophis sibilans*. Anatomisches Anzeiger 116: 124–138.

1149. Kamal, A. M., and H. G. Hammouda. 1965e. Observations on the chon-drocranium of the snake, *Cerastes vipera*. Gegenbaurs Morphologisches Jahr-buch, Leipzig 107: 58–98.

1150. Kamal, A. M., and H. G. Hammouda. 1965f. The chondrocranium of the snake *Eryx jaculus*. Acta zoologica, Stockholm 46: 167–208.

1151. Kamal, A. M., and H. G. Hammouda. 1965g. On the laterosphernoid bone in Ophidia. Anatomisches Anzeiger 116: 116–123.

1152. Kamal, A. M., and H. G. Hammouda. 1969. The structure of the inner ear (membranous labyrinth) and secondary tympanic membrane in a late embryo of the snake *Psammophis sibilans*. Proceedings of the Zoological Society of the United Arab Republic 3: 31–40.

1153. Kamal, A. M., H. G. Hammouda, and F. M. Mokhtar. 1970a. The devel-opment of the osteocranium of the Egyptian cobra. I. The embryonic osteo-cranium. Acta zoologica, Stockholm 51: 1–17.

1154. Kamal, A. M., H. G. Hammouda, and F. M. Mokhtar. 1970b. The devel-opment of the osteocranium of the Egyptian cobra. II. The median dorsal bones, bones of the upper jaw, circumorbital series, and occipital ring of the adult osteocranium. Acta zoologica, Stockholm 51: 19–30.

1155. Kamal, A. M., H. G. Hammouda, and F. M. Mokhtar. 1970c. The devel-opment of the osteocranium of the Egyptian cobra. III. The otic capsule, palate, temporal bones, lower jaw, and hyoid apparatus of the adult osteocra-nium. Acta zoologica, Stockholm 51: 31–42.

1156. Kamal, A. M., and S. K. Zada. 1970. The phylogenetic position of the family Agamidae in the light of the study of the chondrocranium. Anatom-isches Anzeiger 184: 327–335.

1157. Kamal, A. M., and S. K. Zada. 1973. The early development stages of the chondrocranium of *Agama pallida*. Acta morphologica neerlando-scandina-vica 11: 75–104.

1158. Kanagasuntheram, R. 1967. A note on the development of the tubotym-panic recess in the human embryo. Journal of Anatomy, London 101: 731–741.

1159. Kanagasuntheram, R., and C. V. Kanan. 1964. The chondrocranium of a 19 mm c.r. length embryo of *Galago senegalensis senegalensis*. Acta zoologica, Stockholm 45: 107–121.

1160. Kanan, C. V. 1959a. A study of the nasal region in a fully formed chondrocranium of *Ovis orientalis* (Gmelin). Acta zoologica, Stockholm 40: 85–99.

1161. Kanan, C. V. 1959b. Observations on the development of the central stem of the chondrocranium in *Ovis orientalis* Gmelin. Acta morphologica neerlando-scandinavica 2A: 210–219.

1162. Kanan, C. V. 1959c. A study of the development of the auditory capsule of the chondrocranium of *Ovis orientalis* Gmelin. Acta morphologica neerlando-scandinavica 2A: 353–364.

1163. Kanan, C. V. 1960. A preliminary study on the pattern of development of the chondrocranium of *Camelus dromedarius*. Sudan Journal of Veterinary Science 1: 35–41.

1164. Kanan, C. V. 1961. Some observations on the development of the nasal capsule of the chondrocranium in *Camelus dromedarius*. Proceedings of the Royal Society of Edinburgh 68: 91–102.

1165. Kanan, C. V. 1962. Observations on the development of the osteocranium in *Camelus dromedarius*. Acta zoologica, Stockholm 43: 297–310.

1166. Kanazawa, E., and K. Mochizuki. 1974. The time and order of appearance of ossification centers in the hamster before birth. Jikken dobutsu (Experimental Animals), Tokyo 23: 113–122.

1167. Kanazawa, E., and K. Takano. 1979. Studies on the development of the Meckel's cartilage and the mandible in the hamster. Nihon University Journal of Oral Science 5: 88–97.

1168. Kaneko, Y. 1978. Seasonal and sexual differences in absolute and relative growth in *Microtus montebelli*. Acta theriologica 23: 75–98.

1169. Kapoor, A. S. 1970. Development of dermal bones related to sensory canals of the head in the fishes *Ophicephalus punctatus* Bloch (Ophicephalidae) and *Wallago attu* Bl. & Sch. (Siluridae). Zoological Journal of the Linnean Society 49: 69–97.

1170. Kappers, J. 1940. Some topographic relations of the orbits in man and anthropoids during ontogenesis, especially bearing on the ontogenetic development of the "rostrale orbitale." Proceedings, Koninklijke Nederlandse akademie van Wetenschappen, Amsterdam 43: 1199–1211.

1171. Kato, M., S. Isotani, K. Hibino, T. Kato, and T. Kobayashi. 1981. Developmental study on human fetuses by Moire method. 1. Analysis of the frontal and facial regions. Journal of the Medical Society of Toho University 28: 504–528.

1172. Katsavarias, E. G. 1988. The growth of nasal cavities. Odontostomatological Progress 42: 89–100.

1173. Kaufmann, P., H. Leisten, and H. Mangold. 1981. Die Kiemenbogenentwicklung bei Ratte und Maus. I. Zur Entwicklung von Sinus cervicalis und operculum. Acta anatomica 110: 7–22.

1174. Kauri, H. 1964. The influence of post optimal temperatures on the development and ossification of the cranium of *Rana esculenta*. Acta Universitatis lundensis, Lund 59: 1–18.

1175. Kawamata, S. 1988. Effects of calcium preloading on the growth of calcium carbonate crystals in the endolymphatic sac of the tree frog, *Hyla arborea japonica*. Cell and Tissue Research 252: 679–682.

1176. Kay, E. D. 1986. The phenotypic interdependence of the musculoskeletal characters of the mandibular arch in mice. Journal of Embryology and Experimental Morphology 98: 123–136.

1177. Kean, M. R., and P. Houghton. 1987. The role of function in the development of human craniofacial form—a perspective. Anatomical Record 218: 107–110.

1178. Keith, D. A. 1982. Development of the human temporomandibular joint. British Journal of Oral Surgery 20: 217–224.

1179. Keller, R. 1946. Morphogenetische Untersuchungen und Skelett von *Siredon mexicanus* Shaw mit besonderer des Ossifikationsmodus beim neotenen Axolotl. Revue suisse de zoologie 53: 329–426.

1180. Kelley, D., D. Sassoon, N. Segil, and M. Scudder, 1989. Development and hormone regulation of androgen receptor levels in the sexually dimorphic larynx of *Xenopus laevis*. Developmental Biology 131: 111–118.

1181. Kemp, A. 1977. The pattern of tooth plate formation in the Australian lungfish, *Neoceratodus forsteri* Krefft. Zoological Journal of the Linnean Society 60: 223–258.

1182. Kemp, A. 1982. The embryonical development of the Queensland lungfish, *Neoceratodus forsteri* (Krefft). Memoirs of the Queensland Museum 20: 553–597.

1183. Kemp, N. E., and J. A. Hoyt. 1969. Sequence of ossification in the skeleton of growing and metamorphosing tadpoles of *Rana pipiens*. Journal of Morphology 129: 415–444.

1184. Kemp, N. E., and B. L. Quinn. 1954. Morphogenesis and metabolism of amphibian larvae after excision of heart. II. Morphogenesis of heartless larvae of *Amblystoma punctatum*. Anatomical Record 118: 773–787.

1185. Kenny, J. S. 1969. Feeding mechanisms in anuran larvae. Journal of Zoology, London 157: 225–246.

1186. Kent, M. L., S. R. Wellings, W. T. Yasukate, and R. A. Elston. 1987. Cranial nodules associated with cranial fenestrae in juvenile Atlantic salmon, *Salmo salar* L. Journal of Fish Disease 10: 419–421.

1187. Kerr, G. R., J. II. Wallace, C. F. Chesney, and H. A. Waisman. 1972. Growth and development of the fetal rhesus monkey. III. Maturation and linear growth of the skull and appendicular skeleton. Growth 36: 59–76.

1188. Kesteven, H. L. 1940. The osteogenesis of the base of the saurian cranium and a search for the parasphenoid bone. Proceedings of the Linnean Society of New South Wales 65: 447–467.

1189. Kesteven, H. L. 1941. On certain debatable questions in cranio-skeletal homologies. Proceedings of the Linnean Society of New South Wales 66: 293–334.

1190. Kesteven, H. L. 1942a. The ossification of the avian chondrocranium, with special reference to that of the emu. Proceedings of the Linnean Society of New South Wales 67: 213–237.

1191. Kesteven, H. L. 1942b. The ossification of basisphenoid and parasphenoid bones in *Melopsittacus.* Proceedings of the Linnean Society of New South Wales 67: 349–351.

1192. Kesteven, H. L. 1942c. The evolution of the skull and the cephalic muscles: A comparative study of their development and adult morphology. Part II. The Amphibia. Memoirs of the Australian Museum 8: 1–316.

1193. Kesteven, H. L. 1957a. On the development of the crocodilian skull. Proceedings of the Linnean Society of New South Wales 82: 117–124.

1194. Kesteven, H. L. 1957b. Notes on the skull and cephalic muscles of the Amphisbaenia. Proceedings of the Linnean Society of New South Wales 82: 109–116.

1195. Kharitonov, V. M. 1973. A study of the differences in postnatal ontogeny of the skull of modern and fossil primates. Vestnik Moskovskogo Universiteta, Seriya VI, Biologiya Pochvovedemie 28: 96–98.

1196. Kier, E. L., and S. L. G. Rothman. 1976. Radiologically significant anatomic variations of the developing sphenoid in humans. In *Development of the Basicranium,* J. F. Bosma, ed. Bethesda: U.S. Department of Health, Education, and Welfare, pp. 107–140.

1197. Kieser, J. A., and H. T. Groeneveld. 1987. Static intraspecific maxillofacial allometry in the chacma baboon. Folio primatologica 48: 151–163.

1198. Kim, J.-M., and M. Okiyama. 1989. Larval morphology and distribution of *Callanthias japonicus* Franz. Ocean Research, Seoul 11: 1–8.

1199. Kim, Y.-U., and K. H. Han. 1989. Early life history of the marine animals. 1. Egg development, larvae, and juveniles of *Chaenoglobus laevis* (Steindachner). Bulletin of the Korean Fisheries Society 22: 317–331.

1200. King, C. M. 1980. Age determination in the weasel (*Mustela nivalis*) in relation to the development of the skull. Zeitschrift für Saeugetierkunde 45: 153–173.

1201. King, C. M., and J. E. Moody. 1982. The biology of the stoat (*Mustela erminea*) in the national parks of New Zealand. 3. Morphometric variation in relation to growth, geographical distribution, and colonization. New Zealand Journal of Zoology 9: 81–102.

1202. Kirby, M. L. 1989. Plasticity and predetermination of mesencephalic and trunk neural crest transplanted into the region of the cardiac neural crest. Developmental Biology 134: 402–412.

1203. Kirkland, G. L., Jr. 1973. Observations on the degree of ossification in neonatal *Napaeozapus insignis* (Preble). American Midland Naturalist 90: 465–467.

1204. Kishimoto, R. 1988. Age and sex determination of the Japanese serow *Capricornis crispus* in the field study. Journal of the Mammalogical Society of Japan 13: 51–58.

1205. Kjaer, I. 1989. Prenatal skeletal maturation of the human mandible. Journal of Craniofacial Genetics and Developmental Biology 9: 257–264.

1206. Klevezal', G. A., and A. Fedyk. 1978. Adhesion lines pattern as an indicator of age in voles. Acta theriologica 23: 413–422.

1207. Klevezal', G. A., M. Pucek, and E. P. Malafeeva. 1984. Body and skeleton growth in laboratory field voles of different seasonal generations. Acta theriologica 29: 3–16.

1208. Klevezal', G. A., L. I. Uskhovskaya, and S. A. Blokhin. 1986. Determining the age in baleen whales according to annual layers in the bone. Zoologicheskii zhurnal 65: 1722–1730.

1209. Klijn, H. B. 1975. Quantitative and qualitative age and sex criteria of the starling, *Sturnus vulgaris*, in March. Bijdragen tat de Dierkunde 45: 39–49.

1210. Klima, M. 1987. Morphogenesis of the nasal structures of the skull in toothed whales (Odontoceti). In *Morphogenesis of the Mammalian Skull*, H.-J. Kuhn and U. Zeller, eds. Hamburg and Berlin: Verlag Paul Parey, pp. 105–121.

1211. Klima, M., M. Seel, and P. Deimer. 1986a. Die Entwicklung des hochspezialisierten Nasenschädels beim Pottwal (*Physeter macrocephalus*). Teil I. Gegenbaurs Morphologisches Jahrbuch, Leipzig 132: 245–284.

1212. Klima, M., M. Seel, and P. Deimer. 1986b. Die Entwicklung des hochspezialisierten Nasenschädels beim Pottwal (*Physeter macrocephalus*). Teil II. Gegenbaurs Morphologisches Jahrbuch, Leipzig 132: 349–374.

1213. Klima, M., and P. J. H. Van Bree. 1985. Überzählige Skeletelemente im Nasenschädel von *Phocoena phocoena* und die Entwicklung der Nasenregion bei den Zahnwalen. Gegenbaurs Morphologisches Jahrbuch, Leipzig 131: 131–178.

1214. Klimkiewicz, M. K. 1980. Notes from the BBL: Ageing and sexing house finches. North American Bird Banding 5: 96.

1215. Klingener, D., and G. K. Creighton. 1984. Small bats of the genus *Pteropus* from the Phillipines. Proceedings of the Biological Society of Washington 97: 395–403.

1216. Kobayashi, T., S. Kikuyama, A. Kume, J. Okuma, and M. Ohkawa. 1989. 35^s-sulphate uptake by *Xenopus laevis* cartilage: The influence of plasma from the growth hormone–treated animal. Zoological Science 6: 757–762.

1217. Kobrynczuk, F., and H. Kobryn. 1980. Growth rate of selected parameters of the European bison skull (*Bison bonasus*). Folia morphologica, Warsaw 39: 69–78.

1218. Kobrynczuk, F., and T. Roskosz. 1980. Correlation of skull dimensions in the European bison (*Bison bonasus*). Acta theriologica 25: 349–364.

1219. Kodama, G. 1965. Developmental studies on the presphenoid of the human sphenoid bone. Okajimas folia anatomica japonica 1: 159–172.

1220. Kodama, G. 1971a. Developmental studies on the body of the human sphenoid bone. Hokkaido Journal of Medical Science 46: 313–321.

1221. Kodama, G. 1971b. Developmental studies on the orbitosphenoid of the human sphenoid bone. Hokkaido Journal of Medical Science 46: 324–331.

1222. Koh, H. S., and R. L. Peterson. 1983. Systematic studies of deer mice, *Peromyscus maniculatus* Wagner (Cricetidae, Rodentia): Analysis of age and secondary sexual variation in morphometric characters. Canadian Journal of Zoology 61: 2618–2628.

1223. Köhncke, M. 1985. The chondrocranium of *Cryptoprocta ferox*. Advances in Anatomy, Embryology, and Cell Biology 95: 1–89.

1224. Köhncke, M., and H. Schliemann. 1977. Über zwei Foeten von *Cryptoprocta ferox*. Bennett, 1833. Mitteilungen aus dem Hamburgischen zoologischen Museum und Institut 74: 171–175.

1225. Kohno, H., M. Shimuzu, and Y. Nose. 1984. Morphological aspects of the development of swimming and feeding functions in larval *Scomber japonicus*. Bulletin of the Japanese Society for Scientific Fisheries 50: 1125–1137.

1226. Kohno, H., Y. Taki, Y. Ogasawara, Y. Shirojo, and M. Inoue. 1983. Development of swimming and feeding functions in larval *Pagrus major*. Japanese Journal of Ichthyology 30: 47–60.

1227. Koike, H., and T. Shimamura. 1988. Age determination and skeletal growth of Japanese monkey (*Macaca muscata*) using specimens of the Takagoyama T1 troup. Journal of Saitana University, Natural Science 24: 73–85.

1228. Kokich, V. G. 1986. The biology of sutures. In *Craniosynostosis: Diagnosis, Evaluation, and Management,* M. M. Cohen, Jr., ed. New York: Raven Press, pp. 81–104.

1229. Kokich, V. G., P. A. Shapiro, B. C. Moffett, and E. W. Retzlaff. 1979. Craniofacial sutures. In *Ageing in Nonhuman Primates,* D. M. Bowden, ed. New York: van Nostrand Reinhold Co., pp. 356–368.

1230. Kong, Y. C., K. Ko, T. Yip, and S. W. Tsao. 1987. Epidermal growth factor of the cervine velvet antler. Acta zoologica sinica 33: 301–308.

1231. Korablev, P. N. 1988. The secondary bonelets in the moose skull. Byulleten' Moskovskogo Obschchestva Ispytalelei Prkody Otdel Biologicheskii 93: 26–34.

1232. Kordylewski, L. 1977. Anatomical diversity of amphibian superficial mandibular musculature. Acta biologica cracoviensia, Zoologia 20: 107–117.

1233. Korovina, V. M. 1975a. The parietal fontanelles in the chondrocranium of salmon of the genus *Oncorhynchus*. Voprosy Ikhtiologii 15: 629–635.

1234. Korovina, V. M. 1975b. Parietal fontanelae in the chondrocranium of Far Eastern salmon of the genus *Oncorhynchus*. Voprosy Ikhtiologii 15: 703–708.

1235. Kosa, F., and I. G. Fazekas. 1972. The possibilities of determining the age of a fetus from transformations of the bones of the cranial arch. Medecine legale et dommage corporel 5: 339–346.

1236. Kosher, R. A., and M. Solursh. 1989. Widespread distribution of type II colagen during embryonic chick development. Developmental Biology 131: 558–566.

1237. Koski, K. 1975. Cartilage of the face. Birth Defects, Original Article Series 11 (7): 231–254.

1238. Kosyagina, E. B. 1979. Development of structural elements of the middle ear in human osteogenesis. Archives d'anatomie, d'histologie, et d'embryologie 77: 73–79.

1239. Kotlyarov, O. N. 1981. On methods for studying age changes in rodent skull suture. Vestnik Zoologii: 62–63.

1240. Koubek, P., V. Hraba, and M. Horakova. 1989. Postnatal development of the skull of *Rupicapra rupicapra rupicapra* (Mammalia, Bovidae). Folia zoologica 38: 31–44.

1241. Kovacs, G., and M. Ocsenyi. 1981. Age structure and survival of a European hare population determined by periosteal growth lines: Preliminary study. Acta oecologica applicata 2: 241–245.

1242. Kowalska, M. 1974. Studies on the ossification of the skull in the mallard domestic variety (*Anas platyrhynchos* var. *Domestica* L.). Acta ornithologica, Warsaw 13: 451–473.

1243. Kraemer, M. 1974. La morphogenèse du chondrocrâne de *Discoglossus pictus* Otth. (Amphibiens, anoure). Bulletin of Biology 108: 211–228.

1244. Kratochvil, J. 1976. Volume of neurocranium in relation to the craniological criteria in *Felis silvestris* and *Felis lybica* f. *catus*. Zoologicke listy 25: 117–128.

1245. Kratochvil, J. 1981. *Chionomys nivalis* (Arvicolidae, Rodentia). Prirodovedne Prace Untavu Ceskoslovenska Akademie Ved v Brne 15: 1–62.

1246. Kratochvil, J., V. Barus, F. Tenora, and R. Wiger. 1977. The growth of the skull during postnatal development of *Lemmus lemmus* (Mammalia, Rodentia). Prirodovedne Prace Untavu Ceskoslovenska Akademie Ved v. Brne 11: 1–36.

1247. Kratochvil, J., V. Barus, F. Tenora, and R. Wiger. 1979. The wood lemming, *Myopus schisticolor*. Folia zoologica 28: 193–207.

1248. Kratochvil, J., and Z. Kux. 1984. Kraniometrische Untersuchungen an Rehgeissen. Prirodovedne Prace Ceskoslovenska Akademie, n.s., 18: 1–55.

1249. Krebs, S. L., and R. A. Brandon. 1984. A new species of salamander (family Ambystomatidae) from Michoacan, Mexico. Herpetologica 40: 238–245.

1250. Kreiner, J. 1954. Saccus endolymphaticus in *Xenopus laevis* Daud. Folia biologica 2: 271–286.

1251. Krogman, W. M. 1969. Growth changes in skull, face, jaws, and teeth of the chimpanzee. In *The Chimpanzee*, vol. 1, G. H. Bourne, ed. Basel: S. Karger, pp. 104–164.

1252. Krukoff, S. 1980. Croissance comparée de la partie supérieure de la voûte de crâne lignée des hominidéa et celle du chimpanzé (*Pan troglodytes*). Comptes rendus hebdomadaires des séances de l'Académie des sciences, ser. D, Paris 290: 409–412.

1253. Kruska, D. 1979. Comparative investigations on skulls of subadult and adult farm minks, *Mustela vison* (Mustelidae, Carnivora). Zeitschrift für Saeugetierkunde 44: 360–375.

1254. Krylova, T. V. 1978. Age structure of a natural population of the clawed jird *Meriones unguiculatus*. Zoologicheskii zhurnal 57: 1842–1847.

1255. Kuam, T. 1983. Age determination in European *Lynx lynx* (L.) based on cranial development. Fauna norvegica (A) 4: 31–36.

1256. Kubota, K., S. Togawa, K. Nagae, T. Katayama, K. Hosaka, and S. Sibanai. 1986. A developmental aspect of the neuromuscular innervation of the jaw muscles in the northern fur seal embryos. Nova acta Leopoldina 58 (262): 223–242.

1257. Kuehn, D. W., and W. E. Berg. 1983. Use of radiographs to age otters. Wildlife Society Bulletin 11: 68–70.

1258. Kuhn, H.-J. 1971. Die Entwicklung und Morphologie des Schädels von *Tachyglossus aculeatus*. Abhandlungen herausgegeben von der Senckenbergischen Naturforschenden Gesellschaft, Frankfurt am Main 528: 1–224.

1259. Kuhn, H.-J. 1987. Introduction. In *Morphogenesis of the Mammalian Skull*, H.-J. Kuhn and U. Zeller, eds. Hamburg: Verlag Paul Parey, pp. 9–15.

1260. Kuhn, H.-J., and U. Zeller, 1987a. *Morphogenesis of the Mammalian Skull.* Hamburg: Verlag Paul Parey.

1261. Kuhn, H.-J., and U. Zeller, 1987b. The cavum epiptericum in monotremes and therian mammals. In *Morphogenesis of the Mammalian Skull,* H.-J. Kuhn and U. Zeller, eds. Hamburg: Verlag Paul Parey, pp. 51–70.

1262. Kuhn, O., and H. O. Hammer. 1956. Über die Einwirkung des Schilddrüsenhormons auf die Ossifikation. Experientia 12: 231–233.

1263. Kuklina, O. I. 1974. The structure of the cranial flat bones in human fetuses. Archives d'anatomie, d'histologie, et d'embryologie 67: 29–34.

1264. Kuliev, G. K. 1961. Growth of the skeleton and of the internal organs in Azerbaidjan mountain sheep in its stages. Izvestiya Akademii Nauk Azerbaidzhanskai SSR, 5: 83–86.

1265. Kulshrestha, S. K. 1978. Development of osteocranium in *Labeo rohita.* Bioresearch, Ujjain 2: 95–104.

1266. Kummer, B. 1952. Untersuchungen über die Entstehung der Schädelbasisform bei Mensch und Primaten. Verhandlungen der Anatomischen Gesellschaft, Jena 50: 122–126.

1267. Kummer, B. 1953. Untersuchungen über die Entwicklung des Menschen und einiger Anthropoiden. Abhandlungen zur exakten biologie, Berlin 3: 1–44.

1268. Kummer, B., and S. Neiss. 1957. Das Cranium eines 103 mm langen Embryos des südlichen SeeElefanten (*Mirounga leonina* L.). Gegenbaurs Morphologisches Jahrbuch, Leipzig 98: 288–346.

1269. Kunz, T. H., and J. Chase 1983. Osteological and ocular anomalies in juvenile big brown bats (*Eptesicus fuscus*). Canadian Journal of Zoology 61: 365–369.

1270. Kuratani, S. 1987. The development of the orbital region of *Caretta caretta* (Chelonia, Reptilia). Journal of Anatomy, London 154: 187–200.

1271. Kuratani, S. 1989. Development of the orbital region in the chondrocranium of *Caretta caretta.* Reconsideration of the vertebrate neurocranium configuration. Anatomisches Anzeiger 169: 335–349.

1272. Kuts, G. A., N. N. Tkacheva, and N. S. Voskresenskaya. 1975. Specificity of the embryonic development of precoce sheep. Sel'skokhozyaistvennaya biologiya 10: 900–904.

1273. Kuz'min, A. A., and Y. F. Perrin. 1983. The main features of the skull formation in dolphin (Cetacea) during the prenatal period. Zoologicheskii zhurnal 62: 102–112.

1274. Kvinnsland, S. 1971. The sagittal growth of the fetal cranial base. Acta odontologica scandinavica 29: 699–715.

1275. Laitman, J. T., and R. C. Heimbuch. 1984. A measure of basicranial flexion in *Pan paniscus,* the pygmy chimpanzee. In *The Pygmy Chimpanzee: Evolutionary Biology and Behavior,* R. L. Susman, ed. New York: Plenum Press, pp. 49–63.

1276. Laitman, J. T., R. C. Heimbuch, and E. S. Crelin. 1978. Developmental changes in a basicranial line and its relationship to the upper respiratory system in living primates. American Journal of Anatomy 152: 467–482.

1277. Lakars, T. C., and S. W. Herring. 1980. Ontogeny of oral function in hamsters (*Mesocricetus auratus*). Journal of Morphology 165: 237–254.

1278. Lambiris, A. J. L. 1978. Surgery on a captive salamander. British Journal of Herpetology 5: 843–844.

1279. Lammens, E. H. R. R., J. Guersen, and P. J. MacGillivray. 1987. Diet shifts, feeding efficiency, and coexistence of bream (*Abramis brama*), roach (*Rutilus rutilus*) and white bream (*Blicca bjoerkna*) in hypertrophic lakes. In *Fifth Congress of European Ichthyology, Proceedings Commemorating Petrus Artedi (1705–1735)*, S. O. Kullander and B. Fernholm, eds. Stockholm: Department of Vertebrate Zoology, Swedish Museum of Natural History, pp. 153–162.

1280. Lang, C. T. 1952. Über die Ontogenie der Knickungsverhältnisse beim Vogelschädel. Verhandlungen der Anatomischen Gesellschaft, Jena 50: 127–136.

1281. Lang, C. T. 1955. Beitrage zur Entwicklungsgeschichte des Kopfskelettes von *Melopsittacus undulatus*. Gegenbaurs Morphologisches Jahrbuch, Leipzig 94: 335–390.

1282. Lang, C. T. 1956. Das cranium der Ratiten mit besonderer Berücksichtigung von *Struthio camelus*. Zeitschrift für wissenschaftliche Zoologie 159: 165–224.

1283. Langille, R. M., and B. K. Hall. 1986. Evidence of cranial neural crest cell contributions to the skeleton of the sea lamprey, *Petromyzon marinus*. In *New Discoveries and Technologies in Developmental Biology*, pt. B, H. C. Slavkin, ed. New York: Alan R. Liss, pp. 263–266.

1284. Langille, R. M., and B. K. Hall. 1987. Development of the head skeleton of the Japanese Medaka, *Oryzias latipes* (Teleostei). Journal of Morphology 193: 135–158.

1285. Langille, R. M., and B. K. Hall. 1988a. The organ culture and grafting of lamprey cartilage and teeth. In Vitro: Cellular and Developmental Biology 24: 1–8.

1286. Langille, R. M., and B. K. Hall. 1988b. Role of the neural crest in the development of the trabeculae and branchial arches in embryonic sea lamprey, *Petromyzon marinus* (L). Development 102: 301–310.

1287. Langille, R. M., and B. K. Hall. 1988c. The role of the neural crest in the development of the cartilaginous cranial and visceral skeleton of the medaka, *Oryzias latipes* (Teleostei). Anatomy and Embryology 177: 297–305.

1288. Langille, R. M., and B. K. Hall. 1989a. Neural crest–derived branchial arches link lampreys and gnathostomes. Fortschritte der Zoologie 35: 210–212.

1289. Langille, R. M., and B. K. Hall. 1989b. Developmental processes, developmental sequences, and early vertebrate phylogeny. Biological Reviews of the Cambridge Philosophical Society 64: 73–91.

1290. Langille, R. M., D. F. Paulsen, and M. Solursh. 1989. Differential effects of physiological concentrations of retinoic acid *in vitro* on chondrogenesis and myogenesis in chick craniofacial mesenchyme. Differentiation 40: 84–92.

1291. Langston, E. 1973. The crocodilian skull in historical perspective. In *Biol-*

ogy of the Reptilia, vol. 4, C. Gans and T. S. Parsons, eds. London: Academic Press, pp. 263–284.

1292. Lannoo, M. J., D. S. Townsend, and R. J. Wassersug. 1987. Larval life in the leaves: Arboreal tadpole types, with special attention to the morphology, ecology, and behavior of the oophagous *Osteopilus brunneus* (Hylidae) larva. Fieldiana: Zoology, n.s., 38: 1–31.

1293. Laroche, J., M. Peron, and Y. le Gal. 1982. Étude de l'hyperostosé vertébré et cranienne chez deux téléostéens *Trachurus trachurus* et *Trachurus mediterraneus*, par la diffraction des rayons X et l'incorporation de ^{45}Ca. Comptes rendus, Académie des sciences, Paris, ser. 3, 294: 1045–1050.

1294. Laroche, W. A., and S. L. Richardson. 1980. Development and occurrence of larvae and juveniles of the rockfishes *Sebastes flavidus* and *Sebastes melanops* (Scorpaenidae) off Oregon. U.S. National Marine Fisheries Service, Fishery Bulletin 77: 901–924.

1295. Laroche, J., and S. L. Richardson. 1981. Development of the larvae and juveniles of the rockfishes *Sebastes entomelas* and *S. zacentrus* (Family Scorpaenidae) and occurrence off Oregon, with notes on head spines of *S. mystinus*, *S. flavidus*, and *S. melanops*. U.S. National Marine Fisheries Service, Fishery Bulletin 79: 231–257.

1296. Lascelles, A. K. 1959. The time of appearance of ossification centres in the Peppin-type Merino. Australian Journal of Zoology 7: 79–86.

1297. Latham, R. A. 1970. Maxillary development and growth: The septomaxillary ligament. Journal of Anatomy, London 107: 471–478.

1298. Latham, R. A. 1971. The development, structure, and growth pattern of the human mid-palatal suture. Journal of Anatomy, London 108: 31–41.

1299. Latham, R. A. 1972. The different relationship of the sella point to growth sites of the cranial base in fetal life. Journal of Dental Research 51: 1646–1650.

1300. Lau, S. R., and P. L. Schefland. 1982. Larval development of snook, *Centropomus undecimalis* (Pisces: Centropomidae). Copeia: 618–627.

1301. Lauder, G. V., and S. M. Reilly. 1988. Functional design of the feeding mechanism in salamanders: Causal bases of ontogenetic changes in function. Journal of Experimental Biology 134: 219–233.

1302. Lauder, G. V., and H. B. Shaffer. 1985. Functional morphology of the feeding mechanism in aquatic ambystomatid salamanders. Journal of Morphology 185: 297–326.

1303. Lauder, G. V., and H. B. Shaffer. 1988. Ontogeny of functional design in tiger salamanders (*Ambystoma tigrinum*): Are motor patterns conserved during major morphological transformations? Journal of Morphology 197: 249–268.

1304. Lavilla, E. O., and M. Fabrezi. 1987. Anatomia de larvas de *Hyla pulchella andina* (Anura: Hylidae). Physis, Buenos Aires 45: 77–82.

1305. Lawes, I. N. C., and P. L. R. Andrews. 1987. Variation of the ferret skull (*Mustela putorius furo* L.) in relation to stereotaxic landmarks. Journal of Anatomy 154: 157–171.

1306. Layne, J. N. 1966. Postnatal development and growth of *Peromyscus floridanus*. Growth 30: 23–45.

1307. Leamy, L., and R. S. Thorpe. 1984. Morphometric studies in inbred and hybrid house mice: Heterosis, homeostasis, and heritability of size and shape. Biological Journal of the Linnean Society 22: 233–241.

1308. Lebedkina, N. S. 1960. Development of the bones of the palatal arch in the caudate amphibia. Doklady Akademii Nauk SSSR 131: 1206–1208.

1309. Lebedkina, N. S. 1961. Development of the parasphenoid in the caudate amphibia. Doklady Akademii Nauk SSSR 133: 1476–1479.

1310. Lebedkina, N. S. 1963. The development of the preoptic connections of the palatoquadrate cartilage in *Ranodon sibiricus*. Doklady Akademii Nauk SSSR 150: 199–202.

1311. Lebedkina, N. S. 1964a. Development of the dermal bones of the base of the skull in tailed amphibia of the family Hynobiidae. Trudy Zoologicheskogo instituta Akademiya Nauk SSSR 33: 75–172.

1312. Lebedkina, N. S. 1964b. Development of the nasal bones in the caudate Amphibia. Doklady Akademii Nauk SSSR. 159: 219–222.

1313. Lebedkina, N. S. 1968. The development of bones in the skull roof of Amphibia. In *Current Problems of Lower Vetebrate Phylogeny*, T. Ørvig, ed. Stockholm: Almqvist and Wiksell, pp. 317–329.

1314. Lebedkina, N. S. 1979. *Evolution of the Amphibian Skull*. Moscow: Nauka.

1315. Lebedkina, N. S. 1981. Some pecularities of bony skull development in the Ussurian salamander, *Onychodactylus fischeri* Bigr. (Hynobiidae). In *Herpetological Investigations in Siberia and the Far East*, L. J. Borkin, ed. Moscow: Academy of Sciences, USSR, Zoological Institute, pp. 61–65.

1316. Lebedkina, N. S. 1982. Development of the bones at the cranial basis of *Emys orbicularis*. In *Morphofunctional Transformations of Vertebrates during the Conquest of the Land*, E. I. Vorobyeva and N. N. Iodanskij, eds. Moscow: Nauka, pp. 57–75.

1317. Lebedkina, N. S. 1985. The ontogeny and phylogeny of correlative systems. In *Evolution and Morphogenesis*, J. Mlikovsky and V. J. A. Novak, eds. Praha: Academia, pp. 447–452.

1318. Lebedkina, N. S. 1986. The homologies of temporal bones in Amphibia and Reptilia. In *Studies in Herpetology*, Z. Roček, ed. Prague: Charles University, pp. 303–306.

1319. Lebedkina, N. S., T. P. Evgeneva, and T. P. Antipenkova. 1985. Factors determining the form of the frontoparietal bone in the newt *Hynobius keyserlingii* (Urodela). Doklady Akademie Nauk SSSR 281: 757–761.

1320. Leberman, R. C. 1970. Pattern and timing of skull pneumatization in the ruby-crowned kinglet. Bird Banding 41: 121–124.

1321. Le Douarin, N. M. 1982. *The Neural Crest*. Cambridge: Cambridge University Press.

1322. Leghissa, S. 1951. A proposito dello sviluppo del tetto otico nei Teleostei *Salmo fario*. Bollettino di zoologia, pubblicato dell' Unione zoologica italiana, Napoli 18: 355–365.

1323. Leibel, W. S. 1976. The influence of the otic capsule in ambystomid skull formation. Journal of Experimental Zoology 196: 85–104.

1324. Leiby, M. M. 1979a. Leptocephalus larvae of the eel family Ophichthidae. I. *Ophichthus gomesi* Castelnau. Bulletin of Marine Science 29: 329–343.

1325. Leiby, M. M. 1979b. Morphological development of the eel *Myrophis punctatus* (Ophichthidae) from hatching to metamorphosis, with emphasis on the developing head skeleton. Bulletin of Marine Science 29: 509–521.

1326. Leiby, M. M. 1981. Larval morphology of the eels *Bascanichthys bascanium, B. scuticaris, Ophichthus melanoporus,* and *O. ophis* (Ophichthidae), with a discussion of larval identification methods. Bulletin of Marine Science 31: 46–71.

1327. Leiby, M. M. 1984. Ophichthidae: Development and relationships. In *Ontogeny and Systematics of Fishes,* American Society of Ichthyologists and Herpetologists Special Publication no. 1, H. G. Moser, ed. Lawrence, Kans.: Allen Press, pp. 102–108.

1328. Leikola, A. 1976. The neural crest: Migrating cells in embryonic development. Folia morphologica, Prague 24: 155–172.

1329. Leis, J. M. 1977. Development of the eggs and larvae of the slender mola, *Ranzania laevis* (Pisces, Molidae). Bulletin of Marine Science 27: 448–466.

1330. Leis, J. M. 1984. Tetraodontoidei: Development. In *Ontogeny and Systematics of Fishes,* American Society of Ichthyologists and Herpetologists Special Publication no. 1, H. G. Moser, ed. Lawrence, Kans.: Allen Press, pp. 447–450.

1331. Lekander, B. 1949. The sensory line system and the cranial bones in the head of some Ostariophysi. Acta zoologica, Stockholm 30: 1–131.

1332. Le Lièvre, C. S. 1974. Rôle des cellules mésectodermiques issues des crêtes neurales céphaliques dans la formation des arcs branchiaux et du squelette viscéral. Journal of Embryology and Experimental Morphology 31: 453–477.

1333. Le Lièvre, C. S. 1978. Participation of neural crest–derived cells in the genesis of the skull in birds. Journal of Embryology and Experimental Morphology 47: 17–37.

1334. Le Lièvre, C. S., and N. M. Le Douarin. 1975. Mesenchymal derivatives of the neural crest: Analysis of chimeric quail and chick embryos. Journal of Embryology and Experimental Morphology 34: 125–154.

1335. Lemire, R. J. 1986. Embryology of the skull. In *Craniosynostosis: Diagnosis, Evaluation, and Management,* M. M. Cohen, Jr., ed. New York: Raven Press, pp. 105–130.

1336. Lessa, E. P., and J. L. Patton. 1989. Structural constraints, recurrent shapes, and allometry in pocket gophers (genus *Thomomys*). Biological Journal of the Linnean Society 36: 349–363.

1337. Lessertisseur, J., and R. Saban. 1967. Généralités sur le squelette. In *Traité de zoologie: Anatomie, systématique, biologie,* vol. 16(1), *Mammifères: Téguments squelette,* P.-P. Grassé, ed. Paris: Masson et Cie, pp. 334–404.

1338. Lethbridge, R. C., and I. C. Potter. 1981. The development of teeth and associated feeding structures during the metamorphosis of the lamprey, *Geotria australis.* Acta zoologica, Stockholm 62: 201–214.

1339. Leutenegger, W., and T. J. Masterson. 1989a. The ontogeny of sexual dimorphism in the cranium of Bornean orangutans (*Pongo pygmaeus pyg-*

maeus). I. Univariate analyses. Zeitschrift für Morphologie und Anthropologie 78: 1–14.

1340. Leutenegger, W., and T. J. Masterson. 1989b. The ontogeny of sexual dimorphism in the cranium of Bornean orangutans (*Pongo pygmaeus pygmaeus*). II. Allometry and heterochrony. Zeitschrift für Morphologie und Anthropologie 78: 15–24.

1341. Levy, B. M. 1948. Growth of the mandibular joint in normal mice. Journal of the American Dental Association 36: 177–182.

1342. Levy, B. M. 1964. Embryonical development of the temporomandibular joint. In *The Temporomandibular Joint*, B. G. Sarnat, ed. Springfield: C. H. Thomas, pp. 59–70.

1343. Liem, K. F. 1973. Evolutionary strategies and morphological innovations: Cichlid pharyngeal jaws. Systematic Zoology 22: 425–441.

1344. Liem, K. F., and L. S. Kaufman. 1984. Intraspecific macroevolution: Functional biology of the polymorphic cichlid species *Cichlasoma minckleyi*. In *Evolution of Fish Species Flocks*, A. A. Echelle and I. Kornfield, eds. Orono: University of Maine Press, pp. 203–215.

1345. Liem, K. F., and H. M. Smith. 1961. A critical reevaluation of the so-called "angular" in the crocodilian mandible. Turtox News 39: 146–148.

1346. Likhotop, R. I. 1988. On excessive cranial bones in *Erinaceus europaeus*. Vestnik zoologii: 76–77.

1347. Lim, T. M., E. R. Lunn, R. J. Keynes, and C. D. Stern. 1987. The differing effects of occipital and trunk somites on neural development in the chick embryo. Development 100: 525–534.

1348. Limborgh, J. van. 1970. A new view on the control of the morphogenesis of the skull. Acta morphologica neerlando-scandinavica 8: 143–160.

1349. Limborgh, J. van. 1971. The control of the morphogenesis of the skull. Nederlands Tijdschrift vorn Tandheelkunde 78: 44–53.

1350. Limborgh, J. van. 1972. The role of genetic and local environmental factors in the control of postnatal craniofacial morphogenesis. Acta morphologica neerlando-scandinavica 10: 37–47.

1351. Limborgh, J. van. 1982. Factors controlling skeletal morphogenesis. In *Factors and Mechanisms Influencing Bone Growth*, A. D. Dixon and B. G. Sarnat eds. New York: Alan R. Liss, pp. 1–17.

1352. Lincoln, G. A. 1973. Appearance of antler pedicles in early foetal life in red deer. Journal of Embryology and Experimental Morphology 29: 431–437.

1353. Lindahl, P. E. 1946. On some archaic features in the developing central stem of the mammalian chondrocranium. Acta zoologica, Stockholm 27: 91–100.

1354. Lindahl, P. E. 1948. Über die Entwicklung und Morphologie der Chondro-Kranium von *Procavia capensis* Pall. Acta zoologica, Stockholm 29: 281–376.

1355. Linden, H., and R. A. Vaisanen. 1986. Growth and sexual dimorphism in the skull of the Capercaillie *Tetrao urogallus:* A multivariate study of geographical variation. Ornis scandinavica 17: 85–98.

1356. Lochman, J. 1985. Wild deer. Statni Zemedelske Nakladatelstvi Praue: 1–351.

1357. Lombard, R. E. 1977. Comparative morphology of the inner ear in sala-
      manders (Caudata: Amphibia). Contributions to Vertebrate Evolution 2:
      1–140.
1358. Long, C. A. 1975. Growth and development of the teeth and skull of the
      wild North American badger, *Taxidea taxus*. Transactions of the Kansas
      Academy of Science 77: 106–120.
1359. Lopashov, G. V. 1944. Origin of pigment cells and visceral cartilage in te-
      leosts. Doklady Akademii Nauk SSSR 44: 169–172.
1360. Lorch, J. I. 1949a. The distribution of alkaline phosphatase in the skull of
      the developing trout. Quarterly Journal of Microscopical Science 90: 183–
      207.
1361. Lorch, J. I. 1949b. The distribution of alkaline phosphatase in relation to
      calcification in *Scyliorhinus canicula*. Quarterly Journal of Microscopical Sci-
      ence 90: 381–391.
1362. Løvtrup, S. 1977. *The Phylogeny of Vertebrata*. New York: Wiley and Sons.
1363. Lozanoff, S., and V. M. Diewert. 1989. A computer graphics program for
      measuring two- and three-dimensional form changes in developing cranio-
      facial cartilages using finite element methods. Computers and Biomedical Re-
      search 22: 63–82.
1364. Luder, H. U., C. P. Leblond, and K. von der Mark. 1988. Cellular stages in
      cartilage formation as revealed by morphometry, radioautography, and type II
      collagen immunostaining of the mandibular condyle from weanling rats.
      American Journal of Anatomy 182: 197–214.
1365. Luke, D. A. 1970. Development of the secondary palate in man. Acta ana-
      tomica 94: 596–608.
1366. Luke, D. A. 1976. Dental and craniofacial development in the normal and
      growth-retarded human fetus. Biology of the Neonate 29: 171–177.
1367. Luke, D. A. 1989. Cell proliferation in palatal processes and Meckel's car-
      tilage during development of the secondary palate of the mouse. Journal of
      Anatomy 165: 151–158.
1368. Lumer, H. 1940. Evolutionary allometry in the skeleton of the domesticated
      dog. American Naturalist 74: 439–467.
1369. Lumsden, A. G. S. 1987. Neural crest contribution to tooth development in
      the mammalian embryo. In *Developmental and Evolutionary Aspects of the
      Neural Crest*, P. F. A. Maderson, ed. New York: John Wiley and Sons,
      pp. 261–300.
1370. Lumsden, A. G. S. 1989. Multipotential cells in the avian neural crest.
      Trends in Neurosciences 12: 81–82.
1371. Lundelius, E. L., Jr., and B. H. Slaughter. 1976. Notes on American Pleis-
      tocene tapirs. In *Essays in Paleontology in Honour of Loris Shano Russell*,
      C. S. Churcher, ed. Toronto: Royal Ontario Museum of Life Sciences Miscel-
      laneous Publications, pp. 226–240.
1372. Lüps, P. 1974. Investigations on the development of the base of the skull in
      the red fox (*Vulpes vulpes* L.). Zoologischer Jahresbericht Anatomischer 98:
      288–298.
1373. Lüps, P., and A. I. Wandeler. 1983. Weight and size variation in foxes
      (*Vulpes vulpes*) from Swiss midlands. Zoologischer Anzeiger 211: 285–298.

1374. Lutz, H. 1942. Beiträge zur Stammesgeschichte der Ratiten. Vergleich zwischen Emu-Embryo und entsprechendem Carinatenstadium. Revue suisse de zoologie 49: 299–399.

1375. Lutz, B. 1948. Ontogenetic evolution in frogs. Evolution 2: 29–39.

1376. Lyagina, T. N. 1984. On morphological differences of bream and Blicca bjoerkna L. fry. Gidrobiologischeskii Zhurnal 24: 82–83.

1377. Lynch, J. D., and P. M. Ruiz-Carannza. 1985. A synopsis of the frogs of the genus Eleutherodactylus from the Sierra Nevada de Santa Marta, Colombia. University of Michigan Museum of Zoology, Occasional Papers, no. 711:1–59.

1378. Lyne, A. G. 1982. Observations on skull growth and eruption of teeth in the marsupial bandicoot Peramales nasuta (Marsupialia: Paramelidae). Australian Mammal 5: 113–126.

1379. Lyne, A. G., and P. A. Mort. 1981. A comparison of skull morphology in the marsupial bandicoot genus Isodon: Its taxonomic implications and notes on Isodon arnhemenis, new species. Australian Mammal 4: 107–134.

1380. Lynn, W. G. 1942. The embryology of Eleutherodactylus nubicola, an anuran which has no tadpole stage. Contributions to Embryology, Carnegie Institute of Washington, Publication 541: 27–64.

1381. Lynn, W. G., and B. Lutz. 1946a. The development of Eleutherodactylus guentheri Stdnr. 1864. Bollettino dei Musei nazionale, Zoologia 71: 1–46.

1382. Lynn, W. G., and B. Lutz. 1946b. The development of Eleutherodactylus nasutus Lutz. Bollettino dei Musei Nacional, Zoologia 79: 1–30.

1383. Lynn, W. G., and A. M. Peadon. 1955. The role of the thyroid gland in direct development in the anuran, Eleutherodactylus martinicensis. Growth 19: 263–286.

1384. Macalister, A. D. 1955. The development of the human temporomandibular joint: A microscopic study. Australian Journal of Dentistry 59: 21–27.

1385. MacArthur, J. W., and L. P. Chiasson. 1945. Relative growth in races of mice produced by selection. Growth 9: 303–315.

1386. McCann, C. 1976. Notes on the foetal skull of Mesoplodon stejnegeri. Scientific Report of the Whales Research Institute, Tokyo 29: 107–117.

1387. McClain, J. A. 1939. The development of the auditory ossicles of the opossum (Didelphys virginiana). Journal of Morphology 64: 211–265.

1388. McCrady, E., Jr. 1938. The embryology of the Opossum. American Anatomical Memoires 16: 1–226.

1389. McCullogh, C. A. G., H. C. Tenenbaum, C. A. Fair, and C. Birek. 1989. Site-specific regulation of osteogenesis: Maintenance of discrete levels of phenotypic expression in vitro. Anatomical Record 223: 27–34.

1390. McGowan, C. 1986. A putative ancestor for the swordfish-like ichthyosaur Eurhinosaurus. Nature 322: 454–456.

1391. McGowan, C. 1988. Differential development of the rostrum and mandible of the swordfish (Xiphias gladius) during ontogeny and its possible functional significance. Canadian Journal of Zoology 66: 496–503.

1392. Machado-Allison, A. 1986. Aspectos sobre la historia natural del "curito" Hoplosternum littorale (Hancock, 1828) (Siluriformes-Callichthyidae) en el Bajo Llano de Venezuela: Desarrollo, alimentación y distribución espacial. Acta científica venezolana 37: 72–78.

1393. Machado-Allison, A., and C. Garcia. 1986. Food habits and morphological changes during ontogeny in three serrasalmin fish species of the Venezuelan floodplains. Copeia: 193–196.

1394. Macke, T. 1969. Die Entwicklung des Craniums von *Fulica atra* L. Gegenbaurs Morphologisches Jahrbuch, Leipzig 113: 229–294.

1395. McKee, G. J., and M. W. J. Ferguson. 1984. The effects of mesencephalic neural crest cell extirpation on the development of chicken embryos. Journal of Anatomy, London 139: 491–512.

1396. McKeown, M. 1975. The influence of environment on the growth of the craniofacial complex—a study on domestication. Angle Orthodontist 45: 137–140.

1397. MacKinnon, J. 1981. The structure and function of the tusks of babirusa (*Babyrousa babyrussa*). Mammal Review 11: 37–40.

1398. McLeod, M. J., M. J. Harris, G. F. Chernoff, and J. R. Miller. 1980. First arch malformation: A new craniofacial mutant in the mouse. Journal of Heredity 71: 331–335.

1399. McNeil, R. 1967. Concerning the cranial development in the greenish elaenia, *Myiopagis viridicata* (Veillot). American Midland Naturalist 78: 529–530.

1400. McNeil, R., and A. Martinez. 1967. Retarded or arrested cranial development in *Myiornis ecaudatus*. Wilson Bulletin 79: 323–344.

1401. McPhee, J. R., and T. R. Van de Water. 1982. A biochemical profile of the ECM during the sequential stages of otic capsule formation *in vivo* and *in vitro*. In *Extracellular Matrix*, S. Hawkes and J. L. Wang, eds. New York: Academic Press, pp. 189–294.

1402. McPhee, J. R., and T. R. Van de Water. 1985. A comparison of morphological stages and sulfated glycosaminoglycan production during otic capsule formation: *In vivo* and *in vitro*. Anatomical Record 213: 566–577.

1403. McPhee, J. R., and T. R. Van de Water. 1986. Epithelial-mesenchymal tissue interactions guiding otic capsule formation: The role of the otocyst. Journal of Embryology and Experimental Morphology 97: 1–24.

1404. MacPhee, R. D. E. 1977. Ontogeny of the ectotympanic-petrosal plate relationship in strepsirhine prosimians. Folia primatologica 27: 245–283.

1405. MacPhee, R. D. E. 1979. Entotympanics, ontogeny, and primates. Folio primatologica 31: 23–47.

1406. MacPhee, R. D. E. 1987a. Basicranial morphology and ontogeny of the extinct giant lemur *Megaladapis*. American Journal of Physical Anthropology 74: 333–355.

1407. MacPhee, R. D. E. 1987b. The shrew tenrecs of Madagascar: Systematic revision and Holocene distribution of *Microgale* (Tenrecidae, Insectivora). American Museum Novitates, no. 2889: 1–45.

1408. MacPhee, R. D. E., M. Cartmill, and K. D. Rose. 1989. Craniodental morphology and relationships of the supposed Eocene dermopteran *Plagiomeme* (Mammalia). Journal of Vertebrate Paleontology 9: 329–349.

1409. MacPhee, R. D. E., and N. C. Durham. 1981. Auditory regions of primates and eutherian insectivores: Morphology, ontogeny, and character analysis. Contributions to Primatology 18: 1–282.

1410. Maderson, P. F. A., ed. 1987. *Developmental and Evolutionary Aspects of the Neural Crest.* New York: John Wiley and Sons.

1411. Madkour, G. 1982. Skull osteology in some species of bats from Egypt. Lynx, Prague 21: 97–109.

1412. Madkour, G. 1984. Chondral and osteological structures in the cranial region of common Qatarian gerbels. Zoologischer Anzeiger 213: 247–257.

1413. Maeda, K. 1988. Age and sexual variations of the cranial characters in the least horseshoe bat, *Rhinilophus cornutus* Temminck. Journal of the Mammalogical Society of Japan 13: 43–50.

1414. Maeda, N., H. Amano, M. Machino, T. Kaneko, and M. Kumegawa. 1986. L-thyroxine, cortisol, and diet affect the postnatal development of the facial part of the skull in developing rats. Anatomisches Anzeiger 161: 99–104.

1415. Maffei, M. D., W. D. Klimstra, and T. J. Wilmers. 1988. Cranial and mandibular characteristics of the key deer (*Odocoileus virginianus clavium*). Journal of Mammalogy 69: 403–407.

1416. Mahan, C. J. 1979. Age determination of bobcats (*Lynx rufus*) by means of canine pulp cavity ratios. Scientific and Technical Series of the National Wildlife Federation no. 6: 126–129.

1417. Maier, W. 1980. Nasal structures in Old and New World primates. In *Evolutionary Biology of the New World Monkeys and Continental Drift*, R. L. Ciochon and A. B. Chiarelli, eds. New York: Plenum Press, pp. 219–241.

1418. Maier, W. 1983. Morphology of the interorbital region of *Saimiri sciureus*. Folia Primatologica 41: 277–303.

1419. Maier, W. 1987a. The ontogenetic development of the orbitotemporal region in the skull of *Monodelphis domestica* (Didelphidae, Marsupialia), and the problem of the mammalian alisphenoid. In *Morphogenesis of the Mammalian Skull*, H.-J. Kuhn and U. Zeller, eds. Hamburg: Verlag Paul Parey, pp. 71–90.

1420. Maier, W. 1987b. Der processus angularis bei *Monodelphis domestica* (Didelphidae: Marsupialia) und seine Beziehungen zum Mittehorn: Eine ontogenetische und evolutionsmorphologische Untersuchung. Gegenbaurs Morphologisches Jahrbuch 133: 123–161.

1421. Maier, W. 1989a. Ala temporalis and alisphenoid in therian mammals. Fortschritte der Zoologie 35: 396–400.

1422. Maier, W. 1989b. Morphologische untersuchungen an mittelohr der Marsupialis. Zeitschrift für Zoologie und Systematik Evolutionforschung 27: 149–168.

1423. Maier, W., and F. Schrench. 1987. The hystricomorphy of the Bathyergidae, as determined from ontogenetic evidence. Zeitschrift für Saeugetierkunde 52: 156–164.

1424. Maillard, J. 1948. Recherches embryologiques sur *Catharacta skua* Brünn. Revue suisse de zoologie 55: 1–114.

1425. Maisey, J. G. 1986. Heads and tails: A chordate phylogeny. Cladistics 2: 201–256.

1426. Maisey, J. G. 1988. Phylogeny of early vertebrate skeletal induction and ossification pattern. Evolutionary Biology 22: 1–36.

1427. Makeeva, A. P. 1980. Peculiarities of early ontogenesis in the bigmouth buffalo *Ictiobus cyprinella* (Val.) (Catastomidae). Voprosy Ihktiologii 20: 855–874.

1428. Malan, M. E. 1946. Contributions to the comparative anatomy of the nasal capsule and the organ of Jacobson of the Lacertilia. Annals of the University of Stellenbosch 24: 69–137.

1429. Mal'dzhyunaite, S. A. 1957. Age determination and age structure of pine martens in Lithuania. Translated in *Biology of Mustelids: Some Soviet Research* (1975), C. M. King, ed. Boston Spa: British Lending Library Division, pp. 132–144.

1430. Malinowski, A. 1970. The length, width, and cranial index in human fetuses. Folia morphologica, Warsaw 29: 495–501.

1431. Mallatt, J. 1984. Early vertebrate evolution: Pharyngeal structure and the origin of gnathostomes. Journal of Zoology, London 204: 169–183.

1432. Mallory, F. F., R. J. Brooks, and J. R. Elliott. 1986. Variations of skull-body regressions of the lemming (*Dicrostonyx groenlandicus*) under laboratory and field conditions. Zoological Journal of the Linnean Society, London 87: 125–138.

1433. Malloy, R. B. 1973. Assessment of sutural and cranial growth in young guinea pig skulls: A quantitative tetracycline labelling study. Journal of Dental Research 52: 1332–1339.

1434. Manaserova, N. S. 1988. Morphological characteristics of the skull of *Ovis ammon gmelini*. Biologicheskii zhurnal armenii 41: 668–675.

1435. Mandarim de Lacerda, C. A. 1989. Relative growth of the human temporal bone in the prenatal period. Acta morphologica hungarica 37: 65–70.

1436. Mandru, C. V. 1982. The ontogenetic development of the cranium in herons (Ardeidae-Ciconiiformes). Analele stiintifice ale Universitatii A1.I. Cuza din Iasi, n.s., Biol. 28: 101–103.

1437. Mangia, F., and G. Palladini. 1970. Recherches histochimiques sur le mucocartilage de la lamproie pendant son ontogenèse larvaire. Archives d'anatomie microscopique et de morphologie experimentale 59: 283–288.

1438. Mangold, O. 1961. Molchlarven ohne Zentrainervensystem und ohne ektomesoderm. Wilhelm Roux' Archiv für Entwicklungsmechanik der Organismen 152: 725–769.

1439. Mangold, U., A. Dörr, and P. Kaufmann. 1981. Die Kiemenbogenentwicklung bei Ratte und Maus. II. Zur Existenz von Kiemenspalten. Acta anatomica 110: 23–34.

1440. Manikowski, S. 1980. The dynamics of the Chari-Logone population of *Quelea quelea* and its control. In *Proceedings of the Fourth Pan-African Ornithological Congress*, D. N. Johnson, ed. South Africa: Southern African Ornithological Society, pp. 411–421.

1441. Manning, T. H. 1974. Variations in the skull of the bearded seal, *Erignathus barbatus* (Erxleben). Biological Papers of the University of Alaska 16:1–21.

1442. Manzanares, M. C., M. Goret-Nicaise, and A. Dhem. 1988. Metopic sutural closure in the human skull. Journal of Anatomy 161: 203–215.

1443. Marathe, V. B., and D. V. Bal. 1957. The development of the chondrocranium in *Trichopodus trichopterus* (Pall). Proceedings of the Indian Academy of Science 46B: 347–375.

1444. Marathe, V. B., and D. V. Bal. 1960. Observations on the ossification centres of *Trichopodus trichopterus* (Pall). Proceedings of the Indian Academy of Science 51B: 74–81.

1445. Marathe, V. B., and S. K. Suterwala. 1964. The development of the chondrocranium in *Tylosurus crocodilus* (Lesueur). Journal of the University of Bombay, n.s., 31: 61–74.

1446. Marche, C., and J. P. Durand. 1983. Recherches comparatives sur l'ontogenèse et l'évolution de l'appareil hyobranchial de *Proteus anguinus* L., proteidae aveugle des eaux souterraines. Amphibia-Reptilia 4: 1–16.

1147. Marconi, M., and A. M. Simonetta. 1989. The morphology of the skull in neotenic and normal *Triturus vulgaris meridionalis* (Boulenger) (Amphibia Caudata Salamandridae). Monitore zoologico italiano 22: 365–396.

1448. Marinelli, W., and A. Strenger. 1954. Vergleichende Anatomie und Morphologie der Wirbeltiere. I. Lieferung: *Lampetra fluviatilis*. Wien: Franz Deuticke, pp. 1–80.

1449. Marinelli, W., and A. Strenger. 1956. Vergleichende Anatomie und Morphologie der Wirbeltiere. II. Lieferung: *Myxine glutinosa*. Wien: Franz Deuticke, pp. 81–172.

1450. Markens, I. S. 1975. Embryonic development of the coronal suture in man and rat. Acta anatomica 93: 257–273.

1451. Markle, G. E. 1974. On the distribution and development of larval swordfish (*Xiphias gladius* L.) in the western Atlantic. Fisheries Research Board of Canada, Manuscript Report Series no. 1305.

1452. Markowski, J. 1980. Morphometric variability in a population of the root vole (*Microtus oeconomus*). Acta theriologica 25: 155–200.

1453. Martin, B. G. H., and A. d'A. Bellairs. 1977. The narial excrescence and pterygoid bulla of the gharial *Gavialis gangeticus* (Crocodilia). Journal of Zoology, London 182: 541–556.

1454. Martindale, M. Q., S. Meier, and A. G. Jacobson. 1987. Mesodermal metamerism in the teleost, *Oryzias latipes* (the Medaka). Journal of Morphology 193: 241–252.

1455. Martof, B. S., and F. L. Rose. 1962. The comparative osteology of the anterior cranial elements of the salamanders *Gyrinophilus* and *Pseudotriton*. Copeia: 727–732.

1456. Maryanska, T., and H. Osmolska. 1979. Aspects of hadrosaurian cranial anatomy. Lethaia 12: 265–273.

1457. Maryanska, T., and H. Osmolska. 1981. Cranial anatomy of *Saurolophus angustirostris* with comments on the Asian Hadrasauridae (Dinosauria). Palaeontologia polonica, no. 42: 5–24.

1458. Matson, J. O. 1984. Nongeographic variation in the rufous elephant shrew, *Elephantulus rufescens* (Peters, 1878) from Kenya. Mammalia 48: 593–598.

1459. Matson, J. O., and K. A. Shump, Jr. 1980. Intrapopulation variation in cranial morphology in the agouti, *Dasyprocta punctata* (Dasyproctidae). Mammalia 44: 559–570.

1460. Matsumato, M., H. Nishinakagawa, and J. Otsuka. 1984. Morphometrical study of the skull of *Cervus pulchellus, Cervus nippon mageshimae,* and *Cer-*

vus nippon yakushimae. Journal of the Mammalogical Society of Japan 10: 41–54.

1461. Matsuoka, M. 1985. Osteological development in the red sea bream, *Pagrus major.* Japanese Journal of Ichthyology 32: 35–41.

1462. Matsuoka, M. 1987. Development of the skeletal tissues and skeletal muscles in the red sea bream. Bulletin of the Seikai Regional Fisheries Research Laboratory 65: 1–114.

1463. Matsuura, Y., and N. T. Yoneda. 1987. Osteological development of the lophiid anglerfish, *Lophius gastrophysus.* Japanese Journal of Ichthyology 33: 360–367.

1464. Matthes, E. 1938. A tearia vertebral do crânio desde Goethe ate á actualidade. Archivos do Museu Bocage, Lisboa 9: 1–16.

1465. Matveiev, B. S. 1940. Zur Frage der Ontogenese des Knochenschädels der Chondrostei. Doklady Akademii Nauk SSSR 27: 631–634.

1466. May, E. 1978. Zur Kenntnis der Entwicklung des Schädels von *Leposternon microcephalum* Wagler 1824 (Reptilia: Amphisbaenia). Senckenbergiana biologica 59: 41–69.

1467. Mebes, H.-D. 1984. Beobachtungen zur embryogenese des rosenpapageis *Agapornis roseicollis* (Viellot) (Aves, Psittaciformes): Schnabelentwicklung und zehenstellung. Zoologische Garten, Jena 54: 121–127.

1468. Mednick, L. W., and S. L. Washburn. 1956. The role of sutures in the growth of the braincase of the infant pig. American Journal of Physical Anthropology 14: 175–191.

1469. Medvedeva, E. D. 1977a. Intrapopulation variability of chondrocranium and some other osteological characters in the genus *Salvelinus* (Salmoniformes, Salmonidae) on the Bering Island (Commander Islands). Zoologicheskii zhurnal 56: 563–575.

1470. Medvedeva, E. D. 1977b. Intrapopulation variation of some skull membrane bones in *Salvelinus alpinus* (Salmoniformes, Salmonidae) on the Bering Island (Commander Islands). Zoologischeskii zhurnal 56: 725–735.

1471. Medvedeva, I. M. 1959. The naso-lachrymal duct and its relationship to the lachrymal and septomaxillary dermal bones in *Ranodon sibiricus.* Doklady Akademii Nauk SSSR 128: 425–428.

1472. Medvedeva, I. M. 1960a. On the relationship of the developing naso-lachrymal duct to the lachrymal and septomaxillary dermal bones in *Hynobius keyserlingii.* Doklady Akademii Nauk SSSR 131: 1209–1212.

1473. Medvedeva, I. M. 1960b. New material on the form of choanae and choanal canal in Anura. Zoologicheskii zhurnal 39: 567–579.

1474. Medvedeva, I. M. 1961a. Some data on the early development of the lateral lines of the head in the Hynobiidae. Doklady Akademii Nauk SSSR 139: 748–751.

1475. Medvedeva, I. M. 1961b. On the problem of the origin of the choana of Amphibia. Doklady Akademii Nauk SSSR 137: 468–471.

1476. Medvedeva, I. M. 1963. Development and reduction of the nasolachrymal duct in *Pleurodeles waltlii.* Doklady Akademii Nauk SSSR 148: 1215–1217.

1477. Medvedeva, I. M. 1964. Development, origin, and homology of the choana and the choanal canal of Amphibia. Trudy Zoologicheskogo Instituta Akademiya Nauk SSSR 33: 173–211.

1478. Medvedeva, I. M. 1965. Localization of material in the olfactory placode of the caudate amphibians. Doklady Akademii Nauk SSSR 162: 709–712.

1479. Medvedeva, I. M. 1975. *The Olfactory Organ in Amphibians and Its Phylogenetic Significance.* Leningrad: Nauka.

1480. Medvedeva, I. M. 1986a. On the origin of nasolacrimal duct in Tetrapoda. In *Studies in Herpetology,* Z. Roček, ed. Prague: Charles University, pp. 37–40.

1481. Medvedeva, I. M. 1986b. Nasolachrymal canal of Ambystomatidae in the light of its origin in other terrestrial vertebrates. In *Morphology and Evolution of Animals,* E. E. Vorobyeva and N. S. Lebedkina, eds. Moscow: Nauka, pp. 138–156.

1482. Medvedeva, K. D., and K. A. Savvaitova. 1981. Intrapopulation and geographic variability of the skull in charrs. In *Charrs: Salmonid Fishes of the Genus Salvelinus,* E. K. Balon, ed. The Hague: W. Junk, pp. 435–440.

1483. Medvedeva-Vasil'eva, E. D. 1978. Intrapopulational variability of jaw bones and some other bones of the skull in the charr (*Salvelinus alpinus* L.) of the Bering Island in the Komandorskiye Islands. Voprosy Ikhtiologii 18: 399–414.

1484. Mees, G. F. 1985. Nomenclature and systematics of birds from Suriname. Proceedings, Koninklijka Nederlandse Akademie van Wetenschappen, ser. C, Biological and Medical Sciences 88: 75–91.

1485. Meier, S. 1979. Development of the chick embryo mesoblast: Formation of the embryonic axis and establishment of the metameric pattern. Developmental Biology 73: 25–45.

1486. Meier, S. 1981. Development of the chick embryo mesoblast: Morphogenesis of the prechordal plate and cranial segments. Developmental Biology 83: 49–61.

1487. Meier, S. 1982. The development of segmentation in the cranial region of vertebrate embryos. Scanning Electron Microscopy: 1269–1282.

1488. Meier, S., and C. Drake. 1984. Scanning electron microscopy localization of cell-surface-associated fibronectin in the cranium of chick embryos utilizing immunolatex microspheres. Journal of Embryology and Experimental Morphology 80: 175–196.

1489. Meier, S., and A. G. Jacobson. 1982. Experimental studies of the origin and expression of metameric pattern in the chick embryo. Journal of Experimental Zoology 219: 217–232.

1490. Meier, S., and D. S. Packard, Jr. 1984. Morphogenesis of the cranial segments and distribution of neural crest in the embryo of the snapping turtle, *Chelydra serpentina.* Developmental Biology 102: 309–323.

1491. Meier, S., and P. P. L. Tam. 1982. Metameric pattern development in the embryonic axis of the mouse. I. Differentiation of the cranial segments. Differentiation 21: 95–108.

1492. Meinke, D. K. 1982. A light and scanning electron microscope study of microstructure, growth, and development of the dermal skeleton of *Polypterus* (Pisces: Actinopterygii). Journal of Zoology, London 197: 355–382.

1493. Meinke, D. K. 1984. A review of cosmine: Its structure, development, and relationship to other forms of the dermal skeleton in osteichthyans. Journal of Vertebrate Paleontology 4: 457–470.

1494. Meinke, D. K. 1986. Morphology and evolution of the dermal skeleton in lungfishes. Journal of Morphology 1 (suppl.): 133–149.

1495. Mendakov, M. N. 1984. Age variation in skull sizes of the large-toothed souslik on Barsa-Kelmes Island. In *The Species and Its Productivity within its Distribution Range*, pt. 1, *Mammals (Insectivores, Rodents)*, F. V. Kryazhim-skij, ed. Sverdlovsk: Urals Scientific Centre, Academy of Sciences USSR, p. 49.

1496. Menon, C. B. 1965. The interorbital septum in *Tilapia mossambica* (Peters). Zoologischer Anzeiger 174: 351–352.

1497. Menzies, T. I. 1967. An ecological note on the frog *Pseudhymenochirus merlini* Chabanaud in Sierra Leone. Journal of the West African Science Association 12: 23–28.

1498. Merrett, N. R., J. Badcock, and P. J. Herring. 1973. The status of *Benthalbella infans* (Pisces, Myctophoidei): Its development, bioluminescence, general biology, and distribution in the eastern north Atlantic. Journal of Zoology, London 170: 1–48.

1499. Metzmacher, M. 1986. Moineux domestiques, *Passer domesticus,* et Espagnols, *Passer hispaniolensis,* dans une region de l'ouest Algerien: Analyses comparative de leur morphologie externe. Gerfaut 76: 317–334.

1500. Metzner, L., J. D. Garol, H. W. Fields, Jr., and V. G. Kokich. 1978. The craniofacial skeleton in anencephalic human fetuses. III. Facial skeleton. Teratology 17: 75–82.

1501. Meyer, A. 1987. Phenotypic plasticity and heterochrony in *Cichlasoma managuense* (Pisces, Cichlidae) and their implications for speciation in cichlid fishes. Evolution 41: 1357–1369.

1502. Meyer, M. N. 1978. Taxonomic and intraspecific variation of *Microtus* from the Far East of the USSR. Trudy Zoologich Instituta, Leningrad 75: 3–62.

1503. Mezhzherin, V. A., and S. A. Kirichuk. 1988. Seasonal and age changes in the cranium and body weights in small shrew. Vestnik zoologii 1988: 36–40.

1504. Michejda, M. 1971. Ontogenetic changes of the cranial base in *Macaca mulatta:* Histologic study. In *Proceedings of the Third International Congress of Primatology*, vol. 1, *Taxonomy, Anatomy, Reproduction*, J. Biegert and W. Leutenegger, eds. Basel: S. Karger, pp. 215–222.

1505. Michejda, M. 1972a. The role of basicranial synchondroses in flexure processes and ontogenetic development of the skull base. American Journal of Physical Anthropology 37: 143–150.

1506. Michejda, M. 1972b. Significance of basicranial synchondroses in nonhuman primates and man. In *Medical Primatology, 1972. I. General Primatology, Reproduction and Perinatal Studies, Genetics, Phylogenetics, and Evolution*, E. I. Goldsmith and J. Moor-Jankowski, eds. Basel: S. Karger, pp. 372–378.

1507. Michejda, M. 1975. Ontogenetic growth changes of the skull base in four genera of nonhuman primates. Acta anatomica 91: 110–117.

1508. Michejda, M., and D. Lamey. 1971. Flexion and metric age changes of the cranial base in the *Macaca mulatta:* I. Infant and juveniles. Folia primatologica 14: 84–94.

1509. Milaire, J. 1974. Histochemical aspects of organogenesis in vertebrates. Handbuch der Histochemie 8 (suppl. 3).

1510. Miller, J. D. 1985. Embryology of marine turtles. In *Biology of the Reptilia*, C. Gans, F. Billett, and P. F. A. Maderson, eds., vol. 14, Development A. New York: John Wiley and Sons, pp. 269–328.

1511. Miller, J. M., and B. Y. Sumida. 1974. Development and life history of *Caranx mate* (Carangidae). U.S. National Marine Fisheries Service, Fishery Bulletin 72: 497–514.

1512. Minami, T. 1981. The early life history of a sole *Heteromycteris japonicus*. Bulletin of the Japanese Society of Fisheries Science 47: 857–862.

1513. Minkoff, R. 1980a. Regional variation of cell proliferation within the facial processes of the chick embryo: A study of the role of "merging" during development. Journal of Embryology and Experimental Morphology 57: 37–49.

1514. Minkoff, R. 1980b. Cell proliferation and migration during primary palate development. In *Current Research Trends in Prenatal Craniofacial Development*, R. M. Pratt and R. Christiansen, eds. New York: Elsevier/North Holland, pp. 119–136.

1515. Minkoff, R. 1984. Cell cycle analysis of facial mesenchyme in the chick embryo. I. Labelled mitosis and continuous labelling studies. Journal of Embryology and Experimental Morphology 81: 49–59.

1516. Minkoff, R., and R. E. Martin. 1984. Cell cycle analysis of facial mesenchyme in the chick embryo. II. Label dilution studies and development fate of slow cycling cells. Journal of Embryology and Experimental Morphology 81: 61–73.

1517. Mitala, J. J., J. P. Boardman, R. A. Carrano, and J. D. Iuliucci. 1984. Novel accessory skull bone in fetal rats after exposure to aspirin. Teratology 30: 95–98.

1518. Miwa, S., M. Tagawa, Y. Inui, and T. Hirano. 1988. Thyroxine surge in metamorphosing flounder larvae. General and Comparative Endocrinology 70: 158–163.

1519. Miyazaki, N., M. Amano, and Y. Fujise. 1987. Growth and skull morphology of the harbor porpoises in the Japanese waters. Memoirs of the National Science Museum, Tokyo, no. 20: 137–146.

1520. Modrzewski, A., M. Ogrodnik, T. Pawlega, A. Wilgoszynski, and Z. Wojtowicz. 1969. Morphology of some of the cranial bones in *Macacus rhesus*. Folia morphologica, Warsaw 28: 243–262.

1521. Moelle, H. F. 1980. Growth dependent changes in the skeleton proportions of *Thylacinus cynocephalus*. Saeugetierkundliche Mitteilungen 28: 62–69.

1522. Moen, R. C., D. W. Rowe, and R. D. Palmiter. 1979. Regulation of procollagen synthesis during the development of chick embryo calvaria: Correlation with procollagen mRNA content. Journal of Biological Chemistry 254: 3526–3530.

1523. Moffett, B. C. 1957. The prenatal development of the human temporomandibular joint. Contributions to Embryology from the Carnegie Institute of Washington 36 (611): 19–28.

1924. Moffett, B. C. 1964. The development of discs and fibrous articular tissue in the temporomandibular and clavicular joints. Anatomical Record 148: 313.

1525. Moffett, B. C. 1965. The Morphogenesis of joints. In *Organogenesis*, R. L. DeHaan and H. Ursprung, eds. New York: Holt, Rinehart and Winston, pp. 301–313.

1526. Moffett, B. C. 1972. *Mechanisms and Regulation of Craniofacial Morphogenesis*. Amsterdam: Swets and Zeitlinger B.V. Also published in Acta morphologica neerlando-scandinavica 10: 1–150.

1527. Mohr, E. 1937. Revision der Centriscidae (Acanthopterygii Centrisciformes). Dana Reports of the Carlsberg Foundation 13.

1528. Mondolfi, E. 1974. Taxonomy, distribution, and status of the manatee in Venezuela. Memoria de la Sociedad de ciencias naturales, La Salle 34: 5–23.

1529. Montagu, M. F. A. 1943. The mesethmoid-presphenoid relationships in the primates. American Journal of Physical Anthropology 1: 129–141.

1530. Montague, J. J. 1984. Morphometric analysis of *Crocodylus novaeguineae* from the Fly River drainage, Papua, New Guinea. Australian Wildlife Research 11: 395–414.

1531. Mook, D. 1977. Larval and osteological development of the sheepshead *Archosargus probatocephalus* (Pisces: Sparidae). Copeia: 126–133.

1532. Moore, G. C. 1987. Observations on cranial differences between juvenile and adult eastern coyotes, *Canis latrans*. Canadian Field Naturalist 101: 461–463.

1533. Moore, R. N. 1978. A cephalometric and histologic study of the cranial base in foetal monkeys, *Macaca nemestrina*. Archives of Oral Biology 23: 57–68.

1534. Moore, R. N., and P. E. Lestrel. 1979. Modeling of the cranial base. In *Aging in Nonhuman Primates*, D. M. Bowden, ed. New York: van Nostrand and Reinhold Col, pp. 369–377.

1535. Moore, R. N., and C. Philipps. 1980. Sagittal craniofacial growth in the fetal macaque monkey, *Macaca nemestrina*. Archives of Oral Biology 25: 19–22.

1536. Moore, W. J. 1981. *The Mammalian Skull*. Cambridge: Cambridge University Press.

1537. Moore, W. J. 1982. Skull form in hominoids. In *Progress in Anatomy*, vol. 2, R. J. Harrison and V. Navaratnam, eds. London: Cambridge University Press, pp. 49–79.

1538. Moore, W. J. 1985. The use of shape measures in the study of skeletal growth and development. In *Normal and Abnormal Bone Growth: Basic and Clinical Research*, Progress in Clinical and Biological Research, vol. 187, A. D. Dixon and B. G. Sarnat, eds. New York: Alan R. Liss, pp. 495–510.

1539. Moore, W. J., and C. L. B. Lavelle. 1974. *Growth of the Facial Skeleton in the Hominoidea*. London: Academic Press.

1540. Moore, W. J., and B. Mintz. 1972. Clonal model of vertebral column and skull development derived from genetically mosaic skeletons in allophenic mice. Developmental Biology 27: 55–70.

1541. Moore, W. J., and T. F. Spence. 1969. Age changes in the cranial base of the rabbit (*Oryctolagus cuniculus*). Anatomical Record 165: 355–362.

1542. Moore, W. M. O., B. S. Ward, V. P. Jones, and F. N. Bamford. 1988. Sex difference in fetal head growth. British Journal of Obstetrics and Gynaecology 95: 238–242.

1543. Morejohn, G. V., and K. T. Briggs. 1973. Post-mortem studies of Northern elephant seal pups. Proceedings of the Zoological Society of London 171: 67–77.

1544. Moreno, S. 1986. Allometric study of the garden dormouse, Eliomys quercinus (L.) in the Iberian peninsula and north Morocco. Miscelanea zoologica 10: 315–322.

1545. Morii, R. 1976. Biological study of the Japanese house bat, Pipistrellus abramus (Temminck, 1840) in Kagawa Prefecture. Part 1. External, cranial, and dental characters of embryos and litters. Journal of the Mammalogical Society of Japan 6: 248–258.

1546. Morita, S., F. Ohtsuki, K. Hattori, E. Sugawara, and Y. Kaito. 1976. A study of the symmetry in the thickness of human fetal cranial bones. Jikeikal Medical Journal 23: 169–175.

1547. Morris, J. M., and G. A. Bubenik. 1983. The effects of androgens on the development of antler bone. In Antler Development in Cervidae, R. D. Brown, ed. Kingsville, Tex.: Caesar Kleberg Wildlife Research Institute, pp. 123–141.

1548. Morris, S. L., and A. J. Gaudin. 1982. Osteocranial development in the viviparous surfperch, Amphistichus argenteus (Pisces: Embiotocidae). Journal of Morphology 174: 95–120.

1549. Morriss, G., and P. V. Thorogood. 1978. An approach to cranial neural crest cell migration and differentiation in mammalian embryos. In Development in Mammals, vol. 3, M. H. Johnson, ed. Amsterdam: Elsevier/North Holland, pp. 363–412.

1550. Morriss-Kay, G., and S.-S. Tan. 1987. Mapping cranial neural crest cell migration pathways in mammalian embryos. Trends in Genetics 3: 257–261.

1551. Moser, H. G. 1970. Development and geographical distribution of the rockfish, Sebastes macdonaldi (Eidenmann and Beeson, 1893), family Scorpaenidae, off southern California and Baja California. U.S. National Marine Fisheries Service, Fishery Bulletin 70: 941–958.

1552. Moser, H. G., ed. 1984. Ontogeny and Systematics of Fishes, American Society of Ichthyologists and Herpetologists Special Publication no. 1. Lawrence, Kans.: Allen Press.

1553. Moser, H. G., and E. H. Ahlstrom. 1970. Development of lanternfishes (family Myctophidae) in the California Current. Part I. Species with narrow-eyed larvae. Natural History Museum of Los Angeles County, Bulletin 7: 1–145.

1554. Moser, H. G., and E. H. Ahlstrom. 1978. Larvae and pelagic juveniles of blackgill rockfish. Sebastes melanostomus, taken in midwater trawls off Southern California. Journal of the Fisheries Research Board of Canada 35: 981–996.

1555. Moss, M. L. 1955. Relative growth of the human facial skeleton. Annals of the New York Academy of Sciences 63: 528–536.

1556. Moss, M. L. 1957. Premature synostosis of the frontal suture in the cleft palate skull. Plastic Reconstructive Surgery 20: 199–205.

1557. Moss, M. L. 1958. Fusion of the frontal suture in the rat. American Journal of Anatomy 102: 141–166.

1558. Moss, M. L. 1960. Functional analysis of human mandibular growth. Journal of Prosthetic Dentistry 10: 1149–1159.

1559. Moss, M. L. 1961. Rotation of the otic capsule in bipedal rats. American Journal of Physical Anthroplogy 19: 301–317.

1560. Moss, M. L. 1962. Studies on the acellular bone of teleost fish. II. Response to fracture under normal and acalcemic conditions. Acta anatomica 48: 46–60.

1561. Moss, M. L. 1972. New research objectives in craniofacial morphogenesis. Acta morphologica neerlando-scandinavica 10: 103–110.

1562. Moss, M. L. 1973. Functional cranial analysis of primate craniofacial growth. In Craniofacial Biology of Primates, M. R. Zingeser, ed. Basel: S. Karger, pp. 191–208.

1563. Moss, M. L. 1975. Functional anatomy of cranial synostosis. Child's Brain 1: 22–33.

1564. Moss, M. L., and M. J. Baer. 1956. Differential growth of the rat skull. Growth 20: 107–120.

1565. Moss, M. L., and W. C. Feliciano. 1977. A functional analysis of the fenestrated maxillary bone of the rabbit (Oryctolagus cuniculus). Zentralblaat fuer Veterinaermedizin, Reihe C, Anatomia, Histologia, Embryologia 6: 167–187.

1566. Moss, M. L., M.-A. Meehan, and L. Salentijn. 1972. Transformative and translative growth processes in neurocranial development of the rat. Acta anatomica 81: 161–182.

1567. Moss, M. L., L. Moss-Salentijn, H. Vilmann, and L. Newell-Morris. 1982. Neuro-skeletal topology of the primate basicranium: Its implications for the "fetalization hypothesis." Gegenbaurs Morphologisches Jahrbuch 128: 58–67.

1568. Moss, R. 1987. Demography of capercaillie Tetrao urogallus in northeast Scotland [UK]. I. Determining the age of Scottish capercaillie from skull and head measurements. Ornis scandinavica 18: 129–134.

1569. Moss-Salentijn, L. 1976. Cartilage canals and the growth of the spheno-occipital synchondrosis of the human fetus. In Development of the Basicranium, J. F. Bosma, ed. Bethesda: U.S. Department of Health, Education, and Welfare, pp. 93–105.

1570. Mostafa, Y. A., N. H. El-Mangoury, R. A. Meyer, Jr., and R. J. Ioxio. 1982. Deficient nasal bone growth in the X-linked hypophosphatemic (Hyp) mouse and its implications in craniofacial growth. Archives of Oral Biology 27: 311–318.

1571. Mourgue, M. 1940. Activité phosphatasique des os dermiques de la raie cloutée (Raia clavata Rondelet). Comptes rendus des séances de la Société de biologie, Paris 133: 465–467.

1572. Moutou, F., and I. E. Vesmanis. 1986. To the knowledge of the house shrew, Suncus murinus (Linneaus, 1766), from Reunion (Indian Ocean). Zoologische Abhandlungen, Dresden 42: 41–52.

1573. Moy-Thomas, J. A. 1938. The problem of the evolution of the dermal bones in fishes. In *Evolution: Essays on Aspects of Evolutionary Biology*, G. R. de Beer, ed. Oxford: Oxford University Press, pp. 305–319.

1574. Moy-Thomas, J. A. 1941. Development of the frontal bones of the rainbow trout. Nature 147: 681–682.

1575. Müller, H. J. 1961. Über strukturelle Ähnlichkeiten der Orh- und Occipitalregion bei Vogel und Säuger. Zoologischer Anzeiger 166: 391–402.

1576. Muhlhauser, J. 1986. Resorption of the unmineralized proximal part of Meckel's cartilage in the rat: A light and electron microscopic study. Journal of Submicroscopic Cytology 18: 717–724.

1577. Muir, P. D., A. R. Sykes, and G. K. Barrell. 1985. Mineralization during antler growth in red deer. Bulletin of the Royal Society of New Zealand, no. 22: 251–254.

1578. Muir, P. D., A. R. Sykes, and G. K. Barrell. 1987. Growth and mineralization of antlers in red deer (*Cervus elaphus*). New Zealand Journal of Agricultural Research 30: 305–315.

1579. Mullen, K., and H. J. Swatland. 1979. Linear skeletal growth in male and female turkeys. Growth 43: 151–159.

1580. Müller, D. 1981. Beitrag zur Craniogenese von *Saguinus tamarin* Link, 1795 (Platyrrhini, Primates). Courier Forschungsinstitut Senckenberg, Frankfurt am Main 46: 1–100.

1581. Müller, F. 1965. Zur Morphogenese des Ductus nasopharyngeus und des sekundären Gaumendaches bei den *Crocodilia*. Revue suisse de zoologie 72: 647–652.

1582. Müller, F. 1967. Zur embryonalen Kopfentwicklung von *Crocodylus cataphractus* Cuv. Revue suisse de zoologie 74: 189–294.

1583. Müller, F. 1972. Zur stammesgeschichtlichen Veränderung der Eutheria-Ontogenesen: Versuch einer Übersicht aufgrund vergleichend morphologischer Studien an Marsupialia und Eutheria. Revue suisse de zoologie 79: 1–97.

1584. Müller, F., and R. O'Rahilly. 1980a. The human chondrocranium at the end of the embryonic period proper, with particular reference to the nervous system. American Journal of Anatomy 159: 33–58.

1585. Müller, F., and R. O'Rahilly. 1980b. Early development of the nervous system in staged insectivore and primate embryos. Journal of Comparative Neurology 193: 741–752.

1586. Müller, F., and R. O'Rahilly. 1983. The first appearance of the major divisions of the human brain at stage 9. Anatomy and Embryology 168: 419–432.

1587. Müller, F., and R. O'Rahilly. 1986. The development of the human brain and the closure of the rostral neuropore at stage 11. Anatomy and Embryology 175: 205–222.

1588. Müller, F., and R. O'Rahilly. 1987. The development of the human brain, the closure of the caudal neuropore, and the beginning of secondary neurulation at stage 12. Anatomy and Embryology 176: 413–430.

1589. Müller, F., and R. O'Rahilly. 1988a. The development of the human brain from a closed neural tube at stage 13. Anatomy and Embryology 177: 203–224.

512 Brian K. Hall and James Hanken

1590. Müller, F., and R. O'Rahilly. 1988b. The first appearance of the future cerebral hemispheres in the human embryo at stage 14. Anatomy and Embryology 177: 495–511.
1591. Müller, G., G. Wagner, and B. K. Hall. 1989. Experimental vertebrate embryology and the study of evolution: Report of a workshop. Fortschritte der Zoologie 35: 299–303.
1592. Müller, H. E. J. 1987. An effective method for using the degree of skull pneumatization to age living passerines. Beiträge zur Vogelkunde 33: 265–270.
1593. Müller, H. J. 1961. Über strukturelle Ähnlichkeiten der Ohr-und Occipitalregion bei Vogel und Säuger. Zoologischer Anzeiger 166: 391–402.
1594. Müller, H. J. 1963. Die Morphologie und Entwicklung des Craniums von *Rhea americana* Linné. II. Visceralskelett, Mittelohr und Osteocranium. Zeitschrift für wissenschaftliche Zoologie 168: 35–118.
1595. Mungall, E. C. 1978. *The Indian Blackbuck Antelope: A Texas View.* Kleberg Studies in Natural Resources. College Station: Texas Agricultural Experimental Station.
1596. Murray, P. D. F. 1941. Epidermal papillae and dermal bones of the chick sclerotic. Nature 148: 471.
1597. Murray, P. D. F. 1943. The development of the conjunctival papillae and of the scleral bones in the chick embryo. Journal of Anatomy, London 77: 225–240.
1598. Murray, P. D. F. 1963. Adventitious (secondary) cartilage in the chick embryo and the development of certain bones and articulations in the chick skull. Australian Journal of Zoology 11: 368–430.
1599. Murray, P. D. F., and D. B. Drachman. 1969. The role of movement in the development of joints and related structures: The head and neck in the chick embryo. Journal of Embryology and Experimental Morphology 22: 349–371.
1600. Murray, P. D. F., and M. Smiles. 1965. Factors in the evocation of adventitious (secondary) cartilage in the chick embryo. Australian Journal of Zoology 13: 351–381.
1601. Nader, I. A. 1978. Kangaroo rats: Intraspecific variation in *Dipodomys spectabilis* and *Dipodomys deserti.* Illinois Biological Monographs, vol. 49. Chicago: University of Illinois Press.
1602. Nagretskii, L. N. 1971. Some data on linear skeletal growth in *Alopex lagopus beringensis* M. Zoologicheskii zhurnal 50: 1240–1246.
1603. Naito, Y. 1975. Ecology and morphology of *Phoca vitulina largha* and *Phoca kurilensis* in the southern sea of Okhotsk and northeast of Hokkaido, Japan. Rapports et procès-verbaux des réunions, Conseil international pour l'exploration de la mer 169: 379–386.
1604. Nakajima, T. 1987. Development of the pharyngeal dentition in the cobitid fishes *Misgurnus anguillicaudatus* and *Cobitis biwae,* with a consideration of evolution of cypriniform dentitions. Copeia: 208–213.
1605. Nakamura, H., T. Kamimura, Y. Yabuta, A. Suda, S. Ueyanagi, S. Kikawa, M. Honma, M. Yukinawa, and S. Morikawa. 1951. Notes of the life-history of the sword fish, *Xiphias gladius* Linneaus. Japanese Journal of Ichthyology 1: 264–271.

1606. Nammalwar, P. 1976. A note on hyperostosis in the perch *Pomadasys hasta* (Bloch). Indian Journal of Fisheries 23: 247–249.

1607. Naples, V. L. 1982. Cranial osteology and function in the tree sloths, *Bradypus* and *Choloepus*. American Museum Novitates, no. 2739: 1–41.

1608. Nel, P. P. C., and J. H. Swanepoel. 1984. The development of the nasal capsule of the silver carp *Hypophthalmichthys molitrix* (Valenciennes). South African Journal of Zoology 19: 309–313.

1609. Nelson, I., and R. Brandl. 1987. Wachstum und Organentwicklung bei Lachmowennestlinen (*Larus ridibundus*). Journal of Ornithology 128: 431–439.

1610. Nelsen, O. E. 1953. *Comparative Embryology of the Vertebrates*. New York: Blakiston.

1611. Nelson, G. J. 1969. Gill arches and the phylogeny of fishes, with notes on the classification of vertebrates. Bulletin of the American Museum of Natural History 141: 477–552.

1612. Nelson, N. M. 1942. The sclerotic plates of the White Leghorn chicken. Anatomical Record 84: 295–306.

1613. Nelson, T. W., and K. A. Shump, Jr. 1978. Cranial variation and size allometry in *Agouti paca* from Ecuador. Journal of Mammalogy 59: 387–394.

1614. Nemeschkal, H. L. 1982. On the first record of a prearticular bone in pigeons. Zoologische Jahrbücher, Anatomie 107: 609–615.

1615. Nemeschkal, H. L. 1983a. Zur Morphologie und Ontogenie des Os goniale bei tetrapoden Wirbeltieren: Ein System homologer und homoiologer Einzelmerkmale. Gegenbaurs Morphologisches Jahrbuch, Leipzig 129: 181–216.

1616. Nemeschkal, H. L. 1983b. Zum Nachweis eines Os coronoideum bei Vögeln: Ein Beitrag zur Morphologie des Sauropsiden-Unterkiefers. Zoologische Jahrbücher, Anatomie 109: 117–151.

1617. Nemeschkal, H. L. 1983c. On the morphology of the lower jaw skeleton: The sauropsidian dentary bone—an element consisting of two dermal bones (Vertebrata, Sauropsida). Zoologische Jahrbücher, Anatomie 109: 369–396.

1618. Nemeschkal, H. L. 1989. The mandibular fossa with respect to avian ancestry. Fortschritte der Zoologie 35: 467–471.

1619. Nero, R. W. 1951. Pattern and rate of cranial "ossification" in the house sparrow. Wilson Bulletin 63: 84–88.

1620. Nesslinger, C. L. 1956. Ossification centers and skeletal development in the postnatal Virginia opossum. Journal of Mammalogy 37: 382–394.

1621. Neumayer, L. 1938. Die Entwicklung des Kopfskelettes von *Bdellostoma* St. L. Archivio italiano di anatomia e di embriologia, Florence 40 (suppl.): 1–222.

1622. Newbrey, J. W., and W. J. Banks. 1983. Ultrastructural features of the cellular and matrical components of developing antler cartilage. In *Antler Development in Cervidae*, R. D. Brown, ed. Kingsville, Tex.: Caesar Kleberg Wildlife Research Institute, pp. 261–272.

1623. Newgreen, D., and J.-P. Thiery. 1980. Fibronectin in early avian (*Gallus domesticus*) embryos: Synthesis and distribution along the migration pathways of neural crest cells. Cell and Tissue Research 211: 269–292.

1624. Newman, L. M., and A. G. Hendrickx. 1984. Fetal development in the normal thick-tailed bushbaby (*Galago crassicaudatus pananguinus*). American Journal of Primatology 6: 337–355.

1625. Newth, D. R. 1954. Determination of the cranial neural crest of the axolotl. Journal of Embryology and Experimental Morphology 2: 101–105.

1626. Newth, D. R. 1956. On the neural crest of the lamprey embryo. Journal of Embryology and Experimental Morphology 4: 358–375.

1627. Nichols, D. H. 1981. Neural crest formation in the head of the mouse embryo as observed using a new histological technique. Journal of Embryology and Experimental Morphology 64: 105–120.

1628. Nichols, D. H. 1986. Formation and distribution of neural crest mesenchyme to the first pharyngeal arch region of the mouse embryo. American Journal of Anatomy 176: 221–231.

1629. Nichols, D. H. 1987. Ultrastructure of neural crest formation in the midbrain/rostral hindbrain and preotic hindbrain regions of the mouse embryo. American Journal of Anatomy 179: 143–154.

1630. Nicolau-Guillamet, P. 1975. La détermination de l'âge chez les oiseaux. In *Problèmes d'ecologie: La démographie des populations des vertébrés*, F. Bourlière, ed. Paris: Masson and Cie, pp. 129–145.

1631. Nicolls, K. E. 1985. Adenohypophyseal acidophil cells and antler development in immature male mule deer. Bulletin of the Royal Society of New Zealand, no. 22: 279–281.

1632. Niemitz, C., and H. Sprankel. 1974. Early postnatal ossification in *Tarsius bancanus* Horsfield, 1821 (Mammalia, Primates) and its relation to the hypothesis of Nidifugous and Nidicolous animals. Zeitschrift für Morphologie der Tiere 79: 155–163.

1633. Nieuwkoop, P. D., and J. Faber. 1956. Normal table of *Xenopus laevis* (Daudin): A systematical and chronological survey of the development from the fertilized egg until the end of metamorphosis. Amsterdam: North Holland.

1634. Nikolaeva, A. I. 1981. Variability in the relative size of cranial bones and those of the extremities in the water vole (*Arvicola terrestris*) of western Siberia, USSR. Vestnik zoologii 3: 65–72.

1635. Ninov, L. K., and I. V. Krustaleva. 1985. Skeletal morphology of domestic and wild pigs during postnatal ontogenesis. In *Morphology and Genetics of the Boar*, L. V. Davletova, ed. Moscow: Nauka, pp. 122–130.

1636. Nitecki, C. 1985. Trapping of adult black-headed gulls at nests and preliminary data on sex/age criteria. Notaki Ornithology 26: 209–214.

1637. Nitikin, V. B. 1986. On the nasal muscles in Anura and Urodela. In *Studies in Herpetology*, Z. Roček, ed. Prague: Charles University, pp. 251–254.

1638. Noback, C. R. 1944. The developmental anatomy of the human osseous skeleton during the embryonic, fetal, and circumnatal periods. Anatomical Record 88: 91–126.

1639. Noback, C. R., and M. L. Moss. 1953. The topology of the human premaxillary bone. American Journal of Physical Anthropology 11: 181–187.

1640. Noden, D. M. 1978a. The control of avian cephalic neural crest cytodifferentiation. I. Skeletal and connective tissues. Developmental Biology 67: 296–312.

1641. Noden, D. M. 1978b. Interactions directing the migration and cytodifferentiation of avian neural crest cells. In *The Specificity of Embryological Interactions*, D. Garrod, ed. London: Chapman and Hall, pp. 4–49.

1642. Noden, D. M. 1980. The migration and cytodifferentiation of cranial neural crest cells. In *Current Research Trends in Craniofacial Development*, R. M. Pratt and R. L. Christiansen, eds. Amsterdam: Elsevier/North-Holland, pp. 3–25.

1643. Noden, D. M. 1982a. Periocular mesenchyme: Origins and control of development. In *Biomedical Foundations of Ophthalmology*, D. Garrod, ed. New York: Harper and Row, pp. 97–120.

1644. Noden, D. M. 1982b. Patterns and organization of craniofacial skeletogenic and myogenic mesenchyme: A perspective. In *Factors and Mechanisms Influencing Bone Growth*, A. D. Dixon and B. G. Sarnat, eds. New York: Alan R. Liss, pp. 167–203.

1645. Noden, D. M. 1983a. The embryonic origins of avian cephalic and cervical muscles and associated connective tissues. American Journal of Anatomy 168: 257–276.

1646. Noden, D. M. 1983b. The role of the neural crest in patterning of avian cranial skeletal, connective, and muscle tissues. Developmental Biology 96: 144–165.

1647. Noden, D. M. 1984a. Craniofacial development: New views on old problems. Anatomical Record 208: 1–13.

1648. Noden, D. M. 1984b. The use of chimeras in analysis of craniofacial development. In *Chimeras in Developmental Biology*, N. M. Le Douarin and A. McLaren, eds. London: Academic Press, pp. 241–280.

1649. Noden, D. M. 1986. Origins and patterning of craniofacial mesenchymal tissues. Journal of Craniofacial Genetics and Developmental Biology 2 (suppl.): 15–31.

1650. Noden, D. M. 1987. Interactions between cephalic neural crest and mesodermal populations. In *Developmental and Evolutionary Aspects of the Neural Crest*, P. F. A. Maderson, ed. New York: John Wiley and Sons, pp. 89–119.

1651. Noden, D. M. 1988. Interactions and fates of avian craniofacial mesenchyme. Development 103 (suppl.): 121–140.

1652. Noden, D. M., and A. de Lahunta. 1985. *The Embryology of Domestic Animals: Normal Development and Congenital Malformations*. Baltimore: Williams and Wilkins.

1653. Noden, D. M., and H. E. Evans. 1986. Inherited homeotic midfacial malformations in Burmese cats. Journal of Craniofacial Genetics and Developmental Biology 2: 249–266.

1654. Noldus, L. P. J. J., and R. J. J. de Klerk. 1984. Growth of the skull of the harbor porpoise, *Phocaena phocaena* (Linnaeus, 1758), in the North Sea, after age determination based on dentinal growth layer groups. Zoologische Mededelingen, Leiden 58: 213–229.

1655. Norberg, R. A. 1978. Skull asymmetry, ear structure and function, and auditory localization in Tengmalm's owl, *Aegolius funereus* (Linné). Philosophical Transactions of the Royal Society of London 282B: 325–410.

1656. Northcott, M. E., and M. C. M. Beveridge. 1988. The development and structure of pharyngeal apparatus associated with filter feeding in tilapias (*Oleochromis niloticus*). Journal of Zoology, London 215: 133–149.

1657. Northcutt, R. G. 1985. The brain and sense organs of the earliest vertebrates: Reconstruction of a morphotype. In *Evolutionary Biology of Primitive Fishes*, R. E. Foreman, A. Gorbman, J. M. Dodd, and R. Olsson, eds. New York: Plenum Publishing, pp. 81–112.

1658. Northcutt, R. G., and C. Gans. 1983. The genesis of neural crest and epidermal placodes: A reinterpretation of vertebrate origins. Quarterly Review of Biology 58: 1–28.

1659. Novacek, M. 1977. Aspects of the problem of variation, origin, and evolution of the eutherian auditory bulla. Mammal Review 7: 131–149.

1660. Novacek, M. J. 1985. Comparative morphology of the bat auditory region. Fortschritte der Zoologie 30: 149–151.

1661. Novikov, B. V. 1978. Materials on comparative morphology of foxes (*Vulpes vulpes dolichocrania* and *V. v. beringiana*). Zoologicheskii zhurnal 57: 801–805.

1662. Novitskaya, L. I., and N. I. Krupina. 1985. On the ethmoid of Paleozoic dipnoans. Paleontologicheskii zhurnal: 92–100.

1663. Nussbaumer, M. 1978. Biometric comparison of types of topogenesis in skull base of small and medium-sized dogs. Zeitschrift für Tierzuechtung und Zeuchtungsbiologie 95: 1–14.

1664. Nybelin, O. 1982. On the tooth-bearing bone element in the lower jaw of some primitive Recent teleostean fishes. Acta Regiae societatis scientiarum et litterarum gothoburgensis, Zoologica 13: 1–36.

1665. Oelschläger, H. A. 1986a. Tympanohyal bone in toothed whales and the formation of the tympano-periotic complex (Mammalia: Cetacea). Journal of Morphology 188: 157–165.

1666. Oelschläger, H. A. 1986b. Comparative morphology and evolution of the otic region in toothed whales (Cetacea: Mammalia). American Journal of Anatomy 177: 353–368.

1667. Ohtsuki, F. 1976. On the growth of thickness of cranial bones in human fetuses. Jikeikai Medical Journal 23: 47–60.

1668. Ohtsuki, F. 1977. Developmental changes of the cranial bone thickness in the human fetal period. American Journal of Physical Anthropology 46: 141–153.

1669. Okada, E. 1955. Isolationsversuche zur analyse der knorpelbildung aus neuralleistenzellen bei urodelenkeim. Memoirs of the College of Science, Kyoto University 22B: 23–28.

1670. Okada, E., and M. Ichikawa. 1956. Isolationsversuche zur analyse der knorpelbildung aus neuralleistenzellen beim anurenkeim. Memoirs of the College of Science, Kyoto University 23B: 27–36.

1671. Okada, T. S. 1955. Experimental studies on the differentiation of the endodermal organs in amphibia. III. The relation between the differentiation of pharynx and head-mesenchyme. Memoirs of the College of Science, Kyoto University, ser. B, 22: 17–22.

1672. Okada, T. S. 1957. The pluripotency of the pharyngeal primordium in urodelan neurulae. Journal of Embryology and Experimental Morphology 5: 438–448.

1673. Okiyama, M. 1972. Morphology and identification of the young ipnopid, "*Macristiella*," from the tropical western Pacific. Japanese Journal of Ichthyology 19: 145–153.

1674. Okiyama, M. 1984. Myctophiformes: Development. In *Ontogeny and Systematics of Fishes*, American Society of Ichthyologists and Herpetologists Special Publication no. 1, H. G. Moser, ed. Lawrence, Kans.: Allen Press, pp. 206–218.

1675. Okiyama, M., and S. Ueyanaga. 1978. Interrelationships of scombroid fishes: An aspect from larval morphology. Bulletin of the Far Seas Fisheries Research Laboratory, Shimuzu 16: 103–113.

1676. Okutomi, K. 1937. Die Entwicklung des Chondrocraniums des *Polypedates buergeri schlegeli*. Zeitschrift für Anatomie und Entwicklungsgeschichte 107: 28–64.

1677. Oldani, N. O. 1983. Identification and morphology of larvae, juveniles, and adults of *Mylossoma paraguayensis* (Pisces, Characidae). Studies on the Neotropical Fauna 18: 89–100.

1678. Olivier, G. 1973. Asymmetry of the skull bones. Bulletin de l'Association des anatomistes 58: 387–396.

1679. Olivier, G., C. Libersa, and R. Fenart. 1955. Le crâne du Semnopithèque. Mammalia 19: 1–292.

1680. Olney, J. E. 1984. Lampriformes: Development and relationships. In *Ontogeny and Systematics of Fishes*, American Society of Ichthyologists and Herpetologists Special Publication no. 1, H. G. Moser, ed. Lawrence, Kans.: Allen Press, pp. 368–379.

1681. Omarkhan, M. 1949. The morphology of the chondrocranium of *Gymnarchus niloticus*. Zoological Journal of the Linnean Society 41: 452–481.

1682. Omarkhan, M. 1950. The development of the chondrocranium of *Notopterus*. Zoological Journal of the Linnean Society 41: 608–624.

1683. Omura, H., M. Shirakihara, and H. Ito. 1984. A pygmy sperm whale accidentally taken by drift net in the north Pacific. Scientific Reports of the Whales Research Institute, Tokyo 35: 183–193.

1684. Opitz, J. M., R. J. Gorlin, J. F. Reynolds, and L. M. Spano. 1988. *Neural Crest and Craniofacial Disorders: Genetic Aspects*. New York: Alan R. Liss.

1685. O'Rahilly R. 1960. The development of the sclera and choroid in staged chick embryos. Journal of Anatomy 94: 577–578.

1686. O'Rahilly R. 1962. The development of the sclera and the choroid in staged chick embryos. Acta anatomica 48: 335–346.

1687. O'Rahilly R. 1967. The early development of the nasal pit in staged human embryos. Anatomical Record 157: 380.

1688. O'Rahilly R., and E. Gardner. 1972. The initial appearance of ossification in staged human embryos. American Journal of Anatomy 134: 291–308.

1689. O'Rahilly R., and E. Gardner. 1976. The embryology of bone and bones. In *Bones and Joints*, L. V. Ackerman, H. J. Spjut, and M. R. Abell, eds. Baltimore: Williams and Wilkins, pp. 1–15.

1690. O'Rahilly R., and E. Gardner. 1978. The embryology of movable joints. In *The Joints and Synovial Fluid,* vol. 1, L. Sokoloff, ed. New York: Academic Press, pp. 49–104.

1691. O'Rahilly R., and F. Müller. 1984. The early development of the hypoglossal nerve and occipital somites in staged human embryos. American Journal of Anatomy 169: 237–257.

1692. O'Rahilly R., F. Müller, G. M. Hutchins, and G. W. Moore. 1984. Computer ranking of the sequence of appearance of 100 features of the brain and related structures in staged human embryos during the first five weeks of development. American Journal of Anatomy 171: 243–257.

1693. O'Rahilly R., F. Müller, and D. B. Meyer. 1983. The human vertebral column at the end of the embryonic period proper. 2. The occipitocervical region. Journal of Anatomy, London 136: 181–195.

1694. Orr, R. T., J. Schonewald, and K. W. Kenyon. 1970. The California sea lion (*Zalophus californianus californianus*): Skull growth and a comparison of two populations. Proceedings of the California Academy of Science 37: 381–394.

1695. Orton, G. L. 1943. The tadpole of *Rhinophrynus dorsalis.* Occasional Papers of the Museum of Zoology, University of Michigan, no. 472: 1–7.

1696. Orton, G. L. 1949. Larval development of *Nectophrynoides tornieri* (Roux) with comments on direct development in frogs. Annals of the Carnegie Museum 31: 257–277.

1697. Orton, G. L. 1954. Dimorphism in larval mouthparts in spadefoot toads of the *Scaphiopus hammondi* group. Copeia: 97–100.

1698. Orton, G. L. 1963. Notes on larval anatomy of fishes of the order Lyomeri. Copeia: 6–15.

1699. Ørvig, T. 1968. The dermal skeleton: General considerations. In *Current Problems of Lower Vertebrate Phylogeny,* T. Ørvig, ed. Stockholm: Almqvist and Wiksell, pp. 373–397.

1700. Ørvig, T. 1980. Histologic studies of ostracoderms, placoderms, and fossil elasmobranchs. 3. Structure and growth of the gnathalia of certain arthrodires. Zoologica scripta 9: 141–159.

1701. Osborn, J. W., ed. 1981. *Dental Anatomy and Embryology: A Companion to Dental Studies,* vol. 1, bk. 2. Oxford: Blackwell Scientific Publications.

1702. Otten, E. 1981. Vision during growth of a generalized *Haplochromis* species: *H. elegans* Trewavas 1933 (Pisces, Cichlidae). Netherlands Journal of Zoology 31: 650–700.

1703. Otten, E. 1982. The development of a mouth-opening mechanism in a generalized *Haplochromis* species: *H. elegans* Trewavas 1933 (Pisces, Cichlidae). Netherlands Journal of Zoology 32: 31–48.

1704. Otten, E. 1983. The jaw mechanism during growth of a generalized *Haplochromis* species: *H. elegans* Trewavas 1933 (Pisces, Cichlidae). Netherlands Journal of Zoology 33: 55–98.

1705. Otten, E. 1985. Proportions of the jaw mechanism of cichlid fishes: Changes and their meaning. Acta biotheoretica 34: 207–217.

1706. Otten, E. 1986. Vision during growth of the cichlid fish *Astatotilapia elegans.* Nova Acta Leopoldina, no. 262: 287–291.

1707. Otto, H.-D. 1984. The mistake of the theory of Reichert-Gaupp: A contribution to the onto- and the phylogenesis of the temporomandibular joint and the auditory ossicles of the mammals. Anatomischer Anzeiger 155: 223–238.

1708. Oudhof, G. 1975. *Development and Growth of the Cranium: A Quantitative Experimental Study in the Chick Embryo.* Netherlands: Nooy's Drukkerit-Purmerend.

1709. Oudhof, H. A. J. 1982. Sutural growth. Acta anatomica 112: 58–68.

1710. Oudhof, H. A. J., and W. J. Van Doorenmaalen. 1983. Skull morphogenesis and growth: Hemodynamic influence. Acta anatomica 117: 181–186.

1711. Owen, J. G. 1989. Population and geographic variation of *Peromyscus leucopus* in relation to climatic factors. Journal of Mammalogy 70: 98–109.

1712. Oyen, O. J. 1982. Masticatory function and histogenesis of the middle and upper face in chimpanzees (*Pan troglodytes*). Progress in Clinical and Biological Research 101: 559–568.

1713. Oyen, O. J. 1984. Palatal growth in baboons (*Papio cynocephalus anubis*). Primates 25: 337–351.

1714. Oyen, O. J., and R. W. Rice. 1980. Supraorbital development in chimpanzees, macaques, and baboons. Journal of Medical Primatology 9: 161–168.

1715. Ozawa, T., and A. Fukui. 1986. Studies on the development and distribution of the bothid larvae in the western North Pacific. In *Studies on the Oceanic Ichthyoplankton in the Western North Pacific,* T. Ozawa, ed. Fukuoka-shi: Kyushu University Press, pp. 322–419.

1716. Özeti, N., and D. B. Wake. 1969. The morphology and evolution of the tongue and associated structures in salamanders and newts (family Salamandridae). Copeia: 91–123.

1717. Padmanabhan, K. G. 1961. The early development of *Solenostomus cyanopterus.* Bulletin of the Central Research Institute, Trivandrum 80: 1–13.

1718. Pal, G. P. 1987. Anatomical notes: Variations of the interparietal bone in man. Journal of Anatomy, London 152: 205–234.

1719. Pal, G. P., B. P. Tamankar, R. V. Routal, and S. S. Bhagwat. 1984. The ossification of the membranous part of the squamous occipital bone in man. Journal of Anatomy, London 138: 259–266.

1720. Palko, R. J., G. L. Beardsley, and W. J. Richards. 1981. Synopsis of the biology of the swordfish, *Xiphias gladius* Linnaeus. NOAA Technical Reports, NMFS Circular no. 441.

1721. Palomera, I., and P. Rubies. 1977. Descripción de huevos y larvas de *Microchirus ocellatus* y *M. azevia* (Pleuronectiformes, Soleidae) de las costas del NW de Africa. Resultados expediciones cientificas del buque oceanografico, Cornide de Saaredra 6: 211–220.

1722. Panda, S., and P. Mohanty-Hejmadi. 1984. Ossification of chondrocranium during development in the skipper frog, *Rana cyanophyctis.* Pranikee, Journal of the Zoological Society, Orissa 5: 47–50.

1723. Pankakoski, E. 1983. Morphological variation and population structure of Finnish muskrats, *Ondatra zibethica.* Annales zoologici fennici 20: 207–222.

1724. Pankakoski, E. 1985. Epigenetic asymmetry as an ecological indicator in muskrats. Journal of Mammalogy 66: 52–57.

1725. Pankakoski, E., and K. Nurmi. 1986. Skull morphology of Finnish muskrats

[*Ondatra zibethica*]: Geographic variation, age differences, and sexual dimorphism. Annales zoologici fennici 23: 1–32.

1726. Pankakoski, E., R. A. Vaisanen, and K. Nurmi. 1987. Variability of muskrat skulls: Measurement error, environmental modification, and size allometry. Systematic Zoology 36: 35–51.

1727. Parenti, L. R. 1986. The phylogenetic significance of bone types in euteleost fishes. Zoological Journal of the Linnean Society 87: 37–51.

1728. Parenti, L. R. 1987. Phylogenetic aspects of tooth and jaw structure of the Medaka, *Oryzias latipes,* and other beloniform fishes. Journal of Zoology, London 211: 561–572.

1729. Park, A. W., and B. J. A. Nowosielski-Slepowron. 1976. Biology of the rice rat (*Oryzomys palustris natator*) in a laboratory environment. IX. Preweaning growth of the skull. Acta morphologica neerlando-Scandinavica 14: 39–60.

1730. Park, A. W., and B. J. A. Nowosielski-Slepowron. 1980. Aspects of skull and dentition morphology of the mink (*Mustela vison*). Acta morphologica neerlando-Scandinavica 18: 47–65.

1731. Park, Y.-S., and Y. U. Kim. 1987. Studies on the larvae and juveniles of flying fish, *Prognichthys agoo* (Temminck et Schlegel) (Pisces, Exocoetidae). 2. Osteological development of larvae and juveniles. Bulletin of the Korean Fisheries Society 20: 447–456.

1732. Parker, H., H. Ottesen, and E. Knudsen. 1985. Age determination in Svalbard ptarmigan *Lagopus mutus hyperboreas*. Polar Research 3: 125–126.

1733. Parrington, F. R. 1949. A theory of the relations of lateral lines to dermal bones. Proceedings of the Zoological Society of London 119: 65–78.

1734. Parrington, F. R. 1967. The identification of the dermal bones of the head. Zoological Journal of the Linnean Society 47: 231–239.

1735. Parrington, F. R., and T. S. Westoll. 1940. On the evolution of the mammalian palate. Philosophical Transactions of the Royal Society of London 230B: 305–355.

1736. Parsons, T. S. 1959. Studies on the comparative embryology of the reptilian nose. Bulletin of the Museum of Comparative Zoology, Harvard University 120: 101–277.

1737. Parsons, T. S. 1970. The nose and Jacobson's organ. In *Biology of the Reptilia,* vol. 2, C. Gans and T. S. Parsons, eds. New York: Academic Press, pp. 99–191.

1738. Parthow, G. D., D. E. Barrales, and K. R. S. Fisher. 1981. Morphology of a two-headed piglet. Anatomical Record 199: 441–448.

1739. Pashine, R. G., and V. B. Marathe. 1974. Observations on the ossification centers in the skull of *Brachydanio rerio* (Hamilton-Buchanan). Journal of the University of Bombay 42: 53–62.

1740. Pashine, R. G., and V. B. Marathe. 1977. The development of the chondrocranium of *Cyprinus carpio* Linn. Proceedings of the Indian Academy of Science, ser. B, 85: 351–363.

1741. Pashine, R. G., and V. B. Marathe. 1979. Observations on the ossification centers in the skull of *Cyprinus carpio*. Proceedings of the Indian Academy of Science, ser. B, 88: 13–24.

1742. Paterson, N. F. 1939. The head of *Xenopus laevis*. Quarterly Journal of Microscopical Science 81: 161–234.

1743. Paterson, N. F. 1949. The development of the inner ear of *Xenopus laevis*. Proceedings of the Zoological Society of London 119: 269–291.

1744. Paterson, N. F. 1955. The skull of the toad, *Hemipipa carvalhoi* Mir.-Rib. with remarks on other Pipidae. Proceedings of the Zoological Society of London 125: 223–252.

1745. Patterson, C. 1975. The braincase of pholidophorid and leptolepid fishes with a review of the actinopterygian braincase. Philosophical Transactions of the Royal Society of London 269B: 275–579.

1746. Patterson, C. 1977. Cartilage bones, dermal bones, and membrane bones, or the exoskeleton versus the endoskeleton. In *Problems in Vertebrate Evolution*, S. M. Andrews, R. S. Miles, and A. D. Walker, eds. London: Academic Press, pp. 77–122.

1747. Patterson, S. B., and R. Minkoff. 1985. Morphometric and autoradiographic analysis of frontonasal development in the chick embryo. Anatomical Record 212: 90–99.

1748. Patton, J. L., and P. V. Brylski. 1987. Pocket gophers in alfalfa fields: Causes and consequences of habitat-related body size variation. American Naturalist 130: 493–506.

1749. Patton, J. L., and M. A. Rogers. 1983. Systematic implications of non-geographic variation in the spiny rat genus *Proechimys* (Echymidae). Zeitschrift für Saeugetierkunde 48: 363–370.

1750. Pavlinov, I. Y. 1976. Variability of the sagittal crest (Crista sagittalis external) on the skull of the pine marten. Byulletin' Moskovskogo Obschchestva Ispytatelei Prkody Otdel Biologicheskii 81: 28–33.

1751. Pavlinov, I. Y. 1977. Age-related changes in skull indices of *Martes martes* L. (Mammalia: Mustelidae) in the late postnatal period. Byulletin' Moskovskogo Obschchestva Ispytatelei Prkody Otdel Biologicheskii 82: 33–50.

1752. Pavlinov, I. Y. 1980. Anomalies of skull structure in the pine marten (*Martes martes* L.). Byulletin' Moskovskogo Obschchestva Ispytatelei Prkody Otdel Biologicheskii 85: 30–36.

1753. Pegueta, V. P. 1985. Evolution and morphogenesis of cartilage preformed bones. In *Evolution and Morphogenesis*, J. Mlikovsky and V. J. A. Novak, eds. Praha: Academica, pp. 679–686.

1754. Pehrson, T. 1940. The development of dermal bones in the skull of *Amia calva*. Acta zoologica, Stockholm 21: 1–50.

1755. Pehrson, T. 1944a. Some observations on the development and morphology of the dermal bones in the skull of *Acipenser* and *Polyodon*. Acta zoologica, Stockholm 25: 27–48.

1756. Pehrson, T. 1944b. The development of latero-sensory canal bones in the skull of *Esox lucius*. Acta zoologica, Stockholm 25: 135–157.

1757. Pehrson, T. 1945. Some problems concerning the development of the skull in turtles. Acta zoologica, Stockholm 26: 157–184.

1758. Pehrson, T. 1947. Some new interpretations of the skull in *Polypterus*. Acta zoologica, Stockholm 28: 399–455.

1759. Pehrson, T. 1949. The ontogeny of the lateral line system in the head of dipnoans. Acta zoologica, Stockholm 30: 153–182.

1760. Pehrson, T. 1958. The early ontogeny of the sensory lines and the dermal skull in *Polypterus*. Acta zoologica, Stockholm 39: 241–258.

1761. Penaz, M., E. Wohlgemuth, J. Hamackova, and J. Kouril. 1982. Early ontogeny of the tench, *Tinca tinca*. 2. Larval period. Folia zoologica 31: 175–180.

1762. Peris Alvarez, S. J. 1983. Criteria for age determination in the spotless starling (*Sturnus unicolor*): Cranial pneumatization and tarsal colour. Journal für Ornithologie, Berlin 124: 78–81.

1763. Perrin, W. F. 1975. Variation of spotted and spinner porpoise (genus *Stenella*) in the eastern tropical Pacific and Hawaii. Bulletin of the Scripps Institute of Oceanography, University of California, no. 21.

1764. Persson, M. 1973. Structure and growth of facial sutures: Histologic, microangiographic, and autoradiographic studies in rats and a histologic study in man. Odontologisk Revy 24 (suppl. 26): 1–146.

1765. Persson, M. 1983. The role of movement in the development of sutural and diarthrodial joints tested by long-term paralysis of chick embryos. Journal of Anatomy 137: 591–599.

1766. Persson, M., B. C. Magnusson, and B. Thilander. 1978. Sutural closure in rabbit and man: A morphological and histochemical study. Journal of Anatomy, London 125: 313–322.

1767. Persson, M., and W. Roy. 1979. Suture development and bony fusion in the fetal rabbit palate. Archives of Oral Biology 24: 283–291.

1768. Petersen, S., and E. W. Born. 1982. Age determination of the Atlantic walrus, *Odobenus rosmarus rosmarus* (Linnaeus), by means of mandibular growth layers. Zeitschrift für Saeugetierkunde 47: 55–62.

1769. Peterson, R. L., and M. B. Fenton. 1970. Variation in the bats of the genus *Harpyionycteris* with the description of a new race. Royal Ontario Museum of Life Sciences Occasional Papers 17: 1–15.

1770. Petit-Maire, N. 1971. Morphogenesis of the primate skull. Anthropologie, Paris 75: 85–118.

1771. Petit-Maire, N. 1972. Evolution trends and comparative ontogenesis in primate cranium. Journal of Human Evolution 1: 17–22.

1772. Petit-Maire, N., and J. F. Ponge. 1977. Morphogenesis of primate crania: Factorial analysis; taxonomic implications; position and redefinition of the genus *Homo*. Bulletin et mémoires de la société d'anthropologie de Paris 13: 275–285.

1773. Petricioni, V. 1964. Entwicklungsphysiologische Untersuchungen über die induzierbarkeit von Skelettelementen des Anurenschädels durch flüssigen Organextrakt. Wilhelm Roux Archiv für Entwicklungsmechank der Organismen 155: 358–390.

1774. Petrov, A. K. 1964. Ossification of the skeleton in the ontogeny of the elk. Zoologicheskii zhurnal 43: 1837–1847.

1775. Peyer, B. 1950. Goethes Wirbeltheorie des Schädels. Neujahrsblatt herausgegeben von der Naturforschenden Gesellschaft in Zürich 94: 1–129.

1776. Phillips, I. R. 1976a. The embryology of the common marmoset (*Callithrix jacchus*). Advances in Anatomy, Embryology, and Cell Biology 52 (5): 1–47.

1777. Phillips, I. R. 1976b. Skeletal development in the foetal and neonatal marmoset (*Callithrix jacchus*). Laboratory Animals 10: 317–333.

1778. Piatt, J. 1938. Morphogenesis of the cranial muscles of *Amblystoma punctatum*. Journal of Morphology 63: 531–587.

1779. Pichler-Semmelrock, F. 1988. Der einfluss des wachstums auf den bau der Kiemenfilter und die Nahrungsaufnahme des silberkarpfens *Hypophthalmichthys molitrix* Val. (Teleostei, Osteichthyes). Zoologischer Anzeiger 221: 267–280.

1780. Pietsch, T. W. 1984. Lophiiformes: Development and relationships. In *Ontogeny and Systematics of Fishes*, American Society of Ichthyologists and Herpetologists Special Publication no. 1, H. G. Moser, ed. Lawrence, Kans.: Allen Press, pp. 320–325.

1781. Pilleri, G. 1987. Os interparietale and postinterparietal ossicles in a fetus of *Pseudorca crassidens* (Cetacea, Delphinidae). Investigations on Cetacea 19: 36–39.

1782. Pilleri, G., M. Gihr, V. V. Zijganov, and C. Kraus. 1982. Fenestration of the skull in some cetaceans. Investigations on Cetacea 14: 149–193.

1783. Pine, R. H., P. L. Dalby, and J. O. Matson. 1985. Ecology, postnatal development, morphometrics, and taxonomic status of the short-tailed opossum, *Monodelphis dimidiata*, an apparently semelparous annual marsupial. Annals of the Carnegie Museum 54: 195–231.

1784. Pinganaud-Perrin, G. 1973a. Conséquences de l'ablation de l'os frontal sur la forme des os du toit crânien de la truit (*Salmo irideus* Gib, Pisces-Teleostei). Comptes rendus hedbomadaires des séances de l'Académie des sciences, Paris 276: 2809–2811.

1785. Pinganaud-Perrin, G. 1973b. Effets de l'ablation de l'oeil sur la morphogenèse du chondrocrâne et du crâne de *Salmo irideus*. Acta zoologica, Stockholm 54: 209–221.

1786. Pinna, G. 1976. Osteologic study of the skull of the placodont reptile *Placochelyanus stoppanii* (Osswald, 1930) based on a specimen found recently in the Rhaetian of Lombardy, Italy. Atti della Società italiana di scienze naturali, Museo civico di storia naturale di Milano 117: 3–45.

1787. Pinna, G. 1979. The skull of a young placochelid (*Psephoderma alpinum*) from the Upper Triassic of Endenna (Bergamo, Italy) (Reptilia, Placondontia). Atti della Società italiana di scienze naturali, Museo civico di storia naturale di Milano 120: 195–202.

1788. Pirsig, W., B. K. Hall, and M. Silbermann. 1988. International Symposium Report: "The Growing Midface." Journal of Craniofacial Genetics and Developmental Biology 8: 293–295.

1789. Pisano, N. M., and R. M. Greene. 1986. Hormone and growth factor involvement in craniofacial development. IRCS Medical Science 14: 635–640.

1790. Piveteau, J. 1954. Le problème du crâne. In *Traité de zoologie*, vol. 12, *Vertébrés: Généralités, embryologie, topographie, anatomie, comparée*, P. P. Grassé, ed. Paris: Masson et Cie, pp. 553–604.

1791. Plasota, K. 1974a. The development of the chondrocranium, neurocranium, and the mandibular and hyoid arches in *Rana temporaria* (L.) and *Pelobates fuscus* (Laur.). Zoologica poloniae 24: 99–168.

1792. Plasota, K. 1974b. The auditory ossicle of the Anura and the problem of its homology. Przeglad zologiczny 18: 77–83.

1793. Poggesi, M., P. Mannucci, and A. M. Simonetta. 1982. Development and morphology of the skull in the dik-diks (genus *Madoqua* Ogilby, Artiodactylia Bovidae). Monitore zoologico italiano 17: 191–217.

1794. Policansky, D. 1982. The asymmetry of flounders. Scientific American 246: 96–102.

1795. Polulyakh, Y. A. 1980. Pigment cells of the periosteum in some mammals. Doklady Akademie Nauk, Ukranaine SSR, ser. B, Geologiche, Khimistri no. 2: 85–89.

1796. Poplin, C. 1981. Les homologies du pont prootique chez les Osteichthyes. Cybium, ser. 3, 5: 3–17.

1797. Popova-Latkina, N. V. 1971a. On the development of the human cerebral cranium *in utero*. Doklady Akademii Nauk SSSR 197: 225–227.

1798. Popova-Latkina, N. V. 1971b. On the development of the human cerebral cranium *in utero*. Doklady Akademii Nauk SSSR 197: 1445–1447.

1799. Potter, F. E., and S. S. Sweet. 1981. Generic boundaries in Texas cave salamanders and a redescription of *Typhlomolge robusta* (Amphibia: Plethodontidae). Copeia: 64–75.

1800. Potthoff, T. 1974. Osteological development and variation in young tunas, genus *Thunnus* (Pisces, Scombridae), from the Atlantic Ocean. U.S. National Marine Fisheries Service, Fishery Bulletin 72: 563–588.

1801. Potthoff, T. 1980. Development and structure of fins and fin supports in dolphin fishes *Coryphaena hippurus* and *Coryphaena equiselis* (Coryphaenidae). U.S. National Marine Fisheries Service, Fishery Bulletin 78: 277–312.

1802. Potthoff, T., and S. Kelley. 1982. Development of the vertebral column, fins and fin supports, branchiostegal rays, and squamation in the swordfish, *Xiphias gladius*. Fisheries Bulletin of the United States National Ocean Administration 80: 161–186.

1803. Potthoff, T., S. Kelley, and L. A. Collins. 1988. Osteological development of the red snapper, *Lutjanus campechanus* (Lutjanidae). Bulletin of Marine Science 43: 1–40.

1804. Potthoff, T., S. Kelley, H. Moe, and F. Young. 1984. Description of porkfish larvae (*Anisotremus virginicus,* Haemulidae) and their osteological development. Bulletin of Marine Science 34: 21–59.

1805. Potthoff, T., S. Kelley, V. Saksena, M. Moe, and F. Young. 1987. Description of larval and juvenile yellowtail damselfish, *Microspathodor chrysurus,* Pomacentridae, and their osteological development. Bulletin of Marine Science 40: 330–375.

1806. Pratt, C. W. M. 1948. The morphology of the ethmoidal region of *Sphenodon* and lizards. Proceedings of the Zoological Society, London 118: 171–201.

1807. Pratt, R. M., and R. L. Christiansen. 1980. *Current Research Trends in Prenatal Craniofacial Development.* New York: Elsevier/North Holland.

1808. Pratt, R. M., M. A. Larson, and M. C. Johnston. 1975. Migration of cranial neural crest cells in a cell-free hyaluronate-rich matrix. Developmental Biology 44: 298–305.

1809. Precious, D., and J. Delaire. 1987. Balanced facial growth: A schematic interpretation. Oral Surgery, Oral Medicine, Oral Pathology 63: 637–644.

1810. Pregill, G. 1981. Cranial morphology and the evolution of West Indian toads (Salientia: Bufonidae): Resurrection of the genus *Peltophryne* Fitzinger. Copeia: 273–285.

1811. Prershinskaya, N. M. 1983. Changes in the general growth of skull size of Arctic lemming. In *Rodents: Material from the Sixth All-Union Conference Leningrad 25–28 January 1984*, E. M. Gromov, ed. Leningrad: Nauka, pp. 182–184.

1812. Presley, R. 1978. Ontogeny of some elements of the auditory bulla in mammals. Journal of Anatomy, London 126: 428.

1813. Presley, R.1979. The primitive course of the internal carotid artery in mammals. Acta anatomica 103: 238–244.

1814. Presley, R. 1981. Alisphenoid equivalents in placentals, marsupials, monotremes, and fossils. Nature 294: 668–670.

1815. Presley, R. 1983. A shaky foundation in the structure of the skull? Nature 302: 210–211.

1816. Presley, R. 1984. Lizards, mammals, and the primitive tympanic membrane. In *The Structure, Development, and Evolution of Reptiles*, M. W. J. Ferguson, ed. London: Academic Press, pp. 127–154.

1817. Presley, R. 1989. Ala temporalis: Function or phylogenetic memory? In *Trends in Vertebrate Morphology*, Forschritte der Zoologie, vol. 35, H. Splechtna and H. Hilgers, eds. Stuttgart: Gustav-Fischer Verlag, pp. 392–395.

1818. Presley, R., and F. L. D. Steel. 1976. On the homology of the alisphenoid. Journal of Anatomy, London 121: 441–459.

1819. Presley, R., and F. L. D. Steel. 1978. The pterygoid and ectopterygoid in mammals. Anatomy and Embryology 154: 95–110.

1820. Pringle, J. A. 1954. The cranial development of certain South African snakes and the relationships of these groups. Proceedings of the Zoological Society of London 123: 813–865.

1821. Prisyazhnyuk, V. E. 1983. Age changes in craniological characters of aboriginal axis deer. In *Rare Species of Mammals of the USSR and Their Conservation*, V. E. Sokolov, ed. Moscow: A. N. Severtsov Institute of Evolutionary Morphology and Ecology of Animals, pp. 200–201.

1822. Pritchard, J. J., J. H. Scott, and F. G. Girgis. 1956. The structure and development of cranial and facial sutures. Journal of Anatomy, London 90: 73–86.

1823. Prummel, W. 1987. Atlas for identification of foetal skeletal elements of cattle, horse, sheep, and pig. Archaeozoologia 1: 23–30.

1824. Prushinskaya, N. M., V. N. Bolshakov, and E. A. Gileva. 1984. Variation in the correlational structure of the skull of Arctic lemming. In *Population Ecology and Morphology of Mammals*, L. N. Dobrinskij, ed. Sverdlovsk: Academy of Sciences USSR, Urals Scientific Centre, pp. 37–52.

1825. Pucciarelli, H. M. 1974. The influence of experimental deformation on neurocranial Wormian bones in rats. American Journal of Physical Anthropology 41: 29–37.

1826. Pucciarelli, H. M. 1978. Craniofacial development of the rat with respect to vestibular orientation. Acta anatomica 100: 101–110.

1827. Puchkov, V. F. 1963. Effect of the scleral papillae on the development of the bonelets of the eye in the chick embryo. Doklady Akademii Nauk SSSR 152: 494–496.

1828. Pugin, E. 1972. Induction de cartilage, après excision de la cupule otique chez l'embryon de Poulet, par des greffons d'organes embryonnaires de Souris. Comptes rendus hedbomadaires des séances de l'Académie des sciences, Paris 275: 2543–2546.

1829. Purohit, N. R., R. J. Choudhary, D. S. Chouhan, and K. S. Deora. 1987. Congenital deviations of premaxilla and nasal septum in camel. Indian Journal of Animal Science 57: 1294–1295.

1830. Pusey, H. K. 1938. Structural changes in the anuran mandibular arch during metamorphosis with reference to *Rana temporaria*. Quarterly Journal of Microscopical Science 80: 479–565.

1831. Pusey, H. K. 1943. On the head of the leiopelmid frog, *Ascaphus truei*. I. The chondrocranium, jaws, arches, and muscles of a partly-grown larva. Quarterly Journal of Microscopical Science 84: 105–185.

1832. Qui Youxiang. 1987. On the hyobranchial skeleton of the larval *Salamandrella keyserlingii*. Acta herpetologica sinica 6: 74.

1833. Quinones, N. C. 1976. Biology of the Philippine deer (*Cervus philippinus*) in captivity. Sylvatrop 1: 265–296.

1834. Radermaker, F., C. Surlemont, P. Sanna, M. Chardon, and P. Vandewalle. 1989. Ontogeny of the Weberian apparatus of *Clarias gariepinus* (Pisces, Siluriformes). Canadian Journal of Zoology 67: 2090–2097.

1835. Radinsky, L. 1983. Allometry and reorganization in horse skull proportions. Science 221: 1189–1191.

1836. Radinsky. L. 1984. Ontogeny and phylogeny in horse skull evolution. Evolution 38: 1–15.

1837. Rajtová, V. 1969a. The development of the skeleton of the guinea pig. VI. Prenatal and postnatal ossification of the bones of the neurocranium in the guinea pig. Folia morphologica 17: 48–55.

1838. Rajtová, V. 1969b. Development of the skeleton in the guinea pig. VII. Prenatal and postnatal ossification of bones of the splanchnocranium in the guinea pig (*Cavia porcellus* L.). Folia morphologica 17: 56–65.

1839. Rajtová, V. 1971. Les transformations du cartilage de Meckel et l'ossification de la mandible chez *Cavia procellus* L. Part I. Anatomisches Anzeiger 128: 392–401.

1840. Rajtová, V. 1972a. Morphogenesis des Chondrocraniums beim Meerschweinchen (*Cavia porcellus* L.). Anatomisches Anzeiger 130: 176–206.

1841. Rajtová, V. 1972b. Über die Morphogenesis des Chondrocraniums beim Goldhamster (*Mesocricetus auratus* Wrth.). Anatomisches Anzeiger 130: 207–221.

1842. Rak, Y. 1985. Part 2, The voice of today: *Australopithecus* in the forest of hominid trees; sexual dimorphism, ontogeny, and the beginning of differentiation of the robust Australopithecine clade. In *Hominid Evolution: Past, Present, and Future*, P. V. Tobias, ed. New York: Alan R. Liss, pp. 233–237.

1843. Rak, Y., and F. C. Howell. 1978. Cranium of a juvenile *Australopithecus boisei* from the Lower Omo basin, Ethiopia. American Journal of Physical Anthropology. 48: 345–366.

1844. Ramaswami, L. S. 1938. Connections of the pterygoquadrate in the tadpoles of *Philautus variabilis* (Anura). Nature 142: 577.

1845. Ramaswami, L. S. 1940. Some aspects of the chondrocranium in the tadpoles of South Indian frogs. Half-Yearly Journal of Mysore University, sec. B, Science 1: 15–41.

1846. Ramaswami, L. S. 1941a. Pterygoquadrate connections in the embryos of *Ichthyophis glutinosus* (Apoda). Nature 148: 470.

1847. Ramaswami, L. S. 1941b. Some aspects of the cranial morphology of *Uraeotyphlus narayani seilacher* (Apoda). Records of the Indian Museum, Calcutta 43: 143–207.

1848. Ramaswami, L. S. 1941c. Some aspects of the head of *Xenopus laevis*. Proceedings of the Indian Scientific Congress 28: 183–184.

1849. Ramaswami, L. S. 1943a. The segmentation of the head of *Ichthyophis glutinosus* (L.). Proceedings of the Zoological Society, London 112B: 105–112.

1850. Ramaswami, L. S. 1943b. An account of the chondrocranium of *Rana afghana* and *Megophrys*, with a description of the masticatory musculature of some tadpoles. Proceedings of the National Institute of Science, India 2: 43–59.

1851. Ramaswami, L. S. 1943c. An account of the head morphology of *Gegenophis carnosus* (Beddome), Apoda. Half-Yearly Journal of Mysore University, n.s., 3B: 205–220.

1852. Ramaswami, L. S. 1944. The chondrocranium of two torrent-dwelling anuran tadpoles. Journal of Morphology 74: 347–374.

1853. Ramaswami, L. S.1945. The chondrocranium of *Gambusia* (Cyprinodontes) with an account of the osteocranium of the adult. Journal of Mysore University, n.s., 6: 19–45.

1854. Ramaswami, L. S. 1946. The chondrocranium of *Calotes versicolor* (Daud.) with a description of the osteocranium of a just-hatched young. Quarterly Journal of Microscopical Science 87: 237–297.

1856. Ramaswami, L. S. 1948. The chondrocranium of *Gegenophis* (Apoda: Amphibia). Proceedings of the Zoological Society of London 118: 752–760.

1857. Ramaswami, L. S. 1956. "Frontoparietal" bone in Anura (Amphibia). Current Science 25: 19–20.

1858. Ramaswami, L. S. 1957. The development of the skull in the slender loris, *Loris tardigradus lydekkerianus* Cabr. Acta zoologica, Stockholm 38: 27–68.

1859. Randall, F. E. 1943. The skeletal and dental development and variability of the Gorilla. Human Biology, Baltimore 15: 236–254, 307–337.

1860. Randall, F. E. 1944. The skeletal and dental development and variability of the Gorilla (concluded). Human Biology, Baltimore 16: 23–76.

1861. Ranly, D. M. 1988. *A Synopsis of Craniofacial Growth*. 2d ed. Norwalk, Conn.: Appleton and Lange.

1862. Rao, K. S., and K. Lakshmi. 1984. Head skeleton of the marine catfish,

Arius tenuispinis Day (Osteichthyes: Siluriformes: Ariidae). Journal of Morphology 181: 221–238.

1863. Rao, M. K. M., and L. S. Ramaswami. 1952. The fully formed chondrocranium of *Mabuya* with an account of the adult osteocranium. Acta zoologica, Stockholm 33: 209–275.

1864. Rasmussen, G. P., J. Powers, and S. H. Clarke. 1982. Relation of mandible length to age and its reliability as a criterion of sex in white-tailed deer. New York Fish and Game Journal 29: 142–151.

1865. Ratti, P., and K.-H. Habermehl. 1977. Investigation on age estimation and age determination of mountain ibex (*Capra ibex ibex*) in Graubunden Canton. Zeitschrift für Jagdwissenschaft 23: 188–213.

1866. Rauchfuss, A. 1989. Pneumatization and mesenchyme in the human middle ear. Acta anatomica 136: 285–290.

1867. Raunich, L. 1957. Sul comportamento di trapianti dei cercini neurale di Anfibi anuri. Annali, Università di Ferrara, Sezione 13, Anatomia comparata 1: 45–58.

1868. Raunich, L. 1958. Comportamento del materiale dei cercini neurale di Anfibi anuri in condizioni di espianto. Annali, Università di Ferrara, Sezione 13, Anatomia comparata 1: 59–62.

1869. Rauther, M. 1937. Kiemer der Anamnier-Kiemendarmderivate der Cyclostomen and Fische. In *Handbuch vergleichenden Anatomie der Wirbeltiere*, vol. 3. Berlin und Wien: Urban and Schwarzenberg, pp. 212–278.

1870. Ravosa, M. J. 1988. Browridge development in Cercopithecidae: A test of two models. American Journal of Physical Anthropology 76: 535–555.

1871. Raynaud, A., J. Fretey, J. Brabet, and M. Clerque-Gazeau. 1983. Étude, au moyen de la microscopie électronique à labayage, des structures epitheliales annexées aux feutes viscerales chez les embryos de Turtue Luth (*Dermochelys coriacea* V.). Comptes rendus hedbomadaires des séances de l'Académie des sciences, Paris 296: 297–302.

1872. Raynaud, A., J. Fretey, and M. Clerque-Gazeau. 1980. Structures epitheliales d'existence temporaire, portées par les arcs branchiaux chez embryons de tortue luth (*Dermochelys coriacea* L.P.). Bulletin biologique de la France et de la Belgique 114: 71–99.

1873. Reeve, E. C. R. 1940. Relative growth in the snout of anteaters. Proceedings of the Zoological Society of London 110A: 47–80.

1874. Reeve, E. C. R., and P. D. F. Murray. 1942. Evolution in the horse's skull. Nature 150: 402–403.

1875. Regal, P. J. 1966. Feeding specializations and the classification of terrestrial salamanders. Evolution 20: 392–407.

1876. Regel, E. D. 1961a. Traces of segmentation in the chordal region of the chondrocranium of *Hynobius keyserlingii*. Doklady Akademii Nauk SSSR 140: 253–255.

1877. Regel, E. D. 1961b. The palatoquadrate cartilage and its connection to the skull axis in *Hynobius keyserlingii*. Doklady Akademii Nauk SSSR 142: 237–240.

1878. Regel, E. D. 1964a. The development of the axial cartilaginous skull and its connections with the palatoquadrate cartilage in *Hynobius keyserlingii*. Trudy Zoologicheskogo Instituta Akademiya Nauk SSSR 33: 34–74.

1879. Regel, E. D. 1964b. Homology of the antorbital processes in amphibians. Doklady Akademii Nauk SSSR 154: 728–730.

1880. Regel, E. D. 1968. The development of the cartilaginous neurocranium and its connection with the upper part of the mandibular arch in the Siberian salamander *Ranodon sibiricus* (Hynobiidae, Amphibia). Trudy Zoologicheskogo Instituta, Leningrad 46: 5–85.

1881. Regel, E. D. 1970. Ascending process of the palatoquadrate cartilage in urodelans. Doklady Akademii Nauk SSSR 194: 981–984.

1882. Regel, E. D. 1973. Pre-spiracular slits in anura. Doklady Akademii Nauk SSSR 208: 1487–1490.

1883. Regel, E. D. 1979. Peculiarities of development and morphology of olfactory capsules in the Ussurian salamander (*Onychodactylus fischeri* Blgr., Hynobiidae, Urodela) in comparison with other amphibians. Trudy Zoologicheskogo Instituta, Leningrad 89: 71–97.

1884. Regel, E. D., and S. M. Epstein. 1972. Segmentation of inter-auricular skull region in Anura. Zoologicheskii zhurnal 51: 1517–1528.

1885. Reif, W.-E. 1978a. Types of morphogenesis of the dermal skeleton in fossil sharks. Paläontologische Zeitschrift 52: 110–128.

1886. Reif, W.-E. 1978b. Shark dentitions: Morphogenetic processes and evolution. Neues Jahrbuch für Geologie und Paläontologie 157: 107–115.

1887. Reif, W.-E. 1980a. Development of dentition and dermal skeleton in embryonic *Scyliorhynchus canicula*. Journal of Morphology 166: 275–288.

1888. Reif, W.-E. 1980b. A model of morphogenetic processes in the dermal skeleton of elasmobranchs. Neues Jahrbuch für Geologie und Paläontologie 159: 339–359.

1889. Reif, W.-E. 1982. Evolution of dermal skeleton and dentition in vertebrates: The odontode regulation theory. Evolutionary Biology 15: 287–368.

1890. Reilly, S. M. 1986. Ontogeny of cranial ossification in the eastern newt, *Notophthalmus viridescens* (Caudata: Salamandridae) and its relationship to metamorphosis and neoteny. Journal of Morphology 188: 315–326.

1891. Reilly, S. M. 1987. Ontogeny of the hyobranchial apparatus in the salamanders *Ambystoma talpoideum* (Ambystomatidae) and *Notophthalmus viridescens* (Salamandridae): The ecological morphology of two neotenic strategies. Journal of Morphology 191: 205–214.

1892. Reilly, S. M., and G. V. Lauder. 188a. Ontogeny of aquatic feeding performance in the eastern newt, *Notophthalmus viridescens* (Salamandridae). Copeia: 87–91.

1893. Reilly, S. M., and G. V. Lauder. 1988b. Atavisms and the homology of hyobranchial elements in lower vertebrates. Journal of Morphology 195: 237–246.

1894. Reilly, S. M., and G. V. Lauder. 1989. Kinetics of tongue projection in *Ambystoma tigrinum*: Quantitative kinematics, muscle function, and evolutionary hypotheses. Journal of Morphology 199: 223–243.

1895. Reinbach, W. 1939. Untersuchungen über die Entwicklung des Kopfskeletts von *Calyptocephalus gayi* (mit einem Anhang über das Os supratemporale der anuren Amphibien). Jenaische Zeitschrift für Naturwissenschaften, Jena 72: 211–362.

1896. Reinbach, W. 1950. Über den schalleitenden Apparat der Amphibien und Reptilien (zue Schmalhausenschen Theorie der Gehörnknochelchen). Zeitschrift für Anatomie und Entwicklungsgeschichte 114: 611–639.

1897. Reinbach, W. 1951a. Über einen Rest des Parasphenöids bei einem rezenten Säugetier. Zeitschrift für Morphologie und Anthropologie, Stuttgart 43: 195–205.

1898. Reinbach, W. 1951b. Die vordere quadrato-kraniale Kommisur bei den Anuren. Verhlandlungen, Anatomische Gesellschaft, Jena 48: 111.

1899. Reinbach, W. 1952. Zur Entwicklung des Primordialcraniums von *Dasypus novemcinctus* Linné (*Tatusia novemcincta* Lesson). I. Zeitschrift für Morphologie und Anthropologie, Stuttgart 44: 375–444.

1900. Reinbach, W. 1953. Zur Entwicklung des Primordialcraniums von *Dasypus novemcinctus* Linné (*Tatusia novemcincta* Lesson). II. Zeitschrift für Morphologie und Anthropologie, Stuttgart 45: 1–72.

1901. Reinbach, W. 1955. Das Cranium eines Embryos des Gürteltieres *Zaedyus minutus* (65 mm SchSt). Gegenbaurs Morphologisches Jahrbuch, Leipzig 95: 79–141.

1902. Reinbach, W. 1963a. Das Cranium eines menschlischen Feten von 93 mm SchSt Länge: Zur Morphologie des Cranium älterer menschlicher Feten. I. Zeitschrift für Anatomie und Entwicklungsgeschichte 124: 1–50.

1903. Reinbach, W. 1963b. Die lamina alaris (Voit) am Occipitalpfeiler der Säugercraniums sowie eine weitere lamellenförmige Bildung in dieser Region bei *Zaedyus minutus* (Ameghino). Zeitschrift für Anatomie und Entwicklungsgeschichte 124: 51–56.

1904. Reiner, F. 1986. First record of Sowerby's beaked whale from Azores. Scientific Report of the Whales Research Institute, Tokyo, no. 37: 103–107.

1905. Reinhard, W. 1958. Das Cranium eines 35 mm Langen Embryos des Mantelpavians, *Papio hamadyras* L. Zeitschrift für Anatomie und Entwicklungsgeschichte 120: 427–455.

1906. Rempel, J. S. 1943. The origin and differentiation of the larval head musculature of *Triturus torosus* (Rathke). University of California Publications in Zoology 51: 87–116.

1907. Reumer, W. F. 1985. Some aspects of the cranial osteology and phylogeny of *Xenopus* (Anura, Pipidae). Revue suisse de zoologie 92: 969–980.

1908. Rice, R. W., and O. J. Oyen. 1979. Supernumerary molars in baboons (*Papio cynocephalus anubis*). Texas Journal of Science 31: 267–270.

1909. Richany, S., T. H. Bast, and B. J. Anson. 1954. Account of the developmental history of three ossicles. Quarterly Bulletin of the Northwestern University Medical School 28: 17–45.

1910. Richany, S. F., T. H. Bast, and B. J. Anson. 1956. The development of the first branchial arch in man, and the fate of Meckel's cartilage. Quarterly Bulletin of the Northwestern University Medical School 30: 331–355.

1911. Richards, W. J., R. V. Miller, and E. D. Houde. 1974. Egg and larval development of the Atlantic thread herring, *Opisthonema oglinum*. U.S. National Marine Fisheries Service, Fishery Bulletin 72: 1123–1136.

1912. Richardson, G. P., K. L. Crossin, C.-M. Chuong, and G. M. Edelman. 1987. Expression of cell adhesion molecules during embryonic induction. III. Development of the otic placode. Developmental Biology 119: 217–230.

1913. Richardson, S. L., and W. A. Laroche. 1979. Development and occurrence of larvae and juveniles of the rockfishes, *Sebastes crameri, Sebastes pinniger,* and *Sebastes helvomaculatus* (Family Scorpaenidae) off Oregon. U.S. National Marine Fisheries Service, Fishery Bulletin 77: 1–41.

1914. Richman, J. M., and V. M. Diewert. 1987. An immunofluorescence study of chondrogenesis in murine mandibular ectomesenchyme. Cell Differentiation 21: 161–173.

1915. Richman, J. M., and V. M. Diewert. 1988. The fate of Meckel's cartilage chondrocytes in ocular culture. Developmental Biology 129: 48–60.

1916. Richman, J. M., and C. Tickle. 1989. Epithelia are interchangeable between facial primordia of chick embryos and morphogenesis is controlled by the mesenchyme. Developmental Biology 136: 201–210.

1917. Richtsmeier, J. T., and J. M. Cheverud. 1986. Finite element scaling analysis of human craniofacial growth. Journal of Craniofacial Growth and Developmental Biology 6: 289–324.

1918. Richtsmeier, J. T., J. M. Cheverud, and J. E. Buikstra. 1984. The relationship between cranial metric and nonmetric traits in the Rhesus macaques from Cayo Santiago [Puerto Rico]. American Journal of Physical Anthropology 64: 213–222.

1919. Rieppel, O. 1976a. The homology of the laterosphenoid bone in snakes. Herpetologica 32: 426–429.

1920. Rieppel, O. 1976b. Die orbitotemporale Region im Schädel von *Chelydra serpentina* Linnaeus (Chelonia) und *Lacerta sicula* Rafinesque (Lacertilia). Acta anatomica 96: 309–320.

1921. Rieppel, O. 1977. Über die Entwicklung des Basicranium bei *Chelydra serpentina* Linnaeus (Chelonia) und *Lacerta sicula* Rafinesque (Lacertilia). Verhandlungen, Naturforschende Gesellschaft, Basel 86: 153–170.

1922. Rieppel, O. 1978. The phylogeny of cranial kinesis in lower vertebrates, with special reference to the Lacertilia. Neues Jahrbuch für Geologie und Paläontologie 156: 353–370.

1923. Rieppel, O. 1979a. Ontogeny and the recognition of primitive character states. Zeitschrift für Zoologische Systematik und Evolutionsforschung 17: 57–61.

1924. Rieppel, O. 1979b. The braincase of *Typhlops* and *Leptotyphlops* (Reptilia: Serpentes). Zoological Journal of the Linnean Society of London 65: 161–176.

1925. Rieppel, O. 1980. The skull of the Upper Jurassic cryptodire turtle, *Thalassemys moseri,* with a reconsideration of the chelonian braincase. Palaeontographica, Abteilung A, Palaeozoologie-Stratigraphie 171: 105–140.

1926. Rieppel, O. 1984. The upper temporal arcade of lizards: An ontogenetic problem. Revue suisse de zoologie 91: 475–482.

1927. Rieppel, O. 1985. The recessus scalae tympani and its bearing on the classification of reptiles. Journal of Herpetology 19: 373–384.

1928. Rieppel, O. 1987. The development of the trigeminal jaw adductor musculature and associated skull elements in the lizard *Podarcis sicula*. Journal of Zoology, London 212: 131–150.

1929. Rieppel, O. 1988. The development of the trigeminal jaw adductor musculature in the grass snake, *Natrix natrix*. Journal of Zoology, London 216: 743–770.

1930. Rieppel, O., and L. Labhardt. 1979. Mandibular mechanics in *Varanus niloticus* (Reptilia: Lacertilia). Herpetologica 35: 158–163.

1931. Roček, Z. 1981. Cranial anatomy of frogs of the family Pelobatidae Stannius, 1856, with outline of their phylogeny and systematics. Acta Universitatis Carolinae biologica 1980: 1–164.

1932. Roček, Z. 1986. An "intracranial" joint in frogs. In *Studies in Herpetology*, Z. Roček, ed. Prague: Charles University, pp. 49–54.

1933. Roček, Z. 1988. Origin and evolution of the frontoparietal complex in anurans. Amphibia-Reptilia 9: 385–403.

1934. Roček, Z. 1989. Developmental patterns of the ethmoidal region of the anuran skull. Fortschritte der Zoologie 35: 412–415.

1935. Roček, Z., and M. Vesely. 1989. Development of the ethmoidal structures of the endocranium in the anuran *Pipa pipa*. Journal of Morphology 200: 301–320.

1936. Roche, J. 1978. Teething and age data on rock dassies (genus *Procavia*). Mammalia 42: 97–104.

1937. Roeder, U. 1981. Bemerkenswertes an Flachlandgorillas. Saeugetierkundliche Mitteilungen 29: 79–80.

1938. Roehrer-Erti, O. 1989. On cranial growth of orangutan with a note on the role of intelligence in evolution: Morphological study on directions of growth primarily dependent on the age within a population of *Pongo satyrus borneensis* von Wurms 1784 from Skalau, West Bornea [Indonesia] (Mammalia, Primates: Ponginae). Zoologische Abhandlungen, Dresden 44: 9–15.

1939. Rohrs, M. 1986. "Allometrische Betrachtungen" zur Schädelgrösse und Gesichtsschädelgrösse in der Evolution und Domestikation. Nova acta leopoldina 58 (262): 319–333.

1940. Rojas, M. A., B. Morales, F. Estay, and M. A. Montenegro. 1984. Light microscopic and histochemical study on the development of the bovine secondary palate (*Bos taurus*). Archives de biologie, Brussels 95: 475–492.

1941. Romanoff, A. L. 1960. *The Avian Embryo: Structural and Functional Development*. New York: Macmillan Co.

1942. Romanoff, N. S. 1976. Some characteristics of the chondrocranium development in Coho in postembryonic ontogenesis. Biologiya Morya: 13–21.

1943. Romanoff, N. S. 1977. Some aspects of chondrocranial development of the Sockeye in postembryogenesis. Biologiya Morya: 31–40.

1944. Romanoff, N. S. 1978a. Developmental characteristics of the Chum salmon chondrocranium in postembryogenesis. Biologiya Morya: 47–52.

1945. Romanoff, N. S. 1978b. Peculiarities in the development of the chondrocranium of Chum salmon (*Oncorhynchus keta*) in postmbryogenesis. Soviet Journal of Marine Biology 4: 518–522.

1946. Romanoff, N. S. 1983. Relations between Pacific salmon and the genus *Oncorhynchus* and *Salmo* on the basis of studying head skeleton in post-embryonic ontogenesis. In *Morphology, Population Structure, and Problems of Rational Utilization of Salmonoidei*, O. A. Skarlato and E. A. Dorofeeva, eds. Leningrad: Nauka, pp. 176–178.

1947. Romanoff, N. S. 1984. Effect of culture conditions on skull morphology in smolts of the masu salmon *Oncorhynchus masou*. Aquaculture 41: 147–154.

1948. Romanoff, N. S. 1985a. Postembryonic changes in the skull of *Hucho perryi* (Brevoort). In *Morphology and Classification of the Salmonoid Fishes*, O. A. Skarlato, ed. Leningrad: Academy of Sciences, USSR, Zoological Institute, pp. 53–61.

1949. Romanoff, N. S. 1985b. Morphology of the head skeleton of *Hucho perryi* (Brevoort) during postembryonic ontogenesis. In *Biological Studies of Salmon: Collected Works*, S. M. Konovalov, N. S. Romanoff, and A. Y. Semenchenko, eds. Vladivostock: Academy of Sciences, USSR, Far East Science Centre, pp. 106–153.

1950. Romanoff, N. S., and N. I. Krupyanko. 1983. Postembryonic changes in the neurocranium of *Hucho perryi*. In *Morphology, Population Structure, and Problems of Rational Utilization of Salmonoidei*, O. A. Skarlato and E. A. Dorofeeva, eds. Leningrad: Nauka, pp. 178–180.

1951. Romer, A. S. 1956. *Osteology of the Reptiles*. Chicago: University of Chicago Press.

1952. Romer, A. S. 1972. The vertebrate animals as a dual animal: Somatic and visceral. Evolutionary Biology 6: 121–156.

1953. Rosen, D. E. 1971. The Macristiidae, a ctenothrissiform family based on juvenile and larval scopelomorph fishes. American Museum Novitates, no. 2452: 1–22.

1954. Rosen, D. E., and L. R. Parenti. 1981. Relationships of *Oryzias* and the groups of atherinomorph fishes. American Museum Novitates, no. 2719: 1–25.

1955. Rosenberg, K. F. A. 1966. Die postnatale Proportionsänderung der Schädel zweier extremer Wuchsformen des Haushundes. Zeitschrift für Tierzüchtung und Züchtungsbiologie 82: 1–36.

1956. Rosenthal, J., and F. Doljanski. 1961. Biochemical growth patterns of normal and ratiothyroidectomized rats. Growth 25: 347–365.

1957. Roskosz, T., and F. Kobrynczuk. 1986. The variability of the length measurements of chosen parts of the axial skeleton and their correlations in the European bison, *Bison bonasus* (L.). Annals, Warsaw Agricultural University, SGGW-AR, Veterinary Medicine, no. 13: 3–10.

1958. Ross, G. J. B. 1979. Records of pygmy and dwarf sperm whales, genus *Kogia*, from southern Africa, with biological notes and some comparisons. Annals of the Cape Province Museum of Natural History 11: 259–327.

1959. Rossman, C. E. 1980. Ontogenetic changes in skull proportions of the diamondback water snake, *Nerodia rhombifera*. Herpetologica 36: 42–46.

1960. Rossolimo, D. L. 1985. Peculiarities in the interpopulational and geographic correlation of the skull indices of *Alopax lagopus* L. Trudy Biologiscke Nauchno-Issledoval'skogo Instituta, no. 37: 51–60.

1961. Rossolimo, D. L., and I. Y. Pavlinov. 1974. Sex-related differences in the development, size, and proportions of the skull in the pine marten *Martes martes* L. (Mammalia: Mustelidae). Byulleten' Moskovskogo Obschchestva Ispytatelei Prirody Otdel Biologicheskii 79: 23–35.

1962. Roth, G., and D. B. Wake. 1985. Trends in the functional morphology and sensorimotor control of feeding behavior in salamanders: An example of the role of internal dynamics in evolution. Acta biotheoretica 34: 175–192.

1963. Roth-Lutra, K. H. 1982. A pilot study on the differentiating morphogenesis of the skull. Anatomisches Anzeiger 151: 119–125.

1964. Roux, G. H. 1947. The cranial development of certain Ethiopian "insectivores" and its bearing on the mutual affinities of the group. Acta zoologica, Stockholm 28: 165–307.

1965. Rowedder, W. 1937. Die Entwicklung des Geruchsorgans bei *Alytes obstetricans* and *Bufo vulgaris*. Zeitschrift für Anatomie und Entwicklungsgeschichte 107: 91.

1966. Ruch, J.-V. 1985. Epithelial-mesenchymal interactions in formation of mineralized tissues. In *The Chemistry and Biology of Mineralized Tissues*, W. T. Butler, ed. Birmingham, Ala.: Ebsco-Medica, pp. 54–61.

1967. Ruibal, R., and E. Thomas. 1988. The obligate carnivorous larvae of the frog, *Lepidobatrachus laevis* (Leptodactylidae). Copeia: 591–604.

1968. Ruiz I Altaba, A., and D. A. Melton. 1989. Bimodal and graded expression of the *Xenopus* homeobox gene Xhox3 during embryonic development. Development 106: 173–184.

1969. Runner, M. N. 1986. Epigenetically regulated genomic expressions for shortened stature and cleft palate are regionally specific in the 11-day mouse embryo. Journal of Craniofacial Genetics and Developmental Biology 2 (suppl.): 137–168.

1970. Ruple, D. 1984. Gobioidei: Development. In *Ontogeny and Systematics of Fishes*, American Society of Ichthyologists and Herpetologists Special Publication no. 1, H. G. Moser, ed. Lawrence, Kans.: Allen Press, pp. 582–587.

1971. Ruprecht, A. L. 1972. The morphological variability of the *Passer domesticus* skull in postnatal development. Acta ornithologica 23: 36.

1972. Ruprecht, A. L. 1979. Criteria for species determination in the subgenus *Sylvaemus* (Rodentia: Muridae). Przeglad Zologiczny 23: 340–349.

1973. Ruprecht, A. L. 1981. Falle von Selbstausheilung von Unterkieferbruchen bei Kleinsaugern aus dem Lebensraum. Säugetierkundliche Mitteilungen 29: 79–80.

1974. Ruprecht, A. L. 1984. Correlations of skull measurements in the postembryonic development of the house sparrow, *Passer domesticus*. Acta ornithologica, Warsaw 20: 147–158.

1975. Russell, G. J. B., A. E. Mattison, W. T. Easson, D. Clark, T. Sharpe, and J. McGouch. 1972. Skeletal dimensions as an indication of fetal maturity. British Journal of Radiology 45: 667–669.

1976. Ryabov, L. S. 1962. The morphological development of caucasian pine martens and stone martens in relation to age determination. Translated in *Biology of Mustelids* (1975), C. M. King, ed. Boston Spa: British Library Lending Division, pp. 145–157.

1977. Saban, R. 1955. Contribution à l'étude de la genèse et de la croissance de l'os temporal chez le macaque. Mammalia. Morphologie, biologie, systématique des mammifères, Paris 19: 447–458.

1978. Saban, R. 1956. Les affinités du genre *Tupaia* Raffles, 1821, d'après les caractères morphologiques de la tête osseuse. Annales de paléontologie, Paris 42: 170–224.

1979. Saban, R. 1957. Les affinités du genre *Tupaia* Raffles, 1821, d'après les caractères morphologiques de la tête osseuse. Annales de Paléontologie, Paris 43: 1–44.

1980. Saban, R. 1963. Contribution à l'étude de l'os temporal des Primates: Description chez l'homme et les Prosimiens; Anatomie comparée et phylogénie. Mémoires du Muséum national d'histoire naturelle 29A: 1–377.

1981. Saban, R. 1964a. Sur la pneumalisation de l'os temporal des Primates adultes et son développement ontogénique chez le genne *Alouatta* (Platyrhinien). Gegenbaurs Morphologische Jahrbuch, Leipzig 106: 569–593.

1982. Saban, R. 1964b. Aspects modernes de la théorie vertébrale du crâne. Annales de paléontologie 50: 1–21.

1983. Saber, G. M., S. B. Parker, and R. Minkoff. 1989. Influence of epithelial-mesenchymal interactions on the viability of facial mesenchyme *in vitro*. Anatomical Record 225: 56–66.

1984. Sachs, T. 1988. Epigenetic selection: An alternative mechanism of pattern formation. Journal of Theoretical Biology 134: 547–559.

1985. Sadaghiani, B., and C. H. Thiébaud. 1987. Neural crest development in the *Xenopus laevis* embryo, studied by interspecific transplantation and scanning electron microscopy. Developmental Biology 124: 91–110.

1986. Sadaghiani, B., and J. R. Vielkind. 1989. Neural crest development in *Xiphophorus* fishes: Scanning electron and light microscopic studies. Development 105: 487–504.

1987. Sage, R. D., and R. K. Selander. 1975. Trophic radiation through polymorphism in cichlid fishes. Proceedings of the National Academy of Sciences, U.S.A. 72: 4669–4673.

1988. Sägessar, H., and W. Huber. 1962. Der Verkeilung der Frontainaht beim Reh (*Capreolus capreolus*). Revue suisse de zoologie 69: 360–369.

1989. Saiff, E. I. 1981. The middle ear of the skull of birds: The ostrich, *Struthio camelus*. Zoological Journal of the Linnean Society of London 73: 201–212.

1990. Saint Girons, H. 1976. Données histologiques sur les fosses nasales et leurs annexes chez *Crocodylus niloticus* Laurenti et *Caiman crocodilus* (Linnaeus) (Reptilia, Crocodylidae). Zoomorphologie 84: 301–318.

1991. Salmanov, A. V., and M. Kaukaranta. 1987. Osteological peculiarities of the Finnish populations of the Atlantic salmon (*Salmo salar* L.) from the River Simojoki. Trudy Zoologicheskogo Instituta Akademiya Nauk SSSR 162: 22–37.

1992. Salvini-Plawen, L. Van. 1989. Mesoderm heterochrony and metamery in Chordata. Fortschritte der Zoologie 35: 213–219.

1993. Salzmann, H. C. 1977. Body weight, skull dimensions, and growth of horns in Chamois from the Jura Mountains Switzerland and a comparison with other populations. Zeitschrift für Jagdwissenschaft 23: 69–80.

1994. Sampson, W. J., G. C. Townsend, and A. C. Goss. 1987. A cephalometric study of young marmosets (Callithrix jacchus). Journal of Dental Research 66: 1684–1686.

1995. Sandberg, M., H. Autio-Harmainen, and E. Vuorio. 1988. Localization of the expression of Types I, III, and IV collagen, TGF-β1 and c-fos genes in developing human calvarial bones. Developmental Biology 130: 324–334.

1996. Sander, P. M. 1988. A fossil reptile embryo from the Middle Triassic of the Alps. Science 239: 780–783.

1997. Sanz, J. L., and N. Lopez-Martinez. 1984. The prolacertid lepidosaurian Cosesaurus aviceps: A claimed protoavian from the Middle Triassic of Spain. Geobios, Lyon 17: 747–756.

1998. Sapargel'dyev, M. 1987. Morphological features of the Afghan pika. Izvestiya Akademii Nauk, Turkmenskoi SSR Seriya Biologicheskikh, no. 3: 31–37.

1999. Sarkisova, T. B., and I. V. Khrustaleva. 1985. The skeleton of wild and domestic pigs during early ontogenesis. In Morphology and Genetics of the Boar, L. V. Davletova, ed. Moscow: Nauka, pp. 114–122.

2000. Sarnat, B. G. 1964. The Temporomandibular Joint. 2d ed. Springfield: C. C. Thomas.

2001. Sarnat, B. G. 1983. Normal and abnormal craniofacial growth. Angle Orthodontist 53: 263–289.

2002. Sarnat, B. G. 1986. Growth patterns of the mandible: Some reflections. American Journal of Orthodontics and Dentofacial Orthopaedics 90: 221–233.

2003. Sasaki, H., and G. Kodama. 1973. Developmental studies on the postsphenoid of the human sphenoid bone. Hokkaido Journal of Medical Science 48: 167–174.

2004. Sassoon, D., and D. B. Kelley. 1986. The sexually dimorphic larynx in Xenopus laevis: Development and androgen regulation. American Journal of Anatomy 177: 457–472.

2005. Sassoon, D., N. Segil, and D. Kelley. 1986. Androgen-induced myogenesis and chondrogenesis in the larynx of Xenopus laevis. Developmental Biology 113: 135–140.

2006. Sato, G., and Y. Matsuura. 1986. Early development of Thyrsitops lepidopoides (Pisces: Gempylidae). Boletim, Instituto Oceanografico 34: 55–69.

2007. Saunderson, E. C. 1937. The early development of the chondrocranium of Salmo salar. Proceedings of the Nova Scotia Institute of Science, Halifax 19: 121–147.

2008. Savage, R. M. 1955. The ingestive, digestive, and respiratory systems of the microhylid tadpole, Hypopachus aguae. Copeia: 120–127.

2009. Schachner, O. 1989. Raising of the head and allometry: Morphometric study on the embryonic development of the mouse skeleton. Fortschritte der Zoologie 35: 291–298.

2010. Schaeffer, B. 1971. The braincase of the holostean fish Macrepistius, with comments on neurocranial ossification in the Actinopterygii. American Museum Novitates, no. 2459: 1–34.

2011. Schaeffer, B. 1987. Deuterostome monophyly and phylogeny. Evolutionary Biology 21: 179–235.

2012. Schaeffer, B., and K. S. Thomson. 1980. Reflections on agnathan-gnathosome relationships. In *Aspects of Vertebrate History: Essays in Honor of Edwin Harris Colbert,* L. L. Jacobs, ed. Flagstaff: Museum of Northern Arizona Press, pp. 19–33.

2013. Scherschlicht, R. 1973. Mikroskopisch-anatomische Untersuchung der Veränderungen am kopf des Hühnerkeimes nach TEM-Behandlung während der Organogenese. Wilhelm Roux Archiv für Entwicklungsmechanik der Organismen 173: 83–106.

2014. Schinz, H. R., and R. Zangerl. 1937a. Uber die Osteogenese des Skelettes beim Haushuhn bei der Haustaube und beim Haubensteissfuss. Gegenbaurs Morphologisches Jahrbuch, Leipzig 80: 620–628.

2015. Schinz, H. R., and R. Zangerl. 1937b. Beiträge zue Osteogenese des Knochensystems beim Haushuhn, bei der Haustaube und beim Haubensteissfuss. Denkschriften der schweizerischen naturforschenden Gesellschaft 72: 113–164.

2016. Schliemann, H. 1966. Zur Morphologie und Entwicklung des Craniums von *Canis lupus f. familiaris* L. Gegenbaurs Morphologisches Jahrbuch, Leipzig 109: 501–603.

2017. Schliemann, H. 1987. The solum nasi of the mammalian chondrocranium with special reference to the Carnivora. In *Morphogenesis of the Mammalian Skull,* H.-J. Kuhn and U. Zeller, eds. Hamburg: Verlag Paul Parey, pp. 91–103.

2018. Schmahl, W., I. Meyer, H. Kriegel, and K. H. Tempel. 1979. Cartilaginous metaplasia and overgrowth of neurocranium skull after X-irradiation *in utero.* Virchows Archiv A, Pathological Anatomy and Histology 384: 173–184.

2019. Schmalhausen, I. I. 1939. Role of the olfactory sac in the development of the cartilage capsule of the olfactory organ in Urodela. Doklady Akademii Nauk SSSR 23: 395–398.

2020. Schmalhausen, I. I. 1950a. On the attachment of the visceral arches to the skull axis in fishes. Zoologicheskii zhurnal 29: 435–448.

2021. Schmalhausen, I. I. 1950b. Experimental study of the development of the olfactory rudiments in the early stages of Amphibia. Doklady Akademii Nauk SSSR 74: 863–865.

2022. Schmalhausen, I. I. 1951a. Development of oral and branchial apparatus in *Acipenser stellatus.* Doklady Akademii Nauk SSSR 80: 681–684.

2023. Schmalhausen, I. I. 1951b. Functional significance of the modification of the dorsal divisions of the visceral apparatus in the transition from fishes to terrestrial vertebrates. Zoologicheskii zhurnal 30: 149–164.

2024. Schmalhausen, I. I. 1953a. The autostyle and the differentiation of the terminal portions of the first visceral arches in the lower land vertebrates. Zoologicheskii zhurnal 32: 30–42.

1025. Schmalhausen, I. I. 1953b. The first arterial arch and the development of the carotid artery system in Amphibia. Zoologicheskii zhurnal 32: 937–954.

2026. Schmalhausen, I. I. 1953c. Development of the arterial system of the head in urodele Amphibia. Zoologicheskii zhurnal 32: 642–661.

2027. Schmalhausen, I. I. 1954. Development of gills, their blood vessels, and musculature in Amphibia. Zoologicheskii zhurnal 33: 848–868.

2028. Schmalhausen, I. I. 1955a. Development of the visceral musculature in urodele Amphibia. Zoologicheskii zhurnal 34: 162–174.

2029. Schmalhausen, I. I. 1955b. Distribution of the seismosensory organs in urodele Amphibia. Zoologicheskii zhurnal 34: 1334–1356.

2030. Schmalhausen, I. I. 1955c. Development of gills in larvae of the Volga sturgeon. Doklady Akademii Nauk SSSR 100: 605–608.

2031. Schmalhausen, I. I. 1956. Morphology of the sound transmitting apparatus of Urodelea. Zoologicheskii zhurnal 35: 1023–1042.

2032. Schmalhausen, I. I. 1957a. The sound-transmitting mechanism of amphibians. Zoologicheskii zhurnal 36: 1044–1063.

2033. Schmalhausen, I. I. 1957b. On the seismosensory system of urodeles in connection with the problem of the origin of tetrapods. Zoologicheskii zhurnal 36: 100–112.

2034. Schmalhausen, I. I. 1958. Nasolacrymal duct and septomaxillae of Urodela. Zoologicheskii zhurnal 37: 570–583.

2035. Schmalhausen, I. I. 1968. *The Origin of Terrestrial Vertebrates*. New York: Academic Press.

2036. Schmid, P., and Z. Stratil. 1986. Growth changes, variations, and sexual dimorphism of the gorilla skull. In *Primate Evolution: Selected Proceedings of the Congress of the International Primatological Society,* vol. 1, J. G. Else and P. C. Lee, eds. Cambridge: Cambridge University Press, pp. 239–248.

2037. Schmitt, R. J., and S. A. Holbrook. 1984. Ontogeny of prey selection by black surfperch *Embiotoca jacksoni* (Pisces: Embiotocidae): The role of fish morphology, foraging behavior, and patch selection. Marine Ecology Progress Series 18: 225–239.

2038. Schneck, G. H. 1985. Studies of the ontogenetic development of the cranial base in *Hylobates*. Zeitschrift für Morphologie und Anthropologie 76: 37–48.

2039. Schneck, G. H. 1986. Some aspects of the development of the orbitotemporal region in hominoid primates. In *Primate Evolution*, J. G. Else and P. C. Lee, eds. Cambridge: Cambridge University Press, pp. 265–271.

2040. Schneider, K. J. 1981. Age determination by skull pneumatization in the field sparrow. Journal of Field Ornithology 52: 57–59.

2041. Schneider, R. 1955. Zur Entwicklung des Chondrocraniums der Gattung *Bradypus*. Gegenbaurs Morphologisches Jahrbuch, Leipzig 95: 209–307.

2042. Schoen, M. A. 1976. Adaptive modifications in the basicranium of howling monkeys *Alouatta seniculus*. In *Symposium on Development of the Basicranium,* J. F. Bosma, ed. Bethesda: U.S. Department of Health, Education, and Welfare, pp. 664–676.

2043. Schowing, J. 1959a. Influence de l'excision de rhombencéphale et du mésencéphale sur la morphogenèse du crâne chez l'embryon du poulet. Comptes rendus hebdomadaires des séances de l'Académie des sciences, Paris 248: 2391–2392.

2044. Schowing, J. 1959b. Influence de l'excision du mésencéphale et du prosencéphale sur la morphogenèse du crâne chez l'embryon du poulet. Comptes rendus hebdomadaires des séances de l'Académie des sciences, Paris 249: 170–172.

2045. Schowing, J. 1961. Influence inductrice de l'encéphale et de la chorde sur la morphogenèse du squelette crânien chez l'embryon de Poulet. Journal of Embryology and Experimental Morphology 9: 326–334.

2046. Schowing, J. 1968a. Influence inductrice de l'encéphale embryonnaire sur le développement du crâne chez le Poulet. I. Influence de l'excision des territoires nerveux antérieurs sur le développement cranien. Journal of Embryology and Experimental Morphology 19: 9–22.

2047. Schowing, J. 1968b. Influence inductrice de l'encéphale embryonnaire sur le développement du crâne chez le Poulet. II. Influence de l'excision de la chorde et des territoires encéphaliques moyen et postérieur sur le développement cranien. Journal of Embryology and Experimental Morphology 19: 23–32.

2048. Schowing, J. 1968c. Mise en évidence du rôle inducteur de l'encéphale dans l'ostéogenèse du crâne embryonnaire du poulet. Journal of Embryology and Experimental Morphology 19: 88–93.

2049. Schowing, J. 1974. Role morphogène de l'encéphale embryonnaire dans l'organogenèse du crâne chez l'oiseau. Annales de biologie 13: 69–76.

2050. Schowing, J. 1975. Morphogenetic role of the embryonic encephalon in cranial organogenesis. In Chemical and Experimental Embryology: Recent Results, R. Courrier, ed. Paris: Masson et Cie, pp. 69–76.

2051. Schowing, J., and M. Robadey. 1971. Substitution à l'encéphale embryonnaire de Poulet (Gallus gallus) d'un encéphale embryonnaire de Caille (Coturnix coturnix japonica) de même stade. Comptes rendus hebdomadaires des séances de l'Académie des sciences, Paris 272: 2382–2384.

2052. Schuchmann, K.-L. 1985. Morpho- und Thermogenese nestjunger Blaukehlkibris (Lampornis clemenciae). Journal für Ornithologie, Berlin 126: 305–308.

2053. Schuh, W., and G. W. Niebaur. 1982. Zahn- und Zahnbetterkrankungen beim alternden Elch (Alces alces): Ein Beitrag zur vergleichenden Parodontologie. Zeitschrift für Jagdwissenschaft 28: 123–130.

2054. Schüller, H. 1938. Die Entwicklung des Geruchorgans bei der Sturmmöve und der Seeschwalbe. Zeitschrift für Anatomie und Entwicklungsgeschichte 109: 75–98.

2055. Schulter, F. P. 1976. Studies of the basicranial axis: A brief review. American Journal of Physical Anthropology 45: 545–552.

2056. Schultz, A. H. 1969. The skeleton of the chimpanzee. In The Chimpanzee, vol. 1, G. H. Bourne, ed. Basel: Karger, pp. 50–103.

2057. Schultz, L. P. 1957. The frogfishes of the family Antennariidae. Proceedings of the U.S. National Museum: 47–105.

2058. Schumacher, B., K.-U. Schumacher, and T. Koppe. 1989. Funktionelle morphologie des maxillo-mandibularen apparatus beim miniaturschwein minilewe. 9. Metrische untersuchungen am schadel und unterkiefer. Anatomische Anzeiger 168: 27–36.

2059. Schumacher, G. H. 1963. Zur Morphogenese des Osteocraniums der Lariden. Wissenschaftliche Zeitschrift, Universität Rostock 12: 757–797.

2060. Schumacher, G. H. 1973a. The head muscles and hyolaryngeal skeleton of turtles and crocodilians. In *Biology of the Reptilia*, vol. 4, C. Gans and T. S. Parsons, eds. London: Academic Press, pp. 101–199.

2061. Schumacher, G. H. 1973b. Problems of skull morphogenesis. Deutsch Zahn-Mund-und Kieferheilkunde 60: 145–147.

2062. Schumacher, G. H. 1985. Factors influencing craniofacial growth. In *Normal and Abnormal Growth: Basic and Clinical Research*, Progress in Clinical and Biological Research, vol. 187, A. D. Dixon and B. G. Sarnat, eds. New York: Alan R. Liss, pp. 3–22.

2063. Schumacher, G. H., E. Freund, K. Kremp, and T. Krohn. 1972. Über die Morphogenese des Osteokraniums von *Larus ridibundus* L.: Eine vergleichende Studie auf der Basis von Rekonstruktionsmodellen und Aufhellungspräparaten. Gegenbaurs Morphologisches Jahrbuch, Leipzig 118: 589–606.

2064. Schumacher, G. H., H. Kammel, J. Fanghaenel, E. Schultz, and R. Fanghaenel. 1973. Das Skelettsystem des Syrischen Goldhamster, *Mesocricetus auratus* (Waterhouse): V. Der Schaedel als Ganzes: Cranium (Schluss). Zeitschrift für Mersuchstierkunde 15: 122–134.

2065. Schumacher, G. H., E. Wolff, and G. Schultz. 1963. Wachstumsallometrien am Skellet des Goldhamsters (*Mesocricetus auratus* Wtrh). I. Schädel. Gegenbaurs Morphologisches Jahrbuch, Leipzig 105: 205–230.

2066. Schwartz, J. H. 1983. Premaxillary-maxillary suture asymmetry in a juvenile gorilla. Implications for understanding dentofacial growth and development. Folia primatologica 40: 69–80.

2067. Scott, J. H. 1951. The development of joints concerned with early jaw movements in the sheep. Journal of Anatomy, London 85: 36–43.

2068. Scott, J. H. 1953. The cartilage of the nasal septum (a contribution to the study of facial growth). British Dental Journal 95: 37–43.

2069. Scott, J. H. 1954. The growth of the human face. Proceedings of the Royal Society of Medicine 47: 91–100.

2070. Scott, J. H. 1956. Growth at facial sutures. American Journal of Orthodontics 42: 381–387.

2071. Scott, J. H. 1957. Muscle growth and function in relation to skeletal morphology. American Journal of Physical Anthropology 15: 197–234.

2072. Scott, J. H. 1958. The cranial base. American Journal of Physical Anthropology 16: 319–348.

2073. Scott, J. H. 1962. The growth of the cranio-facial skeleton. Irish Journal of Medical Science, 6th ser., 276–286.

2074. Scott, J. H., and N. B. B. Symons. 1974. *Introduction to Dental Anatomy*. 7th ed. Edinburgh: Churchill Livingstone.

2075. Scott, J. P. 1937a. The embryology of the guinea pig. I. A table of normal development. American Journal of Anatomy 60: 397–432.

2076. Scott, J. P. 1937b. The embryology of the guinea pig. III. The development of the polydactylous monster: A case of growth accelerated at a particular period by a semi-dominant lethal gene. Journal of Experimental Zoology 77: 123–157.

2077. Scott, J. P. 1938. The embryology of the guinea pig. II. The polydactylous monster. Journal of Morphology 62: 299–311.

2078. Sedra, S. N. 1949. On the homology of certain elements in the skull of *Bufo regularis* Reuss (Salientia). Proceedings of the Zoological Society of London 119: 633–641.

2079. Sedra, S. N. 1950. The metamorphosis of the jaws and their muscles in the toad *Bufo regularis* Reuss, correlated with the changes in the animal's feeding habits. Proceedings of the Zoological Society of London 120: 405–449.

2080. Sedra, S. N., and M. I. Michael. 1956. The structure of the hyobranchial apparatus of the fully developed tadpole larva of *Bufo regularis* Reuss. Proceedings of the Egyptian Academy of Science 12: 38–46.

2081. Sedra, S. N., and M. I. Michael. 1957. The development of the skull, visceral arches, larynx, and visceral muscles of the South African clawed toad *Xenopus laevis* (Daudin) during the process of metamorphosis (from stage 55 to stage 66). Verhandelingen der Koninklijke nederlandsche akademie van Wetenschaften 51: 1–80.

2082. Sedra, S. N., and M. I. Michael. 1958. The metamorphosis and growth of the hyobranchial apparatus of the Egyptian toad, *Bufo regularis* Reuss. Journal of Morphology 103: 1–30.

2083. Sedra, S. N., and M. I. Michael. 1959. The ontogenesis of the sound conducting apparatus of the Egyptian toad, *Bufo regularis* Reuss, with a review of this apparatus in Salientia. Journal of Morphology 104: 359–375.

2084. Sellman, S. 1946. Some experiments on the determination of the larval teeth in *Ambystoma mexicanum*. Odontologisk Tidskrift 54: 1–128.

2085. Senders, C. W., P. Eisele, L. E. Freeman, and D. P. Sponeberg. 1986. Observations about the normal and abnormal embryogenesis of the canine lip and palate. Journal of Craniofacial Genetics and Developmental Biology 2: 241–248.

2086. Seno T., and P. D. Nieuwkoop. 1958. The autonomous and dependent differentiation of the neural crest in amphibians. Proceedings, Koninklijke nederlandsche akademie van Wetenschaften, ser. C, 61: 489–498.

2087. Sensenig, E. C. 1957. The development of the occipital and cervical segments and their associated structures in human embryos. Contributions to Embryology from the Carnegie Institute, Washington 36: 141–152.

2088. Seshappa, G., and B. S. Bimacher. 1955. Studies on the fishery and biology of the Malabar sole, *Cynoglossus semifasciatus* Day. Indian Journal of Fisheries 2: 180–230.

2089. Seuthe, G. 1980. Neue Erkenntnisse über die Altersbedingte Verknöcherung bei Männlichen cerviden. Zeitschrift für Jagdwissenschaft 26: 230–233.

2090. Severtsov, A. S. 1964. Formation of the tongue in the Hynobiidae. Doklady Akademii Nauk SSSR 154: 731–734.

2091. Severtsov, A. S. 1966. Food-seizing mechanisms in urodele larvae. Doklady Akademii Nauk SSSR 168: 230–233.

2092. Severtsov, A. S. 1968. The evolution of the hyobranchial apparatus of the urodela's larvae. Trudy Zoologicheskogo Instituta Akademiya Nauk SSSR 46: 125–168.

2093. Severtsov, A. S. 1969a. Food seizing mechanism of anuran larvae. Doklady Akademii Nauk SSSR 187: 211–214.

2094. Severtsov, A. S. 1969b. Origin of the basal elements of the hyobranchial skeleton of larvae of amphibians. Doklady Akademii Nauk SSSR 187: 677–680.

2095. Severtsov, A. S. 1971. The mechanism of food capture in tailed amphibians. Doklady Akademii Nauk SSSR 197: 728–730.

2096. Shah, R. M., and A. P. Chaudhry. 1974a. Light microscopic and histochemical observations on the development of the palate in the golden Syrian hamster. Journal of Anatomy, London 117: 1–15.

2097. Shah, R. M., and A. P. Chaudhry. 1974b. Ultrastructural observations on closure of the soft palate in hamsters. Teratology 10: 17–30.

2098. Shah, R. M., K. M. Cheng, R. Suen, and A. Wong. 1985. An ultrastuctural and histochemical study of the development of secondary palate in Japanese quail, *Coturnix coturnix japonica*. Journal of Craniofacial Genetics and Developmental Biology 5: 41–57.

2099. Shah, R. M., and M. W. J. Ferguson. 1988. Histological evidence of fusion between posterior palatal shelves and the floor of the mouth in *Alligator mississippiensis*. Archives of Oral Biology 33: 769–771.

2100. Shapovalov, Y. N. 1979. Morphological characteristics of definitive and provisory structures in the normal human 17-day-old embryo. Archives d'anatomie, d'histologie, et d'embryologie 77: 25–33.

2101. Sharman, G. B. 1973. Adaptations of marsupial pouch young for extrauterine existence. In *The Mammalian Fetus in Vitro*, C. R. Austin, ed. London: Chapman and Hall, pp. 67–90.

2102. Sharpe, P. M., and M. W. J. Ferguson. 1988. Mesenchymal influences on epithelial differentiation in developing systems. Journal of Cell Science 10 (suppl): 195–230.

2103. Shaw, J. H., E. A. Sweeney, C. C. Capuccino, and S. M. Meller. 1978. *Textbook of Oral Biology*. Philadelphia: W. B. Saunders.

2104. Shaw, J. P. 1986. The functional significance of the pterygomaxillary ligament in *Xenopus laevis* (Amphibia: Anura). Journal of Zoology, London 208A: 469–473.

2105. Shaw, J. P. 1988. A quantitative comparison of osteoclasts in the teeth of the anuran amphibian *Xenopus laevis*. Archives of Oral Biology 33: 451–453.

2106. Shaw, J. P. 1989. A morphometric study of bone and tooth volumes in the pipid frog *Xenopus laevis* (Daudin), with comments on the importance of tooth resorption during normal tooth replacement. Journal of Experimental Zoology 249: 99–104.

2107. Shea, B. T. 1983a. Size and diet in the evolution of African ape craniodental form. Folia primatologica 40: 32–68.

2108. Shea, B. T. 1983b. Allometry and heterochrony in the African apes. American Journal of Physical Anthropology 62: 275–289.

2109. Shea, B. T. 1983c. Paedomorphosis and neoteny in the pygmy chimpanzee. Science 222: 521–522.

2110. Shea, B. T. 1985a. Ontogenetic allometry and scaling: A discussion based on the growth and form of the skull in African apes. In *Size and Scaling in Primate Biology*, W. L. Jungers, ed. New York: Plenum Press, pp. 175–206.

2111. Shea, B. T. 1985b. On aspects of skull form in African apes and orangutans with implications for Hominoid evolution. American Journal of Physical Anthropology, ser. 2, 68: 329–342.

2112. Shea, B. T. 1985c. Bivariate and multivariate growth allometry: Statistical and biological considerations. Journal of Zoology, London 206: 367–390.

2113. Shea, B. T. 1985d. The ontogeny of sexual dimorphism in the African apes. American Journal of Primatology 8: 183–188.

2114. Shea, B. T. 1986. On skull form and the supraorbital torus in Primates. Current Anthropology 27: 257–259.

2115. Shea, B. T., and A. M. Gomez. 1988. Tooth scaling and evolutionary dwarfism: An investigation of allometry in human pygmies. American Journal of Physical Anthropology 77: 117–132.

2116. Sheller, B., S. K. Clarren, S. J. Astley, and P. D. Sampson. 1988. Morphometric analyses of *Macaca nemestrina* exposed to ethanol during gestation. Teratology 38: 411–417.

2117. Shimizu, H. 1987. Bone abnormalities of hatchery-reared black porgy— *Acanthopagrus schlegeli* (Bleekea). Bulletin of the Tokai Regional Fisheries Research Laboratory, no. 122: 1–11.

2118. Shinkareva, E. V. 1972. Some interrelations between the structure of the periosteum and osseous tissues of the flat bones of the vault of the human skull. Nauchnye Trudy Irkutskii Meditsinskii Institut 114: 35–41.

2119. Shirota, A. 1978a. Studies on the mouth size of fish larvae. II. Specific characteristics of the upper jaw length. Bulletin of the Japanese Society of Scientific Fisheries 44: 1171–1177.

2120. Shirota, A. 1978b. Studies on the mouth size of fish larvae. III. Relationship between inflection point of the upper jaw growth and morphological-ecological change. Bulletin of the Japanese Society of Scientific Fisheries 44: 1179–1182.

2121. Shrivastava, R. K. 1963. The structure and the development of the chondrocranium of *Varanus*. Part I. The development of the ethmoidal region. Folia anatomica Japonica 39: 53–83.

2122. Shrivastava, R. K. 1964a. The structure and development of the chondrocranium of *Varanus*. II. The development of the orbito-temporal region. Journal of Morphology 115: 97–108.

2123. Shrivastava, R. K. 1964b. The structure and development of the chondrocranium of *Varanus*. Part III. The otic and occipital regions, basal plate, viscerocranium, and certain features of the osteocranium of a juvenile. Gegenbaurs Morphologisches Jahrbuch 106: 147–187.

2124. Shupe, J. L., A. E. Larsen, and A. E. Olson. 1987. Effects of diets containing sodium fluoride on mink. Journal of Wildlife Diseases 23: 606–613.

2125. Shute, C. C. D. 1956. The evolution of the mammalian eardrum and tympanic cavity. Journal of Anatomy, London 90: 261–281.

2126. Shute, C. D. D. 1972. The composition of vertebrae and the occipital region of the skull. In *Studies in Vertebrate Evolution*, K. A. Joysey and T. Kemp, eds. Edinburgh: Oliver and Boyd, pp. 21–34.

2127. Siebert, J. R. 1986. Prenatal growth of the median face. American Journal of Medical Genetics 25: 369–380.

2128. Siebert, J. R., G. A. Machin, and G. H. Sperber. 1989. Anatomic findings in dicephalic conjoined twins: Implications for morphogenesis. Teratology 40: 305–310.

2129. Siegel, M. I. 1979. A longitudinal study of facial growth in *Papio cynocephalus* after resection of the cartilaginous nasal septum. Journal of Medical Primatology 8: 122–127.

2130. Siegel, M. I., and D. Sadler. 1979. An x-ray cephalometric analysis of premaxillary growth in operated and unoperated baboons (*Papio cynocephalus*). Journal of Medical Primatology 8: 187–191.

2131. Siegel-Causey, D. 1989. Cranial pneumatization in the Phalacrocoracidae. Wilson Bulletin 101: 108–112.

2132. Signoret, J. 1960. Céphalogenèse ches le triton *Pleurodeles waltlii* Michah après traitement de la gastrula par le chlorure de lithium. Memoires de la Société Zoologique de France 32: 1–117.

2133. Sikorski, M. D. 1982a. Craniometric variation of *Apodemus agrarius* in urban green areas. Acta theriologica 27: 71–82.

2134. Sikorski, M. D. 1982b. Non-metrical divergence of isolated populations of *Apodemus agrarius* in urban areas. Acta theriologica 27: 169–180.

2135. Silbermann, M., and J. Frommer. 1972. The nature of endochondral ossification in the mandibular condyle of the mouse. Anatomical Record 172: 659–668.

2136. Silbermann, M., and D. Lewinson. 1978. An electron microscopic study of the premineralizing zone of the condylar cartilage of the mouse mandible. Journal of Anatomy, London 125: 55–70.

2137. Silva, D. G., and J. A. L. Hart. 1967. Ultrastructural observations on the mandibular condyle of the guinea pig. Journal of Ultrastructural Research 20: 227–243.

2138. Silver, P. H. S. 1962. *In ovo* experiments concerning the eye, the orbit, and certain juxta-orbital structures in the chick embryo. Journal of Embryology and Experimental Morphology 10: 423–450.

2139. Sim, D. W. 1989. Relationship of the primary choanae and anterior cranial base in the mouse embryo. Acta anatomica 134: 242–244.

2140. Simionescu, V., and M. Tarca. 1984. Study of the intraspecific allometry of the house mouse *Mus musculus* L. Analele stiintifice ale Universitatii A1. I. Cuza din Iasi n.s. (Biol.) 30: 26–32.

2141. Simon, K. H. 1981. Contributions to the craniogenesis of *Callithrix jacchus* (Platyrrhini, Primates). Forschungsinstitut Senckenberg, no. 45: 1–106.

2142. Simonetta, A. 1956. Organogenesi e significato morfologico del sistema intertympanico dei Crocodilia. Archivo italiano di anatomia e di embriologia, Florence 61: 335–372.

2143. Simonetta, A. 1957. Condrocranio e dermascheletro di *Chrysochloris asiatica* (Linnaeus). Monitore zoologico italiano 15: 28–47.

2144. Simons, E. L., and W. Meinel. 1983. Mandibular ontogeny in the Miocene great ape *Dryopithecus*. International Journal of Primatology 4: 331–337.

2145. Simons, E. V. 1974. The effects of experimental unilateral anotia on skull development in the chick embryo. I. Introduction, techniques, and preliminary results. Acta morphologica neerlando-scandinavica 12: 331–344.

2146. Simons, E. V. 1975. The effects of experimental unilateral anotia on skull development in the chick embryo. II. Essentials of the development of the chondrocranium in normal embryos of 7–20 days of incubation. Acta morphologica neerlando-scandinavica 13: 287–304.

2147. Simons, E. V. 1976. The effects of experimental unilateral anotia on skull development in the chick embryo. III. Chondrocranial development in anotic embryos of 7–20 days of incubation. Acta morphologica neerlando-scandinavica 14: 61–78.

2148. Simons, E. V. 1977. The effects of experimental unilateral anotia on skull development in the chick embryo. IV. Development of the bony skull in embryos of 9–20 days of incubation. Acta morphologica neerlando-scandinavica 15: 75–87.

2149. Simons, E. V. 1979a. The effects of experimental unilateral anotia on skull development in the chick embryo. V. The development of the brain and its meningeal envelope in embryos of 9–20 days of incubation. Acta morphologica neerlando-scandinavica 17: 53–63.

2150. Simons, E. V. 1979b. *Control Mechanisms of Skull Morphogenesis: A Study on Unilaterally Anotic Chick Embryos*. Lisse: Swets and Zeitlinger B.V.

2151. Simons, E. V., and J. van Limborgh. 1979. The effects of experimental unilateral anotia on skull development in the chick embryo. VI. Discussion of the results in relation to the problem of the control of skull morphogenesis. Acta morphologica neerlando-scandinavica 17: 81–103.

2152. Singh-Roy, K. K. 1967. On Goethe's vertebral theory of origin of the skull: A recent approach. Anatomisches Anzeiger 120: 250–259.

2153. Sinning, A. R., and M. D. Olson. 1988. Surface coat material associated with the developing otic placode/vesicle in the chick. Anatomical Record 220: 198–207.

2154. Sirianni, J. E. 1985. Nonhuman primates as models for human craniofacial growth. Monographs in Primatology 6: 95–124.

2155. Sirianni, J. E., and L. Newell-Morris. 1980. Craniofacial growth of fetal *Macaca nemestrina*: A cephalometric roentgenographic study. American Journal of Physical Anthropology 53: 407–421.

2156. Sirianni, J. E., L. Newell-Morris, and M. Campbell. 1981. Growth of the fetal pigtailed macaque (*Macaca nemestrina*). 1. Cephalofacial dimensions. Folia primatologica 35: 65–75.

2157. Sirianni, J. E., and D. R. Swindler. 1984. Growth and development of the pigtailed macaque. Boca Raton: CRC Press.

2158. Sirianni, J. E., and A. L. Van Ness. 1978. Postnatal growth of the cranial base in *Macaca nemestrina*. American Journal of Physical Anthropology 49: 329–340.

2159. Sitt, W. 1943. Zur Morphologie des Primordialcraniums und des Osteo-craniums eines Embryos von *Rhinolophus rouxii* von 15 mm Scheitel-Steiß-Länge. Gegenbaurs Morphologisches Jahrbuch 88: 268–342.

2160. Sive, H. L., K. Hattori, and H. Weintraub. 1989. Progressive determination during formation of the anteroposterior axis in *Xenopus laevis*. Cell 58: 171–180.

2161. Skinner, M. M. 1973. Ontogeny and adult morphology of the skull of the South African skink, *Mabuya capensis* (Gray). Annals of the University of Stellenbosch 48: 1–116.

2162. Skoudlin, J. 1975–76. Variability of the skull size of our hedgehog (*Erinaceus europaeus* and *Erinaceus concolor*). Acta Universitatis Carolinae biologica 15: 209–245.

2163. Skreb, N. 1952. Étude des rapports topographiques de la chorde céphalique et de la plaque préchordale chez les Amphibiens. Archives de biologie, Brussels 63: 85–108.

2164. Slaby, O. 1951. Le développement du chondrocrâne du cormorant, *Phalacrocorax carbo* L. au point de vue de l'évolution. Bulletin international, Académie de Prague 52: 1–47.

2165. Slaby, O. 1953. Le développement de chondrocrâne du cormorant (*Phalacrocorax carbo* L.) au point de vue de l'évolution. Bulletin international, Académie de Prague 52: 105–151.

2166. Slaby, O. 1954. Morfogenza epiteliální trubice nosni. O Morphogenese des epithelialen Nasenschlauches und der knorpeligen Nasenkapsel beim Fischreiher, *Ardea cinerea* L. Ceskoslovenská morfologie, Prague 2: 207–227.

2167. Slaby, O. 1956. The morphogenesis and the morphological interpretation of the processes basitrabeculares and infrapolares of the primordial skull of birds. Ceskoslovenská morfologie, Prague 4: 276–293.

2168. Slaby, O. 1959. Stadium zum Problem des segmentaten Ursprungs der Occipitalregion des Vogelschädels. Gegenbaurs Morphologisches Jahrbuch 99: 752–794.

2169. Slaby, O. 1960. Die frühe Morphogenesis der Nasenkapsel beim Menschen. Acta anatomica 42: 105–175.

2170. Slaby, O. 1979a. Morphogenesis of the nasal capsule, the epithelial nasal tube, and the organ of Jacobson in Sauropsida. I. Introduction and morphogenesis of the nasal apparatus in members of the families Lacertidae and Scincidae. Folia morphologica, Prague 27: 245–258.

2171. Slaby, O. 1979b. Morphogenesis of the nasal capsule, the epithelial nasal tube, and the organ of Jacobson in Sauropsida. II. Morphogenesis of the nasal apparatus in *Gecko verticillatus*. Folia morphologica, Prague 27: 270–281.

2172. Slaby, O. 1979c. Morphogenesis of the nasal capsule, the epithelial nasal tube, and the organ of Jacobson in Sauropsida. III. Morphogenesis of the nasal apparatus in a member of the family Varanidae. Folia morphologica, Prague 27: 259–269.

2173. Slaby, O. 1981. Morphogenesis of the nasal capsule, the epithelial nasal tube, and the organ of Jacobson in Sauropsida. IV. Morphogenesis of the nasal capsule, the nasal epithelial tube, and the organ of Jacobson in a member of the family Agamidae. Folia morphologica, Prague 29: 305–317.

2174. Slaby, O. 1982a. Morphogenesis of the nasal capsule, the epithelial nasal tube, and the organ of Jacobson in Sauropsida. V. Contribution to knowledge of the early morphogenesis of the nasal apparatus in Teidae. Folia morphologica, Prague 30: 20–25.

2175. Slaby, O. 1982b. Morphogenesis of the nasal capsule, the epithelial nasal tube, and the organ of Jacobson in Sauropsida. VI. Morphogenesis of the nasal capsule, the epithelial nasal tube, and the organ of Jacobson in *Iguana iguana* Shaw. Folia morphologica, Prague 30: 75–85.

2176. Slaby, O. 1982c. Morphogenesis of the nasal capsule, the epithelial nasal tube, and the organ of Jacobson in Sauropsida. VII. Morphogenesis and phylogenetic morphology of the nasal apparatus in *Calotes jubatus* O.B. Folia morphologica, Prague 30: 238–248.

2177. Slaby, O. 1984a. Morphogenesis of the nasal capsule, the epithelial nasal tube, and the organ of Jacobson in Sauropsida. VIII. Morphogenesis of the nasal apparatus in a member of the genus *Chamaeleon* L. Folia morphologica, Prague 32: 225–246.

2178. Slaby, O. 1984b. Morphogenesis of the nasal capsule, nasal epithelial tube, and organ of Jacobson in Sauropsida. IX. Morphogenesis and evolutionary morphology of the nasal apparatus of the black-headed gull (*Larus ridibundus* L.). Folia morphologica, Prague 32: 361–378.

2179. Slaby, O. 1984c. Morphogenesis of the nasal capsule, the epithelial nasal tube, and the organ of Jacobson in Sauropsida. X. Contribution to knowledge of the nasal apparatus in the little grebe, *Podiceps ruficollis* Pall. Bulletin of the Zoological Society of Czechoslovakia 48: 302–307.

2180. Slaby, O. 1984d. Early morphogenesis of the nasal apparatus in the little grebe (*Podiceps ruficollis*) (Aves). Vestnik Ceskoslovenska Spolecnosti Zoologiske 48: 202–207.

2181. Slaby, O. 1985a. Morphogenesis of the nasal capsule, the epithelial nasal tube, and the organ of Jacobson in Sauropsida. X. Morphogenesis and evolutionary morphology of the nasal apparatus of the black-headed gull *Larus ridibundus* L. 2. A morphological interpretation of individual structures. Folia morphologica, Prague 33: 1–21.

2182. Slaby, O. 1985b. Development and comparative morphology of the nasal apparatus of the rook (*Corvus frugilegus* L.) (Morphogenesis of the nasal capsule, the nasal epithelial tube, and the organ of Jacobson in Sauropsida. XI). Folia morphologica, Prague 33: 48–62.

2183. Slaby, O. 1985c. Contribution to knowledge of the development and comparative morphogenesis of the nasal apparatus of the white pelican *Pelecanus onocrotalus* L. (Morphogenesis of the nasal capsule, the nasal epithelial tube, and the organ of Jacobson in Sauropsida. XII). Folia morphologica, Prague 33: 63–69.

2184. Slaby, O. 1985d. Contribution to the knowledge of the comparative morphogenesis of the nasal apparatus in the white stork, *Ciconia ciconia* L. (Morphogenesis of the nasal capsule, the epithelial nasal tube, and the organ of Jacobson in Sauropsida. XIII). Folia morphologica, Prague 33: 91–98.

2185. Slaby, O. 1985e. Morphogenesis and comparative morphology of the nasal apparatus in the swallow (*Hirundo rustica* L.) (Morphogenesis of the nasal capsule, the epithelial nasal tube, and the organ of Jacobson in Sauropsida. XV). Folia morphologica, Prague 33: 181–191.

2186. Slaby, O. 1985f. On a few embryonic structures forming evolutionary connections between the two Sauropsida classes (Morphogenesis of the nasal capsule, the epithelial nasal tube, and the organ of Jacobson in Sauropsida. XVI). Folia morphologica, Prague 33: 192–200.

2187. Slaby, O. 1985g. On the continuing differentiation of so-called specialized structures. Folia zoologica 34: 43–55.

2188. Slaby, O. 1986a. A few morphological features of interest in development of the nasal apparatus in the magpie (*Pica pica* L.) (Morphogenesis of the nasal capsule, the epithelial nasal tube, and the organ of Jacobson in Sauropsida. XVII). Folia morphologica, Prague 34: 26–35.

2189. Slaby, O. 1986b. "Biometabolische Modi" and heterochrony in the phylembryogenesis of the nasal apparatus of birds. Folia morphologica, Prague 34: 430–438.

2190. Slaby, O. 1986c. Integration and dissociability in the development of specializations in Sauropsida. Folia morphologica, Prague 34: 439–448.

2191. Slaby, O. 1987a. Contribution to a knowledge of the morphogenesis of the nasal apparatus of the dromedary (*Camelus dromedarius* L.). Folia morphologica, Prague 35: 400–409.

2192. Slaby, O. 1987b. Morphological differences between the structure of the nasal apparatus of the swift (*Apus apus* L.) and the common "avian typus" during morphogenesis (Morphogenesis of the nasal capsule, the epithelial nasal tube, and the organ of Jacobson in Sauropsida). Folia morphologica, Prague 35: 436–440.

2193. Slack, H. E., III. 1979. Abnormal maxilla in a tufted titmouse: Probable cause and growth. North American Bird Banding 4: 112.

2194. Slagsvold, T. 1983. Morphology of the hooded crow *Corvus corone cornix* in relation to age, sex, and latitude. Journal of Zoology, London 199: 325–344.

2195. Slavkin, H. C. 1984. Morphogenesis of a complex organ—vertebrate palate development. In *Palate Development: Normal and Abnormal Cellular and Molecular Aspects*, E. F. Zimmerman, ed., Current Topics in Developmental Biology, vol. 19. Orlando: Academic Press, pp. 1–16.

2196. Slavkin, H. C., and L. A. Bavetta. 1972. *Developmental Aspects of Oral Biology*. New York: Academic Press.

2197. Slavkin, H. C., P. Bringas, Jr., O. Y. Sasai, and M. Mayo. 1989. Early embryonic mouse mandibular morphogenesis and cytodifferentiation in serumless, chemically-defined medium: A model for studies of autocrine and/or paracrine regulatory factors. Journal of Craniofacial Genetics and Developmental Biology 9: 185–206.

2198. Slepzov, M. M. 1940. Development of the osteocranium of the Odontoceti during ontogenesis and phylogenesis. Doklady Akademii Nauk SSSR 28: 363–366.

2199. Slipka, J. 1972. Early development of the bursa pharyngea. Folia morphologica, Prague 20: 138–140.

2200. Smeele, L. E. 1988. Ontogeny of relationship of human middle ear and temporomandibular (squamomandibular) joint. 1. Morphology and ontogeny in man. Acta anatomica 131: 338–341.

2201. Smeele, L. E. 1989. Ontogeny of relationship of middle ear and temporomandibular (squamomandibular) joint in mammals. 2. Morphology and ontogeny in insectivores. Acta anatomica 134: 62–66.

2202. Smirnov, S. 1986. The evolution of the urodelan sound-conducting apparatus. In *Studies in Herpetology*, Z. Roček, ed. Prague: Charles University, pp. 55–58.

2203. Smirnov, S. V. 1988. Morphofunctional factors responsible for the diversification of the amphibian sound-conducting apparatus. In *Current Problems in Evolutionary Morphology*, Moscow: Nauka, pp. 117–136.

2204. Smirnov, S. V. 1989. Postembryonic skull development in *Bombina orientalis* (Amphibia, Discoglossidae), with comments on neoteny. Zoologisches Anzeiger 223: 91–99.

2205. Smirnov, S. V., and E. I. Vorobyeva. 1986. The sound-conducting apparatus of anurans and urodeles and the problem of their origin. In *Morphology and Animal Evolution*, E. I. Vorobyeva and N. S. Lebedkina, eds. Moscow: Nauka, pp. 156–179.

2206. Smirnov, S. V., and E. I. Vorobyeva. 1988. Morphological grounds for diversification and evolutionary change in the amphibian sound-conducting apparatus. Anatomischer Anzeiger 166: 317–322.

2207. Smit, A. L. 1949. Skedelmorfologie en Kinese van *Typhlops delalandii* (Schlegel). South African Journal of Science 45: 117–140.

2208. Smit, A. L. 1953. The ontogenesis of the vertebral column of *Xenopus laevis* Daud., with special reference to the segmentation of the metotic region of the skull. Annals of the University of Stellenbosch 29: 79–136.

2209. Smit, A. L., and G. H. Frank. 1979. Aspects of the ontogenesis of the avian columella auris. South African Journal of Zoology 14: 23–35.

2210. Smith, M. M. 1977. The microstructure of the dentition and dermal ornament of three dipnoans from the Devonian of Western Australia: A contribution towards dipnoan interrelationships, and morphogenesis, growth, and adaptation of the skeletal tissues. Philosophical Transactions of the Royal Society, London 281B: 29–72.

2211. Smith, M. M. 1985. The pattern of histogenesis and growth of tooth plates in larval stages of extant lungfish. Journal of Anatomy, London 140: 627–643.

2212. Smith, R. J. 1981. On the definition of variables in studies of primate dental allometry. American Journal of Physical Anthropology 55: 323–329.

2213. Smith, W. P. 1979. Timing of skull ossification in the kinglets. North American Bird Banding 4: 103–105.

2214. Smits-van Prooije, A. E., C. Vermeij-Keers, J. A. Dubbeldam, M. M. T. Mentink, and R. E. Poelmann. 1987. The formation of mesoderm and mesectoderm in presomite rat embryos cultured *in vitro*, using WGA-Au as a marker. Anatomy and Embryology 176: 71–77.

2215. Smits-van Prooije, A. E., C. Vermeij-Keers, R. E. Poelmann, M. M. T. Mentink, and J. A. Dubbeldam. 1985. The neural crest in presomite to 40-somite murine embryos. Acta morphologica neerlando-scandinavica 23: 99–114.

2216. Smits-van Prooije, A. E., C. Vermeij-Keers, R. E. Poelmann, M. M. T. Mentink, and J. A. Dubbeldam. 1988. The formation of mesoderm and mesectoderm in 5-to 41-somite rat embryos cultured *in vitro,* using WGA-Au as a marker. Anatomy and Embryology 177: 245–256.

2217. Smuts, G. L., J. L. Anderson, and J. C. Austin. 1978. Age determination of the African lion (*Panthera leo*). Journal of Zoology, London 185: 115–146.

2218. Sneath, P. H. A. 1967. Trend-surface analysis of transformation grids. Journal of Zoology, London 151: 65–122.

2219. Sohal, G. S. 1976. Effects of reciprocal forebrain transplantation on motility and hatching in chick and duck embryos. Brain Research 113: 35–43.

2220. Sokol, O. M. 1959. Studien an pipiden froschen. I. Die Kaulquappe von *Hymenochirus curtipes* Noble. Zoologisches Anzeiger 162: 154–160.

2221. Sokol, O. M. 1962. The tadpole of *Hymenochirus boettgeri.* Copeia: 272–284.

2222. Sokol, O. M. 1969. Feeding in *Hymenochirus boettgeri.* Herpetologica 25: 9–24.

2223. Sokol, O. M. 1975. The phylogeny of anuran larvae: A new look. Copeia: 1–24.

2224. Sokol, O. M. 1977. The free swimming *Pipa* larvae, with a review of pipid larvae and pipid phylogeny (Anura: Pipidae). Journal of Morphology 154: 357–426.

2225. Sokol, O. M. 1981. The larval chondrocranium of *Pelodytes punctatus,* with a review of tadpole chondrocrania. Journal of Morphology 169: 161–183.

2226. Sokolov, V. E., G. G. Markov, A. A. Danilkin, K. M. Nikolov, and S. Gerasimov. 1985. A comparative craniometric study of the development of the European roe (*Capreolus capreolus* L.) and the tartarian roe (*C. pygargus* Pall.). Doklady Akademii Nauk SSSR 282: 243–247.

2227. Soliman, M. A., H. G. Hammouda, and F. M. Mokhtar. 1972. The development of the osteocranium of a young nestling of *Upupa epops major* (Egyptian hoopoe). I. The membrane bones and the articular. Bulletin of the Faculty of Science, Cairo University 45: 239–270.

2228. Solov'ev, V. A. 1984. Ontogenetic correlations of the skull morphological features in *Castor fiber* in the northeast of the European part of the USSR. Zoologicheskii zhurnal 63: 598–606.

2229. Somasundarum, B., P. E. King, and S. E. Shackley. 1984. Some morphological effects of zinc upon the yolk-sac larvae of *Clupea harengus.* Journal of Fish Biology 25: 333–343.

2230. Soni, D. D., and B. K. Shrivastava. 1985. The paraphyseal/epiphyseal bar in *Mollienisia sphenops.* Folia morphologica, Prague 33: 230–235.

2231. Spatz, W. B. 1964. Beitrag zur Kenntnis der Ontogenese des Cranium von *Tupaia glis* (Diard 1820). Gegenbaurs Morphologisches Jahrbuch, Leipzig 106: 321–416.

2232. Spatz, W. B. 1966. Zur Ontogenese der Bulla tympanica von *Tupaia glis* Diard 1829 (Prosimiae, Tupaiiformes). Folia primatologica 4: 26–50.

2233. Spatz, W. B. 1967. Zur Ontogenese der Cartilago Meckeli und der Symphysis mandibularis bei *Tupaia glis* (Diard 1820): Die distale Verknöcherung des Meckelschen Knorpels als funktionelle Anpassung an den Saugakt. Folia primatologica 6: 180–203.

2234. Spatz, W. B. 1970. Binocular vision and skull form: A contribution to the problem of the alteration of the shape of the primate skull, especially of the skull of Lorisidae. Acta anatomica 75: 489–520.

2235. Sperber, G. H. 1981. *Craniofacial Embryology*. Dental Practitioners Handbook no. 15, 3d ed. Bristol: Wright PGS.

2236. Spillmann, M. J. 1938. Quelques cas de malformations céphaliques chez la carpe. Bulletin de la Société centrale aquiculture et de la pêche 45: 70–73.

2237. Sprankel, H. 1958. Beiträge zur Entwicklungsgeschichte der Praechordalen Region. Verhandlungen der Deutschen zoologischen Gesellschaft, Leipzig 23: 406–418.

2238. Spyropoulos, M. N. 1977. The morphogenetic relationship of the temporal muscle to the coronoid process in human embryos and fetuses. American Journal of Anatomy 150: 395–410.

2239. Srinivasa, R. K., and K. Lakshmi. 1984. Head skeleton of the marine catfish *Arius tenuispinus* Day (Osteichthyes: Siluriformes, Ariidae). Journal of Morphology 181: 221–238.

2240. Srinivasachar, H. R. 1953. The development of the chondrocranium in *Ophicephalus*. Zoological Journal of the Linnean Society 42: 238–259.

2241. Srinivasachar, H. R. 1955. Observations on the development of the chondrocranium in *Vipera*. Anatomischer Anzeiger 101: 219–225.

2242. Srinivasachar, H. R. 1957a. Development of the skull in catfishes. Part I. Development of the chondrocranium in *Silonia, Pangasius,* and *Ailia* (Schilberdae). Proceedings of the National Institute of Science of India, sec. B, Biological Sciences 22: 335–356.

2243. Srinivasachar, H. R. 1957b. Development of the skull in catfishes. Part II. Development of the chondrocranium in *Mystus* and *Rita* (Bagridae). Gegenbaurs Morphologisches Jahrbuch 98: 244–262.

2244. Srinivasachar, H. R. 1957c. Development of the skull in catfishes. Part IV. The development of chondrocranium in *Arius jella* Day (Aridae) and *Plotosus canius* Ham. (Plotosidae) with an account of their interrelationships. Gegenbaurs Morphologisches Jahrbuch 99: 986–1016.

2245. Srinivasachar, H. R. 1958. Development of the skull in catfishes. Part V. Development of the skull in *Heteropneustes fossilis* (Bloch). Proceedings of the National Institute of Science, India 24B: 165–190.

2246. Srinivasachar, H. R. 1961. Development of the skull in catfishes. Part III. Development of the chondrocranium in *Heteropneustes fossilis* (Bloch) (Heteropneustidae) and *Clarias batrachus* (Linn.) (Clariidae). Gegenbaurs Morphologisches Jahrbuch 101: 373–405.

2247. Srinivasachar, H. R. 1962. Development and morphology of the skull of *Rhyacotriton olympicus olympicus* Gaige (Amphibia, Urodela, Ambystomatidae). Gegenbaurs Morphologisches Jahrbuch 103: 263–302.

2248. Srinivasachar, H. R. 1980. Evolution and taxonomy of catfishes of India. Proceedings of the Indian National Science Academy, pt. B, Biological Science 46: 23–26.

2249. Srivastava, H. C. 1977. Development of the ossification centres in the squamous portion of the occipital bone in man. Journal of Anatomy, London 124: 643–649.

2250. Stadtmüller, F. 1937. Das Os parahyoideum (Fuchs) bei *Liopelma hochstetteri* und *Rhinophrynus dorsalis* mit Bemerkungen über der gesamten Zungenbein-Kehlkoff-Apparat dieser seltenen Froschlurche. Gegenbaurs Morphologisches Jahrbuch 78: 1–35.

2251. Starck, D. 1937. Über einige Entwicklungsvorgänge am Kopf der Urodelen. Morphologisches Jahrbuch 79: 358–435.

2252. Starck, D. 1940. Über die rudimentaren Zahnanlagen und einige weitere Besonderkeiten der Mundhöhle von *Manis javanica*. Anatomisches Anzeiger 89: 305–315.

2253. Starck, D. 1941. Zur Morphologie des Primordialcraniums von *Manis javanica* Desm. Gegenbaurs Morphologisches Jahrbuch 86: 1–122.

2254. Starck, D. 1943. Beitrag zur Kenntnis der Morphologie und Entwicklungsgeschichte der Chiropterencraniums: Das chondrocranium von *Pteropus semindus*. Zeitschrift für Anatomie und Entwicklungsgeschichte 112: 588–633.

2255. Starck, D. 1952. Vergleichende Entwicklungsgeschichte der Wirbeltiere (1944–1950, mit Nachträgen aus der Jahren 1940–1943). Fortschritte der Zoologie, Jena 9: 249–367.

2256. Starck, D. 1959. Ontogenie und Entwicklungs Physiologie der Säugetiere. Handbuch der Zoologie, Berlin, Band 22, Teil 9 (7): 1–276.

2257. Starck, D. 1960a. Das Cranium eines Schimpansenfetus (*Pan troglodytes,* Blumenbach, 1799) von 71 mm SchStlg., nebst Bemerkungen über die Körperform von Schimpansenfetus (Beitrag zur Kenntnis des Primatencraniums II). Gegenbaurs Morphologisches Jahrbuch 100: 559–647.

2258. Starck, D. 1960b. Über ein Anlagerungsgelenk zwischen Unterkiefer und Schädelbasis bei den Mausvögeln (Coliidae). Zoologisches Anzeiger 164: 1–11.

2259. Starck, D. 1961. Ontogenetic development of the skull in primates. K. Medelelingen van de Vlaamsche Academie voor Wetenschapen, Letteren en Schoone Kunsten van België, Brussels 1: 205–214.

2260. Starck, D. 1962. Das Cranium von *Propithecus* spec. (Prosimiae, Lemuriformes, Indriidae) (Beitrag zur Kenntnis des Primaten-Craniums III). Bibliotheca primatologica 1: 163–196.

2261. Starck, D. 1963. Die Metamerie des Kopfes der Wirbeltiere. Zoologisches Anzeiger 170: 393–428.

2262. Starck, D. 1964. Über das Entotympanicum der Canidae und Ursidae (Mammalia, Carnivora, Fissipedia). Acta theriologica, Warsaw 8: 181–188.

2263. Starck, D. 1967. Le crâne des mammifères. In *Traité de zoologie: Anatomie, systématique, biologie,* vol. 16(1), *Mammifères, téguments, squelette,* P.-P. Grassé, ed. Paris: Masson et Cie, pp. 404–549.

2264. Starck, D. 1970a. Parallel development with specialisation during the evolution of the bird skull. Annals of the University of Stellenbosch, ser. A, 44: 217–228.

2265. Starck, D. 1970b. Specializations of the skull in mammals. Annals of the University of Stellenbosch, ser. A, 44: 241–249.

2266. Starck, D. 1973. The skull of the fetal chimpanzee: Chondrocranium and development of the osteocranium. In *The Chimpanzee*, G. H. Bourne, ed. Basel: S. Karger, pp. 1–33.

2267. Starck, D. 1975a. The development of the chondrocranium in primates. In *Phylogeny of the Primates*, W. P. Luckett and F. S. Szalay, eds. New York: Plenum Press, pp. 127–155.

1168. Starck, D. 1975b. *Embryologie: Ein Luhrbuch auf allgemein biologischer Grundlage.* 3d ed. Stuttgart.

2269. Starck, D. 1978. Das evolutive plateau Säugetier. Sonderbände des naturwissenschaftlichen Vereins im Hamburg 3: 7–30.

2270. Starck, D. 1979a. Cranio-cerebral relations in recent reptiles. In *Biology of the Reptilia*, C. Gans, R. G. Northcutt, and P. Ulinski, eds. vol. 9A. London: Academic Press, pp. 1–38.

2271. Starck, D. 1979b. *Vergleichende der Wirbeltiere auf evolutionsbiologischer Grundlage*, Band 2, *Das Skeletsystem: Allgemeines, Skeletsubstanzen, Skelet der Wirbeltiere einschliesslich Lokomotionstypen.* Berlin: Springer-Verlag.

2272. Starck, D. 1982a. *Vergleichende Anatomie der Wirbeltiere auf evolutionsbiologischer Grundlage*, Band 3, *Organe des aktiven Bewegungsapparates, der Koordination, der Umweltbeziehung, des Stoffwechsels und der Fortpflanzung.* Berlin: Springer-Verlag.

2273. Starck, D. 1982b. Zur Kenntnis der Nase und des Nasenskeletts von *Tarsius* (Mammalia, Primates, Tarsioidea). Zoologische Garten 52: 289–304.

2274. Starck, D. 1984. The nasal cavity and nasal skeleton of *Tarsius*. In *Biology of Tarsiers*, C. Niemitz, ed. Stuttgart: Gustav-Fischer Verlag, pp. 275–290.

2275. Starck, D. 1989. Considerations on the nature of skeletal elements in the vertebrate skull, especially in mammals. In *Trends in Vertebrate Morphology*, Fortschritte der Zoologie, vol. 35, H. Splechtna and H. Hilgers, eds. Stuttgart: Gustav-Fischer Verlag, pp. 375–385.

2276. Starck, D., and B. Kummer. 1962. Zur Ontogenese des Schimpansenschädels (mit Bemerkungen zur Fetalisationshypothese). Anthropologische Anzeiger, Stuttgart 25: 204–215.

2277. Starrett, P. H. 1973. Evolutionary patterns in larval morphology. In *Evolutionary Biology of the Anurans*, J. L. Vial, ed. Columbia: University of Missouri Press, pp. 251–271.

2278. Steffek, A. J., D. K. Mujwid, and M. C. Johnston. 1979. Scanning electron microscopy of cranial neural crest migration in chick embryos. In *Developmental Aspects of Craniofacial Dysmorphology*, Birth Defects: Original Article Series, vol. 15(8), M. Melnick and R. Jorgensen, eds. New York: Alan R. Liss, pp. 11–22.

2279. Stein, D. L., and C. E. Bond. 1985. Observations on the morphology, ecology, and behaviour of *Bathylychnops exilis* Cohen. Journal of Fish Biology 27: 215–228.

2280. Stempniewicz, L. 1982. Body proportions in adults and fledglings of the little auk, *Plautus alle*. Acta zoologica, Cracow 26: 149–158.

2281. Stensiö, E. A. 1947. The sensory lines and dermal bones of the cheek of fishes and amphibians. Kungliga Svenska vetenskapsakademiens handlingar, Uppsala and Stockholm, ser. 3, 24: 1–195.

2282. Stephenson, A. B. 1977. Age determination and morphological variation of Ontario otters. Canadian Journal of Zoology 55: 1577–1583.

2283. Stephenson, E. M. T. 1951. The anatomy of the head of the New Zealand frog *Leiopelma*. Transactions of the Zoological Society, London 27: 255–305.

2284. Stephenson, E. M. T. 1960. The skeletal characters of *Leiopelma hamiltoni* McCullock, with particular reference to the effects of heterochrony on the genus. Transactions of the Royal Society of New Zealand 88: 473–488.

2285. Stephenson, N. G. 1951. On the development of the chondrocranium and visceral arches of *Leiopelma archeyi*. Transactions of the Zoological Society of London 27: 203–253.

2286. Stephenson, N. G. 1955. On the development of the frog, *Leiopelma hochstetteri* Fitzinger. Proceedings of the Zoological Society of London 124: 785–795.

2287. Stephenson, N. G. 1960. The comparative osteology of Australian geckos and its bearing on their morphological status. Journal of the Linnean Society, Zoology 44: 278–299.

2288. Stephenson, N. G. 1962. The comparative morphology of the head skeleton, girdles and hind limbs in the Pygopodidae. Journal of the Linnean Society, Zoology 44: 627–644.

2289. Stephenson, N. G. 1965. Heterochronous changes among Australian leptodactylid frogs. Proceedings of the Zoological Society of London 144: 339–350.

2290. Stephenson, N. G., and E. M. T. Stephenson. 1956. The osteology of the New Zealand geckos and its bearing on their morphological status. Transactions of the Royal Society of New Zealand 84: 341–358.

2291. Stern, C. D., W. E. Norriss, M. Bronner-Fraser, G. J. Carlson, J. R. Faissner, and M. Schachner. 1989. J1/tenascin-related molecules are not responsible for the segmented pattern of neural crest cells or motor axons in the chick embryo. Development 107: 309–320.

2292. Stettler, M. 1978. About the ontogenetic change in form of the skull of African monkeys: *Perodicticus potto* Mueller, 1766 and *Arctocebus calabarensis* Smith, 1860. Archives suisses d'anthropologie générale 42: 1–4.

2293. Stewart, P. A., and D. J. McCallion. 1975. Establishment of the scleral ossicles in the chick. Developmental Biology 46: 383–389.

2294. Stokely, P. S., and J. S. List. 1954. Progress of ossification in the skull of the cricket frog *Pseudacris nigrita triseriata*. Copeia: 211–217.

2295. Stork, H.-J. 1972. Development of pneumatic cavities in the skull of birds (Aves). Zeitschrift für Morphologie der Tiere 73: 81–94.

2296. Strahan, R. 1958. Speculations on the evolution of the Agnathan head. Proceedings of the Centenary and Bicentenary Congress of Biology, Singapore: 83–94.

2297. Straney, D. O. 1984. The nasal bones of *Chiroderma* (Phyllostomidae). Journal of Mammalogy 65: 163–165.

2298. Stratil, Z., and P. Schmid. 1984. Ontogenese des gorillaschädels. Archives suisse d'anthropologie générale 48: 13–24.

2299. Strauss, R. E., and L. A. Fuiman. 1985. Quantitative comparisons of body form and allometry in larval and adult Pacific sculpins (Teleostei: Cottidae). Canadian Journal of Zoology 63: 1582–1589.

2300. Streeter, G. L. 1949. Developmental horizons in human embryos: A review of the histogenesis of cartilage and bone. Contributions to Embryology from the Carnegie Institute of Washington 33: 151–167.

2301. Stuart, C. T., and T. D. Stuart. 1985. Age determination and development of foetal and juvenile *Felis caracal* Schreber, 1776. Säugetierkundliche Mitteilungen 32: 217–229.

2302. Stuart, L. J., and G. V. Morejohn. 1980. Developmental patterns in osteology and external morphology in *Phocaena phocaena*. Report of the International Whaling Commission, Special Issue no. 3: 133–142.

2303. Sturm, C.-D. 1985. Untersuchungen am Chondrocranium der Schleichkatzengattung *Herpestes* ein Beitrag zur vergleichenden: Anatomie der Carnivora. Mitteilungen aus den Hamburgischen Zooligischen Museum und Institut 82 (suppl.): 1–124.

2304. Sturm, H. 1937. Die Entwicklung des Präcerebralen Nasenskelets beim Schwein (*Sus scrofa domestica*) und beim Rind (*Bos taurus*). Zeitschrift für wissenschaftliche Zoologie 149: 161–220.

2305. Sugimori, F., N. Oka, and Y. Ishibashi. 1985. The degree of skull ossification as a means of aging short-tailed shearwaters. Journal of the Yamashina Institute of Ornithology 17: 159–165.

2306. Sulik, K. K., and G. C. Schoenwolf. 1985. Highlights of craniofacial morphogenesis in mammalian embryos as revealed by scanning electron microscopy. Scanning Electron Microscopy: 1735–1752.

2307. Sulimski, A. 1984. A new Cretaceous scincomorph lizard from Mongolia. Palaeontologia polonica, no. 46: 143–156.

2308. Sülter, M. M. 1962. A contribution to the cranial morphology of *Causus rhombeatus* (Lichtenstein) with special reference to cranial kinesis. Annals of the University of Stellenbosch 37A: 1–40.

2309. Suttie, J. M., and P. F. Fennessy. 1985. Regrowth of amputed velvet antlers with and without innervation. Journal of Experimental Zoology 234: 359–366.

2310. Suttie, J. M., P. F. Fennessy, I. D. Corson, F. J. Laas, S. F. Crosbie, J. H. Butler, and P. D. Gluckman. 1989. Pulsatile growth hormone, insulin-like growth factors, and antler development in red deer (*Cervus elaphus scoticus*). Journal of Endocrinology 121: 351–360.

2311. Suttie, J. M., P. F. Fennessy, C. G. Mackintosh, I. D. Corson, R. Christie, and S. W. Heap. 1985. Sequential cranial angiography of young red deer stags. Bulletin of the Royal Society of New Zealand, no. 22: 263–268.

2312. Suttie, J. M., P. D. Gluckman, J. H. Butler, P. F. Fennessy, I. D. Corson, and F. J. Laas. 1985. Insulin-like growth factor (IGF-1): Antler stimulating hormone? Endocrinology 116: 846–848.

2313. Suttie, J. M., and B. Mitchell. 1983. Jaw length and hind foot length as measures of skeletal development of red deer (*Cervus elephus*). Journal of Zoology, London 200: 431–434.

2314. Sutton, J. F. 1972. Notes on skeletal variation, tooth replacement, and cranial suture closure of the porcupine (*Erethizon dorsatum*). Tulane Studies in Zoology and Botany 17: 56–62.

2315. Swanepoel, J. H. 1970. The ontogenesis of the chondrocranium and of the nasal sac of the microhylid frog *Breviceps adspersus pentheri* Werner. Annals of the University of Stellenbosch 45: 1–119.

2316. Swarup, H. 1951. On the development and morphology of the chondrocranium in *Ophiocephalus punctatus* (Bloch). Journal of the Zoological Society of India 3: 119–120.

2317. Swarup, H. 1954. Development of the chondrocranium in *Ophiocephalus punctatus* (Bloch). Saugar University Journal 1: 61–79.

2318. Swatland, H. J. 1980. Development of carcass shape in Pekin and Muscovy ducks. Poultry Science 59: 1773–1776.

2319. Sweet, S. S. 1977. Natural metamorphosis in *Eurycea neotenes*, and the generic allocation of the Texas *Eurycea* (Amphibia: Plethodontidae). Herpetologica 33: 364–374.

2320. Swindler, D., J. Sirianni, and L. Tarrant. 1973. A longitudinal study of cephalofacial growth in *Papio cynocephalus* and *Macaca nemestrina* from three months to three years. Craniofacial Biology of the Primates 3: 227–240.

2321. Sykora, I. 1961. Die Entwicklung des Schädels der Feldmäuse (*Microtus arvalis* Pall). Prirodovedna Krajské Museum Hradii Kralove 3: 207–226.

2322. Symons, N. B. B. 1951. Studies on the growth and form of the mandible. Dental Record 71: 41–53.

2323. Symons, N. B. B. 1952. The development of the human mandibular joint. Journal of Anatomy, London 86: 326–332.

2324. Symons, N. B. B. 1965. A histochemical study of secondary cartilage of the mandibular condyle in the rat. Archives of Oral Biology 10: 579–584.

2325. Tahara, U. 1988. Normal stages of development in the lamprey, *Lampetra reissneri* (Dybowski). Zoological Science 5: 109–118.

2326. Takagi, M., R. T. Parmley, F. R. Denys, H. Yagasaki, and Y. Toda. 1984. Ultrastructural cytochemistry of proteoglycans associated with calcification of shark cartilage. Anatomical Record 208: 149–158.

2327. Takahama, H., F. Sasaki, and K. Watanabe. 1988. Morphological changes in the oral (buccopharyngeal) membrane in urodelan embryos: Development of the mouth opening. Journal of Morphology 195: 59–70.

2328. Takata, C. 1960. The differentiation *in vitro* of the isolated endoderm in the presence of the neural fold in *Triturus pyrrhogaster*. Embryologia 5: 194–205.

2329. Takeuchi, K. 1987. Classification of late embryonic stages of medaka, *Oryzias latipes*. Japanese Journal of Ichthyology 34: 47–52.

2330. Takisawa, A., and Y. Sunaga. 1951. Über die Entwicklung des M. depressor mandibulae bei Anuren im Laufe der Metamorphose. Okajimas Folia anatomica japonica 23: 273–293.

2331. Tam, P. P. L., and R. S. P. Beddington. 1986. The metameric organization of the presomitic mesoderm and somite specification in the mouse embryo. In *Somites in Developing Embryos*, R. Bellairs, D. A. Ede, and J. W. Lash, eds. NATO ASI Series, vol. 118. New York: Plenum Press, pp. 17–36.

2332. Tam, P. P. L., and S. Meier. 1982. The establishment of a somitomeric pattern in the mesoderm of the gastrulating mouse embryo. American Journal of Anatomy 164: 209–225.

2333. Tam, P. P. L., S. Meier, and A. G. Jacobson. 1982. Differentiation of a metameric pattern in the embryonic axis of the mouse. II. Somitomeric organisation of the presomitic mesoderm. Differentiation 21: 109–122.

2334. Tamarin, A., and A. Boyde. 1977. Facial and visceral arch development in the mouse embryo: A study by scanning electron microscopy. Journal of Anatomy, London 124: 563–580.

2335. Tan, S. S., and G. Morriss-Kay. 1985. The development and distribution of the cranial neural crest in the rat embryo. Cell and Tissue Research 240: 403–416.

2336. Tan, S. S., and G. M. Morriss-Kay. 1986. Analysis of cranial neural crest cell migration and early fates in postimplantation rat chimaeras. Journal of Embryology and Experimental Morphology 98: 21–58.

2337. Tarara, R. P., D. R. Cordy, and A. G. Hendrickx. 1989. Central nervous system malformations induced by triamcinolone in nonhuman primates: Pathology. Teratology 39: 75–84.

2338. Tarasov, S. A. 1983. Features of skeletal growth of *Lagurus lagurus* Pall. and *Microtus gregalis* Pall. during postnatal development. In *Rodents: Material from the Sixth All-Union Conference, Leningrad 25–28 January 1984*, I. M. Gromov, ed. Leningrad: Nauka, pp. 196–198.

2339. Tarsitano, S. F. 1985. Cranial metamorphosis and the origin of the Eosuchia. Neues Jahrbuch für Paleontologie, Abhandlung 170: 27–44.

2340. Taverne, L. 1974. L'ostéologie d'*Elops* Linné, C. 1766 (Pisces Elopiformes) et son intérêt phylogénétique. Memoires de l'Académie royale de medecine de Belgique 41: 1–96.

2341. Taylor, M. J., E. R. Poole, J. S. Robinson, and F. Clewlow. 1983. Measurement of fetal growth in lambs by ultrasound. Research in Veterinary Science 34: 257–260.

2342. Taylor, P. J., J. U. M. Jarvis, T. M. Crowe, and K. C. Davies. 1985. Age determination in the cape molerat *Georychus capensis*. South African Journal of Zoology 20: 261–267.

2343. Taylor, R. G. 1978. Craniofacial growth during closure of the secondary palate in the hamster. Journal of Anatomy, London 125: 361–370.

2344. Tchernavin, V. 1937a. Preliminary account of the breeding changes in the skulls of *Salmo* and *Oncorhynchus*. Proceedings of the Linnean Society of London 14: 11–19.

2345. Tchernavin, V. 1937b. Skulls of salmon and trout: A brief study of their differences and breeding changes. Salmon and Trout Magazine 88: 235–242.

2346. Tchernavin, V. 1938a. The absorption of bones in the skull of salmon during their migration to rivers. Great Britain, Fisheries Board of Scotland, Edinburgh, no. 6.

2347. Tchernavin, V. 1938b. Changes in the salmon skull. Transactions of the Zoological Society of London 24: 103–184.

2348. Tchernavin, V. 1938c. Notes on the chondrocranium and branchial skeleton of *Salmo*. Proceedings of the Zoological Society of London 108B: 347–364.

2349. Tchernavin, V. 1943. The breeding characters of Salmon in relation to their size. Proceedings of the Zoological Society of London 113B: 206–232.

2350. Teaford, M. F., and A. Walker. 1983. Prenatal jaw movements in the guinea pig, *Cavia porcellus:* Evidence from patterns of tooth wear. Journal of Mammalogy 64: 534–536.

2351. Teichmann, H. 1955. Entwicklungsphysiologische Untersuchungen an der Nase des Alpen molches (*Triturus alpestris* Laur.). Wilhelm Roux' Archiv für Entwicklungsmechanik der Organismen 148: 218–262.

2352. Teichmann, H. 1959. Xenoplastischer Austausch der Nasenanlage zwischen Molch, Unke und Kröte. Wilhelm Roux' Archiv für Entwicklungsmechanik der Organismen 151: 280–300.

2353. Teichmann, H. 1961. Gestaltungsprinzipen der Nase von *Triturus*. Embryologica 6: 110–118.

2354. Teichmann, H. 1962. Experimente zur Analyse der Choanenentstehung und Formbildung der Nase bei *Triturus*. Wilhelm Roux' Archiv für Entwicklungsmechanik der Organismen 153: 455–485.

2355. Teichmann, H. 1964. Experimente zur Nasenentwicklung der Regenbogenforelle (*Salmo irideus* W. Gibb). Wilhelm Roux' Archiv für Entwicklungsmechanik der Organismen 155: 129–144.

2356. Tejada-Filores, A. E., and C. A. Shaw. 1984. Tooth replacement and skull growth in *Smilodon* from Rancho La Brea. Journal of Vertebrate Paleontology 3: 114–121.

2357. Teodoreanu, M. 1978. New data concerning the maturation period of muskrat (*Ondatra zibethicus* L.). Studia Universitatis Babes-Bolyai biologia 2: 19–21.

2358. Teodorescu, R. 1942. Contributions à l'étude du développement des larves de sandre (*Lucioperca sandra* Cuv. et Val.) la nutrition et l'ossification du système osseux. Analele, Institutului de cercetâri piscicole al României, Bucharest 1: 29–42.

2359. Teodorescu, R. 1943. Beitrag zur Kenntnis der Entwicklung, Nahrung und Bildung des Knochensystems bei der larve von *Alburnus lucidus* Heckel. Analele Institutului de cercetâri piscicole al României, Bucharest 2: 247–271.

2360. Thangaraja, M., and K. Ramamoorthi. 1983. Studies on the early life history of *Therapon jarbua* (Forshal) from the Vellar Estuary, Porto Novo. Mahasagar 16: 363–369.

2361. Theiler, K. 1972. *The House Mouse: Development and Normal Stages from Fertilization to Four Weeks of Age.* Berlin: Springer-Verlag.

2362. Thesleff, I., T. Kantomaa, E. Mackie, and R. Chiquet-Ehrismann. 1988. Immunohistochemical localization of the matrix glycoprotein tenascin in the skull of the growing rat. Archives of Oral Biology 33: 383–390.

2363. Thibaudeau, D. G., and R. Altig. 1988. Sequence of ontogenetic development and atrophy of the oral apparatus of six anuran tadpoles. Journal of Morphology 197: 63–70.

2364. Thoma, K. H. 1938. Principal factors controlling development of mandible and maxilla. American Journal of Orthodontics 24: 171–179.

2365. Thomot, A., and R. Bauchot. 1987. The organogenesis of the membranous labyrinth of Polypterus senegalus Cuvier, 1829 (Pisces, Holostei, Polypteridae). Anatomisches Anzeiger 164: 189–211.

2366. Thompson, T. J., P. D. A. Owens, and D. J. Wilson. 1989. Intramembranous osteogenesis and angiogenesis in the chick embryo. Journal of Anatomy 166: 55–65.

2367. Thomson, D. A. R. 1986. Meckel's cartilage in Xenopus laevis during metamorphosis: A light and electron microscopic study. Journal of Anatomy, London 149: 77–87.

2368. Thomson, D. A. R. 1987. A quantitative analysis of cellular and matrix changes in Meckel's cartilage in Xenopus laevis. Journal of Anatomy, London 151: 249–254.

2369. Thomson, D. A. R. 1989. A preliminary investigation into the effects of thyroid hormone on the metamorphic changes in Meckel's cartilage in Xenopus. Journal of Anatomy 162: 149–155.

2370. Thomson, K. S. 1965. The nasal apparatus in Dipnoi, with special reference to Protopterus. Proceedings of the Zoological Society of London 145: 207–238.

2371. Thomson, K. S. 1987. Speculations concerning the role of the neural crest in the morphogenesis and evolution of the vertebrate skeleton. In Developmental and Evolutionary Aspects of the Neural Crest, P. F. A. Maderson, ed. New York: John Wiley and Sons, pp. 301–338.

2372. Thomson, K. S. 1988. Morphogenesis and Evolution. New York: Oxford University Press.

2373. Thorogood, P. 1987. Mechanisms of morphogenetic specification in skull development. In Mesenchymal/Epithelial Interactions in Neural Development, J. R. Wolff, J. Sievers, and M. Berry, eds. Berlin: Springer-Verlag, pp. 141–152.

2374. Thorogood, P. 1988. The developmental specification of the vertebrate skull. Development 103 (suppl.): 141–154.

2375. Thorogood, P., J. Bee, and K. von der Mark. 1986. Transient expression of collagen type II at epitheliomesenchymal interfaces during morphogenesis of the cartilaginous neurocranium. Developmental Biology 116: 497–509.

2376. Thorogood, P., and L. Smith. 1984. Neural crest cells: The role of extracellular matrix in their differentiation and migration. In Matrices and Cell Differentiation, R. B. Kemp and J. R. Hinchliffe, eds. New York: Alan R. Liss, pp. 171–186.

2377. Thorogood, P., and C. Tickle. 1988. Preface. Development 103 (suppl.): 1–2.

2378. Tiemeier, O. W. 1950. The os opticus of birds. Journal of Morphology 86: 25–36.

2379. Tigano, C., and L. R. Parenti. 1988. Homology of the median ethmoid ossification of Aphanius fasciatus and other Atherinomorph fishes. Copeia: 866–870.

2380. Tihen, J. A. 1958. Comments on the osteology and phylogeny of ambysto-matid salamanders. Bulletin of the Florida State Museum 3: 1–50.

2381. Timm, S. 1987a. Zur Morphologie und Entwicklung des Craniums von *Felis silvestris* f. *catus* Linne 1758: Ein Beitrag zur vergleichenden Ana-tomie der Carnivora. Teil 1. Entleitung, Materiel und Methoden: Gesamtes cranium und Regio ethmoidalis. Gegenbaurs Morphologische Jahrbuch 333: 411–467.

2382. Timm, S. 1987b. Zur Morphologie und Entwicklung des Craniums von *Felis silvestris* f. *catus* Linne 1758: Ein Beitrag zur vergleichenden Anatomie der Carnivora. Teil 2. Regio orbitotemporalis. Gegenbaurs Morphologische Jahrbuch 333: 605–637.

2383. Timm, S. 1987c. Zur Morphologie und Entwicklung des Craniums von *Felis silvestris* f. *catus* Linne 1758: Ein Beitrag zur vergleichenden Anatomie der Carnivora. Teil 3. Regio otica, Regio occipitalis. Gegenbaurs Morpholo-gische Jahrbuch 333: 687–729.

2384. Timm, S. 1987d. Zur Morphologie und Entwicklung des Craniums von *Felis silvestris* f. *catus* Linne 1758: Ein Beitrag zur vergleichenden Anatomie der Carnivora. Teil 4. Visceralskelet, Deckknochen; zu zammenfassung und Folgerungen: Literatyr. Gegenbaurs Morphologische Jahrbuch 333: 793–835.

2385. Timm, S., H. Schliemann, and C.-D. Sturm. 1989. On the morphology and development of the side wall of the cranium in fissiped carnivora. Fortschritte der Zoologie 35: 401–405.

2386. Tingpalong, M., F. E. Chapple, and W. K. Andrews. 1981. Unilateral hy-poplasia of the palate and associated structures in a white-handed gibbon (*Hylobates lar*). Journal of Medical Primatology 10: 274–278.

2387. Tkachenko, V. S. 1989. Age-related changes in the skull of the red-tailed Libyan jird. Vestnik zoologii, no. 2: 56–59.

2388. Toendury, G. 1942. Über den Bauplan des fetalen Schädels. Revue suisse de zoologie 49: 194–200.

2389. Toerien, M. J. 1950. The cranial morphology of the Californian lizard—*Anniella pulchra* Gray. South African Journal of Science 46: 321–342.

2390. Toerien, M. J. 1963. Experimental studies on the origin of the cartilage of the auditory capsule and columella in *Ambystoma*. Journal of Embryology and Experimental Morphology 11: 459–473.

2391. Toerien, M. J. 1965a. An experimental approach to the development of the ear capsule in the turtle, *Chelydra serpentina*. Journal of Embryology and Experimental Morphology 13: 141–149.

2392. Toerien, M. J. 1965b. Experimental studies on the columella-capsular inter-relationships in the turtle, *Chelydra serpentina*. Journal of Embryology and Experimental Morphology 14: 265–272.

2393. Toerien, M. J. 1966. Eksperimentale studies op sinskapels. South African Akademie Referate: 167–170.

2394. Toerien, M. J. 1967a. Experimental embryology and cranial morphology. South African Journal of Science 63: 278–281.

2395. Toerien, M. J. 1967b. The metotic cartilage and the metotic fissures in the penguin. Zoologica africana 3: 105–110.

2396. Toerien, M. J. 1969. Die ontwikkeling van die inwendige oor van die konyn in kuikenkoppe (The development of the rabbit's internal ear in a chicken's head). Tydskrif vir Natuurwetenskappe, Junie–Sept.: 152–155.

2397. Toerien, M. J. 1971. The developmental morphology of the chondrocranium of *Podiceps cristatus*. Annals of the University of Stellenbosch 46: 1–128.

2398. Toerien, M. J. 1972. Morphological and experimental studies on the development of the posterior wall of the avian foramen magnum. Zoologica africana 7: 473–489.

2399. Toerien, M. J., and R. J. Rossouw. 1977. Experimental studies on the origin of parts of the nasal capsule. South African Journal of Science 73: 371–374.

2400. Tokioko, Y., Y. Ohta, H. Ike, and Y. Suzuki. 1987. Developmental changes of the zygomaticomaxillary suture of the rabbit. Okajimas Folia anatomica japonica 63: 387–392.

2401. Tollmann, S. M., F. E. Grine, and B. D. Hahn. 1980. Ontogeny and sexual dimorphism in *Aulacephalodon* (Reptilia, Anomodontia). Annals of the South African Museum 81: 159–186.

2402. Tonégawa, Y. 1973. Inductive tissue interactions in the beak of a chick embryo. Development, Growth, and Differentiation 15: 57–71.

2403. Tonneyck-Müller, I. 1971a. The growth of eyes and orbits in the chick embryo. IV. The growth of the skull in 11–19 day embryos with experimentally produced unilateral microphthalmia. Acta morphologica neerlando-scandinavica 8: 309–319.

2404. Tonneyck-Müller, I. 1971b. The growth of eyes and orbits in the chick embryo. V. The development of eye and skull primordia with artificially produced unilateral microphthalmia of 3–6 days. Acta morphologica neerlando-scandinavica 9: 57–74.

2405. Tonneyck-Müller, I. 1971–72. Das Wachstum von Augen und Augenhöhlen beim Höhnerembryo. VI. Die Entwicklung der Augen und Schädelanlage bei Embryonen von 7–10 Tagen mit künstlich erzeugter einseitiger Mikrophthalmie. Acta morphologica neerlando-scandinavica 9: 235–252.

2406. Tonneyck-Müller, I. 1974. The growth of eyes and orbits in the chick embryo. VIII. The development of the skull in embryos of 12–17 days with artifically induced bilateral microphthalmia. Acta morphologica neerlando-scandinavica 12: 145–158.

2407. Tonneyck-Müller, I. 1976. Das Wachstum von Augen und Augenhölen beim Höhnerembryo. IX. Die Entwicklung der Augen-und Schädelanlage bei Embryonen von 3–9 Tagen mit künstlich erzeugterdoppelseitiger Mikrophthalmie. Acta morphologica neerlando-scandinavica 14: 139–164.

2408. Tonneyck-Müller, I., and J. van Limborgh. 1970–71. The growth of eyes and orbits in the chick embryo. III. The quantitative relationships between the orbits and the cross-beak in 1–19 days' embryos with artifical unilateral microphthalmia. Acta morphologica neerlando-scandinavica 8: 293–301.

2409. Torre, C., G. Giagobini, and G. Ardito. 1978. Skeletal development of an orang-utan premature newborn: A comparative study. Journal of Human Evolution 7: 143–149.

2410. Tosney, K. W. 1981. The segregation and early migration of cranial neural crest cells in the chick embryo. Developmental Biology 89: 13–24.

2411. Townsend, G. C., J. White, and A. N. Goos. 1983. A comparison of craniofacial growth between two colonies of marmosets (*Callithrix jacchus*). Journal of Medical Primatology 12: 201–208.

2412. Trenouth, M. J. 1984. Shape changes during human fetal craniofacial growth. Journal of Anatomy, London 139: 639–651.

2413. Trenouth, M. J. 1985. Asymmetry of the human skull during fetal growth. Anatomical Record 211: 205–212.

2414. Trevisan, R. A., and R. P. Scapino. 1976a. Secondary cartilages in growth and development of the symphysis menti in the hamster. Acta anatomica 94: 40–58.

2415. Trevisan, R. A., and R. P. Scapino. 1976b. The symphyseal cartilage and growth of the symphysis menti in the hamster. Acta anatomica 96: 335–355.

2416. Trueb, L. 1966. Morphology and development of the skull in the frog *Hyla septentrionalis*. Copeia: 562–573.

2417. Trueb, L. 1970. Evolutionary relationships of casque-headed tree frogs with co-ossified skulls (family Hylidae). Publications of the Museum of Natural History of the University of Kansas 18: 547–716.

2418. Trueb, L. 1973. Bones, frogs, and evolution. In *Evolutionary Biology of the Anurans: Contemporary Research on Major Problems,* J. L. Vial, ed. Columbia: University Missouri Press, pp. 65–132.

2419. Trueb, L. 1985. A summary of the osteocranial development in anurans with notes on the sequence of cranial ossification in *Rhinophrynus dorsalis* (Anura: Pipoidea: Rhinophrynidae). South African Journal of Science 81: 181–185.

2420. Trueb, L. 1989. A synopsis of the development of the skull of *Pipa pipa* (Anura: Pipoidea: Pipidae) and its evolutionary significance. Fortschritte der Zoologie 35: 232–234.

2421. Trueb, L., and P. Alberch. 1983. Miniaturization and the anuran skull: A case study of heterochrony. Fortschritte der Zoologie 30: 113–121.

2422. Truscott, B. L., B. Lionel, and P. H. Struthers. 1941. The embryological development of the middle ear of the field mouse, *Microtus pennsylvanicus*. Journal of Morphology 69: 329–343.

2423. Tschugunova, T. J. 1981. Interfrontalia in *Bombina orientalis* (Blgr.) and *Bombina bombina* (L.). In *Herpetological Investigations in Siberia and the Far East,* L. J. Borkin, ed. Moscow: Academy of Science USSR, Zoological Institute, pp. 117–121.

2424. Tsimmerman, S. 1940. The chondrocranium of *Anguis fragilis*. Archives of Russian Anatomy, Histology, and Embryology 24: 135–173.

2425. Tsui, C. L., and T. H. Pan. 1946. The development of the olfactory organ of *Kaloula borealis* (Barbour) as compared with that of *Rana nigromaculata*. Quarterly Journal of Microscopical Science 87: 298–316.

2426. Tucker, J. W., Jr. 1982. Larval development of *Citharichthys cornutus, C. gymnorhinus, C. spilopterus,* and *Etropus crossotus* (Bothidae), with notes on larval occurrence. U.S. National Marine Fisheries Service, Fishery Bulletin 80: 35–73.

2427. Tumlinson, C. R., and V. R. McDaniel. 1981. Anomalies of bobcat skulls (*Felis rufus*) in Arkansas. Proceedings of the Arkansas Academy of Science 35: 94–96.

2428. Tyler, J. D. 1987. Spotted gar with deformed mandible. Proceedings of the Oklahoma Academy of Science 67: 81.

2429. Tyler, M. J., M. Davies, and A. A. Martin. 1980. Australian frogs of the leptodactylid genus *Uperoleia* Gray. Australian Journal of Zoology 79: 1–64.

2430. Tyler, M. S. 1978. Epithelial influences on membrane bone formation in the maxilla of the embryonic chick. Anatomical Record 192: 225–234.

2431. Tyler, M. S. 1980. Tissue interactions in the development of neural crest–derived membrane bones. American Zoologist 20: 944.

2432. Tyler, M. S. 1983. Development of the frontal bone and cranial meninges in the embryonic chick: An experimental study of tissue interactions. Anatomical Record 206: 61–70.

2433. Tyler, M. S. 1988. Development of osteogenic and chondrogenic potentials along the mediolateral axis of the embryonic chick mandible. Archives of Oral Biology 33: 443–449.

2434. Tyler, M. S. 1989. Promotion of osteogenesis by extra-embryonic epithelia in maxillary mesenchyme of the embryonic chick. Archives of Oral Biology 34: 387–391.

2435. Tyler, M. S., and B. K. Hall. 1977. Epithelial influences on skeletogenesis in the mandible of the embryonic chick. Anatomical Record 188: 229–240.

2436. Tyler, M. S., and D. P. McCobb. 1980. The genesis of membrane bone in the embryonic chick maxilla: Epithelial-mesenchymal tissue recombination studies. Journal of Embryology and Experimental Morphology 56: 269–281.

2437. Tyler, M. S., and D. P. McCobb. 1981. Tissue interactions promoting osteogenesis in chorioallantoic-grown explants of secondary palatal shelves of the embryonic chick. Archives of Oral Biology 26: 585–590.

2438. Ueckermann, E. 1978. Über die Spiesserstufe hinausgehende Geweihentwicklung beim Damhirsch (*Dama dama* [L.]) vom 1. Kopf. Zeitschrift für Jagdwissenschaft 24: 57–63.

2439. Ueyanagi, S. 1963a. Methods for identification and discrimination of the larvae of five istiophorid species distributed in the Indo-Pacific. Reports of the Nankai Regional Fisheries Research Laboratory 17: 137–151.

2440. Ueyanagi, S. 1963b. A study of the relationships of the Indo-Pacific istiophorids. Reports of the Nankai Regional Fisheries Research Laboratory 17: 151–165.

2441. Uotani, I. 1985. The relation between the development of feeding organs and feeding modes of the anchovy. Bulletin of the Japanese Society of Scientific Fisheries 51: 197–204.

2442. Uzzell, T. M., Jr. 1961. Calcified hyoid and mesopodial elements of plethodontid salamanders. Copeia: 78–86.

2443. Valett, B. B., and D. L. Jameson. 1961. The embryology of *Eleutherodactylus augusti latrans*. Copeia: 103–109.

2444. Vandal, D., C. Barrette, and H. Jolicoeur. 1986. An ectopic antler in a male woodland caribou. Zeitschrift für Säugetierkunde 51: 52–54.

2445. Vandebroek, G. 1964. Recherches sur l'origine des mammifères. Annales de la Société royale zoologique de Belgique 94: 117–160.

2446. Van de Graff, K. M. 1973. Comparative developmental osteology in three species of desert rodents, *Peromyscus eremicus, Perognathus intermedius,* and *Dipodomys merriami.* Journal of Mammalogy 54: 729–741.

2447. Van de Kamp, M., and S. R. Hilfer. 1985. Cell proliferation in condensing scleral ectomesenchyme associated with the conjunctival papillae in the chick embryo. Journal of Embryology and Experimental Morphology 88: 25–38.

2448. Van der Klaauw, C. J. 1946. Cerebral skull and facial skull. Archives néerlandaises de zoologie, Leiden 7: 16–37.

2449. Van der Klaauw, C. J. 1948–52. Size and position of the functional components of the skull: A contribution to the knowledge of the architecture of the skull, based on data in the literature. Archives néerlandaises de zoologie, Leiden 9: 1–159.

2450. Van der Merwe, N. J. 1940. Die Skedelmorfologie van *Pelomedusa galeata* (Wagler). Tydskrif vir Wetenskap en Kuns 1: 67–86.

2451. Van der Merwe, N. J. 1944. Die Skedelmorfologie van *Acontias meleagris* (Linn.). Tydskrif vir Wetenskap en Kuns 5: 59–88.

2452. Van der Westhuizen, C. M. 1961. The development of the chondrocranium of *Heleophryne purcelli* Sclater with special reference to the palatoquadrate and the sound-conducting apparatus. Acta zoologica, Stockholm 42: 3–72.

2453. Vandewalle, P. 1971. Comparaison ostéologique et myologique de cinq cichlidae africains et sud-américains. Annales de la Société royale zoologique de Belgique, Brussels 101: 259–292.

2454. Vandewalle, P. 1972. Ostéologie et myologie de *Tilapia guineenis* (Bleeker, 2). Annales du Musée royal de l'Afrique centrale, ser. 8, Zoologie Wetenschaft 196: 1–50.

2455. Vandewalle, P., C. Surlemont, P. Sanna, and M. Chardon. 1985. Interpretation fonctionelle de modifications du splanchnocrâne pendant le développement post-embryonnaire de *Clarias gariepinus* (Teleostens, Siluriformes). Zoologische Jahrbüch, Anatomie 113: 91–100.

2456. Van Dyke, R. H., and S. R. Detwiler. 1958. Further studies on ear and capsule development in *Amblystoma.* Anatomical Record 131: 61–80.

2457. Van Eeden, J. A. 1951. The development of the chondrocranium of *Ascaphus truei* Stejneger with special reference to the relations of the palatoquadrate to the neurocranium. Acta zoologica, Stockholm 32: 41–176.

2458. van Gennep, E. M. S. J. 1986. The osteology, arthrology, and myology of the jaw apparatus of the pigeon (*Columbia livia* L.). Netherlands Journal of Zoology 36: 1–46.

2459. Van Ness, A. L. 1978. Implantation of cranial base metallic markers in nonhuman primates. American Journal of Physical Anthropology 49: 85–90.

2460. Van Prooije, A. E. S., C. Vermeiz-Keers, R. E. Poelmann, M. M. T. Montink, and J. A. Dubbeldam. 1985. The neural crest in presomite to 40-somite murine embryos. Acta morphologica neerlando-scandinavica 23: 99–111.

2461. Van Utrecht, W. L. 1988. Growth in larval and metamorphosed *Eurypharynx pelecanoides* Vaillant, 1882 (Pisces, Anguilliformes, Eurypharyngidae) from the mid-North Atlantic. Bijdragen tot de Dierkunde 58: 12–19.

2462. Varona, L. S. 1985. Modificaciones ontogenicas y dimorfismo sexual en *Mesoplodon gervais* (Cetacea: Ziphiidae). Caribbean Journal of Science 21: 27–37.

2463. Vasilenko, A. V., A. N. Ivanov, and V. A. Belyaev. 1982. Age and growth of Pacific populations of Japanese mackerel *Scomber japonicus* Houttuyn. In *Ecology and Condition of Reproduction of Fish and Invertebrates in Waters of the Soviet Far East and the Northwest Part of the Pacific Ocean*, S. M. Konovalov, V. P. Shuntov et al., eds. Vladivostock: Pacific Ocean Research Institute of Fisheries and Ocean, pp. 36–50.

2464. Vasil'eva, E. D. 1978. Osteology of the neiva (genus *Salvelinus*, Salmoniformes, Salmonidae) from Karrai Lake, Ochota River Basin. Vestnik Moskovskogo Universiteta, ser. 16, Biologiya, no. 4: 3–10.

2465. Vasil'eva, E. D. 1981. Arctic charr, *Salvelinus alpinus*, from the Zarubikha River Basin, Russian SFSR USSR: Charr and trout from the Kola Peninsula, Russian SFSR USSR. Voprosy Ikhtiologii 21: 232–247.

2466. Vasil'eva, E. D. 1983. Variation in craniological characters in salmon and their use in systematics of this group. In *Morphology, Population Structure, and Problems of Rational Utilization of Salmonidei*, O. A. Skarlato and E. O. Dorofeeva, eds. Leningrad: Nauka, pp. 25–26.

2467. Vasil'eva, E. D., and T. G. Daraseliya. 1989. Intraspecific skull variations and divergence of some populations of *Varicorhinus capeota* (Pisces, Cyprinidae) in the Kura Basin [USSR]. Zoologicheskii zhurnal 68: 113–124.

2468. Vazhenina, I. I., and I. G. Kilheeva. 1983. Age changes in correlations between morphometric and craniological characters in populations of bank vole (*Cleithrionomys glareolus* Schred, 1780). In *Rodents: Material from the Sixth All-Union Conference, Leningrad 25–28 January 1984*, I. M. Gromov, ed. Leningrad: Nauka, pp. 63–64.

2469. Veit, O. 1939. Beiträge zur Kenntnis des Kopfers der Wirbeltiere. III. Beobachtungen zur Frühentwicklung des Kopfes von *Petromyzon planeri*. Gegenbaurs Morphologisches Jahrbuch 84: 86–107.

2470. Vermeij-Keers, C., and R. E. Poelmann. 1980. The neural crest: A study on cell degeneration and the improbability of cell migration in mouse embryos. Netherlands Journal of Zoology 30: 74–81.

2471. Verraes, W. 1974a. Discussion of some relations between the form, position, and function of the hyosymplecticum in developmental stages of *Salmo gairdneri* Richardson, 1836 (Teleostei: Salmonidae). Forma et functio 7: 39–46.

2472. Verraes, W. 1974b. Discussion of the shape of the eye and the influence of its size on shape and position of surrounding structures in normal and abnormal conditions during postembryonic development in *Salmo gairdneri* Richardson, 1836 (Teleostei, Salmonidae). Forma et functio 7: 125–138.

2473. Verraes, W. 1974c. Discussion on some functional-morphological relations between some parts of the chondrocranium and the osteocranium in the skull base and the skull roof, and of some soft head parts during postembryonic development of *Salmo gairdneri* Richardson, 1836 (Teleostei: Salmonidae). Forma et functio 7: 281–292.

2474. Verraes, W. 1975. Some functional aspects of ossifications in the cartilaginous ceratohyale during postembryonic development in *Salmo gairdneri* Richardson, 1836 (Teleostei: Salmonidae). Forma et functio 8: 27–32.

2475. Verraes, W. 1976. Postembryonic development of the nasal organs, sacs, and surrounding skeletal elements in *Salmo gairdneri* (Teleostei: Salmonidae), with some functional interpretations. Copeia: 71–75.

2476. Verraes, W. 1977. Postembryonic ontogeny and functional anatomy of the ligamentum mandibulo-hyoideum and the ligamentum interoperculo-mandibulare, with notes on the opercular bones and some other cranial elements in *Salmo gairdneri* Richardson, 1836 (Teleostei: Salmonidae). Journal of Morphology 151: 111–120.

2477. Verraes, W., and M. H. Ismail. 1980. Developmental and functional aspects of the frontal bones in relation to some other bony and cartilaginous parts of the head roof in *Haplochromis elegans* Trewavas, 1933 (Teleostei, Chichlidae). Netherlands Journal of Zoology 30: 450–472.

2478. Verwoerd, C. D. A., and C. G. Van Ooström. 1979. Cephalic neural crest and placodes. Advances in Anatomy, Embryology, and Cell Biology 58: 1–75.

2479. Verwoerd, C. D. A., C. G. van Oosström, and H. L. Verwoerd-Verhoef. 1981. Otic placode and cephalic neural crest. Acta Oto-laryngologica 91: 431–436.

2480. Vicek, E., and J. Benes. 1975. A cranial asymmetry of *Crocuta spelaea* (Goldfuss) due to a unilateral skull injury. Lynx, Prague 15: 31–44.

2481. Vidic, B., H. G. Greditzen, and W. J. Litchy. 1972. The structure and prenatal morphogenesis of the nasal septum in the rat. Journal of Morphology 137: 131–147.

2482. Vig, K. W. L., and A. R. Burdi. 1988. *Craniofacial Morphogenesis and Dysmorphogenesis*. Ann Arbor: Center for Human Growth and Development, University of Michigan.

2483. Vilmann, H. 1972. Osteogenesis in the basioccipital bone of the Wistar albino rat. Scandanavian Journal of Dental Research 80: 410–421.

2484. Vilmann, H. 1982. The mandibular angular cartilage in the rat. Acta anatomica 113: 61–68.

2485. Vilmann, H., and M. Moss. 1979. Spatial position of the lateral semicircular canal in 14–60-day-old rat heads. Scandinavian Journal of Dental Research 87: 171–177.

2486. Vinkka, H. 1982. Secondary cartilages in the facial skeleton of the rat. Proceedings of the Finnish Dental Society 78 (suppl. 7): 1–137.

2487. Virapomgse, C., and M. Sarawar. 1988. Development of the skull. In *Modern Neuroradiology*, vol. 3, *Computed Tomography of the Head and Neck*, T. H. Newton, A. N. Hasso, and W. P. Dillon, eds. San Anselmo: Clavadel Press, pp. 1–20.

2488. Visser, J. G. J. 1961. The cranial anatomy and kinesis of the birdsnake *Thelotornis capensis* (Smith). Annals of the University of Stellenbosch 36: 147–174.

2489. Visser, J. G. J. 1972. Ontogeny of the chondrocranium of the chamaeleon, *Microsaura pumila pumila* (Daudin). Annals of the University of Stellenbosch 47A: 1–68.

2490. Visser, M. H. C. 1963. The cranial morphology of *Ichthyophis glutinosus* (Linne) and *Ichthyophis monochrus* (Bleeker). Annals of the University of Stellenbosch 38: 1–7, 67–102.

2491. Vogel, P. 1973. Vergleichende Untersuchung zum Ontogenesemodus einheimischer Soriciden (*Crocidura russula, Sorex araneus* und *Neomys fodiens*). Revue suisse de zoologie 79: 1201–1332.

2492. von Braunschweig, A. 1980. Brachygnathie (Kurzkiefrigheit) bei einem Rehbock. Zeitschrift für Jagdwissenschaft 26: 45–47.

2493. von Glass, W., and H.-J. Pesch. 1983. Zum Ossifikationsprinzip des Kehlkopfskeletes von Mensch und Saugetieren: Vergleichende anatomische Untersuchungen. Acta anatomica 116: 158–167.

2494. Vorobyeva, E. 1985. On the evolution of cranial structures in crossopterygians and tetrapods. Fortschritte der Zoologie 30: 123–133.

2495. Vorobyeva, E. 1987. Specific features of cranial structure evolution in lower vertebrates. Zoologicheskii zhurnal 66: 955–979.

2496. Vorobyeva, E., and S. Smirnov. 1987. Characteristic features in the formation of anuran sound-conducting systems. Journal of Morphology 192: 1–11.

2497. Vorobyeva, E., and S. Smirnov. 1989. The evolution of the amphibian sound-conducting apparatus. Fortschritte der Zoologie 35: 256–257.

2498. Voronov, G. A. 1984. The ecology and postembryonic development in *Microtus sachalinensis* (Rodentia, Cricetidae). Zoologicheskii zhurnal 63: 1693–1704.

2499. Vorster, W. 1989. The development of the chondrocranium of *Gallus gallus*. Advances in Anatomy, Embryology, and Cell Biology 113: 1–77.

2500. Waddington, C. H. 1937. The determination of the auditory placode in the chick. Journal of Experimental Biology 14: 232–239.

2501. Wagman, I. H., J. R. Loeffler, and J. A. McMillan. 1975. Relationship between growth of brain and skull of *Macaca mulatta* and its importance for the stereotaxic technique. Brain, Behavior, and Evolution 12: 116–134.

2502. Wagner, G. 1949. Die bedeutung der neuralleiste für die kopfgestaltung der amphibienlarven: Untersuchungen an chimaeren von *Triton* und *Bombinator*. Revue suisse de zoologie 56: 519–620.

2503. Wagner, G. 1959. Untersuchungen an *Bombinator-Triton*-chimaeren. Das skellet larvaler *Triton*-kopfe mit *Bombinator* mesektoderm. Wilhelm Roux Archives of Developmental Biology 151: 136–158.

2504. Wainwright, P. C. 1988. Morphology and ecology: Functional basis of feeding constraints in Caribbean labrid fishes. Ecology 69: 635–645.

2505. Wake, D. B. 1963. Comparative osteology of the plethodontid salamander genus *Aneides*. Journal of Morphology 113: 77–118.

2506. Wake, D. B. 1966. Comparative osteology and evolution of the lungless salamanders, family Plethodontidae. Memoirs of the Southern California Academy of Science 4: 1–11.

2507. Wake, D. B. 1980. Evidence of heterochronic evolution: A nasal bone in the Olympic salamander, *Rhyacotriton olympicus*. Journal of Herpetology 14: 292–295.

2508. Wake, D. B. 1982. Functional and developmental constraints and opportunities in the evolution of feeding systems in urodeles. In *Environmental Adaptation and Evolution*, D. Mossakowski and G. Roth, eds. Stuttgart: Gustav Fisher, pp. 51–66.

2509. Wake, M. H. 1978. Comments on the ontogeny of *Typhlonectes obesus*, particularly its dentition and feeding. Papeis avulsos de zoologia 32: 1–13.

2510. Wake, M. H. 1980. The reproductive biology of *Nectophrynoides malcolmi* (Amphibia: Bufonidae), with comments on the evolution of reproductive modes in the genus *Nectophrynoides*. Copeia: 193–209.

2511. Wake, M. H. 1986. The morphology of *Idiocranium russeli* (Amphibia: Gymnophiona), with comments on miniaturization through heterochrony. Journal of Morphology 189: 1–16.

2512. Wake, M. H. 1987. A new genus of African caecilian (Amphibia: Gymnophiona). Journal of Herpetology 21: 6–15.

2513. Wake, M. H. 1989. Metamorphosis of the hyobranchial apparatus in *Epicrionops* (Amphibia: Gymnophiona: Rhinatrematidae): Replacement of bone by cartilage. Annales des sciences naturelles, Zoologie et biologie animale 13 (ser. 10): 171–182.

2514. Wake, M. H., J.-M. Exbrayat, and M. Delsol. 1985. The development of the chondrocranium of *Typhlonectes compressicaudus* (Gymnophiona), with comparison to other species. Journal of Herpetology 19: 68–77.

2515. Wake, M. H., and J. Hanken. 1982. Development of the skull of *Dermophis mexicanus* (Amphibia: Gymnophiona) with comments on skull kinesis and amphibian relationships. Journal of Morphology 173: 203–223.

2516. Wake, T. A., D. B. Wake, and M. H. Wake. 1983. The ossification sequence of *Aneides lugubris*, with comments on heterochrony. Journal of Herpetology 17: 1–22.

2517. Waldo, C. M., and G. B. Wislocki. 1951. Observations on the shedding of the antlers of Virginia deer (*Odocoileus virginianus borealis*). Anatomical Record 88: 351–396.

2518. Walker, A. 1985. The braincase of *Archaeopteryx*. In *The Beginnings of Birds: Proceedings of the International Archaeopteryx Conference, Eichstatt 1984*, M. K. Hecht, J. H. Ostrom, G. Viohl., and P. Wellnhofer, eds. Eichstatt: Freunde des Jura-Museums Eichstatt, pp. 123–134.

2519. Walker, B. E., and J. Quarles. 1976. Palate development in mouse foetuses after tongue removal. Archives of Oral Biology 21: 405–412.

2520. Walker, M. T., and R. Rose. 1981. Prenatal development after diapause in the marsupial *Macropus rufofriseus*. Australian Journal of Zoology 29: 167–188.

2521. Wang, N.-C. 1979. A new Paleoniscidae, *Turfanis vartus*, new species, from the Upper Permian of Sinkiang (China). Annales de paleontologie vertébré 65: 1–33.

2522. Wang Fei, et al. 1987. Preliminary comparative observations on the histological structure of the young pilose antler and antler of red-deer and sika. Chinese Journal of Zoology 22: 25–27.

2523. Warncke, G., and H.-J. Stork. 1977. Biostatische und thermoregulatorische Funktion der Sandwich-Strukturen in der Schädeldecke der Vogel. Zoologische Anzeiger 199: 251–257.

2524. Warren, A. A., and M. N. Hutchinson. 1988. A new capitosaurid amphibian from the early Triassic of Queensland, and the ontogeny of the capitosaur skull. Palaeontology, London 31: 857–876.

2525. Washburn, S. L., and S. R. Detwiler. 1943. An experiment bearing on the problems of physical anthropology. American Journal of Physical Anthropology 1: 171–190.

2526. Washington, B. B., H. G. Moser, W. A. Larochem, and W. J. Richards. 1984. Scorpaeniformes: Development. In *Ontogeny and Systematics of Fishes*, American Society of Ichthyologists and Herpetologists Special Publication no. 1, H. G. Moser, ed. Lawrence, Kans.: Allen Press, pp. 405–428.

2527. Wassersug, R. J. 1984. The *Pseudohemisus* tadpole: A morphological link between microhylid (Orton type 2) and ranoid (Orton type 4) larvae. Herpetologica 40: 138–149.

2528. Wassersug, R. J., and K. Hoff. 1979. A comparative study of the buccal pumping mechanism of tadpoles. Biological Journal of the Linnean Society 12: 225–259.

2529. Wassersug, R. J., and K. Hoff. 1982. Developmental changes in the orientation of the anuran jaw suspension: A preliminary exploration into the evolution of anuran metamorphosis. Evolutionary Biology 15: 223–246.

2530. Wassersug, R. J., and W. F. Pyburn. 1987. The biology of the pe-ret toad *Otophryne robusta* (Microhylidae), with special consideration of its fossorial larva and systematic relationships. Zoological Journal of the Linnean Society 91: 137–169.

2531. Watanabe, T. 1982. Mandible/basihyal relationships in red howler monkeys (*Alouatta seniculus*): A craniometrical approach. Primates 23: 105–129.

2532. Watson, A. G., A. de Lattunta, and H. E. Evans. 1989. Dorsal notch of foramen magnum due to incomplete ossification of supraoccipital bone in dogs. Journal of Small Animal Practice 30: 666–673.

2533. Watson, J. M. 1939. The development of the Weberian ossicles and anterior vertebrae in the goldfish. Proceedings of the Royal Society of London 127B: 452–469.

2534. Watson, W. 1987. Larval development of the endemic Hawaiian blenniid, *Enchelyurus brunneolus* (Pisces: Blenniddae: Omobranchini). Bulletin of Marine Science 41: 856–888.

2535. Watts, E. S. 1986. Skeletal development. In *Comparative Primate Biology*, vol. 3, *Reproduction and Development*, W. R. Dukelow and J. Erwin, eds. New York: Alan R. Liss, pp. 415–439.

2536. Wayne, R. K. 1986. Cranial morphology of domestic and wild canids: The influence of development on morphological change. Evolution 40: 243–261.

2537. Webb, G. J. W., and H. Messel. 1978. Morphometric analysis of *Crocodylus porosus* from the north coast of Arnhem Land, Northern Territory. Australian Journal of Zoology 26: 1–28.

2538. Webb, M. 1957. The ontogeny of the cranial bones, cranial peripheral, and cranial parasympathetic nerves, together with a study of the visceral muscles of *Struthio*. Acta zoologica, Stockholm 38: 81–203.

2539. Webster, D. B. 1974. Temporal bone ontogeny in kangaroo rat. American Zoologist 14: 1276.

2540. Webster, D. B. 1975. Auditory systems of the Heteromyidae: Postnatal development of the ear of *Dipodomys merriami*. Journal of Morphology 146: 377–394.

2541. Wedden, S. E. 1987. Epithelial-mesenchymal interactions in the development of chick facial primordia and the target of retinoid action. Development 99: 341–352.

2542. Wedden, S. E. 1988. Morphogenesis of the head and face: Discussion report. Development 103 (suppl.): 61–62.

2543. Wedden, S. E., J. R. Ralphs, and C. Tickle. 1988. Pattern formation in the facial primordia. Development 103 (suppl.): 31–40.

2544. Wedden, S. E., and C. Tickle. 1986. Facial morphogenesis and pattern formation. In *Progress in Developmental Biology, Part A*, H. C. Slavkin, ed. New York: Alan R. Liss, pp. 335–337.

2545. Wedin, B. 1949. The development of the head cavities in *Alligator mississippiensis* Daud. Acta Universitatis Lundensis, n.f. 45: 1–31.

2546. Wedin, B. 1951. Die Verbindungsstränge zwischen den Prämandibularhöhlen und der Rathke'schen Tasche. Koninklijke Nederlandse Akademie van Wetenschappen, Proceedings of the Section of Sciences, ser. C, Biological and Medical Sciences 54: 75–83.

2547. Wedin, B. 1952. Tissue bridges and tubular connections between the premandibular cavities and Rathke's pouch. Koninklijke Nederlandse Akademie van Wetenschappen, Proceedings of the Section of Sciences, ser. C, Biological and Medical Sciences 55: 416–428.

2548. Wedin, B. 1953. The development of the head cavities in *Ardea cinerea* L. Acta anatomica 17: 240–252.

2549. Wedin, B. 1955. *Embryonic Segmentations in the Head*. Malmö: Luhdgrens Söneraboktr.

2550. Wegner, R. N. 1957. Studies über die Nebenhöhlen des Schädels. 2. Teil. Die Nebenhöhlen der Nase be den Krokodilen. Wissenschaftliche Zeitschrift, Ernst Moritz Arndt-Universitat 7: 1–39.

2551. Weijs, W. A., P. Brugman, and E. M. Klok. 1987. The growth of the skull and jaw muscles and its functional consequences in the New Zealand rabbit (*Oryctolagus cuniculus*). Journal of Morphology 194: 143–161.

2552. Weisel, G. F. 1967. Early ossification in the skeleton of the sucker (*Catostomus macrocephalus*) and the guppy (*Poecilia reticulata*). Journal of Morphology 121: 1–18.

2553. Weiss, A., E. Livne, and M. Silbermann. 1988. Glucocorticoid hormone adversely affects the growth and regeneration of cartilage *in vitro*. Growth, Development, and Aging 52: 67–75.

2554. Weiss, P., and R. Amprino. 1940. The effect of mechanical stress on the differentiation of scleral cartilage *in vitro* and in the embryo. Growth 4: 245–258.

2555. Weisz, P. B. 1945a. The development and morphology of the larva of the South African clawed toad, *Xenopus laevis*. I. The third-form tadpole. Journal of Morphology 77: 163–192.

2556. Weisz, P. B. 1945b. The development and morphology of the larva of the South African clawed toad, *Xenopus laevis*. II. The hatching and the first- and second-form tadpoles. Journal of Morphology 77: 193–217.

2557. Wenham, G. 1981. A radioautographic study of early skeletal development in fetal sheep. Journal of Agricultural Science 96: 39–44.

2558. Wenham, G., C. L. Adam, and C. E. Moir. 1986. A radiographic study of skeletal growth and development in fetal red deer. British Veterinary Journal 142: 336–349.

2559. Wenham, G., and V. R. Fowler. 1973. A radiographic study of age changes in the skull, mandible, and teeth of pigs. Journal of Agricultural Science 80: 451–461.

2560. Wenz, S. 1967. Remarques sur les transformations des os dermiques du museau chez les Actinoptérygiens. Colloque internationale du Centre de la recherche scientific 163: 89–92.

2561. Werner, C. F. 1960. Das Gehörorgan der Wirbeltiere und des Menschen. Leipzig: George Thieme.

2562. Werner, G. 1960. Das Primordialcranium des Gürteltieres Dasypus novemcinctus Linné (Tatusia novemcincta Lesson) von 14mm Sch.-St. Lg. Zeitschrift für Morphologie und Anthropologie, Stuttgart 50: 317–348.

2563. Werner, G. 1962. Das Cranium der Brückenechse, Sphenodon punctatus Gray, von 58 mm Gesamtlänge. Zeitschrift für Anatomie und Entwicklungsgeschichte 123: 323–368.

2564. Westergaard, B. 1988. The pattern of embryonic tooth initiation in reptiles. Memoires du Museum national d'histoire naturelle, ser. C, Sciences de la terre 53: 55–63.

2565. Westergaard, B., and M. W. J. Ferguson. 1986. Development of the dentition in Alligator mississippiensis: Early embryonic development of the lower jaw. Journal of Zoology, London 210: 575–597.

2566. Westergaard, B., and M. W. J. Ferguson. 1987. Development of the dentition in Alligator mississippiensis: Later development in the lower jaws of embryos, hatchlings, and young juveniles. Journal of Zoology, London 212: 191–222.

2567. Westoll, T. S. 1937. On the cheek bones in teleostome fishes. Journal of Anatomy, London 71: 362–382.

2568. Westoll, T. S. 1941. Latero-sensory canals and dermal bones. Nature 148: 168.

2569. Wettstein, O. V. 1931. Crocodilia (1). In Handbuch der Zoologie 7, W. Kükenthal and T. Krumpach, eds. Berlin: De Gruyter, pp. 236–320.

2570. Wettstein, O. V. 1954. Crocodilia (2) In Handbuch der Zoologie 7, W. Kükenthal, T. Krumpach, J. G. Melmcke, and H. V. Lengerken, eds. Berlin: De Gruyter, pp. 321–424.

2571. White, C. M. N. 1948. Skull ossification in certain Passeriformes. Ibis 90: 328–329.

2572. Wible, J. R. 1986. Transformations in the extracranial course of the internal carotid artery in mammalian phylogeny. Journal of Vertebrate Paleontology 6: 313–325.

2573. Wible, J. R., and M. J. Novacek. 1988. Cranial evidence for the monophyletic origin of bats. American Museum Novitates, no. 2911: 1–19.

2574. Wiens, J. J. 1989. Ontogeny of the skeleton of Spea bombifrons (Anura: Pelobatidae). Journal of Morphology 202: 29–51.

2575. Wiig, O. 1982. Bone resorption in the skull of Mustela vison. Acta theriologica 27: 358–360.

2576. Wiig, O. 1985a. Morphometric variation in the hooded seal (*Cystophora cristata*). Journal of Zoology, London 206: 497–508.
2577. Wiig, O. 1985b. Multivariate variation in feral American mink (*Mustela vison*) from southern Norway. Journal of Zoology, London 206: 441–452.
2578. Wiig, O. 1989. Craniometric variation in Norwegian wolverines *Gulo gulo* L. Zoological Journal of the Linnean Society of London 95: 177–204.
2579. Wiig, O., and T. Andersen. 1986. Sexual size dimorphism in the skull of Norwegian lynx (*Lynx lynx*). Acta theriologica 31: 149–158.
2580. Wiig, O., and R. W. Lie. 1979. Metrical and nonmetrical skull variations in Norwegian wild mink (*Mustela vison*). Zoologica scripta 8: 297–300.
2581. Wika, M. 1980. On growth of reindeer antlers. In *Proceedings, Second International Reindeer/Caribou Symposium, Køros Norway*, E. Riemers, E. Goare, and S. Skjinneeberg, eds. Trondheim: Direktoratet Vilt Ferskvannsfisk, pp. 416–421.
2582. Wika, M. 1982. Foetal stages of antler development. Acta zoologica, Stockholm 63: 187–189.
2583. Wilhelm, W. 1984. Interspecific allometric growth differences in the head of three haplochromine species (Pisces, Cichlidae). Netherlands Journal of Zoology 34: 622–628.
2584. Will, L. A., and S. M. Meller. 1981. Primary palate development in the chick. Journal of Morphology 169: 185–190.
2585. Williams, D. F., and J. S. Findley. 1979. Sexual size dimorphism in vespertilionid bats. American Midland Naturalist 102: 113–126.
2586. Williams, J. P. G., and S. M. Hughes. 1979. Growth of the skull in the mutant dwarf mouse. Acta anatomica 105: 461–468.
2587. Williams, S. L., and H. H. Genoways. 1978. Review of the desert pocket gopher, *Geomys arenarius* (Mammalia: Rodentia). Annals of the Carnegie Museum 47: 541–570.
2588. Wilson, D. B. 1979a. Embryonic development of the head and neck. 1. An overview. Head and Neck Surgery 1: 512–518.
2589. Wilson, D. B. 1979b. Embryonic development of the head and neck. 2. The branchial region. Head and Neck Surgery 2: 59–66.
2590. Wilson, D. B. 1979c. Embryonic development of the head and neck. 3. The face. Head and Neck Surgery 2: 145–153.
2591. Wilson, D. B. 1979d. Embryonic development of the head and neck. 5. The brain and cranium. Head and Neck Surgery 2: 312–320.
2592. Wilson, D. B., and A. G. Hendrickx. 1984. Fine structural aspects of the cranial neuroepithelium in early embryos of the rhesus monkey (*Macaca mulatta*). Journal of Craniofacial Genetics and Developmental Biology 4: 85–94.
2593. Wilson, N. H. F., and D. L. Gardner. 1982. The postnatal development of the temporomandibular joint of the common marmoset (*Callithrix jacchus*). Journal of Medical Primatology 11: 303–311.
2594. Wilson, N. H. F., P. M. Speight, and D. L. Gardner. 1982. Growth of the mandible in the common marmoset (*Callithrix jacchus*). Journal of Medical Primatology 11: 242–251.
2595. Winking, H. 1976. Karyology and biology of the two Iberian vole species

Pitymys mariae and *Pitymys duodecimcostatus*. Zeitschrift für Zoologie Systematik und Evolutionsforschung 14: 104–129.

2596. Winkler, L. A. 1987. Sexual dimorphism in the cranium of infant and juvenile orangutans. Folia primatologica 49: 117–126.

2597. Winkler, R. 1972. Pneumatization of the cranium in *Larus argentatus michahellis*. Alauda 40: 272–277.

2598. Winkler, R. 1979. Zur Pneumatisation des Schädeldachs der Vögel. Der Ornithologische Beobachter 76: 49–118.

2599. Wislocki, G. B. 1942. Studies on the growth of deer antlers. I. On the structure and histogenesis of the antlers of the Virginia deer (*Odocoileus virginianus borealis*). American Journal of Anatomy 71: 371–416.

2600. Wislocki, G. B. 1956. The growth cycle of deer antlers. CIBA Foundation Colloquium on Aging 2: 176–187.

2601. Wislocki, G. B., H. L. Weatherford, and M. Singer. 1947. Osteogenesis of antlers investigated by histological and histochemical methods. Anatomical Record 99: 265–296.

2602. Witschi, E. 1949. The larval ear of the frog and its transformation during metamorphosis. Zeitschrift für Naturforschung 4: 230–242.

2603. Wohrmann-Repenning, A. 1985. Besonderheiten der Cartilago paraseptalis und ihre Entwicklung bei Rodentia. Verhandlungen der Deutsche Zoologische Gesellschaft 78: 173.

2604. Wolf, G. L., L. Koskinen-Moffett, and V. Kokich. 1985. Migration of craniofacial periosteum in growing guinea pigs. Journal of Anatomy, London 140: 245–258.

2605. Wolf, L. L. 1977. Species relationships in the avian genus *Aimophila*. Ornithological Monographs 23: 1–220.

2606. Wolpert, L. 1988. Craniofacial development: A summing up. Development 103 (suppl.): 245–250.

2607. Worthington, R. B., and D. B. Wake. 1971. Larval morphology and ontogeny of the ambystomatid salamander, *Rhyacotriton olympicus*. American Midland Naturalist 85: 349–365.

2608. Wouterlood, F. G. 1975. The mutual relations of structures in the growing bill of chick (*Gallus domesticus* L.) and duck (*Anas platyrhynchos* L.) embryos. I. Normal embryonic growth and growth after excision of the prospective upper or lower bill, in terms of external dimensions. Netherlands Journal of Zoology 25: 353–368.

2609. Wouterlood, F. G. 1976. The mutual relations of structures in the growing bill of chick (*Gallus domesticus* L.) and duck (*Anas platyrhynchos* L.) embryos. II. Normal growth of duck embryos (external dimensions); the size, shape, and position of skeletal elements in the heads of chick and duck embryos lacking an upper or lower bill. Netherlands Journal of Zoology 26: 266–294.

2610. Wouterlood, F. G. 1977a. The mutual relations of structures in the growing bill of chick (*Gallus domesticus* L.) and duck (*Anas platyrhynchos* L.) embryos. III. The size, shape, and position of the upper and lower beaks in unilaterally microphthalmic chick embryos. Acta morphologica neerlando-scandinavica 15: 109–128.

2611. Wouterlood, F. G. 1977b. The mutual relations of structures in the growing bill of chick (*Gallus domesticus* L.) and duck (*Anas platyrhynchos* L.) embryos. IV. The size, shape, and position of the upper and lower bills in unilaterally microphthalmic duck embryos. Acta morphologica neerlandoscandinavica 15: 1–23.

2612. Wouterlood, F. G., and W. van Pelt. 1979. The influence of the lower beak on the interorbital septum-prenasal process complex in the chick embryo. Journal of Embryology and Experimental Morphology 49: 61–72.

2613. Wragg, L. E., V. M. Diewert, and M. Klein. 1972. Spatial relations in the oral cavity and the mechanism of secondary palate closure in the rat. Archives of Oral Biology 17: 683–690.

2614. Wright, G. M., L. A. Armstrong, A. M. Jacques, and J. H. Yousson. 1988. Trabecular, nasal, branchial, and pericardial cartilages in the sea lamprey, *Petromyzon marinus*: Fine structure and immunohistochemical detection of elastin. American Journal of Anatomy 182: 1–15.

2615. Wright, G. M., F. W. Keeley, J. H. Youson, and D. L. Babineau. 1984. Cartilage in the Atlantic Hagfish, *Myxine glutinosa*. American Journal of Anatomy 169: 407–424.

2616. Wright, G. M., and J. H. Youson. 1982. Ultrastructure of mucocartilage in the larval anadromous sea lamprey, *Petromyzon marinus*. American Journal of Anatomy 165: 39–51.

2617. Wright, G. M., and J. H. Youson. 1983. Ultrastructure of cartilage from young adult sea lamprey, *Petromyzon marinus* L.: A new type of vertebrate cartilage. American Journal of Anatomy 167: 59–70.

2618. Wright, H. V., C. W. Asling, H. L. Dougherty, M. M. Nelson, and H. M. Evans. 1958. Prenatal development of the skeleton in Long-Evans rats. Anatomical Record 130: 659–672.

2619. Wu, G., D. Yang, and H. Pang. 1984. The characteristics of the early developmental stages of the perch *Lateolabrax japonicus* (Cuvier et Valenciennes). Marine Science, Qingdao: 43–46.

2620. Wunder, W. 1938. Versuche ueber die Ausheilung von Verletzungen beim Karpfen (*Cyprinus carpio* L). Wilhelm Roux' Archiv für Entwicklungsmechanik der Organismen 137: 540–559.

2621. Wünsch, D. 1975. Beiträge zur Kenntnis des Primaten-Craniums Nr. IV. Zur Kenntnis der Entwicklung des Craniums des Koboldmaki, *Tarsius bancanus borneanus* Horsfield, 1821. Zebtrum der Morphologie, Frankfurt.

2622. Wyszynski, M. 1986. Attempt to determine the applicability of various bony elements for estimation of age and growth of hake *Merluccius australis* (Merluccidae) from New Zealand waters. Prace Morskiego Instytutu Rybackiego 21: 61–95.

2623. Yabe, H., S. Ueyanagi, S. Kikawa, and H. Watanabe. 1959. Study on the life-history of the swordfish, *Xiphias gladius* Linnaeus. Report of the Nankai Regional Fisheries Research Laboratory, no. 10: 107–150.

2624. Yao-ting, G. 1983. Current studies on the Chinese yarkand hare. Acta zoologica fennica 174: 23–25.

2625. Yasuda, F., H. Kohno, A. Yatsu, H. Ida, P. Arena, F. L. Greci, and Y. Taki.

1978. Embryonic and early larval stages of the swordfish, *Xiphias gladius*, from the Mediterranean. Journal of Tokyo University of Fisheries 65: 91–97.

2626. Yeatman, H. C. 1967. Artificially metamorphosed neotenic cave salamanders. Journal of the Tennessee Academy of Science 42: 16–22.

2627. Yemel'yanov, I. H., and S. I. Zolotukhina. 1975. The problem of distinguishing age groups in the vole (*Microtus socialis* Pall.). Doklady Akademie Nauk Ukrainskoi SSR, ser. B, Geologiya, Heofizyka Khimiya, Biologiya 7: 657–660.

2628. Yew, D. T., and W. W. Y. Li. 1987. The eyes and the orbits of two species of fishes with "dorsal eyes." Anatomischer Anzeiger 164: 331–343.

2629. Yntema, C. L. 1950. An analysis of induction of the ear from foreign ectoderm in salamander embryo. Journal of Experimental Zoology 113: 211–243.

2630. Yntema, C. L. 1955. Ear and Nose. In *Analysis of Development*, B. H. Willier, P. A. Weiss, and V. Hamburger, eds. Philadelphia: W. B. Saunders, pp. 415–428.

2631. Yntema, C. L. 1968. A series of stages in the embryonic development of *Chelydra serpentina*. Journal of Morphology 125: 219–252.

2632. Young, B. A. 1989. Ontogenetic changes in the feeding system of the red-sided garter snake, *Thamnophis sirtalis parietalis*. I. Allometric analysis. Journal of Zoology, London 218: 365–382.

2633. Youson, J. H., and P. A. Freeman. 1976. Morphology of the gills of larval and parasitic adult sea lamprey, *Petromyzon marinus* L. Journal of Morphology 149: 73–104.

2634. Youssef, E. H. 1964. The development of the skull in a 34 mm human embryo. Acta anatomica 57: 72–90.

2635. Youssef, E. H. 1966. The chondrocranium of the albino rat. Acta anatomica 64: 586–617.

2636. Youssef, E. H. 1969. Development of the membrane bones and ossification of the chondrocranium in the albino rat. Acta anatomica 72: 603.

2637. Youssef, E. H. 1971. The chondrocranium of *Hemiechinus auritus aegypticus* and its comparison with *Erinaceus europaeus*. Acta anatomica 78: 224–254.

2638. Yunick, R. P. 1977. Timing of completion of skull pneumatization in the pine siskin. Bird Banding 48: 67–71.

2639. Yunick, R. P. 1979a. Timing of completion of skull pneumatization of the purple finch and the common redpoll. North American Bird Bander 4: 53–55.

2640. Yunick, R. P. 1979b. Variation in skull pneumatization patterns of certain passerines. North American Bird Bander 4: 145–147.

2641. Yunick, R. P. 1980. Timing of cranial pneumatization of the black-capped chickadee and the red-breasted nuthatch. North American Bird Bander 5: 43–46.

2642. Yunick, R. P. 1981a. Skull pneumatization rates in three invading populations of black-capped chickadees. North American Bird Bander 6: 6–7.

2643. Yunick, R. P. 1981b. Further observations on skull pneumatization. North American Bird Bander 6: 40–43.

2644. Yuodelis, R. A. 1966. The morphogenesis of the human temporomandibular joint and its associated structures. Journal of Dental Research 45: 182–191.

2645. Yvroud, M. 1976. Différenciation in vitro du canal nasolacrymal de *Discoglossus pictus* Otth. (amphibien, anoure). Comptes rendus, Académie des sciences, Paris, ser. D, 282: 109–112.

2646. Yvroud, M. 1980. Le canal nasolacrymal du *Discoglosse* (amphibien anoure): Détermination précoce, différenciation tardive. Bulletin de la Société zoologique de France 105: 227–229.

2647. Yvroud, M. 1984. Différenciation du canal nasolacrymal de *Discoglossus pictus* Otth. (Amphibien, Anoure). Bulletin de la Société zoologique de France 109: 301–313.

2648. Zada, S. K. 1980. The inter-relationship between the neural elements, cartilage, and bone in the embryonic lower jaw. Bulletin of the Faculty of Science of Cairo University 49: 175–186.

2649. Zada, S. K. 1981. The fully formed chondrocranium of the agamid lizard, *Agama pallida*. Journal of Morphology 170: 43–54.

2650. Zakharov, V. M., B. I. Sheftel, and D. Y. Aleksandrov. 1984. Breakdown of stability of development at the phase of peak abundance in a mammalian population. Doklady Akademii Nauk SSSR 275: 761–764.

2651. Zama, A., M. Asai, and F. Yasuda. 1977. Changes with growth in bony cranial projections and color patterns in the Japanese boarfish, *Pentaceros japonicus*. Japanese Journal of Ichthyology 24: 26–34.

2652. Zangerl, R. 1944. Contributions to the osteology of the skull of the Amphisbaenidae. American Midland Naturalist 31: 417–454.

2653. Zavatskii, B. P. 1978. Craniological characteristics of the Yenisei USSR population of the brown bear (*Ursus arctos*). Zoologicheskii zhurnal 57: 308–312.

2654. Zelditch, M. L. 1987. Evaluating models of developmental integration in the laboratory rat using confirmatory factor analysis. Systematic Zoology 36: 368–380.

2655. Zelditch, M. L. 1988. Ontogenetic variation in patterns of phenotypic integration in the laboratory rat. Evolution 42: 28–41.

2656. Zelditch, M. L., and A. C. Carmichael. 1989a. Ontogenetic variation in patterns of developmental and functional integration in skulls of *Sigmodon fulviventer*. Evolution 43: 814–824.

2657. Zelditch, M. L., and A. C. Carmichael. 1989b. Growth and intensity of integration through postnatal growth in the skull of *Sigmodon fulviventer*. Journal of Mammalogy 70: 477–484.

2658. Zeller, U. 1984. Die Ontogenese und Morphologie der Cartilago antorbitalis am Schädel von *Tupaia belangeri*. Verhandlungen der Anatomischen Gesellschaft, Jena 78: 251–253.

2659. Zeller, U. 1985a. Die Ontogenese und Morphologie der Fenestra rotunda und des Aquaeductus cochleae von *Tupaia* und anderen Säugern. Gegenbaurs Morphologisches Jahrbuch, Leipzig 131: 179–204.

2660. Zeller, U. 1985b. The morphogenesis of the Fenestra rotunda in mammals. Fortschritte der Zoologie 30: 153–157.

2661. Zeller, U. 1986a. Ontogeny and cranial morphology of the tympanic region of the Tupaiidae, with special reference to *Ptilocercus*. Folia primatologica 47: 61–80.

2662. Zeller, U. 1986b. The systematic relations of tree shrews: Evidence from skull morphogenesis. In *Primate Evolution*, Selected Proceedings of the Congress of the International Primatological Society, vol. 1, J. G. Else and P. C. Lee, eds. Cambridge: Cambridge University Press, pp. 273–280.

2663. Zeller, U. 1987. Morphogenesis of the mammalian skull with special reference to *Tupaia*. In *Morphogenesis of the Mammalian Skull*, H. J. Kuhn and U. Zeller, eds. Hamburg: Verlag Paul Parey, pp. 17–50.

2664. Zeller, U. 1988. The lamina cribrosa of *Ornithorhynchus* (Monotremata, Mammalia). Anatomy and Embryology 178: 513–519.

2665. Zeller, U. 1989a. The braincase of *Ornithorhynchus*. Fortschritte der Zoologie 35: 386–391.

2666. Zeller, U. 1989b. Die entwicklung und morphologie des schadels von *Ornithorhynchus anatinus* (Mammalia: Protheria: Monotremata). Abhandlungen, Senckenbergische Naturforschende Gesellschaft, no. 545: 1–138.

2667. Zhu, S., and M. Luo. 1979. Age determination and age structure in the population of the squirrel, *Sciurus vulgaris*, at Wuying, Lesser Khing-an Mountains, China. Acta zoologica sinica 25: 268–276.

2668. Zima, J. 1986. Epigenetic variation in the roe Deer (*Capreolus capreolus*). Vertebratologicke Zpravy: 39–40.

2669. Zimka, J. 1972. Studies on cross breeds of canary *Serinus canaria* and serin *Serinus serinus*. Acta ornithologica 6: 73–84.

2670. Zimmerman, E. F., ed. 1984. Palate Development: Normal and abnormal cellular and molecular aspects. Current Topics in Developmental Biology 19: 1–251.

2671. Zimova, I. 1987. Biology of reproduction and postnatal development of the pine vole, *Pitymys subterraneus* (Mammalia: Rodentia) under laboratory conditions. Acta Universitatis Carolinae biologica: 367–417.

2672. Zingeser, M. R., and W. P. McNulty. 1977. A method of relating craniofacial sections to topography in embryos. Stain Technology 52: 327–330.

2673. Ziolkowski, M., and W. Kurlej. 1986. Variability of measurements' features of the neurocranium in human fetuses. Folia morphologica, Warsaw 45: 86–95.

2674. Zozlo, P. G. 1983. Ecological and morphological analysis of the moose population. Nauka i tekhnika: 1–213.

CONTRIBUTORS

William R. Atchley
Department of Genetics
North Carolina State University
Raleigh, North Carolina 27695-7614
U.S.A.

Richard P. Elinson
Department of Zoology
University of Toronto
25 Harbord Street
Toronto, Ontario M5S 1A1
Canada

Brian K. Hall
Department of Biology
Life Sciences Center
Dalhousie University
Halifax, Nova Scotia B3H 4J1
Canada

James Hanken
Department of Environmental, Population, and Organismic Biology
University of Colorado
Boulder, Colorado 80309-0334
U.S.A.

Susan W. Herring
Department of Orthodontics
University of Washington
Seattle, Washington 98195
U.S.A.

Antone G. Jacobson
Department of Zoology
Center for Developmental Biology
University of Texas
Austin, Texas 78712
U.S.A.

David R. Johnson
Department of Anatomy
Medical School
University of Leeds
Leeds, West Yorkshire LS2 9JT
U.K.

Kenneth R. Kao
Department of Zoology
University of Toronto
25 Harbord Street
Toronto, Ontario M5S 1A1
Canada

Robert M. Langille
Department of Anatomy
Health Sciences Center
University of Ottawa
Ottawa, Ontario K1H 8M5
Canada

Robert Presley
Department of Anatomy
University of Wales College of Cardiff
P.O. Box 900
Cardiff CF1 3YF
U.K.

Christopher S. Rose
Department of Organismic and Evolutionary Biology
Museum of Comparative Zoology
Harvard University
Cambridge, Massachusetts 02138
U.S.A.

John O. Reiss
Department of Organismic and Evolutionary Biology
Museum of Comparative Zoology
Harvard University
Cambridge, Massachusetts 02138
U.S.A.

Peter Thorogood
Developmental Biology Unit
Institute of Child Health
30 Guilford Street
London WC1N 1EH
U.K.

INDEX

Chapter 10, Bibliography of Skull Development, 1937–89, contains both subject and systematic indexes and should be consulted along with this general index.